Third Edition

FOUNDATIONS OF EDUCATION

An EMS Approach

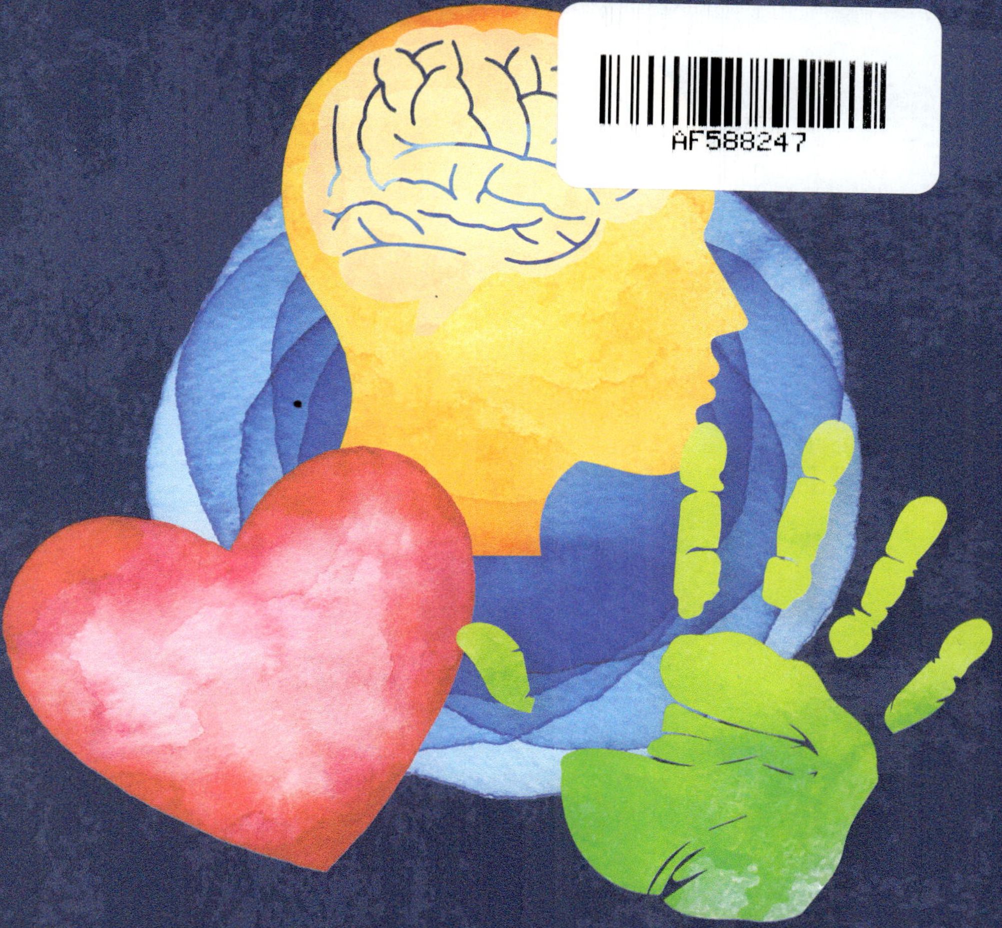

National Association of EMS Educators

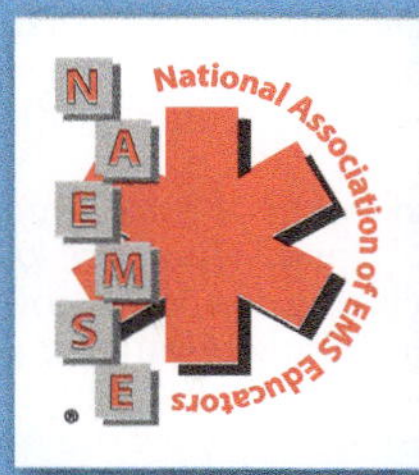

JONES & BARTLETT LEARNING

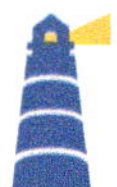

World Headquarters
Jones & Bartlett Learning
5 Wall Street
Burlington, MA 01803
978-443-5000
info@jblearning.com
www.jblearning.com

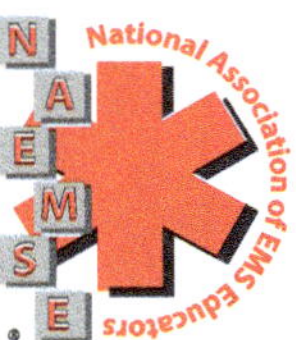

National Association of EMS Educators
250 Mt. Lebanon Boulevard
Suite 209
Pittsburgh, PA 15234
naemse.org

Jones & Bartlett Learning books and products are available through most bookstores and online booksellers. To contact Jones & Bartlett Learning directly, call 800-832-0034, fax 978-443-8000, or visit our website, www.jblearning.com.

Substantial discounts on bulk quantities of Jones & Bartlett Learning publications are available to corporations, professional associations, and other qualified organizations. For details and specific discount information, contact the special sales department at Jones & Bartlett Learning via the above contact information or send an email to specialsales@jblearning.com.

Production Credits
General Manager and Executive Publisher: Kimberly Brophy
VP, Product Development: Christine Emerton
Senior Managing Editor: Donna Gridley
Product Manager: Tiffany Sliter
Senior Editor: Carol B. Guerrero
Editorial Assistant: Alex Belloli
VP, Sales, Public Safety Group: Phil Charland
Senior Project Specialist: Vanessa Richards
Digital Project Specialist: Rachel Reyes
Marketing Manager: Jessica Carmichael
VP, Manufacturing and Inventory Control: Therese Connell
Composition: S4Carlisle Publishing Services
Cover Design: Kristin Parker
Text Design: Scott Moden
Media Development Editor: Troy Liston
Rights & Media Specialist: Rebecca Damon
Cover Image (Title Page, Part Opener, Chapter Opener): Green watercolor texture: © MarinaZakharova/Getty Images; Hand print: © MrsWilkins/Getty Images; Dark blue rough texture: © sntpzh/Getty Images; Orange watercolor texture: © -1001-/Getty Images; Human brain: © image_jungle/Getty Images; Watercolor layered blue dots: © saemilee/Getty Image; Watercolor heart: © saemilee/Getty Images
Printing and Binding: LSC Communications
Cover Printing: LSC Communications

Library of Congress Cataloging-in-Publication Data
Names: National Association of EMS Educators, issuing body.
Title: Foundations of education : an EMS approach / National Association of EMS Educators.
Description: Third edition. | Burlington, MA : Jones & Bartlett Learning, [2020] | Includes bibliographical references and index.
Identifiers: LCCN 2019008558 | ISBN 9781284145168 (pbk.)
Subjects: | MESH: Emergency Medicine--education | Emergency Medical Technicians--education | Teaching
Classification: LCC RA645.5 | NLM WB 18 | DDC 616.02/5071--dc23
LC record available at https://lccn.loc.gov/2019008558

6048

Printed in the United States of America
26 10 9 8

Dedication

To our EMS instructor colleagues, who give so much of themselves to so many students—simply because that is who they are.

—LMA and KMcK

For my sister, Paula, my sons, Ryan and Blake, and grandsons Nathan, Zachary, and Matthew, whose love and encouragement have taught me patience, perseverance, confidence, and courage to live my passion as a healthcare provider and EMS educator.

—LMA

For my family, you are everything.

—KMcK

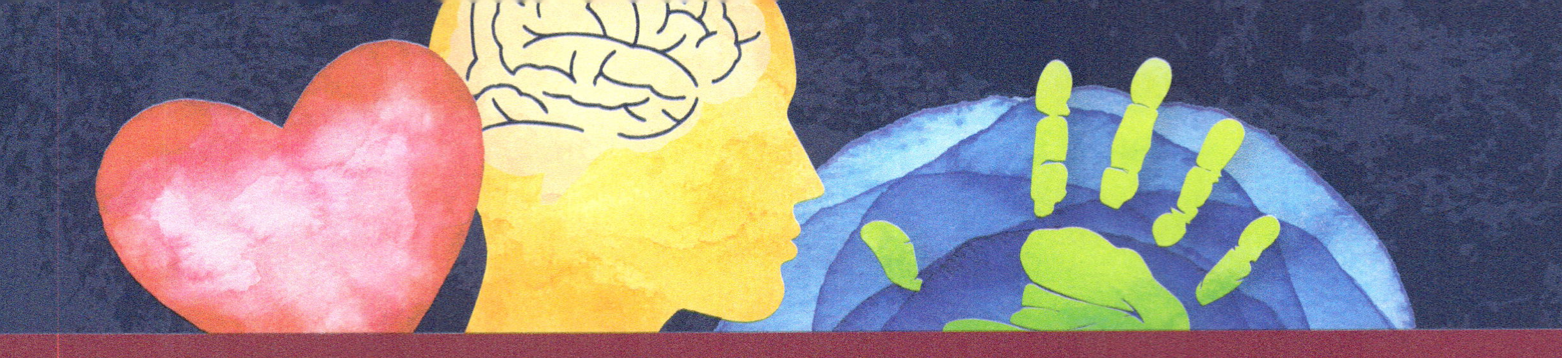

Brief Contents

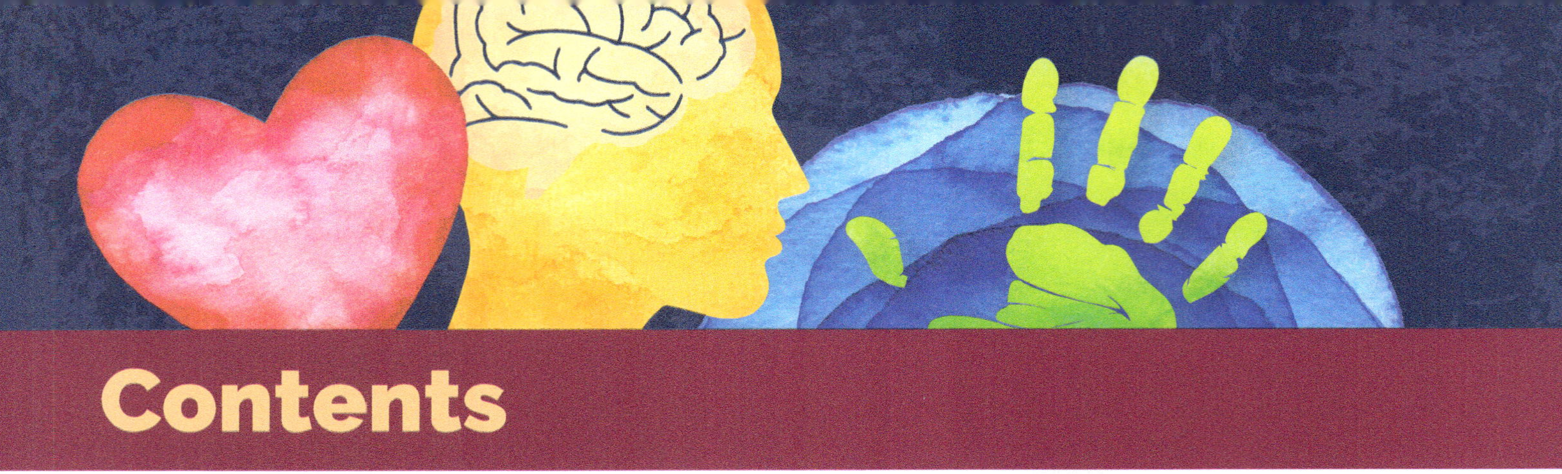

Contents

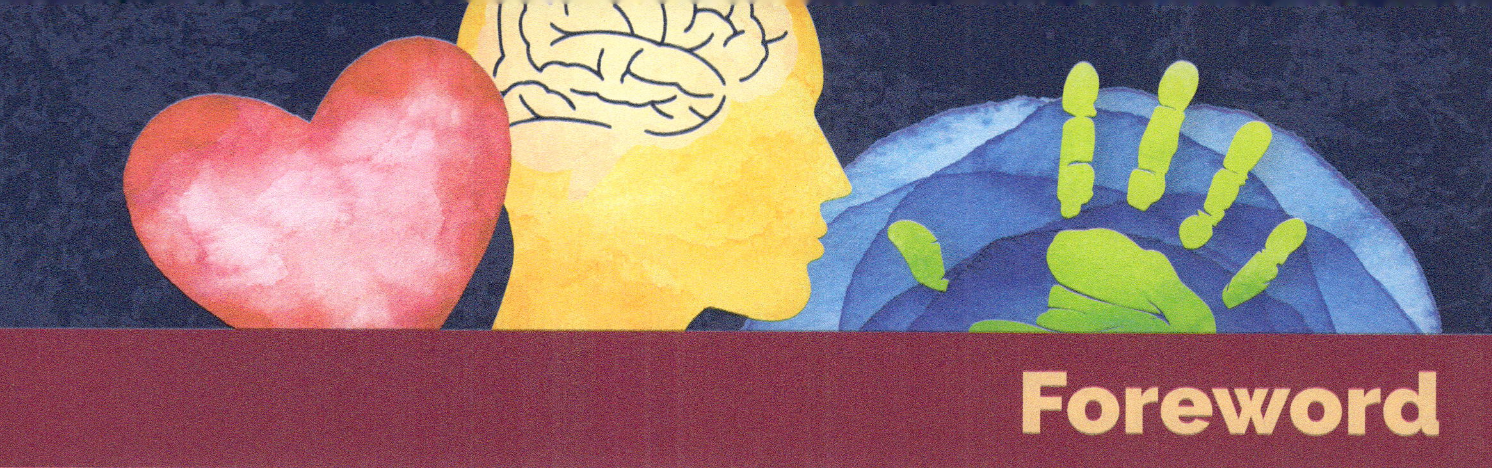

Foreword

The National Association of EMS Educators is very excited about the publication of the third edition of *Foundations of Education: An EMS Approach*. It is hard to believe that it has been 13 years since the publication of the first edition in 2006. It does not take much effort to come up with a long and comprehensive list of everything that has changed in the delivery of prehospital healthcare and the emergency medical services (EMS) classroom during the past 13 years. Provider roles are changing and continuing to evolve at what sometimes feels like a breakneck pace. One can only wonder about the future of EMS, out-of-hospital health care, and the education and training required to prepare and equip the next generation of EMS healthcare professionals.

As EMS and healthcare educators, we are the ones tasked with the responsibility to ensure that classroom, lab, clinical, and field experiences properly educate and prepare our students to enter into the dynamic profession of EMS and out-of-hospital health care. As professional educators, we are at the front line, equipping this next generation of professionals with the knowledge, skills, and behaviors to consistently and compassionately provide quality care. The complexity of these changes and how they are communicated to the provider and student rests on the shoulders of the instructors who choose to take on the rewarding challenge of EMS education. Our students must be properly prepared to care for all patients and respond to situations to which they are called.

The practice of EMS is now being driven by the desire to become fully integrated and recognized as true partners in the healthcare arena. When the first and second editions of *Foundations of Education* were published, who would have thought that there would be a shift in practice from not only providing 911 emergency care and response, to the practice of critical and mobile integrated health care? Who would have imagined that we would be teaching first responders to administer naloxone, a medication once available only in the paramedic tool kit?

The only way EMS can evolve is through the development and implementation of quality education. As emergency medicine and EMS move to more evidence-based practice and education, we will surely see dramatic changes along with new and exciting opportunities no one is even considering today. It will be our responsibility and privilege as educators to address these needs by staying abreast of them and then developing and implementing quality educational opportunities.

EMS education has continued to evolve. Paramedic program accreditation is now mandatory to take the National Registry of EMTs exam; high-fidelity and virtual simulation are increasingly seen in EMS training. Flipped classrooms and the tools provided by social media are much more commonplace. Educational technology is evolving—truly changing and enhancing the way we communicate with our students. We must stay current with available technology and support research to promote best practices in our classrooms and enhance ongoing student success.

Foundations of Education: An EMS Approach, Third Edition is a resource that will continue to provide assistance and guidance that instructors can use every day. As educators, we are committed to lifelong learning and the continued development and mastery of our craft. Education is a calling; EMS educators have a passion for ensuring student success during their education and in their individual practice. The editors and contributing authors of this text bring a wealth of knowledge and expertise in their individual specialties that lends to a unique approach, allowing the reader to hear from many different experts who are all leaders in the field of EMS education.

The entire text has been reviewed and revised by nationally known content experts, and the role of research and the importance of evidence-based practice in the field and in the classroom continue to be emphasized. There are two new chapters in this edition that address paramedic program accreditation and the exciting application of brain-based learning in the classroom. This text is for you, the educator who shares the passion of teaching, inspiring, and forging the next generation of EMS professionals. No matter where or what you teach, this text will serve as an invaluable tool and resource in your continued growth and development as an EMS and healthcare educator.

The mission of the National Association of EMS Educators is to inspire educational excellence. Our vision for the future is a world where EMS lives as an equal partner in the healthcare system. Ultimately, we are committed to the practice of EMS and healthcare education that inspires and enhances the lives of our students. I am confident that this text will serve you well in expanding your educational practice to meet the needs of your students and community. I thank you for your service in education and in answering the call to help prepare and equip the next generation of EMS providers and professionals.

Bryan F. Ericson, MEd, RN, NRP, LP
President, NAEMSE, 2018–2020

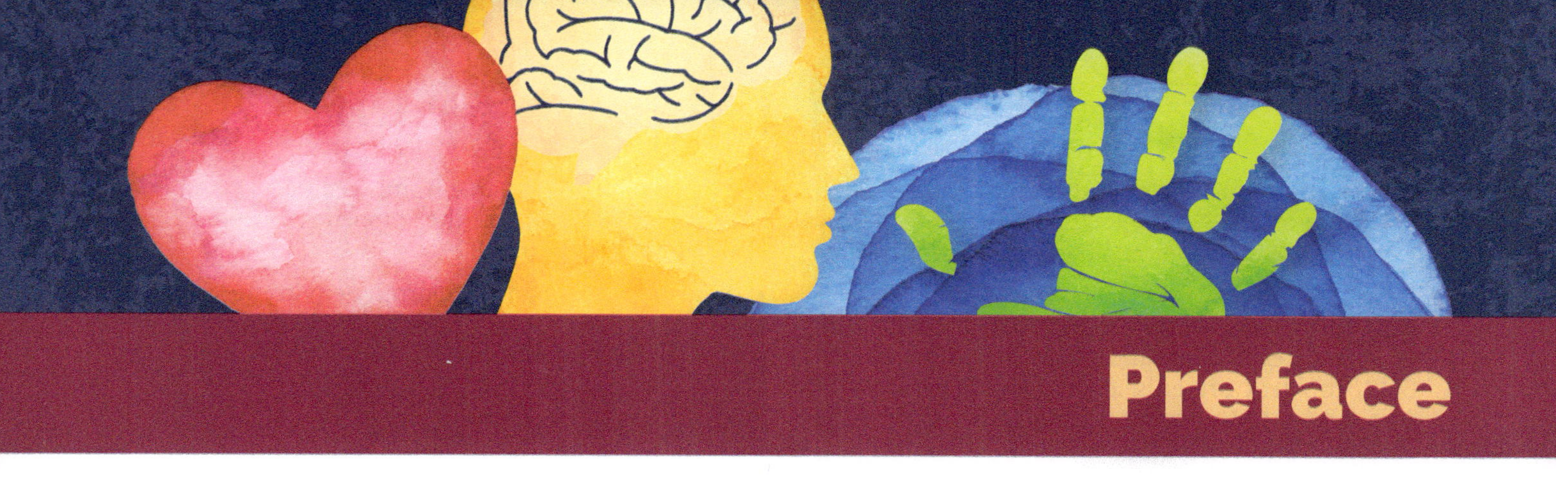

Preface

Foundations of Education: An EMS Approach, Third Edition is designed to provide Emergency Medical Services (EMS) educators with an overview of teaching philosophy, strategy, techniques, and evidence-based adult learning principles. Grounded in this information, EMS educators can promote effective student learning and assessment, regardless of the type of course or setting. The inception of this text was based on the *National EMS Education Standards*. It provides tools to assist instructors in meeting practice guidelines that comply with state and national program-accreditation guidelines.

Organization of This Text

Part I: Instructor Roles and Responsibilities

The introductory chapters outline attributes of instructors and detail the various roles of EMS educators.

Part II: The Student

The chapters in this part cover factors that influence student needs and student learning, such as how the adult human brain learns, and include a discussion of how discoveries in neuroscience inform optimal learning. The importance of classroom culture is also emphasized in this part of the text.

Part III: Education Essentials

Part III introduces instructors to elements in the learning environment that influence effective teaching and learning. It takes instructors through a lesson-planning process based on understanding the need to meet each learning domain and to construct learning objectives that clearly describe the desired outcomes in students in all domains. In addition, it presents the revised Bloom's taxonomy and current concepts such as the flipped classroom and use of evolving technology to enhance student learning.

Part IV: Delivering the Message

Delivering the message elaborates on the many strategies instructors use to promote student learning when they are alone or in groups; or while in the classroom, skills laboratory, or at a distance; or in field and clinical settings. In addition to many other key topics, self-reflection, self-regulated learning, teaching logistics, and use of specific technologies are discussed.

Part V: Student Assessment and Remediation

Significant attention is devoted to elaborating on the methods for sound, reliable, and valid assessment of all domains, including the affective domain. This section also assists instructors in determining the need for and process to implement remediation plans.

Part VI: Administration

The three chapters that comprise this part discuss administration, legal issues, and a overview of various aspects of accreditation. The administration chapter addresses the complexity of planning, delivering, and evaluating educational programs within academic and nonacademic settings, while the legal chapter provides extensive coverage of legal issues in the EMS educational setting. This knowledge will help program directors to ensure programs are managed legally, ethically, and within sound business principles. The new chapter on fundamentals of accreditation is an excellent resource for any program that is seeking or planning to seek accreditation.

Features of This Text

This text is written from an EMS perspective and incorporates features to assist instructors to see how educational principles can be applied within EMS, and specifically, how they might be used within their own educational settings. Although EMS instruction varies from region to region and from institution to institution, some fundamental issues and problems remain the same across the industry. The authors have framed these issues within an EMS context to help readers see how to transition the information directly to their program.

- *By EMS Instructors, for EMS Instructors*: Written specifically for educators teaching EMS and focused on specific challenges and needs of those teaching EMS, this text presents ideas that can be used in a variety of EMS educational settings that include hospital, emergency services-based organizations, and college and university settings.
- *Practical Approach*: "How to" examples blend essential educational theory with practical information applicable to a variety of EMS educational settings and provide a framework for an introductory EMS education curriculum.
- *Case in Point*: Scenarios illustrate how principles or problems are specifically addressed within an EMS setting.
- *Teaching Tips*: These specific examples enable instructors to envision how to apply the concepts directly within their own classrooms.

New to This Edition

- The entire text has been updated to cover new educational theories and techniques, according to recent evidence-based research.
- *New* chapter! Chapter 3: Brain-Based Learning.
- The technology chapter has been completely overhauled to cover cutting-edge teaching techniques and new technologies—from webinars, to open source education, to the flipped classroom, to emerging technologies.
- Updated content on the learning environment discusses personal electronic devices policy, cognitive load, and virtual learning.
- *New* chapter! Chapter 26: Fundamentals of Accreditation and Program Evaluation.
- Two new appendices provide the *NAEMSE Rubric for Quality Online Education*, and key information on *Disabilities in EMS Education*.
- Each chapter includes learning objectives written to Bloom's taxonomy.

NAEMSE Instructor Courses

This text serves as reference for the EMS Educator Courses conducted by the National Association of EMS Educators. The NAEMSE Level I Instructor Course represents the didactic component and practical application of the beginning education process to become an EMS instructor. The NAEMSE Level II Instructor Course is geared toward the experienced instructor and addresses the more administrative roles related to EMS education. All courses are representative of the latest *National Guidelines for EMS Educators*. It provides educators and program directors with the tools and information needed to further build their leadership skills and better evaluate programs, students, and faculty. For more information on these courses, please visit https://naemse.org.

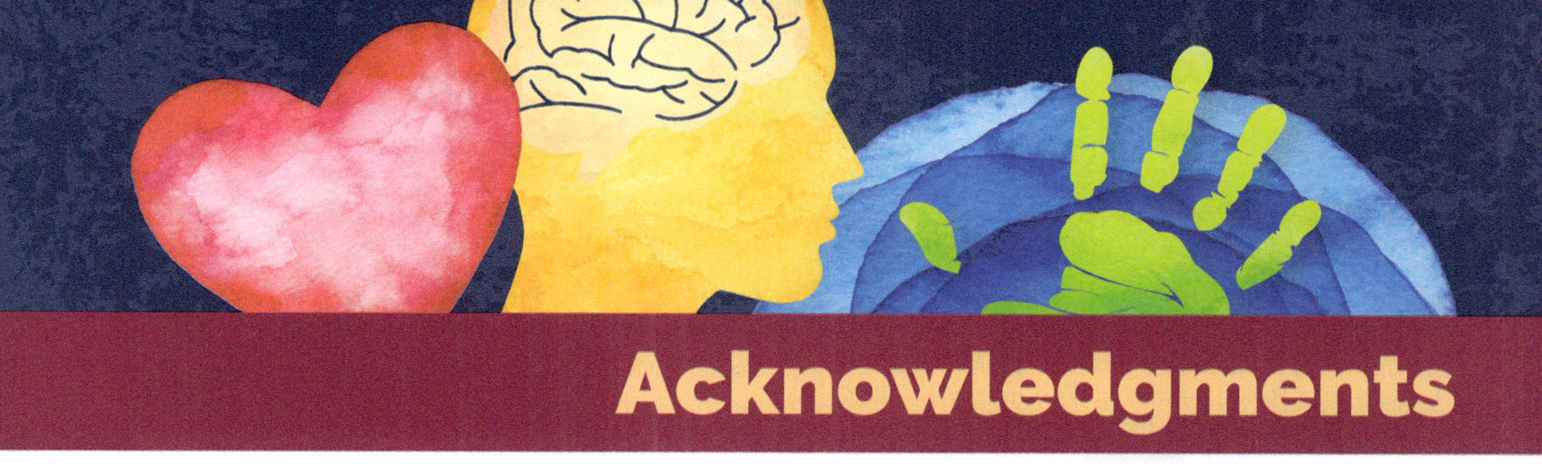

Acknowledgments

About the Editors

Linda M. Abrahamson, MA, ECRN, EMT-P, LI, NCEE

Linda is the paramedic program director for Advocate Christ Medical Center in Oak Lawn, Illinois. Linda is a paramedic, registered nurse, author, and educator. She holds a master's degree in education and training from Governors State University. Linda's leadership in the EMS community has garnered local, state, national, and international recognition. As a charter member of NAEMSE, Linda has served in various leadership roles and is currently national faculty for the NAEMSE Level 1 and Level 2 Instructor Courses. Linda is honored to have served as president of NAEMSE and currently serves as vice president. She has represented providers as an Executive Committee member for NAEMT and served for 10 years as the chair of the Advanced Medical Life Support Course. She currently serves on the National EMS Education Standards Development Team and has contributed to the development of the *2002 National EMS Educator Guidelines*.

Kim D. McKenna, PhD, MEd, BSN, RN, EMT-P

Kim is the director of education for the St. Charles County Ambulance District in St. Peters, Missouri, and the program director for the department's EMT and paramedic programs. Kim has provided emergency care and EMS education for more than 30 years for hospital, fire, and third-service EMS programs. She holds a PhD in education with a focus on educational leadership and policy studies from the University of Missouri–St. Louis. Kim was the emergency medical responder project level leader on the 2009 National EMS Education Standards Task Force. As a former member of the NAEMSE board of directors, she chaired the Publication and Research Committees. Presently Kim serves on the board of advisors for the Prehospital Care Research Forum at UCLA and on the board of directors of the National Registry of EMTs.

About the Authors

Leaugeay C. Barnes, EdD(c), NRP, FP-C, NCEE

Chapter 9: Goals and Objectives

Leaugeay is the paramedic program director at the University of Hawai'i–Kapi'olani Community College and works part time as a fixed-wing flight paramedic for LifeSave Kupono. She earned a bachelor's degree in biomedical science from Texas A&M University, a master's degree in fire and emergency management administration from Oklahoma State University, and is currently working on an EdD degree in interdisciplinary leadership from Creighton University. In 2016, she was awarded the NAEMT *EMS Educator of the Year*. Leaugeay spent 13 years as a helicopter EMS flight paramedic with Tulsa Life Flight in Oklahoma and has experience as a ground provider in Texas and Oklahoma.

Dan Batsie

Chapter 1: Attributes of Effective Educators

Dan serves as EMS chief at Vermont EMS. He has been a paramedic in New York, Maine, and now Vermont for more than 28 years. Prior to working in Vermont, he was a regional education coordinator for the State of Maine and administered the paramedic programs for Eastern Maine and Kennebec Valley Community Colleges. In addition to authoring EMS textbooks, he has written numerous journal articles.

Megan D. Corry, EdD, EMT-P

Chapter 13: Tools for Individual Learning

Megan is the paramedic program director at City College of San Francisco, a board member for the Prehospital Care Research Forum, and a site visitor for the Committee on Accreditation of Educational Programs for the EMS Professions (CoAEMSP).

Alice (Twink) Dalton, MS, RN CNS, NRP

Chapter 5: Learning Styles: Concepts and Controversies

Twink recently retired as the director, EMS division for Mountain View Fire and Rescue and now consults with several EMS agencies. Her varied background includes serving as the EMS education coordinator for the Omaha Fire Department; trauma coordinator for St Joseph's Hospital in Omaha, Nebraska; director of paramedic training program at Creighton University; and emergency department charge nurse at Immanuel Medical Center. She has written EMS-related articles and textbooks, and has participated in field research, with several published studies.

Heather Davis, EdD, NRP

Chapter 11: Introduction to Teaching Strategies

Chapter 12: Teaching in All Domains

Heather is the associate director of the UCLA Center for Prehospital Care and paramedic program director. She holds a doctorate degree in educational psychology from the University of Southern California, where she returned to serve as an adjunct assistant professor, teaching in the graduate programs of the Rossier School of Education. Dr. Davis serves as a board member for the National Registry of EMTs and is a published author and national speaker.

Douglas Gadomski, MA, NRP

Chapter 17: Tools for Distance Learning

Doug is a full-time EMS paramedic/educator at the University of New Mexico School of Medicine. He holds a bachelor's degree in EMS and a master's degree in organizational learning and instructional technology. He has over 4 decades of experience in wilderness, rural, urban, and flight medicine. Doug has a great interest in online learning and use of technology to enhance EMS education.

Rusty Gilpin, BT, NRP

Chapter 14: Tools for Small Group Learning

Rusty is the EMS program director for Gordon Cooper Technology Center's paramedic and EMS programs. He also oversees all other short-term adult allied health program offerings at Gordon Cooper Technology Center. He currently serves as the NREMT representative for the state of Oklahoma, co-chair of the Education Committee for NAEMSE, and chair of the Oklahoma EMS Education Consensus Group. Rusty also sits on the ODCTE Accreditation Advisory Committee, the Seminole State College PT Program Oversight Committee, and the FISDAP advisory board. He is an experienced EMS practitioner, educator, and published author, and a recipient of the *Oklahoma State Capitol Medic of the Day* and *ODCTE PACE Innovation* awards.

Anthony Guerne, MS, NRP, CHSE

Chapter 14: Tools for Small Group Learning

Anthony began his career in the emergency services in 1990 by joining his local volunteer fire department. He became a paramedic in 1994 and began working in New York City. In 2009, he became the simulation specialist for the NY College of Osteopathic Medicine.

After completing his master's degree, he moved to the Adelphi University College of Nursing and Public Health where he remains today. He is still working as a paramedic and is the lead paramedic for the Commack Volunteer Ambulance Corp.

Donna K. Hammaker, JD, MBA

Chapter 25: Legal Issues for EMS Educators

Donna, a health law attorney, holds a faculty appointment in the graduate health services program at Saint Joseph's University and serves as director of the National Institute on Health Care Management/Law. Before entering academia, Donna was the president and chief executive officer of Collegiate Health Care, the nation's first interuniversity managed care organization. She has served on the faculty and taught at Immaculata University, Penn State University, Rutgers University, and Widener University. Donna recently authored *Health Care Management and the Law* (2017) and *Health Care Records and the Law* (2019), and coauthored *Health Care Ethics and the Law* (2018), published by Jones & Bartlett Learning.

Arthur Hsieh, MA, NRP

Chapter 6: Culture in the EMS Classroom

Art has been in the EMS profession since 1982, earning his master's degree in adult education in 2000. He has worked as a volunteer, line medic, educator, and chief officer in private, third-service, and fire-based EMS. He has directed both primary and EMS continuing education programs, and currently is on the faculty and is paramedic program director at Santa Rosa Junior College Public Safety Training Center in California. A past president of the National Association of EMS Educators, and a California *EMS Educator of the Year* awardee, Art has authored several EMS textbooks, and has presented at conferences nationwide.

Yilmaz Kaymak

Chapter 25: Legal Issues for EMS Educators

Yilmaz is a senior manager with Accenture, a global management consulting and professional services company that provides services in strategy, consulting, digital technology, and operations to more than three-quarters of the Fortune Global 500 in more than 120 countries. Kaymak has earned two graduate degrees in finance and in innovation and technology management from the Wharton School of the University of Pennsylvania. Before joining Accenture, Kaymak was helping to develop a proprietary therapy called tumor treating fields with Novocure, a commercial-stage oncology company. Prior to this, Kaymak assisted with the integration of Wyeth into Pfizer Pharmaceuticals.

William J. Leggio, Jr., EdD, NRP

Chapter 2: EMS Educator Roles

William is an assistant professor and paramedic program coordinator at Creighton University. He also has international EMS education experience. As an EMS educator, he served on the technical expert panel for EMS Agenda 2050. In addition to his scholarly contributions to the EMS profession, he still serves on a rural EMS service in Nebraska and practices clinically as a paramedic in an academic, medical, and level 1 trauma center.

Connie J. Mattera, MS, RN, LP

Chapter 24: Administrative Issues

Connie is the EMS administrative director and system coordinator for the Northwest Community EMS System and the director of the Resuscitation and Mobile Integrated Healthcare Departments at Northwest Community Hospital (Arlington Heights, Illinois). She is the EMS program director in affiliation with Harper College (Palatine, Illinois), is the editor for the State of Illinois Trauma Nurse Specialist Course, is a member of the State of Illinois Governor's EMS Advisory Council, and chairs the Illinois EMS Education Committee. She is a frequent presenter at local, state, and national conferences and has published multiple articles in nursing and EMS journals. She is honored to have served on the NAEMSE Board of Directors and is one of the national faculty members for the NAEMSE Level 1 Instructor Course.

Christopher F. Nollette, EdD, NRP, LP

Chapter 3: Brain-Based Learning

Dr. Nollette is a proud Texan who has spent 36 years as an advanced life support street paramedic nationally registered and licensed in four states. He has been an EMS educator for over 31 years, and has established five degreed and nationally accredited EMS college programs. He has his doctorate degree in curriculum and instruction from the University of Houston in adult methodology, with continued studies in the neuroplasticity of the brain and building strategies to reach all learners in a unique and engaging way. He is a former three-time president of NAEMSE, whose leadership cornerstone is being authentic, passionate, courageous, and leading with a servant's heart and vision. Dr. Nolette lives by the words of another famous Texan—Sam Houston—who said, "Do right and risk the consequences."

David Page, MS, NRP, PhD(c)

Chapter 19: Tools for Field and Clinical Learning

Dave is the director of the Prehospital Care Research Forum at UCLA and an active field paramedic with Allina Health EMS in Minneapolis/St. Paul, Minnesota. He serves as the chair of the International Paramedic Registry Assessment and Credentialing Board and has over 33 years of continuous EMS street experience. Dave is an adjunct senior lecturer and PhD candidate at Monash University in Melbourne, Australia. He is a member of the education committee for NAEMT, a site visitor for the Committee on Accreditation of EMS Programs, and senior facilitator for the NAEMSE/CoAEMSP Evaluation Workshop and NREMT Scenario Development Workshop.

William Raynovich, EdD, MPH

Chapter 4: Principles of Adult Learning

Bill recently retired after a career in EMS that began in 1967. He held administrative positions and faculty appointments with the Center for Emergency Medicine, University of Health Sciences at the University of Pittsburgh, Pennsylvania; the Reading Hospital and Medical Center in West Reading, Pennsylvania, now Tower Health; the EMS Academy of New Mexico in Albuquerque, New Mexico; and Creighton University in Omaha, Nebraska. He has served as a member of the board of directors of NAEMSE and as liaison to the board of CoAEMSP. NAEMSE honored Dr. Raynovich with the *Lifetime Achievement Award* in 2012.

Bill Robertson, DHSc, NRP

Chapter 7: The Learning Environment

The chair of emergency healthcare at Weber State University, Bill has over 25 years of experience in EMS and academia. Bill presents around the world, teaches regularly in Africa, and is a site visitor for the Ministry of Education in the UAE. Bill sits on multiple committees, is on the board of directors for NAEMSE, and is an associate of the Prehospital Care Research Forum at UCLA. Bill holds a bachelor's degree in education, a master's degree in health science, and a doctorate degree in global health. As part of his doctorate, Bill interned for a summer in Ghana, completing a practicum in sustainability practices in global healthcare.

Paul L. Rosenberger, EdD, NRP

Chapter 8: Domains of Learning

Paul has over 30 years of EMS experience—in the field as a paramedic and an adult educator. He flew for an aeromedical provider, worked in emergency room and intensive care units, and provided ground paramedic duties for several cities in Texas. Additionally, he has provided leadership in town administration as an assistant to the town manager. He served as a faculty member and assistant program director for UT Southwestern. He is also an instructor for the NAEMSE Evaluating Student Competencies Seminars and has been involved with the instruction of the NREMT's scenario workshops. He currently is the co-chair of the National EMS Education Standards and Instructional Guidelines Revision Team.

Walt Alan Stoy, PhD, EMT-P

Chapter 23: Remediation

Walt is professor and founding director of the Emergency Medicine Program at the University of Pittsburgh and is director emeritus at the Center for Emergency Medicine. He is internationally renowned for his efforts and recognized as a national leader in EMS education. Walt has served as the project director of the 1998 EMT-Intermediate and Paramedic: Revision Project. He served as principal investigator to the 1994 EMT-Basic curriculum, and as project director to the 1995 First Responder curriculum. He has over 45 years of experience in EMS and served as the founding president of the National Association of EMS Educators.

Mark Terry, MPA, NRP

Chapter 20: Assessing Learning

Chapter 21: Written Assessment

Chapter 22: Other Assessment Tools

Mark is the chief certification officer for the National Registry of EMTs. He has been a nationally registered paramedic since 1987, serving in operations and education roles for Kansas City area emergency medical services. Mark served on the American Heart Association national Emergency Cardiovascular Care Committee and helped develop several AHA ECC training programs. He has contributed to projects with the National Association of EMS Educators, the National Association of EMTs, and a variety of state and local initiatives.

Rob Theriault, MET, BHSc, CCP(f)

Chapter 16: Using Technology to Enhance Classroom Learning

Rob is registered paramedic and professor of paramedicine at Georgian College in Ontario, Canada. He has been in the industry since 1984 and is a former critical care flight paramedic with Ontario's air ambulance system. Rob has a bachelor of health sciences degree in paramedicine from Victoria University in Melbourne, Australia, and a master of educational technology degree from the University of British Columbia. Rob is a published author, researcher, blogger, podcaster, and avid extended reality (XR) enthusiast, and speaks at conferences across Canada and internationally.

John Todaro, BA, NRP, RN, TNS, NCEE, CHSE, CHSOS

Chapter 18: Tools for Simulation

John is assistant director of the University of South Florida, College of Nursing, Miller Center for Experiential Learning and Simulation and adjunct EMS faculty at St. Petersburg College. He is a nationally certified EMS educator, healthcare simulation educator, and simulation operations specialist. He holds a bachelor's degree in business administration/healthcare management, and associate's degrees in paramedics and nursing. In August 2009, John was honored by NAEMSE when he was awarded their prestigious *Legends That Walk Among Us* award. He is a charter member and past president of NAEMSE.

Patricia L. Tritt, MA, RN

Chapter 26: Fundamentals of Accreditation and Program Evaluation

Pat is the director of instruction for AMR learning. She has been responsible for the administration of comprehensive EMS education programs for all levels of prehospital providers. Pat is an ICISF faculty member and has trained crisis support teams in a variety of countries. Pat received the *C. J. Shanaberger Award,* recognition for contributions to Colorado EMS; the *9 Who Care Award,* as a leader of volunteer services in Colorado; NAEMT *President's Leadership Award*; the ICISF Award for *Collaborative Outreach in the Field of Crisis Response*; the *Daniel L. Storer, MD Award* for contributions to the EMS professions; the *2012 Swedish Medical Center Leadership Award*; the *Colorado EMSAC Presidents Award*; and NAEMSE *Legends That Walk Among Us* award.

Bruce J. Walz, PhD

Chapter 10: Lesson Plans

Bruce is professor and past chair of the Department of Emergency Health Services at the University of Maryland, Baltimore County (UMBC). He has been in the University System of Maryland since 1979, having served with the Maryland Fire and Rescue Institute until 1987 before joining UMBC.

He was a group leader for development of the National Standard Paramedic and Intermediate Curricula and the National EMS Educational Standards. He is a charter member of NAEMSE and past president. He has authored and contributed to various publications. He has presented at international, national, and regional EMS conferences.

Bill Young, EdD, NRP

Chapter 15: Tools for Large Group Learning

Bill began his EMS career in 1975 with a small fire department near Williamsburg, Kentucky. They began running first responder calls long before the term ever existed. In addition to Kentucky, his career has taken him to Tennessee, Colorado, Georgia, and Kansas. He has served as a street medic, training officer, supervisor, state regulator, and educator. Currently, he is an associate professor and the director of the Department of Paramedicine at Eastern Kentucky University.

Contributors

Along with the editors and authors, we would like to recognize those who contributed this additional engaging content

Todd M. Cage, MEd, NRP, FAEMS
Chapter 19, *A Model for Teaching Team Leadership*
Mayo Clinic
Rochester, Minnesota

Sara K. Houston, JD, EMT-P
Appendix B: Disabilities in EMS Education
Doane University
Crete, Nebraska
Nebraska City Fire and Rescue
Nebraska City, Nebraska

The NAEMSE Educational Technology Committee
Appendix A: Rubric for Quality Online Education

Dean Vokey, MAdEd, BEd, ACP
Chapter 19, *Cultivating Preceptors: Developing a Culture of Preceptorship*
Quality and Learning Department
Emergency Health Services
Nova Scotia, Canada

Reviewer Acknowledgments

A special thank you to our reviewers, whose meticulous review of the technical content offered valuable insight for the development of the third edition.

Chuck Allias, MS, NRP
Indiana University of Pennsylvania
Indiana, Pennsylvania

Jennifer Anderson Warwick, MA
Accreditation Consultant, CoAEMSP
Oconomowoc, Wisconsin

Stephanie Ashford, MEd, CCP-C, NCEE
St. Charles County Ambulance District
St. Peters, Missouri

Kenneth E. Ashley, MS, LAT, ATC, AEMT
Prince Edward County High School
Farmville, Virginia

Leaugeay C. Barnes, MS, NRP, NCEE, FP-C
Kapi'olani Community College
Honolulu, Hawaii

Ryan Batenhorst, MEd, NRP, EMSI
Southeast Community College
Lincoln, Nebraska

Alan M. Batt, MSc, PhD(c), CCP
Professor, Fanshawe College
Ontario, Canada

Rob Bozicevich, BS, NRP
Metro Atlanta EMS Academy
Marietta, Georgia

Todd M. Cage, MEd, NRP, FAEMS
Mayo Clinic
Rochester, Minnesota

Scott J. Corcoran, MS, CIC, Paramedic
Erie Community College
Orchard Park, New York

Rommie L. Duckworth, BS, LP
New England Center for Rescue and Emergency Medicine
Sherman, Connecticut

Bob Elling, MPA, EMT-P
High Quality Endeavors, Ltd.
Lake Placid, New York

William Faust, MPA, NRP
Haywood Community College
Clyde, North Carolina

Ron Feller, Sr., MBA, NRP
Oklahoma City Community College
Oklahoma City, Oklahoma

James W. Fogal, MA, NRP
Auburn University
Auburn, Alabama

José K. Fuentes, BS, BA, CRCR
Saint Joseph's University
Philadelphia, Pennsylvania

Edward Gannon, AS, EMT-P
New England EMS Institute
Manchester, New Hampshire

Rodney Geilenfeldt II, BS, EMT-P
Paramedic Program Coordinator
EMSTA College
Santee, California

Daniel R. Gerard, MS, RN, NRP
Alameda Fire Department
Alameda, California

George W. Hatch, Jr., EdD, LP, EMT-P
Executive Director, CoAEMSP
Rowlett, Texas

Phil Head III, MS, BHS, NRP, FP-C, CP-C
Greenville Health System Division of Prehospital Medicine
Greenville, South Carolina

Gary Heigel, BA, Paramedic
Department Chair of Emergency Services
Rogue Community College
White City, Oregon

Louis D. Horvath, MA, FACHE
Director, Graduate Health Services
Saint Joseph's University
Philadelphia, Pennsylvania

Steven J. Howell, BS, CCEMTP/PNCCT, NRP
New Hanover Regional EMS
Wilmington, North Carolina

Joseph L. Hurlburt, BS, NRP
Instructor Coordinator
North Flight Wexford County EMS
Manton, Michigan

William Johnston, BA (Hons), AEMCA
Fanshawe College
London, Ontario, Canada

Sahaj Khalsa, NRP, BS, NM I/C
Santa Fe Community College
Santa Fe, New Mexico

Gordon A. Kokx, PhD, NRP
Associate Director, CoAEMSP
Rowlett, Texas

Matthew D. Kostinas, MHA
Saint Joseph's University
Philadelphia, Pennsylvania

Chris Kroboth, MS, CCEMT-P, NRP
Fairfax County Fire and Rescue
Fairfax, Virginia

Elisa P. Laird-Metke, JD
Samuel Merritt University
Oakland, California

Ron Lawler, BUS, NRP
Sanford Health EMS Education
Fargo, North Dakota

Edward "Ted" H. Lee, EdS, NRP, CCEMT-P
Missouri Southern State University Department of EMS
Joplin, Missouri

Michael McDonough, MSHS, NRP
Cuesta College
San Luis Obispo, California

Shelly McLaughlin, MS, EMT-I
University of New Mexico
Albuquerque, New Mexico

Scott J. Meagher, BA, NRP, REMT-B, I/C
Massasoit Community College
Middleborough, Massachusetts

Christopher Metsgar, MBA, MS, PM, NCEE
University of Iowa Hospitals and Clinics
Emergency Medical Services Learning Resources Center
Iowa City, Iowa

Michael T. Oaster, MBA, BS, Paramedic
Sinclair Community College
Dayton, Ohio

Jim O'Connor, Paramedic
Columbus Division of Fire, Columbus, Ohio
Ohio Fire Academy
Reynoldsburg, Ohio

Keito Ortiz, Paramedic, NAEMSE Level II
Pre-Hospital Care Training Coordinator
Jamaica Hospital Medical Center
New York, New York

Vanessa V. Palazzolo, EMT, CLI, EMD, EPD, EFD Certified
Communications Specialist
Northwell Health Center for EMS
Adjunct EMS Educator
Suffolk County EMS
Yaphank, New York

Casey B. Quake, LP, NCEE, EMS-I
EMStar Ambulance
Poughkeepsie, New York

Jose V. Salazar, MPH, CEMSO, CTO, NRP
Loudoun County Fire and Rescue
Leesburg, Virginia

Tammy Samarripa, MPH, BA, EMT-LP
Central Texas College
Killeen, Texas

Elise Scanlon, JD
Elise Scanlon Law Group
Washington, District of Columbia

Holly A. Scribner, MSEd, BAS, AS, AAS, Paramedic
Biddeford Regional Center of Technology, Biddeford, Maine
North Berwick Rescue
North Berwick, Maine

Priscilla R. Simmons, EdD, MSN, RN
Professor Emeritus, Department of Nursing
Eastern Mennonite University
Lancaster, Pennsylvania

Rick Slaven, MPS, NRP, CCP, I/C
Lincoln Memorial University–DeBusk College of Osteopathic Medicine
Harrogate, Tennessee

Douglas R. Smith, MAT, EMT-P, I/C
Platinum Educational Group, LLC
Grandville, Michigan

Mark Spiezio, Paramedic, CIC
Regional Faculty, Program Coordinator
Hudson Valley Community College
Troy, New York
Mountain Lakes Regional EMS
Queensbury, New York

Boniface Stegman, PhD, MSN, RN
Catherine McAuley School of Nursing
Myrtle E. & Earl E. Walker College of Health Professions
Maryville University
St. Louis, Missouri

Nerina J. Stepanovsky, PhD, MSN, CTRN, Paramedic
Owner/Freelancer/Consultant
Caduceus Educational Consulting LLC, Parrish, Florida
Retired EMS Program Director
St. Petersburg College
St. Petersburg, Florida

Michael Tarantino, MAS, BA
Director, Bergen County EMS Training Center
Paramus, New Jersey

Leah M. Tilden, MA, AEMT
Durham Technical Community College
Durham, North Carolina

Blake J. Tobias, Jr.
Reading Hospital–Tower Health
Reading, Pennsylvania

William H. Turner, MS, NRP, FF
Assistant Professor
Director, Emergency Medical Technology
Shawnee State University
Portsmouth, Ohio

Sara Walker, MS, EMTP
Arkansas State University
Jonesboro, Arkansas

Brittany Williams, DHSc, REMT-P, RRT-ACCS, RRT-NPS
Santa Fe College
Gainesville, Florida

Tiffany A. Young, BA
Saint Joseph's University
Philadelphia, Pennsylvania

Photography Acknowledgments

Thank you to the following individuals and institutions who contributed to the photography.

John Grant McKenna
St. Louis, Missouri

Kim D. McKenna, PhD, MEd, BSN, RN, EMT-P
St. Charles County Ambulance District
St. Peters, Missouri

Richard A. Nydam, AS, NREMT-P
Training and Education Specialist, EMS
UMass Memorial Paramedics—Worcester EMS
Worcester, Massachusetts

UMass Memorial Paramedics—Worcester EMS
Worcester, Massachusetts

Introduction

Since its grassroots "pass the hat" inception in 1995, the National Association of EMS Educators (NAEMSE) has been committed to providing resources to develop the practice of EMS education as reflected in its mission statement, which is to inspire educational excellence.

As the association has grown in numbers and maturity, so has our collective knowledge and experience in education. Most of the authors of *Foundations of Education: An EMS Approach* came into EMS education the same way we did—from clinical practice. Fortunately we had wise educators who willingly shared educational principles at conference sessions and whetted our appetite to learn more, and even inspired some of us to go back for more formal education in issues related to teaching. NAEMSE has provided programs and educational resources that have inspired over 12,000 EMS instructors to become better educators through EMS instructor courses taught nationally. One of the foundational documents for the NAEMSE courses is the 2002 National Guidelines for Educating EMS Instructors.[1] Both new and seasoned instructors from a variety of educational venues have utilized this text and consequently enhanced their teaching role. Many have been reenergized with evidence-based ideas, techniques, and methodologies.

This text's first edition was written in service to NAEMSE's mission[2] and has provided a foundational resource for novice and expert educators since its publication in 2005 and subsequent revision in 2013. This edition continues to deliver a framework for excellence to all EMS educators, regardless of whether they teach in an ambulance service, fire district, military branch, hospital, private entity, or within a college or university system.

Much has transpired in the world of EMS education since the publication of the first edition of *Foundations of Education: An EMS Approach*. Most of these changes reflect implementation of the key elements of the industry vision document, the 2000 *EMS Education Agenda for the Future: A Systems Approach*.[3] The Institute of Medicine nudged the agenda forward in their 2006 report, *EMS: At the Crossroads*,[4] with recommendations for a uniform national *EMS Scope of Practice*,[5] which subsequently was published in 2007 and revised in 2019, and national paramedic program accreditation tied to national certification, which was implemented in 2013. The *National EMS Education Standards* followed in 2009 and are being revised even as this edition is published.[6] The Standards represented a large shift in how EMS educators approach the design of education. The bedrock for a solid EMS program design based on the Standards is competent educators.

The continuous evolution in EMS policy profoundly influences whom we teach, how we teach, what we teach, and the accountability to our students, to our schools, and to our community for the quality of the instructional programs. All of these changes further the need for us to practice as professional educators who are knowledgeable about teaching and learning strategies, classroom management, assessment and evaluation, technology in learning, legal implications in education, program infrastructure design, and administering programs of excellence to meet state and national accreditation guidelines.

These changes are coupled with other advances in evidence about teaching and learning. With this new science, instructors can harness knowledge about the brain and how students learn. New advances in technology and distance learning strategies are enhancing education and providing tools that instructors must curate to maximize student learning.

This edition was written with those specific challenges and opportunities in mind. Each author's content builds on the contributions of the earlier editions to reflect how current educational knowledge and theory uniquely apply to EMS students, educators, and programs. Specific examples highlight how to apply solid educational principles to meet the challenges of today's EMS classroom. *Foundations of EMS Education: An EMS Approach, Third Edition* was written by experienced EMS educators from diverse regions and backgrounds, acknowledging that, although our practice may vary, we all have common needs and face similar challenges in our attempt to promote excellence in EMS education delivery.

Editors
Linda M. Abrahamson, MA, ECRN, EMTP, LI, NCEE
Kim D. McKenna, PhD, MEd, BSN, RN, EMT-P

References

[1] National Highway Traffic Safety Administration. 2002. *National Guidelines for Educating EMS Instructors*. Washington, DC: U.S. Department of Transportation.

[2] National Association of EMS Educators. n.d. "Core Values." Accessed April 26, 2019. https://naemse.org/page/core.

[3] National Highway Traffic Safety Administration. 2000. *Emergency Medical Services Education Agenda for the Future*. Washington, DC: U.S. Department of Transportation.

[4] Institute of Medicine (IOM). 2006. "Emergency Medical Services: At the Crossroads." In *Future of Emergency Care*, edited by Committee on the Future of Emergency Care in the United States Health System. Washington, DC: IOM.

[5] National Highway Traffic Safety Administration. 2007. *National EMS Scope of Practice Model*. Washington, DC: U.S. Department of Transportation.

[6] National Highway Traffic Safety Administration. 2009. *National EMS Education Standards*. (DOT HS 811 077A). Washington, DC: U.S. Department of Transportation.

Additional Resource

National Highway Traffic Safety Administration. 2005. *Emergency Medical Services Core Content*. Washington, DC: U.S. Department of Transportation.

Instructor Roles and Responsibilities

A career as an educator is one of the most noble and challenging callings. Few individuals possess all of the qualities that are required to become a great educator, including the knowledge, aptitude, ethics, self-motivation, leadership skills, and empathy that are necessary to make a meaningful contribution to the profession. Educators play vital roles in the advancement of their professions, and many emergency medical services (EMS) educators also face the onerous challenge of teaching critical content with limited time and resources. EMS students not only must acquire considerable knowledge and skills, they must also master the concepts so they can apply them quickly and accurately, often in uncontrolled and unpredictable environments. The instructor's goal, therefore, is to teach students the knowledge, skills, and professional behaviors required of a competent practitioner.

The EMS educator is the essential facilitator of this complex learning process. As with any long and challenging journey, the path to becoming an excellent educator begins with the first step. This first part of the text outlines the attributes of effective EMS educators and explains their roles and responsibilities. As experience and knowledge are acquired and teaching becomes more refined, it may be of value to return to the chapters in Part I to reflect on how these concepts contribute to professional growth and formation of mastery in education.

CHAPTER 1

Attributes of Effective Educators

OBJECTIVES

At the conclusion of this chapter, the educator will be able to:

Cognitive Domain

1. Ident ify educator attributes that motivate students to be lifelong learners.
2. Discuss characteristics of an educational philosophy that empower student success.
3. Define strategies that support fair and accurate assessment of student achievement.
4. Define student rights that contribute to a positive learning environment in classroom, lab, clinical, and field environments.
5. Discuss the value of inclusion in a diverse culture of students that promotes trust and advocacy.
6. Identify the value of mentoring by implementing strategies to facilitate student learning and professional growth.
7. Discuss the challenges associated with effective mentoring that affect student-centered learning opportunities.
8. Compare and contrast positive and negative professional attributes of an educator that improve or inhibit student outcomes.
9. Identify strategies that promote student curiosity to learn by embracing creative approaches to content delivery.
10. Discuss the advantages of identifying a career pathway that identifies a personal vision for professional growth.

Psychomotor Domain

There are no psychomotor objectives for this chapter.

Affective Domain

1. Value the behaviors that set the standards of professionalism for healthcare providers and educators through the inclusion of assessing the affective domain.
2. Defend educational design that includes the cognitive, affective, and psychomotor domains of learning.
3. Value professionalism through leadership and role modeling by demonstrating positive ethical behaviors.
4. Defend the value of an educator's commitment to continuing professional development and evidence-based medicine and teaching strategies through investigation of current research.

"Education is not the filling of a pail but the lighting of a fire."

~ William Butler Yeats

CHAPTER GOAL This chapter will inspire all levels of educators to utilize attributes that develop a teaching philosophy to become effective educators.

The future of emergency medical services (EMS) will be defined by those willing to stand up and guide it. Considering that most clinicians will never stand before a class, the decision to join the ranks of a proud tradition of EMS educators is one worthy of congratulations. Although the climb toward excellence as an educator is not easy, the rewards are truly abundant. Achieving this goal will be a path paved by hard work, long hours, frustrating moments, and sometimes failure; but in the end, no other group or professional organization will ever have as much influence on the direction of the EMS profession as will educators.

Envision a model of EMS in its perfect state. What are the crucial elements of the profession? How should practitioners act, speak, and model themselves? These are essential questions, because as of the first class taught, *the EMS educator* is the first and most important role model for the next generation. Beyond the first class, continuing education requirements will have an ongoing influence not only on individual students, but also on how EMS defines its own culture. Students observe instructor behavior, mimic their worst flaws, and carry forward much of the vision instructors describe. If there is any doubt that this is true, EMS educators should consider the influences in their own EMS careers. What effect did initial educators and field training officers have on their own professional development? Although charting the course for students to be inspired to learn may be perceived as a heavy burden, it is also an incredible opportunity.

As educators chart their path, it is important to take stock of the core values that have brought them to this moment. Although there are many reasons for choosing to teach, at some level, that choice must have involved a desire to improve the quality of the profession. And while clinical objectives will certainly be the focus, educators should never forget that truly great medicine involves more than a single dimension of care. While it is hoped that most students come to class ethically and morally prepared to do right, it is also the responsibility of educators to explicitly demonstrate those expectations of the profession.

Great education is more than just the recitation of facts. More importantly, the education of excellent providers does not end in the classroom. In future chapters, lesson plans and class objectives are discussed; but here and now, consider a vision for EMS education and imagine the opportunity educators have in front of them to inspire the traits of a lifelong learner. Beyond certification examinations, new practitioners will require tools to remain competent in an ever-changing world of health care. They will need examples of compassion, forgiveness, and patience. They will need opportunities to find appropriate mentors to help them in their journey. They will look to their educators' example to find those tools. The enthusiasm, passion, and creativity they find in the classroom will be their roadmap.

All educators will have highs and lows. There are great responsibilities, and no one is suggesting that the road will be an easy one. It is important to consider from the earliest moments how to navigate the challenges that will inevitably emerge.

It is a pivotal time to be an EMS educator. Now more than ever, the EMS profession needs innovators, champions, and global thinkers. New educators should consider themselves sculptors ready to wield the chisel. They should dare to think greatly. Most importantly, they should use this text not as simply a set of instructions, but rather to guide their creativity.

The first step in that creativity should be a consideration of educational philosophy.

Creating an Educational Philosophy

Creating an **educational philosophy** dates as far back as to the teachings of Plato and simply refers to the set of beliefs that defines the purpose of education. These beliefs form the foundation for the role as an educator and the application of a curriculum.[1] One's educational philosophy is guided by the standards of the EMS profession but also is strongly rooted in an individual's own core values, ethics, and experiences. Creating an educational philosophy that purposely utilizes attributes to become an effective educator supports the desired outcome of producing excellent EMS practitioners.

The Values of the EMS Profession

The values of the EMS profession can be identified from a wide range of sources. From the National Highway

Traffic Safety Administration (NHTSA) EMS Agenda 2050[2] to the NHTSA National EMS Education Standards (referred to as the Standards),[3] there are ample documents that reflect a lively conversation on the key attributes of a healthy EMS system. While many of these resources reflect a high-level viewpoint, there are explicit core values expressed that are particularly meaningful to the EMS educator. Take for example, the Standards' 11 professional clinical behaviors and judgments of emergency responders.[3]

The Standards is the document that serves as the foundation of an EMS course curriculum and creates the framework for important continuing education. The Standards identify key attributes and expectations of competent practitioners. These attributes include the following:

- Integrity
- Empathy
- Self-motivation
- Neat appearance and personal hygiene
- Effective communication
- Self-confidence
- Effective time management
- Teamwork and diplomacy
- Respect
- Patient advocacy
- Careful delivery of services

Take note that although most EMS curricula are weighted heavily in favor of clinical and factual content, the clear majority of the attributes just listed reflect affective and compassionate care characteristics. If a class offers little more than question and answer recall of facts, where will tomorrow's practitioner learn the elements considered important enough to publish as professional standards?

It must be recognized that many of these attributes reflect leadership and effective teamwork. In an age where as many as 210,000 people may die annually because of medical error,[4] these attributes—that together form the basis for crew resource management—must be not only considered, but held as core values. Concepts such as these are outlined in detail in the Strategy for a National EMS Culture of Safety document.[5]

The origins of EMS leadership qualities remain an elusive topic among the published values of the EMS profession. Although stated frequently in stakeholder conversations, there are few clearly delineated requirements or quantified attributes attached to EMS education. Nonetheless, a wide array of subtopics embraces their importance. From culture of safety, to high performance cardiac arrest care, to recruitment and retention, leadership is acknowledged as a vital attribute for EMS practitioners. And although it may not be formally scripted, standards of practice are rapidly moving to uphold its value. For example, the National Registry of Emergency Medical Technicians' paramedic psychomotor examination now evaluates leadership in its Integrated Out-of-Hospital Scenario evaluation.[6] Furthermore, the Committee on Accreditation of Educational Programs for the Emergency Medical Services Professions (CoAEMSP) has recently updated their standards for paramedic programs to include team leadership evaluation as a required element of a paramedic program curriculum.[7] What this effectively means is that although leadership is not explicitly stated, its value in EMS education should not be underestimated. Key leadership components should be integrated at all levels of EMS education, not just those with specific evaluation requirements.

The professional expectations of EMS are constantly updated. In an age where the total amount of medical information doubles every 73 days,[9] standards must change, and expectations must be adjusted to reflect the new norms. Excellent educators and field training officers must be prepared to adjust, adapt, and maintain their own currency among a growing tide of change.

Common Leadership Characteristics[8]

In his doctoral dissertation, Dr. Michael Miller used a grounded theory evaluation of EMS students to identify 15 common leadership characteristics. They are as follows:

- Adapt-Improvise-Creative
- Calm
- Collaborate-Cooperative
- Communication (effective)
- Critical thinking
- Decisive
- Delegate-Direct-Coordinate-Organize
- Honesty
- Knowledgeable
- Listen
- Mentor-Teacher
- Respectful
- Self-confident
- Self-reflective
- Trust

EMS Agenda 2050

The EMS Agenda 2050 is a vision for the future that identifies EMS systems as people-centered. The vision for EMS systems is based on these major priorities:

- Inherently safe care for patients and practitioners. Effective care is evidence-based.
- Integrated with all stakeholders who provide and receive services, in order to provide seamless care.
- Sustainable resources for services and practitioners, in order to provide efficient services.
- Reliable access to EMS services that are prepared for day-to-day activity as well as unplanned large-scale events.
- Socially equitable access to quality care for all communities.
- Adaptability to effectively implement new technologies and educational programs with innovative leadership.

The Values of the EMS Educator

Any educational philosophy will be grounded in the values and beliefs of the EMS educator. These elements are developed over time and reflect myriad influences from caregivers, education, and religion, to simple life experiences. As an educator, these values guide the interpretation of content and heavily influence the manner in which it is presented. Educators should reflect on personal experiences and remember those moments that have served best—not only EMS practice, but also in life. In most cases, this reflection will lead to the discovery of themes and practices that have been associated with success.

Ethics

Defined by Merriam-Webster as the system of moral principles that govern an individual or group,[10] ethics are a common attribute associated with both interpersonal and vocational success. People want and deserve to be treated fairly and be free from discrimination. Any educational philosophy should hold ethical behavior as a key tenant. Unfortunately, the culture of public safety far too often falls short. Consider the 2014 National Report Card on Women in Firefighting. It noted that of 675 respondents, 31.9% of female firefighters reported being verbally and/or sexually harassed.[11] More than a third were discriminated against! It is incongruent in a time when recruitment and retention are among the highest priorities of most departments for our professional culture to be, in effect, shunning a large portion of those wishing to join its ranks. Although this is a limited study, EMS educators must consider the opportunity to learn from such potential shortcomings and do their part to mold a culture that will be held to a higher ethical standard.

Empowerment

Success is most often linked with the idea of being empowered. This concept relates to encouragement, confidence, self-esteem, and strength. As a concept, these themes are frequently described using the term **self-efficacy**. Self-efficacy has been previously defined as an individual's belief in their capacity to execute behaviors necessary to produce specific performance attainments.[12] Self-efficacy and empowerment enable students to seize opportunity and afford them resilience in the face of failure.[13] Academic environments that empower students foster inquisitive tendencies and push students toward leadership roles. Conversely, situations that leave students feeling disenfranchised and powerless lead to apathy, disengagement, and fear of failure. Unfortunately, empowerment is another trait that is not universally valued in public safety. Public safety has historically structured organizations in a paramilitary model and has bred a top-down leadership style. The "do what I say or else" transactional leadership style empowers a small minority while removing power from the greater majority. Fundamentally, this inhibits the development of future leaders.[14] Top-down leadership instills the flawed notion that empowering others takes power away from leaders. Some experts would suggest that this, in turn, breeds bullying and exclusivity among our profession. More study is needed, but it is interesting to consider that the two professions that, statistically, have the highest rate of workplace bullying are hospital-based health care and public service (including fire and EMS).[15]

Learning Experiences

Specific learning styles will be discussed later in this text, but when developing an educational philosophy, educators should reflect on the experiences that led to personal learning success. In general, past experiences stir passion and enthusiasm that can be harnessed in the classroom, and these positive traits are most commonly linked to learner success. However, while past experiences should not be ignored, it is equally important to remember that not every student learns the same way; the experiences that worked for one, may indeed not benefit all. In addition to learning success,

CASE in Point

"Mary" is one of the few female EMTs in her large urban EMS department. Although she has not experienced active discrimination, she often feels excluded and isolated among her male peers. She is a good provider and works hard to improve her knowledge and skills. She struggles, however, to find opportunities to get ahead.

Each year Mary's service requires annual department continuing education classes. During the class in which the agency's human resources policies were being reviewed, Mary's male instructor, a more senior paramedic on the service, reads aloud the city's sexual harassment policies. However, he makes no attempt to hide his participation in obviously sexist conversations with other employees during breaks. The instructor consistently allows his male students to dominate class discussions and makes no attempt to correct obviously inaccurate comments regarding the department's approach to gender issues. Mary feels like she has little chance for success.

These inequities are repeated not just in human resources policy reviews, but in most department-sponsored continuing education classes. Consistently, male voices are loudest and male employees are first to be selected for scenario-based leadership positions. Mary becomes discouraged and begins to shy away from scenarios because she feels the instructor does not think she "has what it takes" to be a leader. She is struggling.

educators should reflect also on their own negative learning experiences. What common traits made learning more difficult?

Life Experience

When developing an educational philosophy, educators should consider their own life experiences. It is easy to appreciate the idea of a classroom filled with unbending rules and standards set so high as to "weed out" the undeserving. However, filtered through one's own life experiences, it becomes clear that such an approach is not particularly reasonable. Most EMS students are adult learners and carry a full load of life's extraneous baggage. Work requirements, family life, and just plain hard luck all influence the capabilities of today's students. Although this does not mean instructors need to abolish standards, it does mean that policies and expectations should be framed around the idea that sometimes life can be difficult.

Educators' values and experiences influence almost every aspect of their career. These elements serve as the foundation for who they are and what they want to be. Lessons from one's history are the most important barometer for the choices an individual will make. It is important to understand, however, that these values are just one element of a larger educational philosophy. Educators must always learn, adapt, and improve. In fact, transitioning those experiences into quality practice is exactly the path taken by excellent educators.

Transitioning from Philosophy to Practice

An educational philosophy is truly effective only if it can be transitioned from theory to practice. The first step toward becoming an excellent educator is to transfer these experiences, lessons, and values into a meaningful philosophy that can be used in the classroom. Educators should reflect on the key elements that define them as a person and incorporate those elements into an educational strategy. But there is more to excelling as an educator than simply reflecting on and totaling past experiences. In fact, just being a good person or a good practitioner does not always translate into being an excellent educator. Experiences must be translated to an educational model, and the skills of the accomplished educator need to be cultivated.

In *The Skillful Teacher*, Stephen Brookfield suggests that instructors "adopt a critically reflective stance towards their practice."[16] This stance, developed as a teaching philosophy, gives direction and purpose to actions and decisions made while designing learning or when teaching in the classroom. Lindeman supports this when he says, "The person who is vividly aware of his activity, as well as the goal toward which the activity is directed, becomes conscious of his powers and limitations."[17] A philosophical statement can guide an instructor in the same way the mission, vision, and values of an organization drive its key actions, decisions, and strategies. A well thought-out philosophy provides a framework for reflection on action when teaching. It is important to recognize that a teaching philosophy is not a static document. As instructors grow and gain experience, their teaching philosophy will change to reflect their changing views about themselves and their relationships to students, to learning, and to teaching.

Lorraine Zinn suggests that, while defining a working philosophy of education, the first step is to examine what the educator believes about the adult learners, the overall purpose of education, the content or subject, and the learning process. Examining one's beliefs about the role of the adult educator is another

Developing a Teaching Philosophy[19]

David Royse, in his text *Teaching Tips for College and University Instructors*, proposes that all educators should construct a teaching philosophy that represents what is most important to them as educators. In identifying his own philosophy, Royse considered the instructors who had influenced him positively, both personally and professionally, as well as those who had affected him with poor teaching and interpersonal skills. His philosophy of important issues includes the following:

- Create a sense of community in the classroom. Students learn more and enjoy learning when they feel connected to one another and to the instructor.
- Ensure that education is a two-way, interactive process. The instructor is neither infallible nor an authority on all matters.
- Give respect to each individual person in the classroom.
- Be accountable to the students. Make sure to prepare appropriately and be on time for class, as well as to offer timely, high-quality feedback to students.
- Make sure that learning is fun. Include humor as part of all classes.
- Apply learning to issues and problems in the world today.
- Hold lifelong learning as a goal.

important step.[18] There is no "perfect" teaching philosophy; the differences in instructional philosophy mirror the rich diversity seen in great EMS educators. See an example of David Royse's approach in the text box "Developing a Teaching Philosophy."

The Educator as a Role Model

Daniel Tosteson, a longtime dean credited with reshaping Harvard Medical School, said, "We must acknowledge that the most important, indeed the only, thing we have to offer our students is ourselves. Everything else they can read in a book."[20] Today's students have a world of knowledge at their fingertips and the speed at which that knowledge changes is beyond comprehension. The difference between a Web search and a classroom is the presence of the educator. A smartphone cannot impress upon them the value of the information they seek. A computer cannot demonstrate the benefits of experience. In this way, the application of an educational philosophy becomes an invaluable component in creating EMS practitioners who understand and appreciate more than just facts and figures. An excellent educator provides information, but also filters that information through past experiences and core values. As such, graphs and charts become more than just memorization, they become useful tools that students can find relevant and meaningful.

For most students, their educator is the first model of what an EMS provider should be. Similar to the influence of childhood caregivers, EMS educators serve as the first frame of reference for how new information is interpreted. This first snapshot is critically important, as it will powerfully influence the student's core values. Certainly, educators are role models as experienced clinicians and teachers. Keep in mind that they are also role models for ethical behavior.

Learning from role models involves both observation and reflection, and is a complex mix of both conscious and unconscious activities.[21] Students learn not only from their educators' clinical competence and knowledge base, but also from their educators' demeanor, attitude, and engagement. This means that educators must be ever vigilant to display the attributes this profession values the most.

Ethics as an Educator

Central to the EMS profession is the sacred trust shared with patients and their families. A practitioner's integrity ensures that in their worst moments, practitioners will serve as patient advocates who deliver competent, compassionate care. At the core of patient trust is the notion that EMS responders will behave with an ethical standard and deliver care free from bias or discrimination. EMS carries this ethical standard further to ensure that in this profession, practitioners are treated with respect and afforded opportunities based on merit—not race, creed, age, sexuality, gender, or disability. Employers expect the same ethical accountability from their employees, who are daily charged with operating equipment, handling medications, and interfacing with patients. Ethics form the cornerstone of EMS core values, and as such education must reflect this importance.

More than just a lesson or two on "medical-legal" concepts, ethics need to be integrated into each and every class. The lessons of right or wrong are formed in the classroom, and educators should control these lessons.

As role models, educators must be prepared for the daily demonstration of ethical and nonethical behavior. An educator's actions, or inactions, toward these

CASE in Point

The following message was posted to a class message board: "The other night in class our instructor made a joke about homosexuals. I was glad to see him let his hair down a little. I think everyone knew he was just kidding, and the joke was kind of funny. I'm really glad we can have a class where everyone isn't so uptight all the time." What message do you think the instructor's action sent, not just to this student, but to all the students in class?

behaviors will weigh heavier than any reading assignment or quiz. Educators must adhere to the highest professional standards and never waiver. Although this is a heavy burden, recall that educators are both consciously and unconsciously imprinting lasting impressions with every decision they make.

Consider that an EMS educator is a member of two professions, teaching and healthcare practice, and must comply with the requirements and standards of each. An EMS practitioner is subject to the local and state laws of professional ethics and the policies of the services for which they work. Members of the teaching profession are subject to the regulations and ethical guidelines of the institutions or facilities where they teach.

Following best practices concerning ethical and professional responsibility can guide new educators and remind experienced ones of the basic ethical standards of their profession. Of course, more explicit and specific guidelines should be presented in a formal disciplinary code or policy handbook, but the basis and relevance of any guideline is based on the example an educator sets.

Ethical Responsibilities to Students

As educators, scholars, counselors, and mentors, EMS educators can profoundly influence students' attitudes concerning professional competence and responsibility. Educators must help students recognize the liability that surrounds the accountability and responsibility they have to their profession and to the community at large.

Educators should aspire to excellence in teaching and to mastery of the theories and practices of the subjects they teach. Furthermore, they should prepare conscientiously for class and employ teaching methods appropriate for the subject matter and objectives of the courses. For example, accountability and credibility are demonstrated when classes start and end on time.

Explaining the meaning and implications of the syllabus and policies and procedures holds everyone accountable to each other. Policies should be reviewed with the class, ensuring that each student fully understands them and has the opportunity to ask questions. It is advisable to have students sign a contract acknowledging receipt of the handbook and syllabus and acceptance of its contents.

Educators enjoy relative academic freedom and autonomy in the classroom. However, academic freedom and autonomy do not mean that standards of practice and accountability for performance can be ignored or altered. Educators must adhere to educational and clinical practice standards at the institutional, state, and national levels. The best way to ensure that educators are upholding standards of practice is to have a well-developed peer-review process in place (**FIGURE 1.1**).

Several methods are commonly used to develop a peer-review process. The key is to have as many different perspectives as possible from which feedback is obtained. Peer review is different from student evaluation of a program or faculty. Although student evaluations are an important feedback tool, they come from a relatively unsophisticated audience. Having the head of the department or program sit in on a classroom session and provide feedback is the most common form of peer review. Equally valuable, and sometimes less intimidating, is having a peer instructor provide this service. Note that the instructor doing the peer evaluation does not have to be a subject matter expert, but the person should be an experienced educator.

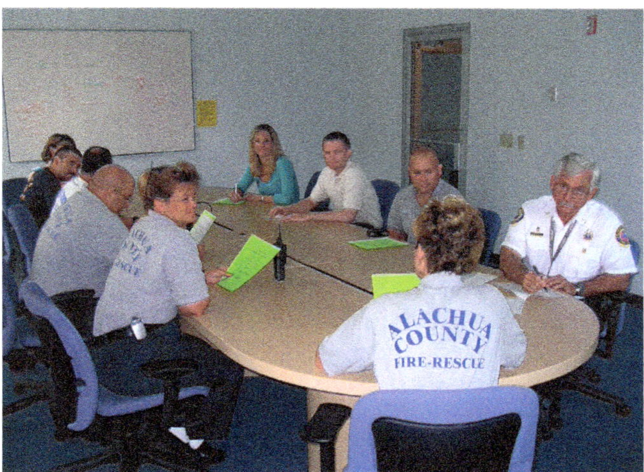

FIGURE 1.1 An advisory group can provide valuable input for the educational program, thus enhancing the value of the program to the community.

Courtesy of L. Charles Smeby, Jr., University of Florida.

Another means of procuring peer review is to obtain feedback from state or national testing organizations. Still another type of peer review is feedback that can be obtained from agencies that employ graduates from the course. Lastly, do not forget to talk with instructors and field and clinical preceptors. They are invaluable sources of information regarding student strengths and weaknesses. The ideal is for each of these peer-review feedback processes to become formal and routine aspects of every school's evaluation process.

Terminology: Assessment versus Evaluation

The terms *assessment* and *evaluation* can be confusing and are sometimes used interchangeably. In general, in the higher education arena, the terms are used as follows:

- **assessment** Measuring student learning
- **evaluation** Measuring program or faculty performance

The Ethics of Student Assessment

EMS educators and field training officers have a fundamental obligation to fairly, accurately, and constructively assess student work. This is a crucial aspect of respecting and nurturing students.

Exams and assignments should be designed to meet the expectations of student performance, and assessment materials should match learning objectives and stated goals. Moreover, student work should be assessed with impartiality. The instructor may enhance impartiality by blinding the review of student material—that is, the student is not identified until after the review has been completed. Another way to achieve impartiality with essay-type exams is by using a **rubric**, or *grading template*, that outlines all of the important points that must appear in the student's written work. (See Chapter 22, *Other Assessment Tools*.)

The standards for assigning grades should be consistent with standards recognized within the facility or institution. Students should be informed about assessment methods in the syllabus with a clearly defined basis on which grades are assigned. Instructors should offer an explanation if students ask why they received a certain grade. In addition, instructors should grade and provide feedback to students in a timely fashion. When assessment criteria are clearly defined and followed by the instructor, students will typically not win an appeal for a failing grade.

The Ethics of Counseling

Timely and accurate counseling is an essential element of developing student success. As an educator, you should make yourself reasonably available to your students to discuss academic, career, and professional concerns.

Confidentiality is the ethical cornerstone of counseling. Students should feel safe sharing sensitive information and be comfortable that the information will not be disclosed. If your institution or local laws require specific counseling disclosures (such as in the case of a student who intends to commit self-harm or harm others), this policy should be stated in your handbook or syllabus and discussed prior to any counseling session.

EMS educators should make every attempt to limit student counseling activities to performance, attitudes about their learning, and suggestions for improvement. Educators should avoid venturing into the counseling arenas of mental health, marital, and other significant life issues and know when and how to direct students to more specialized counseling resources.

The Ethics of Personal Relationships with Students

The small, community-like nature of the EMS profession makes personal relationships difficult to avoid. In EMS, everyone knows everyone, and everyone knows everyone's business. However, as an educator, personal relationships with students can create significant ethical liability and crisis. From outright sexual **harassment** policy violations to the perception of conflict of interest, allowing students to get too close is a significant ethical dilemma. Although most educators wish to be perceived as friendly and maintain a collegial classroom environment, there must be a clear line between the educator and student. It is especially important that the educator not engage in a personal relationship. The perception or reality of harassment of a student has federal law implications and has the potential to end an educator's career. Harassment should be defined in student and faculty policies. Ethically, an educator has professional responsibility for all students while teaching, evaluating, supervising, mentoring, or advising. There are also ethical responsibilities when working with peer instructors.

An educator who is closely related to a student by blood or marriage, or who has a preexisting close relationship with a student, generally should avoid any role involving professional responsibility for that student. There should be full disclosure of any conflict of interest, in documented form.

Maintaining appropriate and ethical relationships may be particularly difficult when an educator is called upon to teach or assess within their own department. Frequently, field training, performance improvement, and continuing education roles can place educators in situations where they are called to teach and assess their peers (and often personal friends). When accepting these roles, an educator must make sure clear, well-documented policies exist that define the scope and expectations of their positions. Furthermore, educators should realize that accepting such positions may temporarily or permanently alter their ability to maintain previous personal relationships and must weigh these consequences before accepting such responsibility. Most importantly, educators should be open, honest, and forthcoming any time the professional/personal line becomes blurry and should err on the side of caution.

Rights of Learners[22]

Learners have a right to the following:

- A clear indication of expectations for a course or program
- Reasonable access to the instructor and resources
- Due process when challenging the judgments and actions of the instructor
- Treatment with dignity and respect at all times
- A learning environment that is fair, safe, and productive

Responsibilities of Educators[22]

Educators have a responsibility for the following:

- Accurately represent the work of others (avoiding plagiarism)
- Maintain professional, vocational, or academic competence
- Maintain confidentiality in matters related to evaluation and assessment
- Ensure that what is taught matches what was promised
- Ensure that what is tested or assessed matches what was taught

The Ethics of Diversity

Educators must make the learning environment a hospitable community and comfortable setting for all students. Discriminatory conduct based on race, color, religion, national origin, sex, sexual orientation, disability, age, or political beliefs is unacceptable in the education community. It is important for educators to be sensitive to the harmful consequences of instructor or student conduct, or comments in classroom discussions or elsewhere that perpetuate stereotypes or prejudices. Educators must put bias, discrimination, and conflict of interest aside. Students will model the collaborative behavior and tolerance if the educator consistently models that behavior.

More importantly, diversity in the classroom enhances the education experience (**FIGURE 1.2**). By celebrating rather than discriminating, educators can weave different backgrounds, experiences, and cultures into the learning process. Too often bigotry is caused by ignorance. In a diverse and equal learning environment, experience challenges assumptions and truth debunks stereotypes. Chapter 6, *Culture in the EMS Classroom,* discusses diversity in the learning environment in detail.

The Ethics of Scholarship

As a community, EMS educators have a basic responsibility to refine, extend, and transmit knowledge regarding the teaching and practice within their specific discipline. Educational institutions and programs also have a responsibility to maintain an atmosphere of

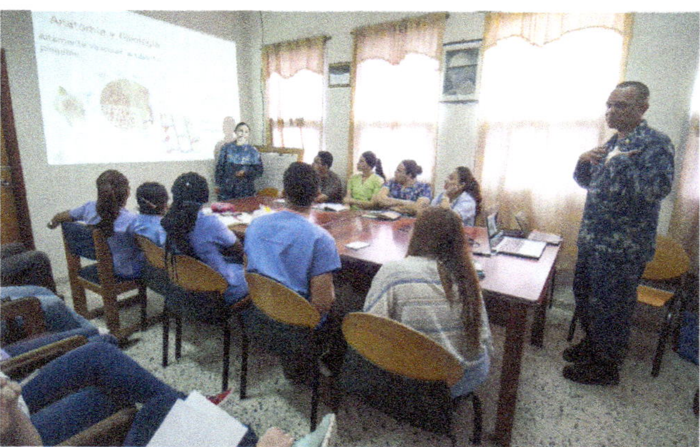

FIGURE 1.2 A diverse classroom enhances the education experience by offering first-hand interaction and perspectives a student may not otherwise have experienced.

freedom and tolerance in which knowledge can be sought and shared. This continuous intellectual exchange ultimately improves knowledge and benefits the profession.

An open exchange of information does however require intellectual honesty. Although an educator should feel free to criticize another's work, distortion or misrepresentation is always unacceptable. When using any intellectual work of another author—whether that of another educator or a student—the original author must be acknowledged every time the ideas are used or transmitted. Appropriate ways to acknowledge contributions of others is through shared authorship, attribution by footnote or endnote, or discussion of the original author's contributions within the main text or within a presentation.

An educator has a responsibility to preserve the integrity and independence of research and to promote the development of new knowledge. Sponsored or compensated research activities or presentations should always be acknowledged with full disclosure of any personal interests. Conflicts of interest should be acknowledged and brought forward for discussion among educators and students. It is best to err on the side of conservatism when addressing conflict of interest situations. If an instructor believes there might be a conflict, there probably is; it is wise to disclose the possibility to others with whom or for whom the instructor is working.

The Educator as a Professional

It is in the best interest of EMS educators to further the professionalization of the industry. The grounding of the attributes of professionalism in education is, by definition, one of the ways EMS as an industry will emerge as unique and valuable

Epstein and Hundert describe the attributes of professionalism in medicine as "the habitual and judicious use of communication, knowledge, technical skills, clinical reasoning, emotions, values, and reflection in daily practice for the benefit of the individual and community being served."[23]

When considering EMS educators as role models, it is important to identify how these key elements translate into classroom attributes.

Dr. Herbert Swick, a physician and executive director of the Institute of Medicine and Humanities at Saint Patrick Hospital and the University of Montana, has done extensive research on professionalism in medicine. His work has distilled distinct elements and attributes of professionalism that can be helpful to educators (see the box, *Swick's Elements of Professionalism*).[24]

Finally, another element of professionalism is creating a nonpolitical classroom environment. Refrain from discussing politics with students and peers in an educational setting.

Swick's Elements of Professionalism[24]

1. Professionals subordinate their own interest to the interest of others.
2. Professionals adhere to the highest ethical and moral standards.
3. Professionals respond to social needs, and their behaviors reflect a social contract with the communities served.
4. Professionals demonstrate core humanistic values, including honesty, integrity, caring, compassion, altruism, empathy, respect for others, and trustworthiness.
5. Professionals exercise accountability for themselves and for their colleagues.
6. Professionals demonstrate a continuing commitment to excellence.
7. Professionals exhibit a commitment to scholarship and to advancing their field of study.
8. Professionals deal with high levels of complexity and uncertainty.
9. Professionals reflect on their actions and decisions.

TEACHING TIP

Prove Me Wrong

Instructors should encourage students to develop their own ideas and opinions by reading and researching. When new evidence or contrary opinions emerge, do not shun them—celebrate them through discussion and classroom sharing.

The Educator as a Leader

From both a professional and operational mindset, role modeling leadership skills is essential to the educator.

How best to teach and demonstrate leadership is a vast topic and well beyond the scope of this chapter, but in general, there are some key concepts that can be easily integrated and make a profound difference. Examples include the following:

- Has the educator defined the attributes of their leadership style? Are these attributes reflected in class values or affective objectives? Are they evaluated?

- Are students placed into leadership roles within the classroom? Are students placed in squads or teams that work consistently together? These can be scenario evolutions, role-playing situations, or even simple class groups with specific goals and objectives.
- Do students feel empowered to assume leadership roles? Is leadership initiative rewarded? How are students mentored as team members and team leaders?
- Are leadership opportunities distributed equally among candidates?

Role modeling must also consider the attributes of effective leaders. Educators should ask themselves if during classroom management they are demonstrating the following:

- Calmness and confidence?
- Willingness to collaborate?
- Effective communication?
- Decisiveness?
- Honesty, trustworthiness, and respect?
- Listening?
- Self-reflectiveness?

These attributes, while seemingly simple, not only demonstrate best practice in managing difficult classroom situations, but also demonstrate the very attributes that are valuable to impart upon students. If it is the expectation that students will learn leadership skills within the classroom, then they must experience quality leadership behaviors by educators.

Swick, in his elements of professionalism, notes that professionals respond to social needs, and their behaviors reflect a social contract with the communities served.

The EMS profession expects practitioners to exhibit, as Swick puts it, "core humanistic values," including honesty, integrity, caring, compassion, altruism, empathy, respect for others, and trustworthiness. Where will students learn these? Students must be able to see their instructors, whether the guest lecturer or practical lab preceptor, working together effectively and respectfully as a team of educators. Not all affective lessons occur in scripted scenarios. Educators have ample opportunities daily to display these attributes through basic classroom management. Even though the lessons may not be explicit, the unconscious evaluation by students of their instructor's behavior creates lasting effects.

Any profession best meets its obligations when its members attend actively to community and social needs. Sullivan's concept of civic professionalism stresses the importance of social leadership.[25] One way in which EMS educators can begin to fulfill their social contract is to form advisory groups from within the community to help guide educational services. It is not enough that educators think they know what is best for the community they serve; they must actively seek out the opinions of those within the community. This involves gathering information on the scheduling of courses, the number and type of courses offered, and suggested additions and deletions to the curriculum. In addition, continuing education and case study reviews, as part of the larger performance management system, can offer timely, agency-specific topics in an effort to improve practice.

It is reasonable to include instructor-facilitated discussions about problematic events or patient situations, to give the student the opportunity to critically think and collaborate on how they can find solutions. Examples of issues might include first responder suicide or domestic violence. Taking an affirmative stand might risk polarizing some students, but it also demonstrates empathy, embracing diversity, and the kind of leadership the EMS profession needs.

TEACHING TIP

The most effective way to impart to students the values of honesty, integrity, caring, compassion, altruism, empathy, respect for others, and trustworthiness is for the instructor to be a good role model for these values by living them every day and in every interaction.

The Educator as a Mentor

It is easy to step into a role as an educator and envision oneself as the hero. The educator is the person with the knowledge and information students seek. In actuality, the educator role is less about being the hero and far more about being a **mentor**. The educator is the supporting actor, and the student is the star. One of the most important roles an educator serves is as the facilitator of learning. The purpose of mentoring is to provide opportunity for professional growth, whether it be for a new faculty member or a student.

Sharing power does not necessarily take power away from the educator. Rather than demanding performance, mentors role-model results. The role of the mentor is to guide, advise, and coach the new instructor.[26] Mentoring involves a willingness to inspire, motivate, and empower students to value learning.

For mentorship to be active, classroom design must be student centered, not instructor centered. A mentoring environment is centered around mutual trust and respect. It is a shared responsibility. This trust builds an interdependent relationship between the mentee and mentor, which may last a lifetime. While interdependency may be a novel concept in regard to mentoring, it is the foundation to observe the student's or faculty member's progressive learning.

As a lead instructor or program director, leadership involves mentoring students as well other faculty. Mentoring new instructors, whether for a lecture or lab, ensures that the information shared is what the student needs to know to be successful. It is reasonable to set high expectations and standards, but these must emerge from open communication and proven support. Educators who mentor effectively demonstrate student advocacy and consider facilitation of student success the highest priority.

Mentoring is also an exceptionally important role for field training officers and continuing education instructors. The world of public safety has many flaws, and practitioners are exposed every day to the worst of what this culture offers. There has never been a stronger need for leaders to emerge and demonstrate excellence. Mentoring offers not only ongoing support, but a constant source of cultural improvement.

Engaged, empathetic mentors show students and new instructors that exploring new ideas or sharing concerns and frustrations results in opportunities to learn new ways to problem-solve, without fear of retribution or failure. Mentors provide support through active listening, collaboration, problem solving, and new challenges. This is done to encourage mentees to be curious and to inspire them to accept the challenge of learning new ideas, skills, and strategies. It also instills the importance of evidence-based practice and a desire to learn throughout their career.

Aspects of Mentorship

Navigating the highs and lows of an educational career requires help. Few can go it alone; education is a team sport. Finding a support system that includes mentors is an essential component of developing a plan for success. Mentors have experienced similar challenges and similar low points, and can provide ongoing motivation to defeat negativity. Most importantly, mentors offer reminders in disillusioned times that educators are not alone, and even the most significant difficulties can be overcome. Fellow EMS educators can offer the unique insight of having shared such challenges, along with suggestions on how to overcome them.

An educator with more experience can help a novice instructor avoid mistakes commonly made by beginners. Fellow educators can also help navigate the sometimes-complex world of EMS education. For example, new instructors can learn from shadowing EMS educators who serve as ambassadors to local educational institutions and systems. Effective mentors can assist with lesson-plan development, syllabi, or other learning activities. Creating a list of colleagues with special knowledge in a particular area of the curriculum facilitates identification of those who can assist in lesson plan building and teaching. The experienced instructor can also direct novice faculty to other resources within the facility and familiarize them with the culture of the institution.

Most importantly, the mentor serves as a sounding board as new instructors reflect on successes and failures in their new role. As professionals, educators should be open to lending time to the newest initiates. Veteran educators must adopt an altruistic approach and recognize that by helping one another, they are in fact helping themselves. In fact, mentors also learn from their role; through actively observing, a mentor may learn new and different approaches to solving a problem or integrating a new skill.

Numerous studies demonstrate a positive correlation between the presence of mentors and an educator's longevity;[27] others identify a link between mentors and job satisfaction.[28] As such, the novice educator should make early efforts to seek out willing professionals to assist with professional development.

Finding a Mentor

Finding a mentor can be a challenge. Most students and new instructors do not feel comfortable or know how to find a person to mentor them. They may worry that the act of seeking out a mentor suggests they are incompetent or lack the ability to be successful on their own. The opposite is actually true. All instructors have experienced successes and failures in their professional career, as either clinicians or instructors.

There is a tendency for people to reflect themselves in their choices of mentors.[29] People tend to gravitate not only toward similar race and gender, but also toward those who share similar experiences, philosophies, and opinions.[30] What opportunity will this provide? This tendency allows for less growth than that afforded by advice from someone who sees the world from a different perspective.

Rather than seeking those who share similar opinions, educators should seek to challenge their own status quo by seeking mentors who offer honesty in the face of difficult decisions. Educators should look for mentors who can challenge their commonly held beliefs and offer ideas that broaden current views. The desired relationship is one based on give and take. Both mentor and mentee must actively listen, dialogue, and share ideas.

Mentors must also be selected for their willingness and ability to dedicate time and energy to their mentees. While altruism is important, it is equally important that an educator be realistic about their own availability. Prospective mentors must ensure that they can schedule the required amount of time to be an effective mentor.

In a large qualitative study conducted at two teaching hospitals, physicians quantified both successful and unsuccessful mentoring relationships. In relationships that led to job satisfaction and longevity, mentors were described as "honest, respectful, active listeners, and willing to dedicate time." Successful mentees were described as "open to feedback, active listeners, respectful of input, and respectful of time." Conversely, the most common terms used to describe failed mentor relationships were "poor communication, inability to listen, and lack of commitment."[31]

New educators need to actively seek out mentors. Waiting passively for one to appear is a failed strategy. If the school does not assign a mentor, the educator should seek one or more colleagues to assist integration into the new teaching setting. Mentors are extremely important to both field training officers and continuing education instructors. In these contexts, an educator might consider turning to more senior employees within the agency to find mentors. They might also consider looking to outside peers or even educator groups like the National Association of EMS Educators (NAEMSE) for assistance.

Mentor roles vary, and in some cases new educators may have more than one mentor in order to gain expertise in a variety of areas.

Even experienced instructors seek career mentors to develop interests or to broaden professional knowledge. An external mentor is someone who is experienced, influential, and well respected in the field. Educators should find someone in the profession who has somewhat more experience, who has succeeded in gaining respect and advancement, and who can provide guidance and support.

Mentors are also important for providing contacts and opportunities in the field. In seeking career mentors, educators should look beyond their organization to the full professional network. Other healthcare professionals can be vital links to gaining important feedback and providing invaluable resources for developing curriculum content. A program advisory committee is an example of how educators work with stakeholders of diverse backgrounds to guide programmatic vision. In a similar way, diverse mentors with differing experiences can help enhance personal growth and development.

Even students can serve as mentors to an educator. If a student has expertise in a given area, consideration could be given to using that student as a resource.

CASE in Point

For a member of a minority community, finding a mentor can be particularly challenging. Consider the case of women in public safety. In a survey conducted in 2012, there were only 174 women in all of the United States employed full time by a fire department at the level of battalion chief or higher.[32] This suggests that a potential mentee, looking to find a female mentor possessing experience at a senior administrative position in the fire service will likely encounter significant difficulty. More than likely, this potential mentee will be forced to turn to a population with very different past experiences compared to her own. Different mentors are not unilaterally bad and many men flourish with guidance from female mentors (and vice versa); however, crossing that cultural barrier is fraught with misperceptions, stereotypes, and other ill-informed notions that can make simply identifying a mentoring opportunity difficult. As a profession, EMS needs to welcome the diversity that exists in the culture and strive to extend mentoring opportunities to deserving candidates based on no other expectation than merit.

Professional Development

The world of emergency care is complex. It requires constant **scholarship**, continuing education, and repetitive training to excel at a high level. The path to excellence as an EMS educator is truly a lifelong journey. Education, experience, coaching, and failure contribute to the EMS educator's ongoing professional development.

Commitment to Excellence and Scholarship

Swick notes that professionals demonstrate a continuing commitment to excellence, commitment to scholarship, and ability to deal with high levels of complexity and uncertainty.[24] These elements are essential behaviors that an EMS educator must model. By role modeling the professional attributes of commitment to excellence and ongoing scholarship, faculty offer students the tools to succeed once they leave class. Although many curricula focus on facts and regurgitation of knowledge, far more important is the quest for that knowledge. In time, answers will change, but what will persist is the need to seek out and obtain that new set of knowledge. Successful practitioners recognize the evolution of their knowledge set and understand how to obtain new and better information.

One of the most important answers an educator can ever offer is simply "I don't know." Many new educators feel pressured to portray themselves as all-knowing and are threatened by the vulnerability of being stumped. However, true professionals understand that no practitioner can ever know everything, and that a moment of vulnerability is not failure, but rather an incredibly important teaching moment that demonstrates the complexity of emergency medicine. Instead of hemming and hawing, "I don't know" should simply be followed by "Let's find out." More importantly, the admission of being stumped should be followed by a demonstration of how a true professional explores the question and obtains the missing information. Once again, the quest for knowledge is more important than the answer.

A commitment to excellence should also demonstrate an appreciation of new information, new research, and novel ideas. These traits should be demonstrated regularly in every classroom. A commitment to scholarship improves an educator's capabilities. Quality, evidence-based continuing education ensures that educational content will always be current.

Continuing Professional Development

Specific core building blocks and key concepts will serve as an excellent foundation for mastery and should be considered in any educator's development plan. From the earliest stages, EMS educators should integrate these key steps into an action plan to help maximize their success.

The term *continuing professional development* encompasses a wide range of activities that can improve an EMS instructor's knowledge, enhance the chance for advancement, and promote job satisfaction. It incorporates three broad areas:[33]

1. Self-directed learning
2. Formal professional development
3. Organizational development

Through lifelong learning, the educator can ensure that they are always employable by constantly developing and maintaining expertise demanded by the marketplace.

Self-Directed Learning

Most of an educator's continuing professional development is self-directed and occurs on a day-to-day basis. This self-directed learning occurs as an instructor prepares a lesson, participates in curriculum planning, teaches, conducts research, participates on committees, and reads professional materials. Ongoing scholarship, experiential learning, mentoring, and clinical development all contribute to the ongoing success of an educator. These techniques form the basis of self-directed learning.

Formal Professional Development

The availability of formal professional development programs is generally broad. It includes Web-based, local, national, and international continuing education seminars and conferences. Topics available through this format vary widely. An instructor's ability to attend this type of education may depend on financial support from their employer if travel is involved. Professional development may also include furthering one's own formal education by obtaining a specialty certification, degree, or advanced degree.

Organizational Development

Organizational (or staff) development is targeted education designed to improve or change performance within an institution. The amount and quality of organizational development varies widely by institution.

Maintaining Clinical Competency

Unfortunately, there is an expiration date on both the clinical information EMS educators have been taught and the educational theory presented in this text. No one knows the exact expiration date or what parts of the information will become incorrect, but it is inevitable that educators will need continuing education to stay current. This can be challenging for both instructors and students. The paired need to simultaneously learn new information and "un-learn" incorrect knowledge is frustrating, but it represents the complex nature of the EMS profession. Managing this complexity is an important attribute of professionalism. Educators should ask themselves how they will stay current as they step away from their original courses.

Clinical competency is perhaps the easiest of the professional attributes to maintain. Like no other point in history, medical information and learning opportunities are readily available at most anyone's fingertips. The Internet, social media, and availability of information have revolutionized continuing education. The biggest obstacle is no longer access, but rather motivation. Dedication to professionalism requires discipline, and that discipline is the key to maintaining clinical currency. Excellent practitioners and educators find time each week to spend on improving themselves in their

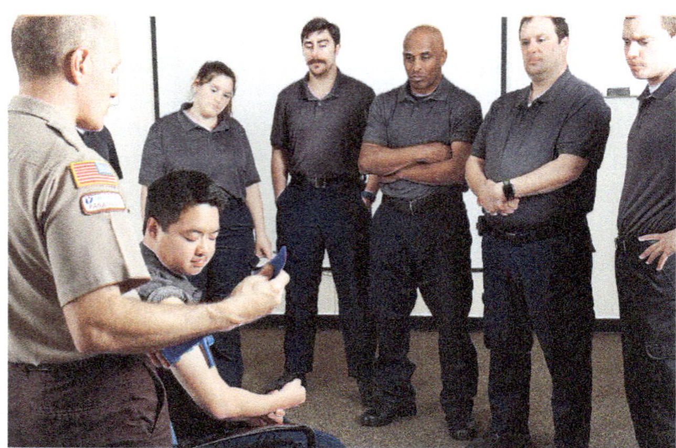

FIGURE 1.3 Mentoring students, shadowing students, and demonstrating skills (as shown here) all contribute to maintaining competency.

field of specialty. Reading, listening, and practicing are activities that can be integrated into a regular schedule.

Continuing to work in health care in a clinical environment or shadowing students in the clinical and field setting can help with maintenance of skill competency. When students see their instructor functioning in the workplace alongside them as a mentor, it helps to establish credibility. Actively performing skill demonstrations within lectures or facilitating in a practical teaching station also contributes to maintenance of skills (**FIGURE 1.3**).

The Free Open Access Meducation (FOAM) movement has been a boon to those looking to stay clinically current. This movement, which is mostly made up of emergency medicine practitioners of all levels, seeks to distribute topical medical information laterally via social media platforms. Readers must apply a scrutinizing eye to information posted on social media, but FOAM is an excellent resource to identify emerging trends in emergency medicine.

Educational Resources

Much like maintaining clinical competency, improving as an educator involves a combination of active participation in education, continuing coursework, and reading.

Many educational resources are readily available to both new and seasoned instructors to improve teaching skills. These resources include other educators' materials, government agencies or professional associations, and periodicals. A list of examples of each is provided in this section, but this is only a start. It would be impossible to list all of the resources available to instructors.

Numerous educators post their materials on the Internet. The instructor can readily find images, scenarios, blogs, PowerPoint presentations, test questions, classroom exercises, screencasts, videos, and other classroom-management tools. One effective way to search for these materials is to search for the medical topic of interest with the suffix "PowerPoint," "lecture," or "video" added to the topic. Another approach is to search the specific educational tool needed, such as "medical math problems," "teaching medical math," "drug calculations," and so on. Be sure to check copyright status before using material found online; some uses constitute copyright infringement, depending on the situation.

Membership in professional organizations is essential for keeping up with the developments of the profession and networking with peers who share problems and solutions. Membership in professional associations, such as NAEMSE, not only provides networking opportunities; it offers a direct connection to the ever-changing national landscape of the profession of clinician and educator. Awareness of those changes allows the educator to be proactive, rather than reactive, to changes in the content itself or methods of content delivery in the classroom.

Professional association, manufacturer, and government websites often have position statements, presentations, videos, and screencasts, or other current, accurate information that can be used to develop lessons. The Trading Post of NAEMSE contains EMS-specific educator resources. The NHTSA office of EMS publishes many vision and position documents, educational resources, research, National EMS Education Standards, and educator guidelines. The National Association of EMS Officials' website houses rich resources, including the National Model EMS Clinical Guidelines. The website and publications of the Centers for Disease Control and Prevention have up-to-date, accurate information related to diseases, EMS trauma triage guidelines, other trauma issues, disasters, and terrorism. Many other agencies and associations have valuable information that can be used as references for lesson preparations, as foundations for discussion assignments, and as resources for student projects.

Finally, there are a number of periodicals to which instructors can subscribe. They include educational journals such as *Domain3*, *Journal of Simulation*, *Adult Education Journal*, and *Adult Education Quarterly*. These journals present the latest research on instructional techniques. EMS and medical journals also include policy statements, articles, or research on education or instructional techniques relevant to EMS education. Referring to these journals informs evidence-based practice for both instructors and students. They include *Prehospital Emergency Care (PEC), EMS World, Journal of Emergency Medical Services (JEMS), Annals of Emergency Medicine, Pediatric Emergency Care, Academic Emergency Medicine, Journal of Emergency Primary Health Care, Circulation,* and many others.

EMS Association and Government Resources

- American College of Emergency Physicians (ACEP)
- American Heart Association (AHA)
- Commission on Accreditation for Prehospital Continuing Education (CAPCE)
- Committee on Accreditation of Educational Programs for the Emergency Medical Services Professions (CoAEMSP)
- Emergency Medical Services for Children (EMSC)
- Federal Emergency Management Agency (FEMA)
- Federal Interagency Committee on EMS (FICEMS)
- Individual state EMS Office websites
- International Association of Fire Chiefs (IAFC)
- International Association of Fire Fighters (IAFF)
- National Association of EMS Physicians (NAEMSP)
- National Association of EMTs (NAEMT)
- National Association of State EMS Officials (NASEMSO)
- National EMS Advisory Council (NEMSAC)
- National Highway Traffic Safety Administration (NHTSA)
- National Institutes of Health (NIH)
- National Registry of EMTs (NREMT)
- Office of EMS
- Society for Academic Emergency Medicine (SAEM)

Research

All professionals should be strongly committed to supporting research within their area of study. This requires the following:

- A functional knowledge of research methods
- The ability to conduct literature searches or reviews
- Evaluation of research for use in the classroom
- Presentation of research to students to instill a commitment in the next generation of professionals

Without formal and informal opportunities in which instructors can routinely gather and share knowledge, any profession is severely limited in its ability to advance. Introducing students to research early in their program provides a foundation upon which an educator can build a learning environment where evidence-based practice is emphasized and valued.

The Prehospital Care Research Forum (PCRF) at UCLA is an excellent resource for educators. As part of its mission to advance prehospital research, it offers articles, podcasts, workshops, and other resources to assist EMS educators and clinicians to participate in and analyze field research.

The EMS educator should subscribe to at least one professional peer-reviewed journal and one professional educational journal. Educators must be strong advocates with their administrators and librarians to ensure that funds for the appropriate professional journals for their professions are included in their institutional budget. In addition to periodicals, there are a number of excellent Web-based blogs, message boards, and news feeds dedicated to emergency medicine and healthcare topics. These blogs are often free and can be found in the form of podcasts and Internet videos, which makes access even more convenient. These are good sources of current clinical debates and topical clinical conversations. Of course, when accessing non-peer-reviewed material, the educator must be a critical consumer, but the value of this contemporary information is often very high.

TEACHING TIP

Require every student in every course to turn in two articles from clinical or educational peer-reviewed journals. The purpose of this exercise is for students to familiarize themselves with professional journals, including how to access them. Also, require students to provide the address of one website resource. In addition to the learning opportunity that this activity provides to students, instructors generally receive numerous interesting articles to read, along with 10 to 15 new Web addresses per class.

Conferences

Educators have a responsibility to learn current patient care methods and teaching strategies, and conferences provide the perfect learning opportunity. EMS educators should not limit themselves to local, regional, or even state conferences, but should attend national conferences as often as possible. Furthermore, educators should not limit themselves to discipline-specific conferences. There are wonderful national conferences on distance education, how to give presentations, technologies in education, testing and measurement, and student counseling (**FIGURE 1.4**). There are many benefits to attending national conferences that go beyond learning new instructional methodologies or learning about new treatment modalities and clinical practices. These include opportunities for career networking and the "cross pollination" of programs. The networking

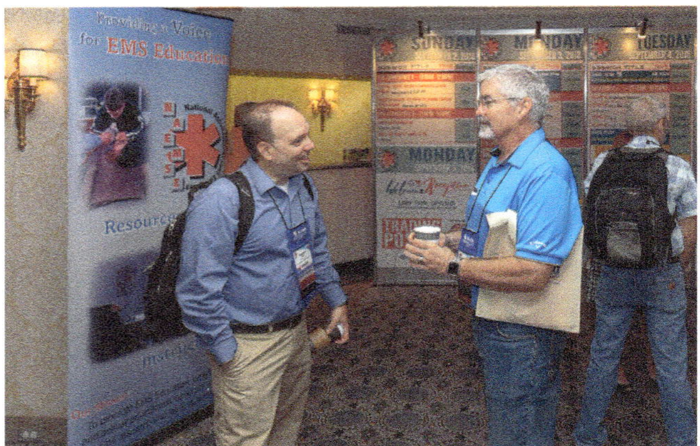

FIGURE 1.4 Instructors can keep abreast of new clinical topics, as well as educational techniques, by networking at conferences.

Courtesy of the National Association of EMS Educators.

opportunities provide avenues for contacts to recruit instructors and for contacts for future possible positions in other locations and institutions. Being tied into a national network is invaluable for assisting educators, students, and colleagues with job searches, and, often, when the time comes to relocate for career advancement, it provides contacts to find the best possible position in the best location.

Factors That Influence Professional Development

According to Zinn, throughout an educator's career there are four main influences that can either support or serve as barriers to an educator's success and satisfaction.[33] They are as follows:

1. Interpersonal relationships
2. Institutional structure
3. Personal considerations
4. Commitments, and intellectual and psychosocial characteristics

If absent, the supporting factors within each of these areas can become barriers. In some cases, the instructor can influence these factors to promote success, while in others they will be out of the instructor's control and the only solution may be a job change.

Interpersonal Relationships

Positive interpersonal relationships are essential for job satisfaction and success. They include demonstrating positive relationships with coworkers and administrative staff in a manner that models respect, recognizes achievement, and provides encouragement. They promote a supportive work environment. The educator should model these behaviors.

Institutional Structures

Institutional structures can influence the educator's success and development. Institutional factors that promote success in education include providing resources and time for the educator to attend professional development. An important institutional attribute is a climate that promotes collaboration and collegiality rather than competition among faculty.

Personal Considerations

Personal factors play a substantial role in an educator's professional development and can determine progress to a successful career. Having a strong network of family and friends to provide support for long and irregular work hours, travel, or interruptions for student crises can help performance. Major life crises such as deaths, divorce, or significant illness can have short- or long-term career implications.

Commitments, and Intellectual and Psychosocial Characteristics

The educator's individual, intellectual, and personal characteristics powerfully impact development. A strong work ethic with a commitment to excellence is essential. Instructors must believe in themselves and that their actions make a difference. The educator's ability to see where their role fits within the success of their students, their school/agency, and their field is critical. Just as important is the enjoyment of challenge and change, because both are essential to learn and grow as educators.

Becoming a Better EMS Educator

Excellence as an EMS educator is the sum of many important parts. Truly great educators combine elements of stage performance and oration with a blend of clinical competency and expertise and, finally, effective program and course design. However, beyond performance, they must also combine these skills with team building, inspirational leadership, and an acumen for interpersonal relationships. No one part is more important, and excellent educators remain flexible enough to apply the right measure of their skill set to the challenge at hand.

Chickering and Gamson reviewed 50 years of research on effective teaching and identified seven common principles of good teaching practice. These principles were later validated by additional research findings. They concluded that effective teaching involves the following:[34]

- Frequent contact between students and faculty
- Encouragement and cooperation among students
- Use of active-learning techniques
- Prompt feedback
- Emphasis on time on task
- Communication of high expectations
- Respect for diverse talents and ways of learning

Future chapters will provide greater depth on specific principles, but as educators consider their own path to excellence, they should plot their tactics around these points. Consider the importance of communication, empowerment, and feedback as they pertain to developing leadership skills. Consider respect for diversity as it pertains to ethics. These are not novel concepts, but rather reflect the core values the EMS profession should stand for.

It is also important to consider the common negative attributes of educators. Reflecting on these can help an educator navigate away from them as they plan development strategies.

Negative Characteristics of Educators

- **Dominating instructors** have difficulty organizing and running discussions. They demonstrate low levels of participation in student activities, especially if they do not learn to control this negative characteristic.
- **Noncurrent (out-of-touch) instructors** have difficulty clarifying issues, beliefs, and problems. They also tend to have problems explaining, informing, and demonstrating.
- **Egocentric (the world revolves around them) instructors** have difficulty referring students to other people and offices. They try to be their students' only source of information. In addition, these instructors find it almost impossible to defend other faculty, course directors, or agencies. They lay blame for any problem in the course to some external source, rather than taking responsibility.
- **Burned-out instructors** find it nearly impossible to motivate or encourage students.
- **Curriculum-based versus student-based (those who place more importance on the curriculum than on the student) instructors** find it very difficult to clarify questions and to construct tests. They have trouble getting into a student's head and seeing the class from the student's perspective.

TEACHING TIP

The best ways to avoid developing negative teaching characteristics are as follows:

- Equally balance decisions between what is good for the course and what is good for the students.
- Be a student. This, more than anything else, helps instructors to see things from the students' perspective.
- Remember that students need different levels of support at different times in the class.
- Be constantly alert to pressures in one's outside life that may creep into the classroom.
- Do not overcommit. It is better to say no to teaching a class than to teach it poorly.

Inspirational Delivery of Content

At the heart, any great educator is an effective communicator. Inspiring learning means first getting the message across; far too few educators truly understand the value of properly preparing their delivery methods. Great teaching is more than spitting out bullet points from a ready-made slide set. Great teaching encompasses honing presentation skills, applying the proper presentation style to best suit the message, selecting the appropriate method to teach specific content, and, of course, preparing.

It is important to note that in Chickering and Gamson's seven characteristics of effective teaching, they noted active learning as a key element. For years EMS education has focused on lecture, when in fact active strategies are more effective. That is not to say that lecture is always ineffective, but the educator should consider more than just one style of communicating.

Practice and experience (both good and bad) will help improve communication skills. Make no mistake though, these capabilities are learned behaviors that must be developed and practiced.

Active learning will be discussed in much greater detail later in the text, but when considering the general concept of self-improvement, it is important to reflect on the broad strategies that will make success more likely.

Creativity in Teaching

According to Thomas L. Schwenk and Neal Whitman, all effective instructors have one attribute in common—they present creative lessons that stimulate their students and make learning easier.[35] An educator can achieve this kind of creativity by starting with the lesson plan and asking if there is something they can do to make the learning more effective by being more creative.

Creativity is defined as any activity that is novel and useful and results in contributions to human experience. Novel approaches in the classroom may involve the use of interesting modalities of communication, the application of inventive or unorthodox teaching techniques, and the provision of memorable and meaningful educational experiences through graphic demonstrations or imagery. Useful approaches may include providing correct, up-to-date, and relevant information, along with opportunities to develop good problem-solving skills and good patient care attitudes.

Creative educators are both novel and useful. They reveal the "inner relevance" of what they teach.[36] Creative instructors exhibit three characteristics:

1. They are selective in choosing their teaching methodologies.
2. They pay attention to delivery.
3. They teach beyond the printed material—beyond the textbook.

On the opposite side of the spectrum of creative and excellent educators, there are ineffective educators, such as charlatans and pedantic bores.

- **Charlatan.** Instructors can be **charlatans**—persons who claim knowledge or skill that they do not possess—when they focus more on being novel, entertaining, and well-liked than on transmitting essential information and designing a meaningful learning experience. Students generally love charlatans. As a result, all will appear to be going well until students have to take the state or national exam. That is when students discover that their instructor has not adequately prepared them for the exam.

  One sign that an instructor is a charlatan is that they excessively use "war stories." Additionally, charlatans rarely have prepared teaching materials and rely more on personal interaction than on content. Moreover, charlatans can be spotted by the fact that they rarely take responsibility for their students' failures—failure is always someone else's fault. Charlatans focus on themselves rather than on meeting the students' learning needs.
- **Pedantic bore.** The term **pedantic bore** describes an instructor who is so concerned with the details, comprehensiveness, and accuracy of a lesson that the content becomes overwhelming and tedious to students. It is certainly better to be a pedantic bore than a charlatan; at least students receive useful information from a pedantic bore. Rarely is anyone who is interested in teaching in health care an unredeemable pedantic bore. Pedantic bores are

TEACHING TIP

Instructors should not attempt to lecture on something they do not really own. If instructors have enough time to thoroughly prepare to present a topic, they will tend to become excited and will start to employ the creative process.

CASE in Point

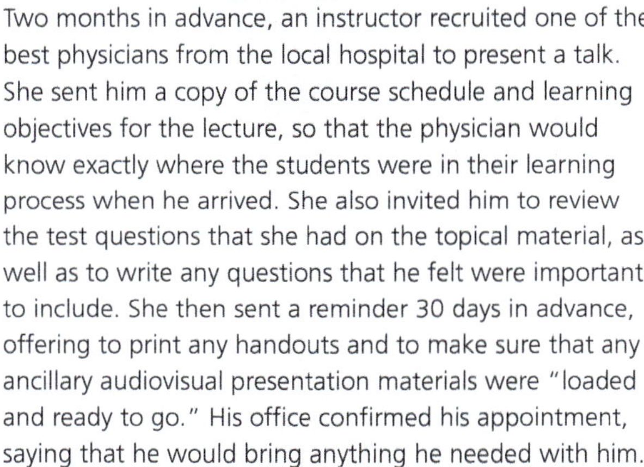

Two months in advance, an instructor recruited one of the best physicians from the local hospital to present a talk. She sent him a copy of the course schedule and learning objectives for the lecture, so that the physician would know exactly where the students were in their learning process when he arrived. She also invited him to review the test questions that she had on the topical material, as well as to write any questions that he felt were important to include. She then sent a reminder 30 days in advance, offering to print any handouts and to make sure that any ancillary audiovisual presentation materials were "loaded and ready to go." His office confirmed his appointment, saying that he would bring anything he needed with him.

The surgeon arrived on time and in good spirits. His lecture was entertaining and filled with valuable clinical tips and anomalies. He spoke of fascinating complications and tragic deaths due to occult anomalies. He brought alive the imagery of the heroic clinical team working feverishly to save the lives of those *in extremis*. The class gave him a warm applause and stood in line to speak with him after the lecture.

The instructor sat and listened in dismay. The guest physician ignored the content objectives. She would have to squeeze another 1-hour lecture into the already full course. The physician had been entertaining and charming, but if the students took their national board examinations based on the lecture, they would be certain to fail. However, the students loved the lecture and his evaluations were excellent.

made, not born. The primary reason that educators may be boring is that they truly find the material boring, or they may be so overbooked that they are simply trying to survive.

The Stages of Creativity

By acting more creatively, an instructor can actually become more creative.[37] Instructors should not be afraid to try new methods in the classroom, or even to fail. Creativity may be viewed more as a process than as a product.[38] In fact, the four stages of this process have been identified as preparation, incubation, illumination, and verification.

In the *preparation stage*, the instructor investigates the subject, deciding on what they want students to value or know. It is often helpful for instructors to brainstorm with other instructors at this point. The more possibilities one explores, the more likely one is to discover effective and creative approaches to presentation.

During the *incubation stage*, the instructor does not devote conscious thought to teaching the assignment but continues to work at the subconscious level. Not allowing oneself time for the incubation stage of the process defeats the creative process. The educator must allow time for doing the subconscious and deliberative creative work, and this process cannot be rushed. Instructors who chronically overbook themselves can expect to do less than their best work.

In the *illumination stage*, the creative instructor becomes aware of how the topic can be presented. It is at this point that the organization of the content is combined with a plan on how to present it.

In the *verification stage*, the instructor teaches and then the validity of the instruction is tested. At this point, the reflective educator should contemplate whether or not they had the desired impact on the students.

FIGURE 1.5 gives an example of these four stages put into action.

TEACHING TIP

The number-one way educators sabotage themselves is by not allowing themselves sufficient time to prepare. When they do not schedule adequate time to be creative, update their material, or simply review their lesson plans before presenting, they give students less than their best.

Charting a Successful Career Path

Every individual goes through life and career cycles. Educators experience exhilarating triumphs and thrills during the first day of a new class, or at a graduation ceremony when an at-risk student graduates and gets a job with a premier employer. At other times, the administrative burdens of lesson planning, preparing routine reports, getting ready for an accreditation inspection, teaching a class of seemingly disinterested students, or hearing endless excuses and appeals, can take a toll and wear down a dedicated and well-balanced instructor. Educators can help chart a path to career success that avoids a downward cycle of apathy and burn out.

It is important for educators to establish a clear set of career goals and produce quality work. Every educator should constantly cultivate a professional image. This begins with learning the structure, mission, and goals of the organization. Educators need to identify available resources and stay visible, while avoiding petty political spats and gossip. It is also advisable to realize that it is not healthy or productive to stay in a job that is not meeting the educator's needs for career growth and satisfaction.

It should be no surprise that, for most educators, job satisfaction is linked to salary, benefits, and long-term job security.[39] Other extrinsic rewards that promote

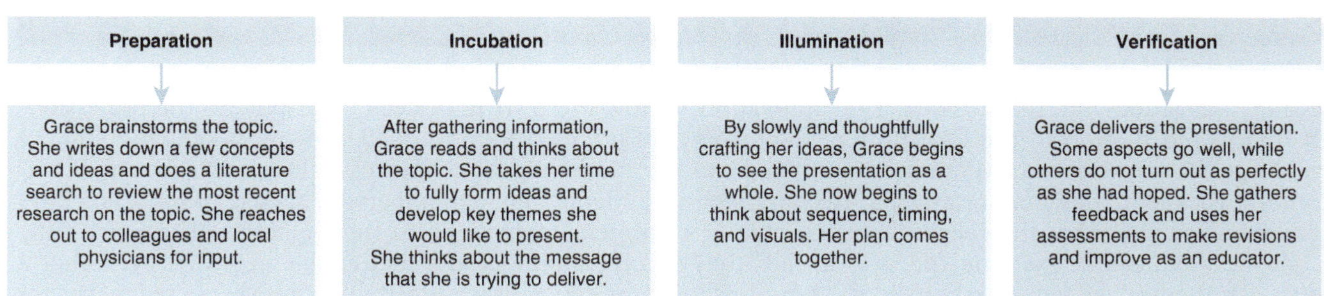

FIGURE 1.5 The four stages of creativity: preparation, incubation, illumination, and verification. In this example, Grace is an educator who has been assigned to teach a continuing education topic to her department. The steps shown describe the process she might use in the development and delivery of the class.

job satisfaction include publications, presentations, and grant funding. There are, however, intrinsic motivators that are equally important to job satisfaction in education. Satisfying one's personal ideals, such as a passion for high-quality teaching, is linked to job satisfaction. New instructors experience stress related to a heavy workload, isolation, scholarly inactivity, perceived lack of support and collegiality, and uncertainty about institutional requirements.[26,40] As mentioned, these stressors can be lessened through mentorship by experienced faculty.

Enhancing one's knowledge through continuing professional development is a strategy to lessen stress and promote excellence and career advancement. Professional development, even in the middle of an educator's career, improves faculty knowledge, behaviors, and satisfaction.[26]

Changing Jobs to Manage Career

For some EMS educators, remaining in the same satisfying job for a prolonged period can be rewarding, and there is no desire or need to change. Other educators enjoy the challenge of job change to learn new skills or to take on new opportunities. In other cases, job dissatisfaction related to conflict or misalignment with institutional goals may lead to a desire for change. Staying in an unsatisfactory position for a prolonged period of time can lead to poor performance. Regardless of the reason for job change, it should be planned in a thoughtful manner.

Vertical promotions are not the only way to advance careers. There are a limited number of higher positions available in EMS education. This can create a "bottle-neck" effect. Lateral moves, even within an organization, such as from one department to another, or from a proprietary company or a municipal agency to a college or university, can enrich the educator's experience portfolio. It may be possible to find a niche in a different type of organization or find a preference for teaching continuing education over primary education. Advancing up the career administrative ladder can also distance an educator from students and teaching as administrative duties increase. It is not for everyone.

The best career-advancement opportunities may occur in other organizations. This makes sense because career opportunities and progressive changes occur all the time, all over the world. The number of especially prestigious or exciting positions available at any given time in any profession is generally small. Thus, being willing or able to relocate to where an opportunity presents itself makes it more likely that an educator will find an appealing position. The EMS educator should be careful about seeking a similar position in the same community with a competing agency. First, it is quite likely that the exploration, and even considering the position, may quickly or eventually get back to the educator's employer. Second, once the move to the competing agency has been made, it must be the right decision and a good fit, as a return to the original employer likely will not be possible.

There is more to being successful than just doing a good job. Career advancement does not happen by luck or chance for most people, but rather through opportunities they as individuals have created through the careful artistry of career development.

Summary

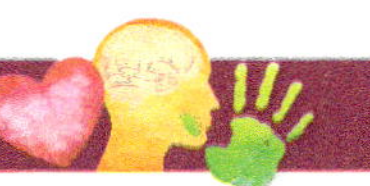

For all the things that are wrong with the EMS profession, education has the answer. The innovation, creativity, and passion of the educators of tomorrow will forge the vision of the EMS profession for years to come. It is exceptionally important that they are welcomed and supported as they begin their journey.

As new educators examine the task ahead, they must ask themselves key questions like, "How will I make a difference?" Although there is no simple answer to that question, future chapters will assist in the development of strategies and style. As these new initiates look to the future, they must think carefully about the attributes they hope to develop and consider how these attributes can contribute to the professionalism of EMS. Most of all, they must keep in mind the ethical obligations they owe their colleagues and their students and remember the sacred promise all EMS professionals make to their patients. These are truly the building blocks that enable greatness. Whether a new educator just starting out or a seasoned instructor wishing to improve, the journey is far from complete. Development as an educator is a lifelong experience; challenges abound, but educators must remember the rewards. If nothing else, remember to have fun.

Glossary

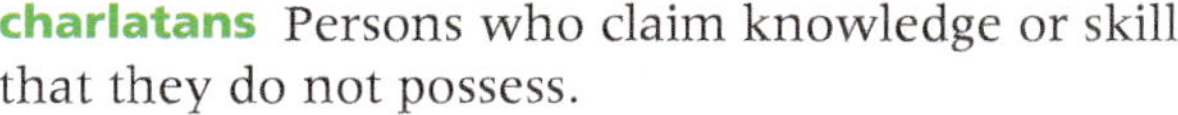
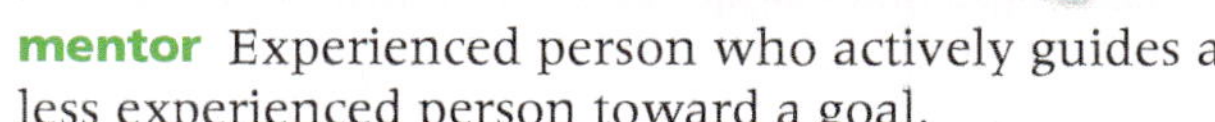

charlatans Persons who claim knowledge or skill that they do not possess.

creativity Activity that is novel and useful and results in contributions to human experience.

educational philosophy Set of beliefs that defines the purpose of education.

harassment Conduct that creates a situation that is hostile or unpleasant, or which makes a person believe they are unsafe; examples include making unwelcome advances, requesting sexual favors, using position or status to intimidate another, insulting another person, interfering with another's ability to do their job, and engaging in bullying behaviors.

mentor Experienced person who actively guides a less experienced person toward a goal.

pedantic bore Instructor who is so concerned with the details, comprehensiveness, and accuracy of a lesson that their content becomes overwhelming and tedious to students.

rubric Structured grading tool that outlines specific assignment criteria and the value assigned if each is completed.

scholarship High standards and/or quality of academic achievement.

self-efficacy Belief in one's own ability to perform or achieve a goal.

References

[1] Frankena, William K., Nathan Raybeck, and Nicholas Burbules. 2002. "Philosophy of Education." In *Encyclopedia of Education*, 2nd ed., edited by James W. Guthrie. New York: Macmillan Reference.

[2] Delbridge, Theodore R., Bob Bailey, John L. Chew, Alasdair K. T. Conn, Jack J. Krakeel, Dan Manz, David R. Miller, et al. 1998. "EMS Agenda for the Future: Where We Are . . . Where We Want to Be. EMS Agenda for the Future Steering Committee." *Annals of Emergency Medicine* 31, no. 2: 251–63.

[3] National Highway Traffic Safety Administration. 2009. "National Emergency Medical Services Education Standards." [DOT HS 811 077A]. Accessed January 15, 2019. https://www.ems.gov/pdf/National-EMS-Education-Standards-FINAL-Jan-2009.pdf.

[4] James, John T. 2013. "A New, Evidence-Based Estimate of Patient Harms Associated with Hospital Care." *Journal of Patient Safety* 9, no. 3: 122–8. http://dx.doi.org/10.1097/PTS.0b013e3182948a69.

[5] EMS.gov. 2013. "Strategy for a National EMS Culture of Safety." Accessed January 15, 2019. https://www.ems.gov/pdf/Strategy-for-a-National-EMS-Culture-of-Safety-10-03-13.pdf.

[6] National Registry of EMTs. 2016. "Integrated Out-of-Hospital Scenario Skill Sheet." Accessed January 15, 2019. https://content.nremt.org/static/documents/Draft%20NREMT%20Integrated%20Out-of-hospital%20Scenario.pdf.

[7] Committee on Accreditation of Educational Programs for the Emergency Medical Services Professions (CoAEMSP). 2018, February 5. "CoAEMSP Interpretations of the CAAHEP 2015 Standards and Guidelines for the Accreditation of Educational Programs in the EMS Professions." Accessed January 15, 2019. https://coaemsp.org/Documents/CoAEMSP%20Interpretations%20of%20the%202015%20CAAHEP%20Standards%202018.02.05.pdf.

[8] Miller, Michael. 2014. "Exploring Paramedic Student Leadership Characteristics in Emergency Medical Services Education Programs: A Grounded Theory Study." Doctoral dissertation, Creighton University. Accessed February 5, 2019. https://dspace2.creighton.edu/xmlui/handle/10504/62743.

[9] Densen, Peter. 2011. "Challenges and Opportunities Facing Medical Education." *Transactions of the American Clinical and Climatological Association* 122: 48–58.

[10] "Ethics." 2018. Merriam Webster online dictionary. Accessed January 15, 2019. https://www.merriam-webster.com/dictionary/ethic.

[11] Hulett, Denise M., Mark Bendick, Jr., Sheila Y. Thomas, and Francine Moccio. 2008, April. "National Report Card on Women in Firefighting." International Association of Women in Fire and Emergency Services. Accessed January 15, 2019. https://i-women.org/wp-content/uploads/2014/07/35827WSP.pdf.

[12] Bandura, Albert. 1977. "Self-Efficacy: Toward a Unifying Theory of Behavioral Change." *Psychological Review* 84, no. 2: 191–215. http://dx.doi.org/10.1037/0033-295X.84.2.191.

[13] Glasser, William. 1990. *Quality School Managing Students without Coercion*. New York: Harper and Row.

[14] Bass, Bernard M. 1996. *A New Paradigm of Leadership: An Inquiry into Transformational Leadership*. Alexandria, VA: U.S. Army Research Institute for the Behavioral and Social Sciences.

[15] Farina, Ann Marie. 2016, April 25. "The Tragedy and Disgrace of Bullying in EMS and Fire." Accessed January 15, 2019. https://www.ems1.com/ems-management/articles/84557048-The-tragedy-and-disgrace-of-bullying-in-EMS-and-fire/.

[16] Brookfield, Stephen D. 2006. *The Skillful Teacher: On Technique, Trust, and Responsiveness in the Classroom*, 2nd ed., 24. San Francisco: Jossey–Bass.

[17] Lindeman, Eduard C. 1926. *The Meaning of Adult Education*, 1961 ed., 33. New York: New Republic.

[18] Zinn, Lorraine M. 2004. "Exploring Your Philosophical Orientation." In *Adult Learning Methods*, 2nd ed., edited by Michael W. Galbraith, 39–74. Malabar, FL: Krieger Publishing.

[19] Royse, David. 2001. *Teaching Tips for College and University Instructors*. Boston: Allyn & Bacon.

[20] Tosteson, Daniel C. 1979. "Learning in Medicine." *New England Journal of Medicine* 301: 690–4. http://dx.doi.org/10.1056/NEJM197909273011304.

[21] Cruess, Sylvia. 2008. "Role Modelling—Making the Most of a Powerful Teaching Strategy." *BMJ* 336: 718. https://doi.org/10.1136/bmj.39503.757847.BE.

[22] Pratt, Daniel D. 2004. "Ethical Reasoning in Teaching Adults." In *Adult Learning Methods*, 2nd ed., edited by Michael W. Galbraith, 173. Malabar, FL: Krieger Publishing.

[23] Epstein, Ronald M., and Edward M. Hundert. 2002. "Defining and Assessing Professional Competence." *JAMA* 287, no. 2: 226–35. https://psycnet.apa.org/doi/10.1001/jama.287.2.226.
[24] Swick, Herbert M. 2000. "Toward a Normative Definition of Medical Professionalism." *Academic Medicine* 75: 612–6.
[25] Sullivan, William M. 1995. *Work and Integrity: The Crisis and Promise of Professionalism in America*. New York: Harper Collins.
[26] Lumpkin, Angela. 2009. "Follow the Yellow Brick Road to a Successful Professional Career in Higher Education." *The Educational Forum* 73: 200–14. https://doi.org/10.1080/00131720902991251.
[27] Moir, Ellen. 1999. "The Stages of a Teacher's First Year." In *A Better Beginning: Supporting and Mentoring New Teachers*, edited by Marge Scherer, 19–23. Alexandria, VA: Association for Supervision and Curriculum Development.
[28] Fleig-Palmer, Michelle M., and Cheryl Rathert. 2015. "Interpersonal Mentoring and its Influence on Retention of Valued Health Care Workers: The Moderating Role of Affective Commitment." *Health Care Management Review* 40, no. 1: 56–64. http://dx.doi.org/10.1097/HMR.0000000000000011.
[29] Johnson, W. Brad, and Charles R. Ridley. 2015. *The Elements of Mentoring*, 2nd ed., New York: St. Martin's Press.
[30] Athey, Susan, Christopher Avery, and Peter Zemsky. 2000. "Mentoring and Diversity." *American Economic Review* 90, no. 4: 765–86. http://dx.doi.org/10.1257/aer.90.4.765.
[31] Straus, Sharon E., Mallory O. Johnson, Christine Marquez, and Mitchell D. Feldman. 2013. "Characteristics of Successful and Failed Mentoring Relationships: A Qualitative Study across Two Academic Health Centers." *Academic Medicine* 88, no. 1: 82–9. http://dx.doi.org/10.1097/ACM.0b013e31827647a0.
[32] Crandall, Scott E. 2012, October 8. "Bullying on the Job: A New Threat to the Fire Service. *Fire Engineering*. Accessed January 15, 2019. http://www.fireengineering.com/articles/2012/10/bullying-on-the-job-a-new-threat-to-the-fire-service.html.
[33] Caffarella, Rosemary S., and Lynn F. Zinn. 1999. "Professional Development for Faculty: A Conceptual Framework for Barriers and Supports." *Innovative Higher Education* 23, no. 4: 241–54.
[34] Chickering, Arthur W., and Zelda F. Gamson. 1987. "Seven Principles for Good Practice in Undergraduate Education." *American Association of Higher Education (AAHE) Bulletin* 39: 3–7.
[35] Schwenk, Thomas L., and Neal A. Whitman. 1987. *The Physician as Teacher*. Baltimore, MD: Williams & Wilkins.
[36] Kestin, Joseph. 1970. "Creativity in Teaching and Learning." *American Science* 58: 250–7.
[37] Stein, Morris Isaac. 1974. *Stimulating Creativity, Vol 1: Individual Procedures*. New York: Academic Press.
[38] Whiting, Charles S. 1958. *Creative Thinking*. New York: Reinhold Press.
[39] American Society for Healthcare Engineering (ASHE). 2007. "Community College Faculty: Overlooked and Undervalued." *ASHE Higher Education Report* 32, no. 6: 1–161.
[40] Reybold, L. Earle. 2005. "Surrendering the Dream: Early Career Conflict and Faculty Dissatisfaction Thresholds." *Journal of Career Development* 32, no. 2: 107–21. https://doi.org/10.1177/0894845305279163.

Additional Resource

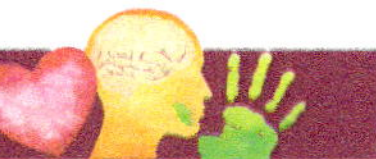

Kokx, Gordon. 2016. "Dissertation on an Exploration of Program Director Leadership Practices in National Accreditated Paramedic Education Programs." Dissertation, University of Idaho. https://eric.ed.gov/?id=ED571934.

CHAPTER 2

EMS Educator Roles

OBJECTIVES

At the conclusion of this chapter, the educator will be able to:

Cognitive Domain

1. Compare and contrast the responsibilities of a medical director, program director, lead instructor, clinical coordinator, and contract/adjunct faculty in primary or continuing education sessions.
2. Identify the student expectations of faculty in the learning environment.
3. Discuss the importance of organizational and leadership skills in the planning of primary and continuing education sessions.
4. Identify the administrative responsibilities of the primary or lead instructor in the development of the syllabus, budget, assessment tools, policies/procedures, curriculum objectives, clinical and field rotations, documentation, and records to support positive outcomes.
5. Describe the advantages of networking with peers, advisory councils, medical directors, and professional associations in the development of programs.
6. Identify the institutions of accountability by the program director and/or lead instructor at the local, state, and national levels of emergency medical services (EMS) education.

Psychomotor Domain

There are no psychomotor objectives for this chapter.

Affective Domain

1. Value consistent and effective communication by the program director, lead instructor, and continuing education coordinator with contract/adjunct faculty in all EMS learning environments by collaboration in session or course development.
2. Value collaboration with professional peers for strategies in tutoring, ADA accommodation, and resources to assist with student success and career development.

"We teach to change the world. The hope that undergirds our efforts to help students learn is that doing this will help them act toward each other and their environment with compassion, understanding, and fairness."

~ Dr. Stephen Brookfield

CHAPTER GOAL This chapter explores EMS educator roles and responsibilities.

The roles of EMS educators encompass far more than simply teaching students in classrooms and practical laboratories. EMS educators must have a thorough understanding of the broader scope of educator responsibilities, one of which is teaching with a team mentality. Although an educator may spend considerable time as the only instructor in the classroom, a team approach is essential in EMS education programs as hospital and field personnel play important roles in paramedic education. The team approach also enriches the quality and breadth of EMS learning experiences. To facilitate a team approach to teaching, it is important to identify the common titles and collaborative roles of the other team members and ensure that they are fully committed and involved in the educational process.

EMS Educator-Specific Roles

Nearly every higher level institution and almost all larger EMS education programs have EMS educators filling all or most of the positions listed here; however, in many moderately sized or smaller programs, several positions may be combined. All of the EMS educator-specific roles fall into four broad general categories:

Program director: The EMS educator with overall responsibility for the program. The program director is accountable to the institutional administrators, state agencies, accreditation bodies, and students. The program director is ultimately responsible for getting the program approved (authorized) by the institution, the state or local regulatory agencies, and the accreditation body, when necessary. The program director is responsible for securing the facility, equipment, supplies, instructors, clinical and field training sites, and funding. The program director is also responsible for selecting and evaluating faculty, ensuring the quality of the instruction, and complying with all regulatory and accreditation standards.

Program medical director: The qualified physician responsible for medical oversight of the program, thus reviewing and approving the curriculum; monitoring, either directly or indirectly, the quality of instruction; and ensuring terminal competency through monitoring, testing, and program evaluation.

Primary (lead) instructor: A person who possesses the appropriate academic or healthcare credentials, an understanding of the principles and theories of education, and the required teaching experience necessary to provide quality instruction to students. This instructor is often identified as the lead instructor.

Secondary instructor: A person who possesses the appropriate academic or healthcare credentials and an understanding of the principles and theories of education, and who may have *limited* teaching experience or a limited teaching role within the program. Secondary instructors are responsible for assisting primary instructors and providing instruction to students. In some situations, they may be responsible for lab sessions in which students practice psychomotor skills. Secondary instructors may even conduct classes on specific topics within their realm of expertise. The teaching skills that secondary instructors possess determine their specific responsibilities within the classroom. In some programs the faculty member in this role is defined as an adjunct or contract instructor.

The titles and roles of the faculty within a program vary based on state or regional statutes or institutional accreditation entities. These regulations may include those of a community college or hospital accreditation body.

Other instructor roles, such as lab or continuing education instructors, that may be found in an EMS education program depend on the size, nature, and resources of the institution that offers the training. In smaller programs, these roles are often combined. They may include the following:

Program (course) coordinator: The educator responsible for all program logistics, such as scheduling facilities, ensuring ready and properly staged equipment, ensuring adequate available supplies, scheduling secondary instructors, and seeing that all other routine functions of the program operate smoothly. In many programs, these responsibilities fall within the responsibility of the program director.

Lecturer: A content expert who presents didactic instruction in traditional instructional settings.

Practical lab instructor: An expert field and hospital practitioner—for example, an experienced paramedic, nurse, or other health professional—who teaches in laboratory settings, most often in psychomotor skills labs and practical scenarios.

Clinical coordinator: The person who schedules and tracks hospital and other clinical training rotations, communicates with clinical programs, and monitors student clinical progress.

Field coordinator: The person who schedules and tracks field EMS rotations, communicates with field clinical programs, and monitors student field clinical progress. In many programs, clinical and field coordinating is performed by the same person.

Simulation coordinator: The person who assists in coordination of simulation opportunities for students. The individual who navigates the technology during the simulation exercise.

Preceptor (field training officer): Practicing paramedics or other health professionals who teach EMS students in the hospital or field clinical setting by (1) demonstrating clinical procedures, (2) coaching the performance of clinical procedures through increasing stages of competency, (3) assessing clinical performance, and (4) assisting with determining or recommending terminal competency. (See Chapter 19, *Tools for Field and Clinical Learning*, for additional information.)

The National Association of State EMS Officials (NASEMSO) provides slightly modified definitions of EMS instructor roles and qualifications in a National EMS Education Standards transition document (**TABLE 2.1**).[1]

Responsibilities of the Program Director

The program director represents a specific category of instructor. The Committee on Accreditation of Educational Programs for the Emergency Medical Services Professions (CoAEMSP) has set the following responsibilities and qualifications for EMS program directors.

Responsibilities: The program director should be employed full time and is responsible for the program overall. Specific responsibilities include (but are not limited to) the following:[2]

- Administration, organization, and supervision of the educational program
- Continuous quality review and improvement of the educational program
- Long-range planning and program development
- Effectiveness of the program, including instruction and faculty, with systems in place to demonstrate the effectiveness of the program
- Cooperative involvement with the medical director
- Orientation, training, and supervision of clinical and field internship preceptors
- Effectiveness and quality of fulfillment of responsibilities delegated to another qualified individual

Qualifications: CoAEMSP requires that program directors meet specific education and experience qualifications. Requirements are as follows:[2]

- Possess a minimum of a bachelor's degree but recommend having a master's degree to direct a paramedic program, and a minimum of an associate's degree to direct an Advanced Emergency Medical Technician (AEMT) program, from an accredited institution of higher education.
- Have appropriate medical or allied health education, training, and experience.

TABLE 2.1 NASEMSO EMS Instructor Roles

Role	Expectations	Experience	Education/Licensure
Program Director	Administrate, plan, coordinate, develop curricula, supervise	Director/manager 2 years of field experience EMS instructional experience	Master's degree from post-secondary school Education degree
Lead Faculty	Deliver content, skills instruction, remediation	2 years of field experience Experience in other instructional role	Post-secondary degree Instructional methods education
Adjunct Faculty (Subject matter expert/content expert)	Deliver targeted content, skills instruction	1 year of experience at level taught or in specific discipline	High school diploma
Assistant Instructor	Skills instruction	1 year of experience at level taught	High school diploma

Modified from National Association of State EMS Officials. 2010, December. "EMS Instructor Qualifications. A Template to Assist States with Implementing the EMS Education Agenda for the Future: A Systems Approach." Accessed November 2, 2018. https://nasemso.org/wp-content/uploads/EMS-Instructor-Qualifications-Template.pdf.

- Be knowledgeable about methods of instruction, testing, and assessment of students.
- Have field experience in the delivery of out-of-hospital emergency care.
- Have academic training and preparation related to EMS at least equivalent to that of program graduates.
- Be currently certified in the United States to practice out-of-hospital care and currently certified by a nationally recognized certifying organization at an equal or higher level of professional training than that for which training is being offered.
- Be knowledgeable concerning current national standards, national accreditation, national registration, and the requirements for state certification or licensure.

The program or course director is often the one responsible for developing program and course policies and procedures. Course and program policies and procedures may govern activities such as the selection and screening of students, student discipline, course or program evaluation, and responses to data regarding outcomes such as pass rates, employer feedback, and feedback from graduates.

The program director and primary or lead instructor may be the same person in a small program. Typically the program director has a reduced teaching load to address the many demands of running the program that are not associated with the direct duties of teaching.

Responsibilities of the Primary (Lead) Instructor

The primary EMS instructor may be called on to provide leadership or supervision over a series of courses, or even over an entire EMS education program. Additionally, this instructor may be called on to provide the coordination of individual courses within a program.

Qualifications: CoAEMSP requires that lead instructors meet specific education and experience qualifications. They require that the lead instructor possess the following:[2]

- An associate's degree at minimum; a bachelor's degree is preferred
- Professional healthcare credentials
- Experience in emergency medicine or prehospital care
- Knowledge of instructional methods
- Teaching experience in content delivery, instruction of skills, and remediation

Frequently, primary instructors are responsible for documenting student progress and course work progression. They have a responsibility to provide timely feedback to students concerning their progress toward successful completion of the courses. In some circumstances, student progress and feedback (with the student's written permission) may be shared with others, such as the student's employer, parents, or sponsors. This information may not be shared with anyone without a student's specific written permission. (See Chapter 25, *Legal Issues for EMS Educators*.)

Course coordination, an important role of primary instructors, may include coordinating guest instructors or special topic instructors, and scheduling and supervising all secondary instructors. Moreover, the primary instructor maintains responsibility for the development, maintenance, and instructional quality of the class regardless of who is teaching.

Additionally, the primary instructor is often asked to identify sources of disciplinary problems and to suggest solutions. In such situations, the instructor must be able to work closely with the medical director, program director, other faculty, and students to resolve problems in the classroom or clinical setting.

Finally, primary instructors are frequently involved in determining the need for and type of remedial instruction students will receive or be required to undergo, and they may also be involved in providing the remedial instruction themselves. Thus, they must be able to assess both the students and their situations to identify the root causes of problems, and then be able to develop workable strategies to help the students succeed.

Responsibilities of the Program Medical Director

The program medical director represents a specific category of leadership and accountability in an EMS program. CoAEMSP has set the following responsibilities and qualifications for medical directors.

Responsibilities: The program medical director is responsible for medical oversight of the program, including (but not limited to) the following:[2]

- Reviewing and approving the educational content of the program curriculum for appropriateness, medical accuracy, and reflection of current evidence-informed prehospital or emergency care practice
- Reviewing and approving the minimum numbers for each of the required patient contacts and procedures listed in the National EMS Education Standards[3]
- Reviewing and approving the instruments and processes used to assess students in didactic, lab, clinical, and field experiences

- Reviewing the progress of each student throughout the program, and assist in the determination of appropriate corrective measures, when necessary
- Ensuring the competence of each graduate of the program in the cognitive, psychomotor, and affective domains
- Engaging in cooperative involvement with the program director
- Ensuring the effectiveness and quality of any medical director responsibilities delegated to another qualified physician
- Ensuring educational interaction with students in a variety of settings, such as lecture, laboratory, and clinical and field internships

Qualifications: CoAEMSP requires that program medical directors meet specific education and experience qualifications. Requirements for the program medical director are as follows:[2]

- Must be a physician currently licensed and authorized to practice in the location of the program, with experience and current knowledge of emergency care of the acutely ill and injured patients
- Must have adequate training or experience in the delivery of out-of-hospital emergency care, including the proper care and transport of patients, medical direction, and prehospital quality improvement
- Must be an active member of the local medical community and participate in professional activities related to out-of-hospital care
- Must be knowledgeable about the education of the EMS professions, including professional, legislative, and regulatory issues regarding the education of the EMS professions

CoAEMSP describes the program medical director as having an active and collaborative leadership, instructional, and professional role in EMS education. A program medical director may delegate responsibilities to an associate or assistant medical director. Associate and assistant medical directors have requirements and educational roles similar to those of the program medical director.

Responsibilities of the Secondary Instructor

The roles of secondary instructors are defined by the primary instructor. Their scope of assigned responsibilities usually involves direct teaching in the classroom and labs, and may extend to clinical instruction in the hospital and the field. The two main responsibilities of secondary instructors are to provide instruction to students and to support primary instructors as needed and assigned. Secondary instructors may be required to possess entry-level teaching competencies and are often not expected to perform with the same proficiency as the program's more experienced instructors. Because the primary instructor often sets the tone for the class, the secondary instructor must be aware of course expectations, lesson plans, acceptable presentation styles, and both formal and informal "rules and regulations" that have been established by the primary instructor for the class. The optimal relationship between the primary and the secondary instructor is one in which mentoring and professional growth take place for both individuals (**FIGURE 2.1**).

While the primary instructor, training officer, or continuing education coordinator has overall responsibility for the learning experience, together, the primary and secondary instructors are expected to work as a team to deliver the curriculum, mentor and support each other, and ensure the program and the students continually strive to meet high standards. The breadth of responsibility assigned to both levels of instructors reinforces the need for participation in a program of teaching instruction before one enters the field of education.

Continuing Education and Service-Based Educators

Another category of instructor is the continuing education (CE) instructor (also referred to as *in-house instructor, service-based instructor*, or *training officer*). While the responsibilities of a CE instructor are similar to

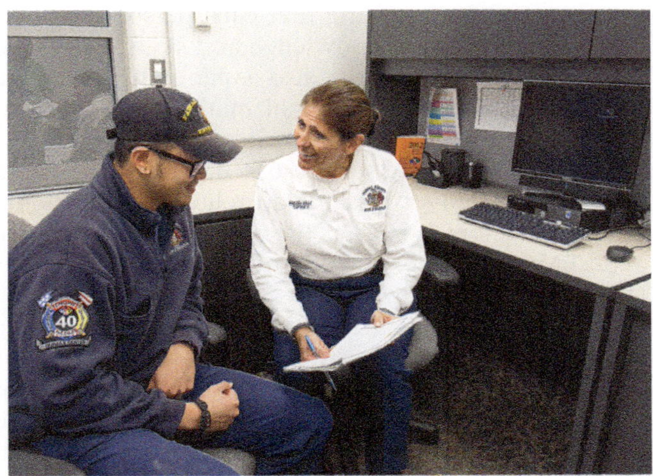

FIGURE 2.1 Mentoring a new instructor is a rewarding experience for both primary and secondary instructors.

those of an instructor teaching entry-level EMS programs, the focus of content and the stressors of the classroom are very different. Entry-level program instructors must teach according to national education standards. Typically, they are preparing students for an independent third-party examination. Such examinations reference questions and skills to nationally accepted standards and are not focused on local protocols. Entry-level instructors must be familiar with the National EMS Education Standards[3] as well as the content of the major certification courses: Advanced Cardiac Life Support, Pediatric Advanced Life Support, Basic Life Support, and Prehospital Trauma Life Support, or International Trauma Life Support, as examples. CE and service-based educators focus on local protocols, identified system quality problems, and national or state recertification or relicensure requirements as well as new equipment, medications, and evidence-based changes in practice. Monitoring peer-reviewed and professional publications to identify current research relevant to prehospital emergency care helps the CE instructor teach according to current scientific evidence.

Service-based educators and training officers are often tasked with onboarding new employees and ensuring continued competence of employees. They must ensure that employees, or other EMS professionals for whom they are accountable, meet or maintain minimum education requirements for relicensure and for other critical competencies identified within their system.

Service-based educators ensure clinical proficiency, evidence-based changes to practice, and quality improvement processes. They are responsible for introducing information related to new standards of care, new policies, and new equipment within their system, and for verifying that each person has mastered the associated knowledge and skills. Often the service-based educator is also assigned to remediate employees when the internal quality improvement process identifies deficiencies in their knowledge or skill. Finally, CE and service-based educators need to organize or deliver sessions on relevant professional nonclinical topics, such as the business of health care and EMS, affective domain and behaviors, and leadership development.

Institutional instructors typically do not have the added pressure of having to instruct as well as test their fellow employees. This can be an unexpected source of stress if not addressed well before the beginning of the course. It is important that management, instructional staff, and students have clearly defined expectations addressing successful completion prior to the start of the in-house courses and education activities.

Student Expectations of Educators

Erving Goffman wrote extensively about student expectations of educators and the ways that educators can sabotage themselves by failing to meet these expectations. The following information about role expectations is adapted from his work.[4]

All EMS students have certain reasonable expectations of their instructors. Because every new and seasoned educator was once a student and likely returns to that role time and again, it would seem that the instructor would have a solid understanding of student expectations. However, when one is taking on the role of educator, it is always helpful to reflect on those basic expectations that students have and keep them in mind when preparing to enter the classroom (**TABLE 2.2**).

The educator's level of experience, training, and position give the educator a different worldview than that of the students. In accordance with this, educators are generally expected to suppress their feelings and

TABLE 2.2 Synthesis of Traditional and Nontraditional Student Expectations

Clarity	Concise and straightforward instruction that is easily understood Clear expectations Detailed syllabi Clear learning objectives that are explained Organized and consistent structure
Recognition	Respect for student contributions in the classroom Demonstrated care for student needs and expectations Following deadlines with timely grading or feedback
Intentional education	Assigning meaningful and appropriate amount of coursework Displaying a personal interest in what is being taught Being approachable, personable, and professional Facilitating delivery of content, then allowing for application

Data from Bourdeaux, Renee, and Lindsie Schoenack. 2016. "Adult Student Expectations and Experiences in an Online Learning Environment." *Journal of Continuing Higher Education 64*: 152–61. https://doi.org/10.1080/07377363.2016.1229072. Houser, Marian L. 2005. "Are We Violating Their Expectations? Instructor Communication Expectations of Traditional and Nontraditional Students." *Communication Quarterly 53*, no. 2: 213–28. https://doi.org/10.1080/01463370500090332.

to convey a professional demeanor that is stoic, pleasant, and welcoming. This is analogous to the expectation that the caregiver will comfort a dying patient by touching the patient's hand and saying something such as, "We are going to do everything that we can to take good care of you."

Educators have many ways to express themselves and convey their role in addition to the words that they speak. Facial expressions, posture, and tone of voice and inflection are just as powerful as words, or even more powerful, to communicate the educator's attitude and set the tone for the course. The expressive repertoire also includes the insignias of office or rank, uniforms or clothing, age, and grooming. Just as the EMT dresses in uniform for quick identification and acceptance by patients, so should the EMS educator dress for respect and professionalism.

Students expect educators to have the ability to effectively communicate the course content. Educators can spoil the impression they want to make by forgetting content, appearing nervous or self-conscious, being unprepared, or giving way to inappropriate outbursts of laughter or anger. Additionally, students expect their instructors to provide them up front with an uncomplicated and straightforward view of the course and all essential materials.

Educators can sabotage themselves in a number of ways when trying to establish their role and authority within the classroom. Most notably, students easily sense when an educator is not personally invested in their success; they may react negatively to the educator's perceived indifference. Moreover, students neither expect nor need their educators to be on the same social plane that they are on. Thus, an educator's appearance and manner should set the instructor apart from students. Confusion is likely to occur if instructors *appear* to have greater professional status than their students but *act* in an egalitarian, intimate, or even apologetic manner.

Students expect educators to behave as educators at all times. Educators are never "offstage" or "off the record" when students are present. Educators must be aware of the environments, or regions, in which they perform their roles. Front regions, such as classrooms and offices, are areas where educators perform formal roles for the observation of their students. But even in back regions, such as hallways, faculty lounges, and out-of-class community settings, where educators may wish to relax and express their "true feelings," they must remember that they are always subject to student expectations and are never truly "offstage." The *Case in Point* on this page demonstrates how a primary instructor and a teaching assistant violated the boundary expectations between students and instructors.

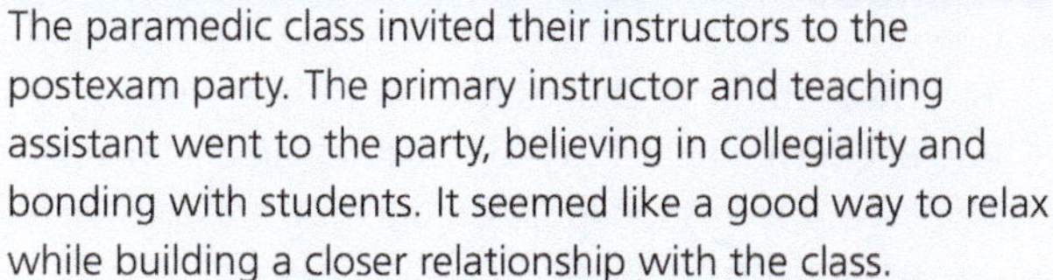

The paramedic class invited their instructors to the postexam party. The primary instructor and teaching assistant went to the party, believing in collegiality and bonding with students. It seemed like a good way to relax while building a closer relationship with the class.

One student at a distant table and out of sight of the instructors began drinking straight shots of alcohol and drank excessively. Two other students, sitting near the instructors, were becoming argumentative over a personal matter. The lead instructor maintained composure and suggested that they hold off on any arguments while the party was going on. The two students looked at the instructor and resented what they perceived as a look of disapproval. A third student, an attractive young student, began openly flirting with the teaching assistant, who was flattered and enjoyed the attention but kept a professional bearing and dismissed the attention with an innocent smile. After all, it was just a harmless party. It was time to relax.

Everyone left an hour later and drove home. Fortunately, there were no crashes, and no traffic violations were received.

Three days later, the lead instructor was called into the dean's office and was confronted about the party. "I understand that you went out and socialized with the class after the exam. Is that correct?"

"Yes, it is," the lead instructor responded, growing nervous. "Is something wrong? Did something happen?"

The dean leaned forward and spoke in a very deliberate, controlled voice. "Yes, something happened. You drank socially with students. You were involved in an argument between two students. You have a complaint filed against you and your teaching assistant for inappropriate conduct. You have very likely compromised your ability to lead this class any further. At minimum, you have compromised your ability to keep this class on a professional plane. You will need to write a letter of explanation to be considered by the faculty review committee. I do not know what the outcome will be."

No formal action was ever taken. The verbal warning was sufficient. It was a hard lesson.

Educator Responsibilities

Many new educators assume that the bulk of their time will be spent in preparing and delivering lectures. The reality is that educators have many additional

Dr. Harry Wong's Tips for the First Days of School[5]

1. Greet students "honestly" and with energy.
2. Begin with an activity to facilitate name learning.
3. Have information (policies, outlines, etc.) posted or ready to hand out.
4. Give the class the idea that you are a person.
5. Give them your expectations, rules, and class policies.
6. Have an activity planned to give them a feel for what is ahead.
7. Establish good control.
8. Know (a) what you are doing, (b) your classroom procedures, and (c) your professional responsibilities.
9. Know that positive and high expectations come from *attitude*.
10. Create a classroom climate for both your students and yourself.
11. Celebrate the first day of school.
12. Dress appropriately and professionally to model success.
13. Use your students' names and correct pronunciations.
14. Practice effective classroom management—*from the beginning*.
15. Initiate a task-oriented and predictable environment.
16. Have your classroom ready.
17. Stress large-group organization and student procedures.
18. Make the first assignment on the first day interesting, short, easy, and successful.
19. Two things are important to state: your name and your expectations.
20. Teach student behaviors: (a) discipline, (b) procedures, and (c) routines.
21. Have a hard copy of your plan and follow it (discipline plan).
22. Introduce the discipline plan on the first day of school; post it and give a copy to each student.
23. Spend more time discussing consequences than rules.
24. Consequences should be reasonable and logical.
25. Communicate your discipline plan effectively (tell students why the rules are needed).
26. Establish your procedures.

duties and must have the skills and characteristics to adapt to these other responsibilities. Although it is true that whenever an instructor teaches a new class, they can expect to dedicate considerable time and effort toward the preparation and delivery of course materials, this "advance" work will decrease each time the class is taught. Additional administrative duties and responsibilities will generally increase and expand and will increasingly consume a large part of the educator's time.

Preparing for the Class

Good teaching appears effortless. This is true of performances in sports, the arts, and clinical care. Professional competence is smooth and seamless. Amateur performances appear jerky and difficult.

How do professional athletes, musicians, and clinicians make their performances look so easy? They prepare in advance with countless hours of practice and preparation. To achieve the appearance of effortless and smooth instruction, the educator needs to prepare a game plan and build a resource collection well in advance of the first class session.

Developing Class Materials and Handouts

Nearly every accredited higher education institution formally credits full-time educators with 3 hours of work, or activities, for each hour of instruction. The 2 extra hours are for preparatory and follow-up time. Preparation includes reviewing the material to be taught in advance and keeping up with current practices and literature, as well as a period of time for mental preparation, as it is educationally unsound for an instructor to "walk in cold" when presenting. Follow-up time includes returning equipment and supplies, meeting with students to answer questions, and grading assignments. Adjunct instructors, those not working as full-time educators with the institution, are often paid a flat rate for each hour they teach. For the adjuncts, the 3:1 hourly rate is included in the flat hourly rate for teaching. Tasks associated with developing and maintaining class instructional materials and handouts should take much more time than it takes to deliver the material. It is essential that the educator's schedule allows sufficient time for this work every semester. When teaching a topic for the first time, a good general rule is to schedule at least three times as much time for preparation as for instruction. After the first time, it may be sufficient to schedule 1 hour of preparation for each hour of instruction. However, instructors who teach the same lecture with the same materials year after year eventually find themselves the object of student scorn. Updates and revisions are essential, particularly in the healthcare field.

Developing Adjunct Materials to Stimulate Class Discussion and Learning

It is helpful for the instructor to have preplanned scenarios, discussion topics, activities, and quizzes that have been developed and made available well before the first class meets. These adjunct materials should support and coordinate lessons that are being taught. Audiovisual materials, for example, can be used to support lectures and presentations; however, they may take a surprising amount of time to develop. The Internet is an excellent source for images and videos; however, use of online content may require permission from the rightsholder; reusing or editing the content may constitute copyright infringement or plagiarism. Creating a collection of supporting classroom activities for each area of course material is time intensive but worthwhile. Each year the collection should be revisited to ensure that the content is keeping pace with current evidence-based practice.

EMS educators can consider using technology, such as a virtual learning environment (VLE) or learning management system (LMS), to create a **flipped classroom**. Flipping the classroom is a pedagogical model in which the typical lecture and homework elements are reversed, which can increase educator–student interaction, but must be planned and carefully implemented to support effective learning. Flipping the classroom potentially improves student self-direction and encourages students to take responsibility for their own education.[6] When flipping an EMS classroom, it is important for the educator to research educational theory on this practice and decide how to best integrate it into the course. Flipped class time should be tailored to the needs of students while being creative and effective time spent learning. Because flipped classrooms are different, it is important to prepare students for the activity. It is important to remember that flipping the classroom takes time and requires organization, and the educator must decide on how this approach will be evaluated. However, a flipped classroom has positive features of more engaged and active learning during class time.

Ordering and Operating Equipment

A surprising amount of time and effort can go into ordering, maintaining, and cleaning equipment. Anything that can be done to help minimize this work, time, and energy spent will be helpful. For instance, an instructor may set up a routine for periodic ordering of new supplies and equipment; assign students to help clean, repair, and move equipment and supplies on a schedule; and acquire adequate room to store, organize, and maintain the equipment (**FIGURE 2.2**).

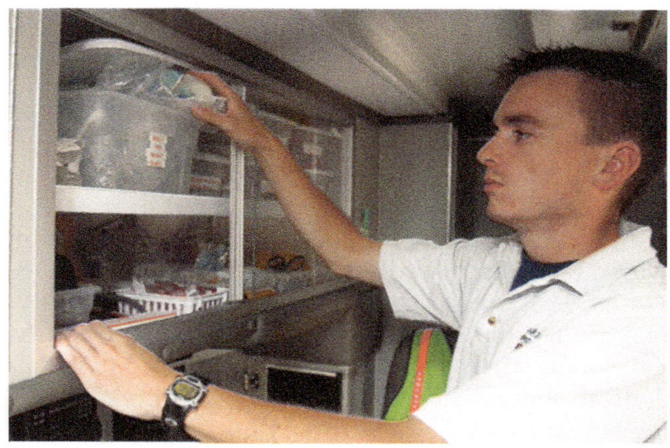

FIGURE 2.2 The instructor may need to assume responsibility for ordering equipment and supplies.

Teaching the Class

The role of today's teacher involves much more than showing up and delivering a "canned" lesson. All programs should have written goals and intended learning outcomes consistent with needs and expectations of stakeholders and the program's advisory committee. Teaching to promote maximal student learning is a planned, purposeful event that includes consideration of advanced assignments, appropriate content delivery methods, student-centered learning activities, and assessment methods. Once the plan is determined, the instructor must coordinate assembly of appropriate resources to execute the lab, lecture, discussion, assessment, or other activity that is planned. The instructor must diligently prepare each time the lesson is repeated and make revisions based on (1) effectiveness of prior strategies; (2) new knowledge, equipment, or evidence that alters content; or (3) the learning needs of the specific students within the current classroom.

TEACHING TIP

The role of educator has many facets. Remember that the ultimate role is student learning.

Organizing and Leading Discussion Sessions

It is important that a portion of each class be devoted to discussion of the learning session. Two of the most valuable and effective ways of achieving this are (1) to start each lecture or session with a brief overview of the learning objectives and (2) to follow each session with a brief summary of the key learning points. (See Part IV, *Delivering the Message*, for a more in-depth coverage of teaching methods.) As mentioned previously, developing an engaging discussion that prompts students to share their ideas and views is a time consuming but worthy investment.

Preparing for Lab Procedures and Assignments

In EMS clinical education, practical sessions, or "labs," tend to account for approximately half of the total amount of time spent in the course. These should include practical skills workshops, patient assessment exercises, and patient care scenarios. Developing relevant lab experiences is just as time intensive as developing lectures. Preparing for invasive labs, such as intravenous and medication administration workshops, generally takes much more time than inexperienced educators may imagine. It is always a good idea to have additional instructors participating to minimize incidents and allow for closer supervision of students when learning invasive procedures. Instructors should allot enough time to obtain and set up the necessary equipment and supplies, and to schedule and brief any secondary instructors. If secondary instructors are paid employees, then additional recruitment and hiring time may be needed. The hiring and orientation process can take months in some cases.

Simulated education requires additional training. Advanced planning is needed to ensure that the appropriate simulated cases are developed to meet the objectives and expected higher-level learning outcomes. To ensure simulation is effective, educators need the appropriate equipment, training, and resources.[7] If live patients are used for simulation, they will need to be coached prior to the education setting to accurately portray the desired patient situation. EMS educators need to consult with their institute if a release of liability is required when using live patients in simulation. In addition, simulated physical injuries or conditions may need to be moulaged prior to the lab session. If a high-fidelity manikin is used, selected vital signs and patient findings may be preprogrammed. Clear direction should be provided regarding the setting, patient presentation, treatment expectations, and patient outcomes based on either optimal or poor treatment. (See Chapter 18, *Tools for Simulation*.)

Managing the Classroom

An important part of teaching is managing the classroom. This includes activities such as starting class on time, using classroom time appropriately, monitoring the class climate, and nipping bullying in the bud, among others. Establishing standards with regard to professional behavior at the beginning of the program or session, along with the consequences for infractions, gives the students guidance and accountability for the expected behavior. New instructors can fail if they do not understand that this is their responsibility; therefore, it is important to prepare for these tasks just as is done for other aspects of the instructor role. Seeking out a mentor can assist the new instructor with strategies on behavior policy development.

Developing and Grading Tests

The development of reliable and valid tests is a highly specialized skill. A great deal of time, energy, and expense goes into ensuring that a test is valid. (See Part V, *Student Assessment and Remediation*, for more information on assessment.) The test should be based on the desired learning outcomes and on the content that has been presented to meet the associated lesson plan objectives. There should be a clear link between the standards, the objectives, the content, and the assessment. The educator should ensure that the right number of questions, at the right level of Bloom's taxonomy, are assessed for any given topic. Asking only recall questions that depend on rote memory will not serve an EMS student well when the outcomes require higher levels of performance. If educators have experience in constructing test questions, they can develop their own bank of test questions from which to generate their tests. EMS educators should not craft trick questions.[8] Instead, questions should focus on using appropriate vocabulary, positive instead of negative stems, and avoiding "all of the above" answers, among other item-writing guidelines.[8] Item analysis and statistics, such as point biserial, should be used to determine the reliability of each question and overall exam validity. Although this takes considerable time and expertise, high stakes examinations must be validated and updated.

Reviewing for Tests

It is common in EMS education for educators to conduct review sessions before tests are given. Review sessions can be conducted in-person or using electronic conferencing technologies. However, students rarely come to these review sessions prepared with questions. To avoid teaching directly to the test, the instructor might require that only student questions will be answered during the review. An alternative would be to consider preparing a number of challenging applied-patient problems for students to discuss. In this way, the instructor will be able to facilitate a thorough review without giving away the specific material included on the test.

Assessing Student Performance

It is time consuming for the educator to develop fair and effective criteria for grading student performance, critical thinking capabilities, and clinical reasoning. Developing grading criteria is a process rather than a single event; the educator should never stop trying to improve the assessment process. Good educators have multiple performance references to use in assessing their students' performance—participation, test scores, practical skills scores, projects, and scenario testing, for example. Developing, reassessing, refining, recording, and providing feedback on these different reference points takes time and effort. The State of EMS Education Research Project (SEERP)[9] found it troubling that attendance was used as a factor in measuring student performance by over half of the educators who were surveyed. Attendance alone does not indicate competency. Grading should be structured to measure student achievement of specific, measurable learning outcomes. The instructor should communicate results of student assessment to students confidentially and in a timely manner to allow them the opportunity to adjust their performance if necessary.

Improving Performance through Assessment (Feedback)

The EMS educator has the responsibility and capacity to ensure a positive and constructive learning environment. Students are typically focused only on their grade point average and goal of passing the course; however, they may voice complaints about aspects of the program. The instructor should spend time listening to the students' concerns and the concerns of fellow educators, with an open mind. By listening and thus communicating to students the importance placed on their concerns, educators will be able to channel the energy in the program toward an open dialogue and ultimately program improvement.

Teaching Psychomotor Skills

When a competent instructor demonstrates and explains procedures, most students readily comprehend them and feel comfortable with what they have seen. However, that does not mean that most students will be able to perform the procedure themselves. Teaching students a procedure requires that each step be broken down, demonstrated, explained, and followed as soon as possible by student performance of each step with careful monitoring and coaching. Once students master the steps, they should be coached through several complete sequences throughout the program to ensure competency over time. Finally, they should be given the chance to perform the skill in the context of patient care scenarios prior to performing skills and interventions on patients in the clinical and field environments.

Teaching Team Leadership and Membership

Team leadership and membership are essential components of EMS practice; EMS care is typically provided by at least a primary and secondary provider. EMS educators have many opportunities to enhance their students' leadership skills and understanding of team dynamics.[10] The following have been identified as components of team leadership in EMS:[11]

1. Creates an action plan
2. Communicates
3. Receives, processes, verifies, and prioritizes information
4. Reconciles incongruent information
5. Demonstrates confidence, compassion, maturity, command presence, and trustworthiness
6. Takes charge
7. Is accountable for team actions and outcomes
8. Assesses the situation and resources and modifies the plan
9. Leaves ego and rank at the door

The following have been identified as components of team membership in EMS:[11]

1. Demonstrates followership
2. Maintains situational awareness
3. Demonstrates/appreciates inquiry
4. Does not freelance
5. Is an active listener
6. Accurately performs tasks in a timely manner
7. Is safety conscious and advocates for safety at all times
8. Leaves ego and rank at the door

Each of these action-oriented components can be formulated into a competency and integrated into classroom, lab, clinical, and field settings. The use of simulations allows for assessments of a student's leadership and membership behaviors, and allows the student to be placed in a variety of leadership circumstances.[10] Experiential learning in field and clinical settings is foundational to EMS education and allows leadership and membership behaviors to be learned in the actual environments for which they are being educated.[10] It is important to ensure students are learning behaviors and attributes that are in line with those expected in medicine, the EMS profession, and the education program. Educators should teach, mentor, and display attributes of leadership and team dynamics during all aspects of the program, which includes with students, peer educators, supervisors, and clinical and field representatives. Strategies for achieving this include effective communication skills, respect for others, and adherence to the same affective behavior standards expected of students. Assessing the affective domain behaviors of the students by reviewing preceptor comments and observation of behaviors in the classroom and lab can provide valuable input on professional behaviors in a variety of settings. Ongoing student evaluation of faculty, staff, and program performance provides input on the overall learning environment.

Administrative Tasks and Duties

Although the primary role of an instructor is to be in the classroom or clinical or field setting, administrative tasks comprise an essential secondary function. The number of administrative tasks assigned to instructors depends on their position and the type of teaching setting. The program director is often tasked with the greatest number of administrative duties; however, each instructor has essential duties in this area.

Holding Instructor Meetings

Departmental meetings, whether formal or informal, are a necessary part of staying connected with the broader picture (**FIGURE 2.3**). The educator should eagerly participate in faculty meetings, as curriculum development and educational design are best accomplished collaboratively. Sharing information about student progress and performance is also important, so that problems can be identified and a plan of action initiated. Collaboration with fellow instructors can ensure that key content areas are being reinforced throughout the curriculum.

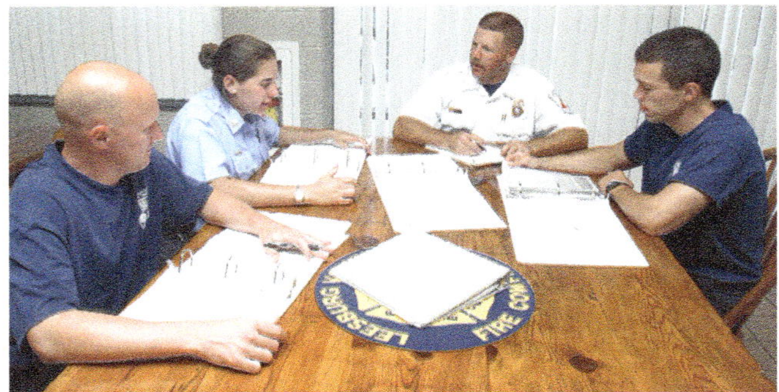

FIGURE 2.3 It is important to hold faculty meetings to discuss important topics, such as student progress, curriculum development, and exam item development.

Additionally, clinical issues or procedures may need to be reviewed together to promote instructor consistency. Last but not least, staff meetings must be documented; this documentation is an element of paramedic program accreditation.

Developing a Budget

Education is a business. Facilities, instructional materials, and instructors cost money. Sources of revenue are required to fund an educational program. Thus, developing and maintaining a budget is a significant part of the education administrator's responsibilities. This often means seeking out external sources of funding, such as grants and donations. Educators should determine who the experts are in these areas within their institution or community for assistance. This may be the public relations department or dean's office. Each instructor has a role in ensuring budget accountability by using resources carefully, monitoring student class size to make sure an excess number of faculty have not been scheduled, and documenting expenses accurately.

Evaluating Personnel

Scheduling times for evaluating and providing frequent feedback for educators and any educational support personnel is a vital and necessary part of the EMS education administrator's job. The administrator's role includes working with primary and secondary instructors to ensure that they are developing appropriate skills as educators. It may also be helpful for the administrator to periodically clarify and revise job responsibilities.

Maintaining Departmental Records and Reports

Records of enrollment, curricula, counseling, schedules, attendance, grades, attrition, and successful completion are all critical to the educational institution. These constitute fundamental legal documentation. Reports to various agencies are also required and may seem endless. CoAEMSP requires documentation of student progress and evaluation in all areas of the program. Additionally, CoAEMSP requires an annual report from accredited programs to document their outcome evaluation of the program's success toward achievement of program goals and objectives. Accreditation is fully discussed in Chapter 26, *Fundamentals of Accreditation and Program Evaluation*.

Attending Committee Meetings

In addition to the vital role of teaching, most educators in academic institutions are expected to improve the overall environment of the organization and the community. This includes serving on a variety of educational committees whose work can range from long-term curriculum development to admissions, to academic affairs of the college, and to the handling of student grievances. These committees may be at the local and state levels. Attendance by educators demonstrates leadership in the form of participation, understanding, and implementation of changes that may occur as a result of committee decisions.

Attending Advisory Committee Meetings

All EMS programs, especially paramedic programs, should have an advisory committee that meets at least annually. Program directors should strive to ensure that the membership of the advisory committee is representative of all stakeholders in their EMS community, as defined in the CoAEMSP standards. Two groups that are often overlooked are students in the program and the lay public. Individuals who are involved on an advisory committee should include representatives of employers of graduates, hospital personnel, regulatory agency representatives, graduates, members of the local medical community, current student representatives, and consumers. Program personnel, such as program director or course coordinator and medical director, as well as program faculty, are also included but are usually *ex officio* members. An *ex officio* member provides a specific area of expertise and serves in an advisory capacity. Specifically, the goal of the advisory committee is to make recommendations for improvement and to provide feedback on the program and on how it is meeting the community's expectations of EMS education. Program challenges, such as requesting major funding for capital investments and recommending changes in admission requirements, are more likely to succeed and are often less contentious when put forward with advisory committee involvement.

Programs seeking CoAEMSP accreditation will be required to show input from their advisory committees as part of their accreditation reporting. This includes annual meetings and documentation of approved changes and revisions in the program.

Participating in State and Local Rule-Making Committees

Educators who do not participate in their EMS regulatory committees at the local, state, or national level lose their ability to effectively voice their concerns and opinions on many vital issues. Also, most, if not all, accredited higher education institutions place great value on involvement with national, state, and regional leadership, regulatory, and accreditation agencies and activities. Furthermore, regulators, who do not have the involvement of the educators when they are developing regulations, may adopt rules that are inappropriate or that present great problems to the educational programs that otherwise might have been avoided.

Maintaining Clinical Expertise

A difficult task, particularly for full-time educators, is maintaining clinical competency. Although educators can attend classes or read journals to keep abreast of new technology and cutting-edge content, clinical skills may be more time consuming to maintain. Often, the educator can work or volunteer part time for an EMS service to maintain patient care skills. Some academic institutions encourage instructors to work clinically by having a 35-hour work week or a 9-month contract. When possible, some educators participate actively with students in hospital and field settings, thus maintaining a level of clinical interaction.

Participating in Professional Associations

It is critically important that educators participate in professional activities outside the educational organization. Professional associations and conferences provide an excellent way for educators to stay current both in content-related areas and in new teaching methods and strategies. Technology has facilitated this effort with the advent of podcasts, webinars, virtual conference rooms, and document sharing capabilities. Professional networking can also contribute significantly to a program's success through the sharing of resources and ideas. Every EMS educator should consider joining local, state, and national EMS educator associations. In addition, every EMS educator should block off uninterrupted time to engage in peer review of publications related to the EMS profession, as well as information disseminated from professional organizations.

Student Issues

Instructors must prepare to spend considerable time outside of regular classroom time to perform other student-centered duties. Time devoted to student-related issues can include meeting with students to review progress or discuss performance issues, providing referrals for life crises, motivating them toward success, or writing letters of recommendation.

Student Conferences

Some students, particularly those who are not progressing satisfactorily, need one-on-one time for feedback, tutorial help, and counseling (**FIGURE 2.4**). Each student should, at minimum, have the opportunity to talk with the primary instructor privately at the course midpoint to discuss their progress. If the student is progressing satisfactorily, this meeting can be brief. On the other hand, if the student is failing to meet minimum class standards, the educator must be prepared to give the student specific information pertaining to their performance deficits, along with concrete examples of how to improve this performance. Records of these meetings must be placed in students' files.

Clear guidelines regarding how to reach the instructor outside of class should be established. Students should know how and when it is appropriate to contact faculty and how quickly a response should be expected. A back-up contact should be made available for an emergency contact, particularly when students are in clinical rotations.

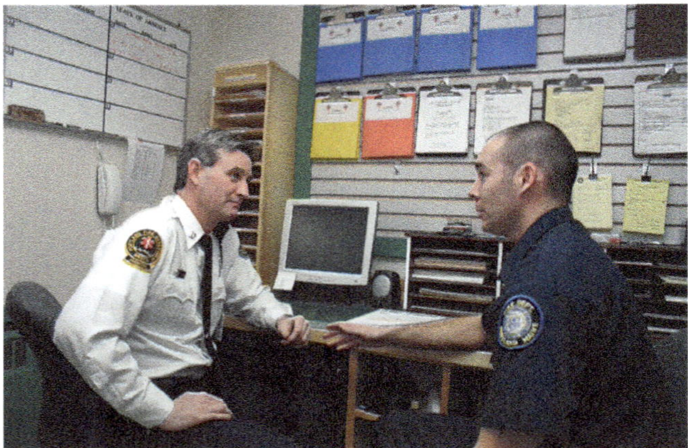

FIGURE 2.4 Student–teacher conferences provide students with valuable feedback about their performance.

Student Advisement

Students need routine advisement in all three domains of learning: cognitive, psychomotor, and affective. Frequent assessment of and advisement in these three domains is the gold standard that programs strive for but rarely reach. While this may seem an impossible goal, there are several proven techniques that greatly increase individual and programmatic ability to advise students.

The use of grading rubrics is a powerful tool. A rubric is a table that clearly defines the grading criteria for a given task. Rubrics can be used for providing feedback in all three domains. Providing feedback in the affective domain can be challenging. Using a rubric can assist the instructor and student to identify key behavioral characteristics to measure to provide feedback in the affective domain. A rubric can also be used to measure and provide feedback for scenario testing in a lab setting. The advantages of using a rubric for grading are as follows:

- It clearly defines the grading criteria.
- It forces the instructor to look at all students exactly the same way.
- It makes grading more objective.
- It allows students to select their grades and make informed decisions on where their focus should be.
- It helps eliminate the emotional aspect of grading.
- It can be done almost instantaneously.

If rubrics are developed for grading and providing feedback on all appropriate aspects of the class and program and used to review students' daily progress, advisement becomes a continuous process rather than a spot check.

There are many websites with premade rubrics or templates that can be used in constructing a rubric tailored to a class. Simply typing in the search term "rubric" yields many free websites with sample grading templates.

Referring Students to Other People and Offices

Another role of the educator is to refer students to appropriate counseling resources or potential employers. Educators have a responsibility to be aware of available student-centered services. The educator might refer a student to a career opportunity, to remedial classes, or for diagnostic testing, as might be the case with a student with a suspected learning disability.

Counseling Students on Personal Issues

Because the educator instills respect and trust, some students will approach their instructor for personal advice and guidance. Sometimes, even when not seeking advice and guidance, a student may bring personal issues to the instructor. Most educators spend a small part of their week dealing with student personal issues. It is paramount that the educator respect the student's feelings and confidentiality in these matters. It is also critically important that privacy is provided for these discussions. Developing a list of internal and community resources and having them readily available for making referrals is also essential. Common issues that can be expected include pregnancies, work terminations, loss of housing, physical abuse, depression, anxiety, other mental health issues, personal illness, illness of a loved one, loss of financial aid, substance abuse, harassment from other students, learning disabilities, and conflicts in schedules. Knowing the institution's policies and resources on these issues goes a long way in helping the educator to determine their role in these issues. It is also critically important that the educator know the responsible professional limits and liabilities of acting in the role of counselor. The profession of counseling is licensed in most states, and several levels of professional counseling licenses are available, including Licensed Mental Health Counselor and Licensed Professional Clinical Counselor. An educator who means well might offer counseling and comfort to a student who later attempts suicide or commits some violent act; the educator could be liable for practicing as a counselor without a license. The instructor must also notify the student of the limits of confidentiality. In instances where the student discloses information that represents a threat of harm to themselves or to others, the educator has an obligation to take appropriate action according to institutional policies.

Motivating Students to Complete Class Assignments

Some students do not require motivation to complete class assignments on time, but many do. Educators must take time and energy from their already busy schedules to devise strategies that encourage students to meet performance requirements, rather than simply nagging them to do so. Enforcing deadlines, and dealing with students who do not meet deadlines, requires time and energy initially, but pays off in the long run. Educators can include two items in the curriculum to assist this effort. First, every assignment and due date should be printed on the course syllabus that is distributed and reviewed on the first day of class. Second, the consequences of missing the deadlines must be clearly explained and appear in written form in a syllabus or policy and procedure document. Many educators are very clear about the assignments in their syllabus, but do not explain the consequences of failing to complete assignments, making a faulty leap in logic that suggests that students will intuitively understand the ramifications. Implementing a student contract, signed by the student, that indicates understanding and willingness to adhere to policies can help to eliminate misunderstanding. Finally, every student must be treated in the same way. If one student receives extra time to complete an assignment, then all other students in the class must receive the same.

Writing Letters of Reference

It is appropriate for students to request letters of reference or recommendation from their educators. An instructor may wish to set guidelines that determine what type of recommendation will be provided. Recommendation procedures should follow policies established by the school. A good place to publish these criteria is in the course syllabus. Some common requirements for letters of reference include a student's taking more than one course with the educator, earning above-average grades (generally a B or better), exhibiting positive, professional learning attitudes, having no disciplinary problems, and doing something to contribute positively to the class or program (e.g., helping with a research project or guest lecturing).

When writing a recommendation, include the following elements:

- The name of the person to whom the application is being sent. Encourage the student requesting the letter of recommendation to supply this name. Avoid addressing letters of recommendation: To whom it may concern. If the student requests a generic letter for possible future use, offer to write the letter at a later date when the student has all the appropriate information.
- When writing an academic or employment letter of recommendation, writers should first state the relationship they have to the student, including how long they have known the student and in what capacity, for example, director, advisor, instructor, or friend. Next, the instructor should describe the moral character, dedication, maturity, and types of skills of the student. In an academic context, focus

on ambition or desire to learn, a passion or drive for the field of teaching or clinical care, leadership skills and experiences, dedication to coursework, and so on. If the letter is for employment, focus on those attributes that indicate the student will make a good employee. Include comments on attendance, being a team member, coping with change, and self-motivation.

- The letter writer should back comments up with concrete examples, via anecdotes of how a student performed in class, on tests, in the lab, and so on. Honors and awards could be mentioned in the context of overall academic performance. Admissions committees want to see candidates who stand out from the crowd, so do not hesitate to use superlatives to describe the student. Was she the most organized in the class? Most willing to work as part of a team? Most curious? The writer should quantify such statements: "Mary was in the top 5% of the class when it came to lab work." Some selection committees request a ranking of the student.

A good letter of recommendation typically has several characteristics. Someone who knows the person fairly well and who is familiar with the student's academic history, personal traits, and goals should write the letter. For example, it could be a professor or other faculty member, an advisor, a college administrator, a teacher, and sometimes an employer—especially if the job or internship is related to the person's academic and career pursuits.

Academic letters of recommendation illustrate a student candidate's leadership skills, character, integrity, intellect, initiative, drive, and readiness to excel amid myriad pressures. The best reference letters present a picture of a student who is not one-dimensional, but instead, well rounded.

Advising Students on a Career

In most cases, students take EMS courses in hopes of obtaining a job. A vital part of the EMS educator's job is developing contacts within the local EMS community to help place students. Hosting career days is another way some schools meet this need. Educators must stay current on various job requirements, salaries, and employment practices. Students also seek information on further education and options for advancement and the instructor should be ready to provide information at the institution or elsewhere.

Tutoring Students

A few general approaches can be taken to providing remedial tutoring. One is to set aside time on a regular basis each week. A second ideal approach is to seek available tutorial resources within the institution or larger community. A third approach is to assign tutorial responsibilities to a secondary instructor, if one exists.

Some precautionary notes apply to providing tutoring, however. The first is to be careful to set limits on the time that services will be provided, as some students have a need that is impossible to fill. If unlimited tutoring is offered, some students will take up that offer. Instructors should consider requiring the student to bring a list of questions to the session. This process helps with student accountability and helps the student reflect on exactly what they do not understand. If there is no accountability by the student in the learning process, not only will the educator's time be drained, but the student may still fail, and the failure becomes the responsibility of the educator. A second cautionary note is that it is best to tutor only in open groups, never by private or exclusive appointment. There may be peer tutoring leadership opportunities available to help classmates who are struggling in a particular area. If in-class, program tutoring, and other institutional resources are not sufficient, students may be referred to fee-for-service tutoring. The program faculty should not provide this paid service, as it could represent a conflict of interest.

Encouraging the Class

Nearly every class hits a slump at some point. This usually occurs about three-quarters of the way through the class. Remember that a major role of the educator is that of coach. Many educators find that they give motivational talks to nearly every class at some point, if not several points, during the class duration. If time permits, introduce a motivational or team-building activity at this point in the program. Consider inviting former graduates to return and discuss their careers. Plan graduation activities if the class is nearing the end of the program. Keeping their eye on the end goal is often a strong motivator for students whose motivation is waning.

Clarifying Issues, Beliefs, and Problems

No matter how brilliant the lectures, no matter how well-crafted the syllabus, key points and policies must be reiterated multiple times. This is a matter of human nature. There is no point in being despondent over the need to do this. Use diverse strategies to reinforce key material. Supplement reading and lecture with other activities such as discussion groups, games, scenarios, or case studies that allow students to integrate the knowledge in higher-level contexts. This not only increases retention, it promotes transfer of learning to the practice of EMS.

TEACHING TIP

Anything worth saying is worth repeating three times—especially to tired, overloaded, overwhelmed students.

Common Role Adjustments

Overall, the educator is expected to handle the teaching load and to continue on the path toward growth and scholarly excellence. Perhaps the most challenging aspect is balancing one's professional and personal lives. The second most challenging aspect is maintaining one's clinical abilities and ensuring they are in keeping with current evidence in EMS practice.

The roles and expectations of the beginning EMS educator are new and very different from those of the EMS care provider. These new roles and expectations are more than just an extension of those clinical roles. They require a new set of assertive behaviors, because the power structure and length of relationships with students are completely different from those between care provider and patient. These new roles and expectations challenge and test the educator's teaching abilities.

One of the first and most important challenges facing the new educator is that of establishing authority and credibility in the classroom. After establishing authority, the educator must be able to exercise that authority prudently. This textbook and other education literature offer effective guidelines for establishing and exercising authority as an educator; however, there are no foolproof guidelines that apply in every situation. Each class, as a group, and each educator, individually, are unique.

Four characteristics of the educator help establish authority in the classroom: experience, expectations, knowledge, and goals.

Experience versus Authority

In general, an older educator relies more on teaching experience than on the authority of a title or position. Often, new educators learn the hard way that the title of instructor does not automatically impart esteem or credibility in a class. New instructors often learn that humility and deferential behaviors are typically more powerful with students than is authoritarian bluster. The educator's ability to deal with the thousand and one challenges of teaching far outweighs any badge of authority that goes with the title of instructor. This same phenomenon can be seen in the streets, where respect for EMS caregivers is earned through competent performance.

Expectations versus Discipline

Seasoned educators inspire students to follow professional behavior simply by their professional demeanor—the way that they impart their knowledge and understanding. As with experience versus authority, it is this expectation of leadership and performance more than any badge of authority that will maintain order and discipline in the classroom. The seasoned educator rarely needs to resort to disciplinary action for misconduct in the classroom. Setting high

CASE in Point

The new EMS educator recently hired by the local community college had 10 years of experience in EMS and had been a practicing paramedic for seven of those last years. She was highly respected for her clinical skills and for having a great personality to go with it. This new educator was perfect for the instructor position at the local community college. Today was her first day in class.

The new educator was a little nervous as she walked into class as lead instructor for the first time to face 23 students. She was more nervous than she had ever imagined, realizing the responsibility for maintaining course continuity, covering the entire curriculum, covering for guest lecturers who did not show up, resolving disputes, counseling, providing discipline, developing and administering exams, and assigning grades. It hit her for the first time—what it meant to be the lead instructor—just as she introduced herself in her new role.

With genuine humility, a professional demeanor, and a little humor, she won over the class. She began with, "Hello, this is my first day of class. You have a lot to teach me. I hope that we enjoy our journey of learning together. We're going to begin by introducing ourselves to one another. I'll start by telling you a little bit about my background, and why these folks asked me to come here to be your lead instructor."

CASE in Point

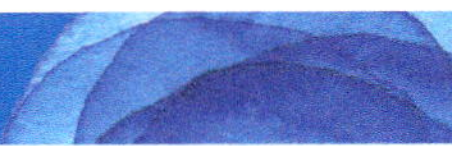

An EMS provider with 7 years of experience in a high-volume system signed up to deliver continuing education on respiratory emergencies. This was the provider's first time delivering continuing education and he was nervous on the day of the presentation. He knew this session was going to be attended by supervisors, field training officers, and colleagues. This certainly added a feeling of uncomfortable pressure to perform well.

The instructor started his session on time by introducing himself and introducing the topic and learning objectives. During the session, the instructor remained mindful to his uneasiness of presenting to this group by keeping a good pace and remaining on topic. He felt comfortable because, as part of his preparation, he took time to learn the science behind the content and he had practiced his well-developed presentation. He asked questions that solicited input from attendees of all levels. When a participant offered a personal story of experience, he acknowledged the importance of experience while refocusing the conversation back to the content and learning objectives.

Shortly after his session, a well-respected colleague came up to him and shared how engaging his presentation was and how they appreciated the obvious effort the instructor put into his presentation. In the end, this acknowledgment washed away all doubt, and the instructor felt empowered to deliver more educational sessions.

professional and academic expectations early in the course will prove to be a valuable strategy in avoiding the use of discipline. Most caregivers have witnessed similar scenarios in the field. Crews may naturally follow a senior paramedic or EMT whom they respect, regardless of rank or title; other supervisors or chiefs become frustrated when they are unable to lead their subordinates.

TEACHING TIP

Remember that it is always better to set high expectations at the beginning of a class, and then be willing to back down a little, than to try to raise expectations later. Students will continually surprise their instructors, if given the chance to strive for high goals.

Knowledge versus Insignia

No title, rank, or uniform will make up for a lack of content knowledge. It is hopeless for educators to hide behind a title or position when faced with a question they cannot answer. Seasoned educators know that students will ask questions they cannot answer. They expect these questions and honor them. Indeed, no EMS educator or any educator in any profession is expected to know every answer to every possible question. Educators who feel confident are not intimidated or threatened by questions that they cannot answer. When a question arises that they cannot immediately answer, they feel confident in telling students that they will get back to the class with the answer as soon as possible. It is also acceptable to inquire whether another student has the answer, or to assign a student to research the answer and report back to the class. Novice educators—those not yet confident in their authority or abilities—will often make up an answer or try to deflect the question. Both of these strategies leave students frustrated, and the educator's authority is undermined as a result.

TEACHING TIP

An effective strategy in dealing with difficult questions is to address them on the first day of class. The instructor might say that occasionally students will ask a question that the instructor will not be able to immediately answer. When that happens, the instructor will write the question in the corner of the whiteboard, and it will stay there until, together, they find the answer to the question.

This approach does three things. First, it validates the students' right to ask questions. Second, it keeps the instructor off the pedestal of "infallible." Lastly, it keeps the educator honest and reliable in the promise to find answers to student questions.

Goals: Firm Grasp versus Cookbook

Experienced EMS providers know what they want to accomplish for each patient, and they generally know several ways to go about it. The same is true for experienced educators. What worked in one class may not work in another. It is more important that educators have their own teaching philosophy and a clear understanding of what students need to learn than merely a series of lesson plans in "cookbook" fashion. Educators should keep the educational goals in mind and should constantly ask whether what they are teaching today brings them closer to those goals.

Summary

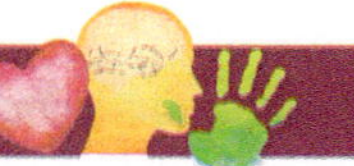

It is paramount that educators be well grounded and comfortable in the content that they are expected to teach. Many other issues will place demands on their time and energy, but educators must ensure they remain strong in their core content areas. Educators also must realize that teaching is a team sport; new instructors should actively seek out resources outside the classroom to help them address some of the issues that may otherwise overwhelm them. Secondary instructors can be a valuable addition to any class, but they may not intuitively know what to do. When an educator works with secondary instructors, the time taken to mentor them will be returned many times. Finally, new educators must seek a balance between teaching obligations and personal commitments, as well as the need to maintain current clinical skills and ensure they are in keeping with current evidence related to EMS practice. Attention to this balance must be a high priority and should begin on the first of day of class.

Glossary

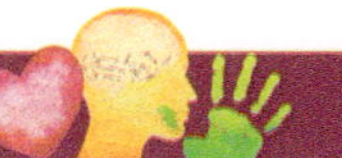

clinical coordinator Person who schedules and tracks hospital and other clinical training rotations.

field coordinator Person who schedules and tracks field EMS rotations.

flipped classroom Pedagogical model in which the typical lecture and homework elements are reversed, for example through the use of technology such as a virtual learning environment or learning management system.

lecturer Content expert who presents selected didactic material.

practical lab instructor Person who teaches in laboratory settings.

preceptor (field training officer) Practicing paramedic or health professional who instructs EMS students in a hospital or the field clinical setting.

primary (lead) instructor Person who is qualified to provide leadership or supervision over a series of courses or entire EMS program.

program (course) coordinator Educator responsible for program logistics.

program director Person who assumes overall responsibility for program.

program medical director Physician responsible for medical oversight of the program and for ensuring terminal competency through monitoring testing and program evaluation.

secondary instructor Person who possesses the appropriate academic or healthcare credentials and an understanding of the principles and theories of education, and is responsible for assisting primary instructors and providing instruction to students.

simulation coordinator Person who assists in coordination of simulation opportunities for students. The individual who navigates the technology during the simulation exercise.

References

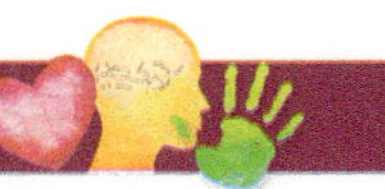

[1] National Association of State EMS Officials. 2010, December. "EMS Instructor Qualifications. A Template to Assist States with Implementing the EMS Education Agenda for the Future: A Systems Approach." Accessed November 2, 2018. https://nasemso.org/wp-content/uploads/EMS-Instructor-Qualifications-Template.pdf.

[2] Commission on Accreditation of Allied Health Education Programs (CAAHEP). 2015. "Standards and Guidelines for the Accreditation of Educational Programs in the Emergency Medical Services Professions." Accessed March 16, 2018. https://www.caahep.org/CAAHEP/media/CAAHEP-Documents/EMSPStandards2015.pdf.

[3] National Highway Traffic Safety Administration. 2009. "National Emergency Medical Services Education Standards." [DOT HS 811 077A]. Accessed January 15, 2019. https://www.ems.gov/pdf/National-EMS-Education-Standards-FINAL-Jan-2009.pdf.

[4] Goffman, Erving. 1959. *Presentation of Self in Everyday Life*. New York: Anchor Books.

[5] Wong, Harry K., and Rosemary T. Wong. 2009. *The First Days of School: How to Be an Effective Teacher*. Mountain View, CA: Harry K. Wong Publications.

[6] Moffett, Jennifer. 2015. "Twelve Tips for 'Flipping' the Classroom." *Medical Teacher* 37, no. 4: 331–6. https://doi.org/10.3109/0142159X.2014.943710.

[7] McKenna, Kim D., Elliot Carhart, Daniel Bercher, Andrew Spain, John Todaro, and Joann Freel. 2015. "Simulation Use in Paramedic Education Research (SUPER): A Descriptive Study." *Prehospital Emergency Care* 19, no. 3: 432–40. https://doi.org/10.3109/10903127.2014.995845.

[8] Haladyna, Thomas M., Steven M. Downing, and Michael C. Rodriguez. 2002. "A Review of Multiple-Choice Item-Writing Guidelines for Classroom Assessment." *Applied Measurement in Education* 15, no. 3: 309–34. https://doi.org/10.1207/S15324818AME1503_5.

[9] Judith A. Ruple, Gregory H. Frazer, Arthur B. Hsieh, William Bake, and Joann Freel. 2005. "The State of EMS Education Research Project: Characteristics of EMS Educators." *Prehospital Emergency Care* 9, no. 2: 203–12. https://doi.org/10.1080/10903120590924807.

[10] Miller, Michael G. 2013, Winter. "Teaching and Assessing Leadership Skills in the Emergency Medical Services Classroom." *Domain3: NAEMSE*, 19–24.

[11] Crowe, Remle P., Robert L. Wagoner, Severo A. Rodriguez, Melissa. A. Bentley, and David Page. 2017. "Defining Components of Team Leadership and Membership in Prehospital Emergency Medical Services." *Prehospital Emergency Care* 21, no. 5: 645–51. https://doi.org/10.1080/10903127.2017.1315200.

PART II

The Student

Emergency medical services (EMS) students are as different from one another as are the patients they will eventually treat. They span a spectrum from working adults looking for a second career to high school students who are still discovering themselves. They come from diverse backgrounds with varying levels of knowledge and life experience. Yet, each must grasp concepts and apply information that is often expected of physicians, anesthesiologists, social workers, and even psychiatrists.

This part of the text provides valuable information about the general attributes of today's EMS learners. It explores how new discoveries in neuroscience can inform educational practices to maximize learning. Likewise, it introduces knowledge of how adults learn and progress from novice to expert. An understanding of the basic principles of adult education, including information about their students' various learning preferences and factors to develop a supportive learning environment, helps educators meet their teaching goals and, ultimately, produce effective, well-rounded EMS personnel.

Remember that all EMS students are unique individuals, each with their own strengths and weaknesses, and each deserving of respect. By harnessing the science of learning and respecting the individuality of each student, their strengths, and their weaknesses, educators can help students achieve their learning objectives and, in return, earn and expect their respect.

CHAPTER 3

Brain-Based Learning

OBJECTIVES

At the conclusion of this chapter, the educator will be able to:

Cognitive Domain

1. Identify the function of various structures in the brain that stimulate long-term memory.
2. Compare and contrast the structures in the limbic system that involve short-term memory, long-term memory, and executive function that impact learning.
3. Discuss classroom strategies that engage the brain and stimulate learning for successful student outcomes.
4. Describe current research by neuroscientists that describes the benefits of physical activity and active participation in a classroom and lab environment that stimulate the brain during learning.
5. Describe the benefits of developing creative classroom strategies that blend theory with application to encourage student understanding and relevance of content.
6. Compare and contrast various classroom strategies that promote student participation to stimulate student critical thinking and problem-solving skills.
7. Discuss the impact of constructive feedback in building student confidence in a safe learning environment.

Psychomotor Domain

1. Design and implement creative classroom and lab strategies that promote problem-solving and teamwork through consistent scenario performance opportunities.

Affective Domain

1. Value positive interpersonal communication skills that model professional behaviors and motivate students to learn.
2. Value effective student teamwork and the impact on learning by providing constructive feedback on student performance during activities and scenarios.
3. Value utilization of intrapersonal and interpersonal communication skills development in the classroom to provide more empathetic interaction with patients.

"Tell me, and I forget. Teach me, and I may remember. Involve me, and I learn."

~ Benjamin Franklin

pain, and stimulation of touch. Most researchers agree that this area of the brain can organize complex visual materials or activities such as putting together puzzles. With practice, this region of the brain, like all areas of the brain, can be strengthened by using novelty and by creating challenges for the brain.

Glial Cells: The Glue

Eric Jensen notes that while Einstein had an average size brain, his brain had "more than average glial cells" and was therefore a heavier, more densely compacted brain.[2]

Glial cells have an important role in learning. They come together with neurons and create an intellectual symphony that makes learning possible. The power seems to come from the nutrition they provide, the myelin for the axons, regulation and strengthening of the immune system, and support of the blood–brain barrier. Recent studies have shown that these structures keep harmful substances away from the neurons. New glial cells, called astrocytes, help filter and improve neural signaling, making the nerves more efficient. With a healthy supply of these protective, strengthening, and supportive cells, brain function seems to be a smoother and easier process as it relates to learning.

Neurons: The Bowstring

The word *neuron* originated from the Greek term for bowstring or sinew. It is the basic structure that makes up the nervous system. The human brain contains around 100 billion neurons. The cell body, or **soma**, extends an outward projection called an **axon** that connects to an inbound feeder system known as the **dendrites**. Neurons change the electrical impulse into a chemical code that leaps the gap separating the cells. This ability to create changeable connections lets the brain adapt to changing situations and environments. The firing of 250 to 2,500 impulses per second transmits signals and releases chemicals stored in synaptic vesicles at the end of the axon, interacting with over 100 different neurotransmitters.

Mirror Neurons: Predict Behavior

Mirror neurons help in survival as they predict the intentions of others and allow a person to respond to their environment. These neurons are critical in allowing humans to have empathy for others and "feel their pain." This is a basic human emotion; being in contact with this information in a correct way can lead to "fitting in socially." When someone smiles, without thinking, the recipient smiles back; this is an incredibly important tool in helping to navigate social interactions. It is not enough to have these nerve cells; they need to be exercised. The more students interact and pay attention to each other, the better their interactions with patients in the field will be. Interpreting intention incorrectly can have dire consequences when interacting with patients; it can lead to misunderstanding a patient's facial affect, body language, or openness to establishing a positive interaction.

Brainstem: Reptilian Brain

The brainstem is located where the brain meets the spinal cord. The spinal cord termination is about 1 inch into the lower brain and is known as the **medulla oblongata**, where motor and sensory nerves cross over as they move to the cerebrum. As they pass over the **pons** (bridge), the bundles link these parts of the brain together so communication can take place and important functions such as the heartbeat, respirations, temperature, and digestion are monitored and controlled. Another key function in this area is the **reticular activating system (RAS)**, which is responsible for keeping the brain alert by heightening awareness to respond to stimuli related to the sympathetic nervous system for the "fight or flight" response. The brainstem is the area where the terminating junction for 11 of the 12 body nerves occurs.

TEACHING TIP

The brain has attention cycles that revolve around the rhythms of rest and activity. The best time to present new information is in the morning when the brain is fresh. Likewise, testing late in the afternoon may catch students on the downhill side of their rhythms. It is preferable to test students when their brains are fresher. Educators should save the later part of the day for more hands-on activity to keep the brain active.

The Limbic System: The Mammalian Brain

The limbic system is the oldest area of the brain and helps maintain focus. The limbic system interacts with many different areas of the brain and is important for memory and learning. The limbic system can be divided into four parts: **thalamus**, **hypothalamus**, **hippocampus**, and **amygdala**.

Thalamus: Inner Chamber. All incoming information except the sense of smell goes through the thalamus from outside areas. Signals are then processed and sent to other areas of the brain, including the cerebrum and cerebellum for additional processing and subsequent action. Memory and much of our cognitive activities are organized in this area of the brain.

Hypothalamus: The Internal Thermostat. The hypothalamus maintains **homeostasis** by regulating temperature, sleep, and nutrient intake through internal monitoring. Damage to the hypothalamus weakens the immune system and its response to viruses or germs; stimulation to this area boosts immunity.

Hippocampus: The Sea Horse. The hippocampus moves learning from short-term memory into long-term memory. This is critical to learning, storing, and retrieving new information for later use. It is now realized that this area of the brain can produce new neurons, a process called **neurogenesis**. Encouraging students to sleep between 6.5 and 8 hours per night, remain well hydrated, exercise regularly, and eat a well-balanced diet can play a large part in helping the limbic system.

Amygdala: The Almond. The amygdala influences intrapersonal and interpersonal interactions (emotions) and how a person deals with learning at every level. When students experience emotions during learning, they imprint the long-term memory, meaning they remember the emotion and remember the experience. This powerful area of the brain is not understood by many educators. The stronger the emotion, the longer the learning event will be imprinted and the easier it can be recalled. This is why clinical and field training can be so powerful in helping students remember treatment modalities and begin to develop muscle memory with a well-trained and educated preceptor. Educators have long concentrated on the cognitive domain (knowledge) and psychomotor domain (skills) but have not understood the power of the affective domain (feelings). Students can learn to model and modify their behavior under stressful situations by tapping into this powerful part of the brain.

Assessing the Affective Domain

Classroom application for reaching the affective domain is often overlooked in the assessment of the EMS classroom. The greatest change that can happen between an educator and a student is not the elevation of a grade, but elevation of the spirit and the motivation to learn. When employers are asked what they consider the most important skill in public safety, the number one reply is positive behavioral attributes. This has driven employers, accreditation organizations, and national testing to spend more time assessing this area of learning. Graduating students who have the cognitive ability and the psychomotor ability is important in the creation of a competent and compassionate entry-level provider. Too often educators fail to concentrate on building the student's affective ability, thereby ignoring the most powerful part of the learning process. To build affective ability, it is important that educators understand how the brain drives a person to take charge of their lives. Every educator must set the tone, model the proper behaviors, and bring the right attitude to the classroom before expecting the student to follow. If educators have no expectations, then as Benjamin Franklin once said, "Blessed is he who expects nothing, for he shall receive it." Educators and students must set high expectations for themselves and the profession. Thoughts become reality—good or bad.

Communicating Neurons: Cascade of Interaction

Hemorrhaging Intellect

It is important for educators to understand that students may have exceptional cognitive ability, perhaps even to the level of a genius. However, external and internal factors may be working to drain this intelligence. When intellectual hemorrhage occurs, an educator may lose a viable student if intervention does not occur. With some emergent and preventive measures, educators may salvage a larger number of students from the brink of disaster.

Mullainathan and Shafir note that stressors can create a "scarcity in the brain that diminishes IQ and self-control."[7] The brain is held hostage to stressors that create scarcity of attention and ability to focus on targeted areas of life. While students worry about their children, bills, the car breaking down, and deadlines for paperwork submission, a price is paid for attending to these areas, leaving less cognitive capacity to deal with other intellectual requirements. This creates a scarcity of intellect, reducing the student's ability to have a healthy bandwidth, which directly affects intellectual performance. Neuroscientists have noted that when bandwidth is taxed, the student enters the "bandwidth blues."

Bandwidth Blues

A student's ability to solve problems, retain information (cognitive capacity), reason and solve problems (fluid intelligence), and initiate and inhibit actions (executive control) are all possible with enough capacity of **bandwidth**—space in the brain. When students are under constant stress, intellectual functions are diverted to deal with the emergent stress. This leaves less bandwidth room, creating an environment of scarcity that is commonly referred to as the bandwidth blues. Raven's Progressive Matrices, named for the British psychologist John Raven and developed in the 1930s, is a universally accepted measure of fluid intelligence. Several studies using this matrix showed that when participants were put under stress, their IQ lowered dramatically and they had a greater chance of increasing impulsive behavior.[7] Educators see this daily in their classrooms and in themselves as they juggle jobs and families. It is no surprise that students are under equal or greater stress, which can affect their ability to balance their lives and their studies. Identifying students' stressors helps stem the intellectual hemorrhage. Simple measures can help counteract the effects that sap the brain of precious intelligence when stressors come to the forefront (**TABLE 3.1**).

TABLE 3.1 Tips for Maximizing Student Brain Power

Sleep	Sleep is one of the most important first steps to improve cognition. Benefits can be seen quickly. The brain punishes those who fail to listen to its warning signs.
Finances	Encourage students to budget, help guide them to financial aid or other resources, and show them the value of savings and budgeting their limited resources.
Exercise	Encourage students to work out, maybe with a friend. Allot time in the classroom to get them on their feet. Encourage them to go outside for a walk during breaks or lunch.
Work	Encourage students to take time off, be with their family, plan a trip after the big test, and to get away to "recharge their batteries."
Family	Encourage students to have a date night once a week to stay connected at home, or to plan a family day once a week if they have children.
Food	Students need to eat smarter and increase their fluid intake, staying away from highly caffeinated and sugary drinks. Water is best.

The simplicity of this research is surprising, but the impact is real and ever present. It is the responsibility of every educator to address these areas and teach students better coping mechanisms so that together, healthier minds can be achieved. If real learning is to take place, educators need to take this piece of common sense and reverse the scarcity while increasing the bandwidth of the mind.

In his book, *Thinking for a Change*, John Maxwell challenges the reader to master the process of intentional thinking.[8] Educators must teach students how to think intentionally, because it matters in their personal and professional lives. **Intentional thinking** empowers the educator, who then can empower the student to reach their full potential. Is that not the goal of education and of the educators who are entrusted to bring about change? Maxwell provides a simple formula that can move educators in the right direction to improve themselves and their classrooms.

Memory-Making Moments

Short-Term Memory

To create memory-making moments, there must be a balance between the short-term and long-term memory. Memory-making begins in short-term memory where the hippocampus, amygdala, and **cerebral cortex** each play a role in converting memories to long-term memories. Many areas of the brain are involved in this conversion, and two types of memory are created in this process: declarative and nondeclarative.[9]

Declarative memories are those of which a person is consciously aware, such as Texas is a state, cars are for transportation, and the sky is blue. Declarative memories are known to be true, can be seen, and can be measured as fact. Short-term memory is used when obtaining a patient history and interpreting the meaning of the information collected. It is the moment of reflection. **Nondeclarative memories** are those of which one is not consciously aware, but which are used to perform motor skills such as throwing a ball, riding a horse, or driving a car.

In a matter of seconds, memories must be encoded. The earlier this is done, the stronger the memory will be, and the greater the chance a long-term memory will be created. Researchers have also noted that increased *CREB* genes allow a neuron to be activated more easily and thus help create a new memory.[10] While researchers are searching for ways to enhance the *CREB* gene, it is known that stimulating emotions

TEACHING TIP

Reinforce important points in many different ways: individual testing, group interaction, practical application, clinical and field experiences, etc. Teaching a subject by involving all the senses and in different unique ways can help transfer important information from short-term to long-term memory.

(amygdala) and using repetition can help a memory form. In the classroom, providing repetition of knowledge and skills by simulating a real situation with associated emotions can create pattern recognition so that information is remembered and transferred into long-term memory.

Long-Term Memory

While most memories disappear within minutes, those that survive strengthen with time.[9] The hippocampus and the cortex work together and communicate to form the possibility that the memory will survive into long-term memory. The new memories provide information that mingles with existing memories and stores them together. Adding new memories builds mental models of information upon information and strengthens the connections, thereby making the memory last longer or even for a lifetime depending on how it is repeated. The repetition process must be present in a variety of ways to ensure that the bonds are being strengthened in intervals over time. So, how does one make, process, encode, store, and retrieve memories as needed? Getting the brain ready to learn by providing a variety of challenging, unusual, repetitive, and rich experiences can and will make all the difference.

Brain-Based Learning and the Educator

Public safety and allied health educators work in a dynamic and fast-paced setting, striving for momentum to engage students in the classroom and lab, monitor ongoing competency, and challenge the efficiency and effectiveness of the classroom experience. In many cases, educators must navigate with fewer resources and consistently do more with less. Many educators serve in other jobs in addition to the role of educator, while also managing a family and a personal life. Educators must take time to slow down for a quiet moment to recharge and refresh the brain (**FIGURE 3.3**).

Often educators are type A personalities and, to varying degrees, must feel in control. This may partially explain why many educators do not use vacation time, or when they do, they bring their laptop on vacation to complete more work. How can educators avoid burnout? How can educators serve as effective leaders and role models to the next generation?

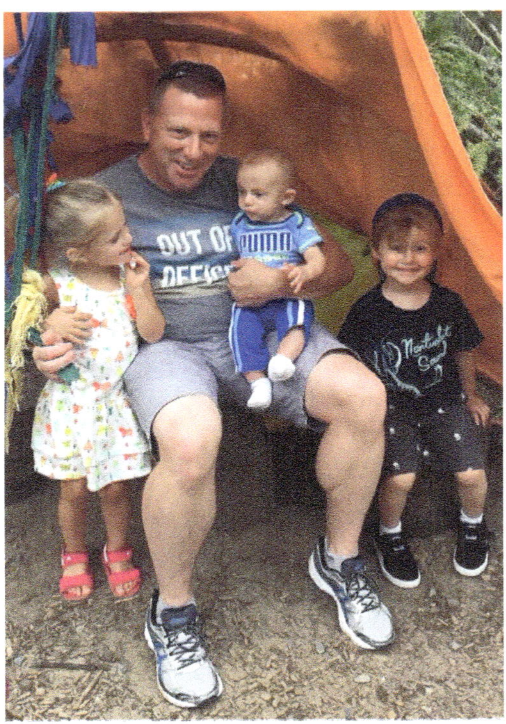

FIGURE 3.3 Although it may be especially difficult in a demanding environment, it is critical for educators to schedule time to recharge, refresh, and take care of themselves.

Courtesy of Richard Nydam.

Ego

Rein in your ego.
Give employees some control.
Take the weekends off.
Use carrots, not sticks.[11]

TEACHING TIP

- Set some time aside daily with students and faculty to brainstorm solutions.
- Treat students as stakeholders, not tourists, in the education process.
- Use the 5-minute meditation to sit quietly and meditate—clear your mind.
- Take the weekends off to recharge your battery.
- Have weekly conversations with staff and students.

Educators need to encourage themselves and their students to begin a process of slowing down. By taking a moment to breathe, educators can build on the science of creating more time for thinking and create a brain that has resilience. Many would question whether this is the job of the educator and whether educators have time to accomplish such moments. With an increase in suicides, divorces, drug usage, and generally an increase in just feeling disconnected, can anyone afford not to train and educate on these important skills?

Educators can cultivate consciousness that centers around mindfulness, which strengthens neural networks. The process of slowing down can help create a brain that can go from a one-dimensional to a multidimensional level of thinking, which can lead to a more attentive state.[12] An attentive state is critical to maintaining an edge and performing in stressful environments. One strategy to keep students attentive is to have students stand when they answer or ask a question (**FIGURE 3.4**). Just by getting students on their feet, the educator moves blood from the lower extremities back into core circulation while increasing the heart by 10 to 20 beats per minute. More blood means more oxygen, fewer blood clots, and a neurological system firing at a faster rate.[2] As another example, an educator can have the class stand when someone walks into the room. Coming to their feet as a class helps create novel stimulation, increases situational awareness, and makes students more accountable for their environment. Give it a try and see if students maintain greater vigilance in the classroom, which may transfer to the street environment.

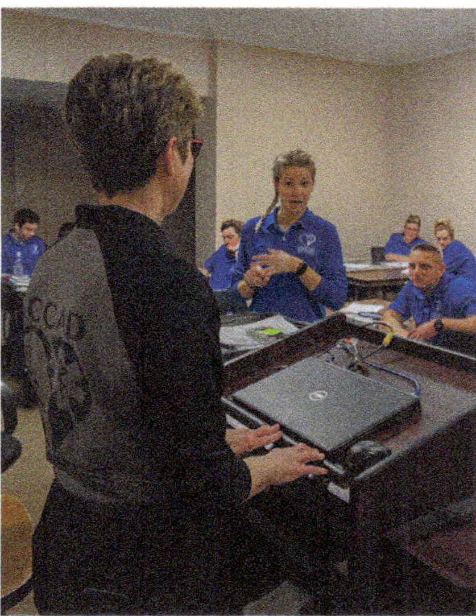

FIGURE 3.4 Educators should incorporate opportunities for students to physically move during class, for example, by standing up when answering a question.

Courtesy of St. Charles County Ambulance District.

In-Flight Corrections

One of the most difficult strategies for educators to employ is the art of change. No one likes change, and those who say they do ask others to go first, for it is an uncomfortable process.

Classroom teachers in grades K-12 have been educated and trained to make "in-flight corrections" because not all strategies work for everyone at all times. Like the science of learning, students change, and educators must be prepared to change with the times. Consider how most Americans were taught in the past, and compare that with how students are taught today; change is a part of a results-driven education. The best strategy is to seek out a mentor, stay in touch with new and evolving research, prepare to update teaching methods and, more importantly, try new strategies in the classroom.

Preparation for each semester should take into account what worked and what could have been improved from the previous semester. This process keeps the educator and the teaching process fresh and relevant.

Creating a Brain Ready for Learning

Educators understand that stress in moderation is good for learning, but stress over long periods of time is harmful. Finding balance for the right amount of stress is critical to create an environment where learning can flourish. To do this, educators must create an environment that balances stress and engagement. Public safety positions (EMS, fire, and law enforcement) along with allied health professions are high-stress jobs. It is the job of all educators to create a safe, challenging, and realistic environment where the application of stress can be applied in measured doses, and to help students acclimate to this stress over time. Human brains were not built for formal education; they were built for survival, and educators must take this into account. Time must be taken to arm students with the knowledge and tools to face harsh situations. Healthcare professionals must make decisions and treat patients in an unforgiving environment; many times they are racing against the clock while a life hangs in the balance.

The following steps provide the educator with strategies to create a classroom that is brain ready.

Team building. No matter what the teaching environment, students must be assigned to teams so that

Teamwork

Keep squads small and manageable—four to eight people seems to work best. Assigning jobs helps a squad run smoothly and gives everyone some responsibility. Examples of such assignments include squad leader, assistant squad leader, lab officer, time management officer, curriculum officer, and morale officer. Rotating roles within the established group empowers every student to practice leadership in the various roles in the work force.

Make sure that the group is given a grade, and keep the group together for the semester or course. Grading students shows that teamwork is important, and keeping them together builds structure and support, and creates a team bond that can reduce stress and increase performance.

every person has a responsibility to and an investment in the team's success. Students need to learn how to problem-solve together, trust one another, and understand that medicine is a team sport. They can rotate the roles of responsibility, but teams should stay together to form trust and encourage each other to complete the mission. The U.S. military has been practicing this for over 2 centuries to help mold the best teams in the world. Lt. Col. Grossman outlines many similarities between the military, fire, EMS, and police.[13]

Create more oxygen in the classroom. Casinos across the world understand how important it is to oxygenate the gaming areas by pumping oxygen into these areas to keep people awake, alert, and energized for longer periods of time. America's astronauts have incorporated over 17 different oxygen-producing plants into their training room to help clean, oxygenate, and negatively ionize the area.[2] Educators must follow suit for all the same reasons to make the classroom a more energetic and cleaner place to learn. Various types of plants can help maximize oxygenation; many educators have found bamboo plants less expensive and easier to find.

Plants in the Classroom

Educators can have students bring in plants to help oxygenate and ionize the classroom. Researchers have shown that this reduces fatigue and illness, while improving concentration. Educators must seek out natural ways to improve the classroom environment and help drive student success.

TEACHING TIP

Use bright-colored slide backgrounds. Avoid blues, as blue has a sedating effect on students.[15] Put up bright, colorful posters with positive messages to stimulate the brain[16] and create a positive environment. Involve the students to work in teams to breathe some life into the environment. They can bring color and excitement to even the dullest of places, and it will be a great team-building exercise.

Add more color to engage the brain. Many educators feel that black and white slides and handouts capture the attention of the learner. While black and white materials initially capture attention, attention is quickly lost because the brain looks for novelty and colors. In 1999, a study spoke to the importance of colors in the learning environment.[14] Avoid dark colors (blue, brown, etc.), as these relax and lower blood pressure. Instead, use bright pastels that engage and excite the brain—the best are bright colors, such as orange and yellow.[15]

Turn the thermostat down to 70°F (21°C). Keep the brain a little cooler to maximize learning.[17] According to Ornstein, "a rise of 1 or 2 degrees in brain temperature above normal is enough to disturb brain functions."[18] Eric Jensen notes in *Brain Based Learning* that the optimal temperature setting is around 70°F (21°C) for more technical studies; a cooler brain does better.[2] How do students respond when the classroom heats up a bit? Are they groggy or sluggish? Educators will find that it is harder for students to learn new concepts or skills in this condition.

Getting students to be more active turns the brain on so learning can begin. **Brain-derived neurotrophic factor (BDNF)** is a natural substance released by the brain to improve cognition (thinking) and boost how neurons talk with one another.[2] Neuroscientists at the University of California in Irvine found that physical activity enhances the ability of neurons to talk with one another, which leads to a more efficient brain.[19] The simplest way is to get students on their feet because activity engages a release of BDNF, which leads to more efficient learning. Activity and an enriching environment create neurogenesis (growth of neurons) and acceleration of connections, encouraging the learning process.[3] Try lecturing for 20 to 30 minutes, then have the students get up to do a patient assessment for 15 to 20 minutes, then turn back to lecture, then to another out-of-seat activity; keep repeating this process throughout the day. The more

TEACHING TIP

Take out the chairs in the lab—students need to be active and engaged. Have students stand in the classroom to answer and ask questions. When lecturing, *stop* every 30 minutes to get students out of their seats with an activity that reinforces what is being taught.

movement and activity, the more the students retain relevant information and learning.

Other ideas have also been found to be effective. While they are based on some basic and older learning principles, they are worth mentioning and worth utilizing in the classroom.

Greet the students. Greet students as they come into the classroom. In some cases, this sadly may be the only positive interaction in their lives, and they need to know the instructor is glad to see them. This lets them know their attendance and participation is valued. Thank them for their contribution in class personally and as a class before they leave.

Create a schedule. Create an agenda for how the class will proceed so students can see the flow and feel a sense of consistency.

Use music as a tool to engage and excite students' brains. Any music will do, according to the research, but try a variety and have a certain music for certain activities, for example, music to start the day, music to time a break, etc. Music has been shown to be an effective tool to calm and sometimes frustrates a brain, so listen to student input concerning the playlist, amount of time music is used, and volume during class.

Move outside of the classroom; take field trips. If this cannot be done, then the educator can take students outside for mini labs. Sunshine may provide some needed vitamin D and refreshment for the brain. This keeps students active and moving, which is important for learning.

Review what the educator did in the previous session. This informs students of what they should have learned. Integrate past knowledge with new information that students have learned. Assign them a battle buddy (as in military training) to reinforce material that they did not know or understand. Research and common sense come into play when educators use the power of peer tutoring. Using peer pressure in a positive way can be effective and can help the learner establish a lifeline in the classroom. Learning can be fun and engaging when teaching lifesaving concepts. The goal is to make learning last well beyond the classroom doors. The goal is to have the brain release mood elevators—**serotonin**, vasopressin, and dopamine. This surge of chemicals will help keep a brain that is built for survival and not formal education become more focused on learning.[20] Passive classrooms do not challenge students, and students who are not challenged cannot master the information. Instructors should keep students active and let them work together so they may gently push each other in the right direction. Nothing is more powerful than positive peer pressure and a sense that everyone is moving in the same direction. Half of the battle in learning is seeing that the information is relevant and useful to the learner. How can students argue with their own results when they are being successful?

The Whiteboard Method

Review with students in the morning using the whiteboard method. Begin by having students find a partner (a pair of two students is best, but a group can include three if necessary). Using an erasable board and marker, ask the students a question from the content covered in the last session. The instructor counts to five, then has the students write the answer on the whiteboard. If they do not know the answer, the instructor has them draw a sad face (emotional tie) on the board. At the end of the 5 seconds, the instructor has them turn around and s hare their answer with their team member(s). The instructor then calls out the correct answer. If they miss the answer, the team must ask each other this question three times during the day to ensure they have the concept down. In a 10-minute time frame, it is possible to review 15 to 20 concepts.

Exercise the Brain: Practice the Way We Play

There was a time in history when law enforcement officers were trained to unload the brass casings from their guns after shooting—to put them in their pocket or in a bag attached to the shooting stand—then load new bullets. In the field when under fire, some officers who emptied their gun in a shoot-out were found to be taking care of their brass unconsciously before reloading and continuing the fight. While they went through the elaborate exercise of unloading their brass casings, many officers died in shoot-outs; during the late 1960s to early 1970s officers died with brass in their hand or in their pocket.[13] Training and education matter. More time must be devoted to reading and analyzing the research to become better educators.

Why do educators continue to have students start lab training sessions by saying, "The scene is safe. . . .

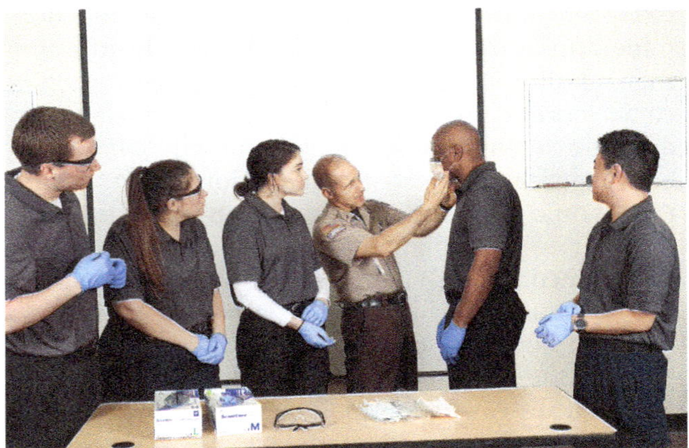

FIGURE 3.5 Students should practice and be tested on the actions they will perform in the field—not verbalization of the actions.

I am wearing standard precautions. . . ." What does this teach students? Saying is not doing; educators are teaching students habits that become muscle memory that may be problematic in a real-world application. Students must train the way they are going to perform in the field; actions must replace talk. Approach all scenes the same way: wear gloves and glasses in every lab session; if outside, ensure students are wearing their helmets and reflective vests, goggles, masks, etc. (**FIGURE 3.5**). It is critical that students practice the same way they will perform if they want to instinctively respond to a dynamic and changing environment. Educators must also veer away from automatically telling students the scene is safe. Instead, allow students to critically assess the scene and make a determination as they would in the field setting. A young marine of the Second Marine Division said it best when he stated, "My old Gunny taught me that in combat you do not rise to the occasion, you sink to the level of your training."[13]

Practicing for Real-Life Performance

Students need to wear all safety equipment and have all equipment available (jump bags) in all training scenarios. Never let students hold up their hands and pretend to wear gloves or safety glasses. Whatever an educator expects students to do on the street must be accomplished in classroom and lab activities; otherwise, educators are teaching them something else entirely. The goal is to get students to think at a higher level, and this can be lost if the educator thinks for them.

Too many classrooms utilize "pretend" as a methodology, which fails to teach students the true essence of what must be learned. The moulage and orchestration of the scenario play an important part in helping the students increase their situational awareness. Students must not only have working equipment, but also the setting in which they practice needs to be authentic. When a high-technology simulation center or staged physical scenario is not possible, take students out to the mall, a local business, or another realistic setting for practice and training. In the end, the more real the training and education become, the more the brain sees the relevance and the more the learning is remembered and modeled in the future.

Practicing in a Real Environment

Get the students out of the classroom to do scenarios. It is more realistic to run a scenario where the public can mingle, where environmental factors can become a factor (night, rain, cold, heat, wind), and where real sounds make communication, assessments, and interventions more challenging. Mirror the elements and relevance of the work environment that students will experience in their career.

CASE in Point

After giving students a lecture on stress and strategies to control stress, an educator sets up the following scenario for the students. Cardiac holter monitors are placed on each student in the scenario. After a baseline has been reached, for example, a heart rate between 60 and 80 beats per minute, the students run through a timed and stressful cardiac arrest or trauma scenario. The instructors monitor the heart rates of each student participating in the team. As the students' heart rates start to climb over 170 beats per minute, the instructors tell the students to start using some of the strategies to control their stress and lower their heart rates. At the point where students' heart rates climb over 170 beats per minutes, instructors note that the students are making more mistakes as their heart rate goes faster, supplying less blood to the brain.

Teaching students how to lower their stress and breathe properly may help them overcome the devastating effects that researchers see when the pulse is so fast that cognitive and psychomotor skills are impaired. The result is diminished higher-level thinking, causing errors, forgetfulness, and clumsiness. This training will remind students to take a few breaths, communicate with each other, or employ any strategy that can get them back on track.

Stephen Covey notes a habit that all educators want to foster: to start with the end in mind.[21] Too many educators run complex scenarios that have no real teaching outcome. Educators must be clear when deciding what they wish to accomplish, then move forward with clear expectations and benchmarks. Everything that educators do must be centered on a lesson that ties the learning together. The more real the situations are, the more students can learn from their mistakes so they sweat more in the classroom than during an emergency situation on the streets. If the educator's goal is to put stress on students to see their reactions under pressure, then the educator must be aware of the research as it pertains to raising heart rates. Educators can learn a lot from soldiers who enter a combat situation; think of law enforcement, fire, and EMS as the warriors of the home front, who must get in the mental zone to make the right decisions.

Lt. Col. Dave Grossman states, "There is a zone that exists, generally between 115 and 145 beats per minute, when you are at your optimal survival and combat performance level."[13] When soldiers reach heart rates at or above 175 beats per minute, there is a *decrease* in physical agility and mental focus, which can lead to a catastrophic set of events. No educator can argue that stress and failure are important parts of learning. However, the stress needs to be regulated and the purpose in training must be clear to the instructors and to the students. Educators must work out strategies with their students to bring down the stress to levels that can be dealt with to accomplish the mission. The power of controlled breathing is well known; in this technique, a person focuses on an object to reduce stress levels. Educators must seek the latest research techniques to find ways to reduce stress in students before and after educational activities, including cognitive and psychomotor testing.

TEACHING TIP

Have instructors and other students take the pulse of the student who is under pressure and note if the pulse is in the danger zone. Teaching students how to lower their stress and breathe properly may help them overcome the devastating effects that researchers see when the pulse is so fast that cognitive and psychomotor skills are impaired. This results in decreased situational awareness and decision-making ability that can be hazardous for both the patient and the providers.

Lt. Col. Dave Grossman relates a story that happened in Florida, where two detectives chased down a suspect, handcuffed the man, and put his rifle in their trunk. The officers had a sympathetic nervous system dump of adrenaline during this time and after securing the prisoner in the back seat of their car, they both sat in the front relaxing as they drove the suspect to jail. Unknown to these officers, the suspect had a handcuff key on a chain around his neck that he used to free himself from the cuffs. The suspect then attacked one of the officers, obtained his service gun, and shot and killed both seasoned detectives. The suspect then got his rifle and used it to kill a state trooper and take a hostage at a gas station. This event only came to an end when the suspect killed himself rather than surrender.[13] This story highlights the power of emotion after a traumatic event. Whereas the officers relaxed after they handcuffed the suspect, the suspect did not; his amygdala was running high, giving him the advantage, which ended tragically for the slain officers and their families. It is the educator's job to train students regarding how powerful the brain and body can be when working in a heightened state.

Educators must concentrate on the concept of practicing the way they want students to perform in real life. An educator's language, dress, equipment, actions, and authenticity of the learning experience create opportunities to succeed. Students need help dealing with the emotions and stress of working in EMS. The real danger is that students will relax during a difficult call and become vulnerable to making a mistake that could hurt them, their partner, or the patient.

Engage the Brain

How to engage the brain is not a secret, but it seems to evade many educators. While theory is important, theory without application has little or no meaning to a brain trying to understand its relevance. Engaging the brain makes learning possible, and this positions the student to understand the value in the information. Educators need to prepare the foundation and preplan the strategies to engage the brain in meaningful and dynamic ways so that learning occurs.

When teaching a medical subject, it can be effective to show relevance by showing real patients who have suffered from the illness or injury and their outcomes. Medical shows about medical examiners, forensics, or true stories from the emergency department can be used to present relevant patients with real illnesses and injuries. The educator can introduce topics by showing a 15- to 20-minute patient segment and then integrating this scenario into their lecture. This style of interaction can lead to higher-level thinking

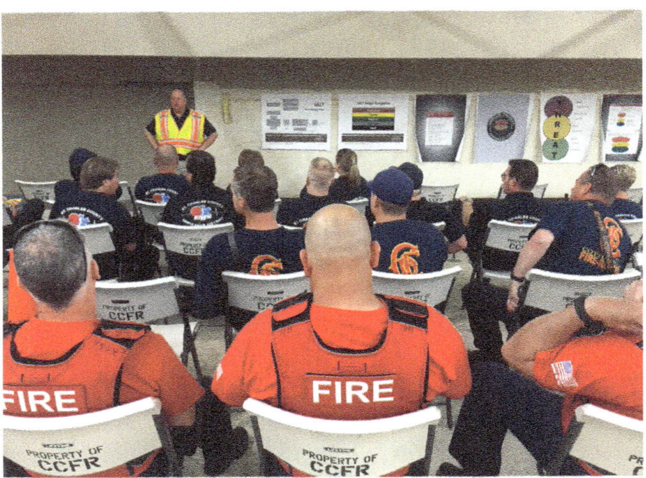

FIGURE 3.6 Educators can engage students by altering the format, for example, by inviting a guest speaker to talk or by taking students out of the classroom to an unfamiliar space.

Courtesy of St. Charles County Ambulance District.

Open the Day Right

Try starting the day with a neural sponge to engage the brain. As students filter into the classroom, play something on the screen. For example, show the TV series *Emergency!*; many episodes are relevant to actual classroom and field application (with some medical modifications and updating). Brains become engaged and learning relevant when minds are curious and interested in learning. Researchers say that students should not walk into a classroom that is quiet; quiet, in this context, is considered an intellectual morgue.

and encourage discussion and treatment plans that are student driven.

An educator can bring in guest speakers who have survived a heart attack to share a first-hand account of what happened to them and how they felt about the rescuers who came to help. What did public safety do that was comforting and helpful? What did they do that could be improved? If possible, the educator can take the students out of the classroom to hear the guest speaker via a field trip to a hospice center, nursing home, or pediatric center. These strategies are effective ways to engage the brain and build relevance into the classroom, blending theory and application together (**FIGURE 3.6**).

Energize the Brain

Energizing the brain requires interest, movement, and emotion to be truly effective. Many strategies have been found to be highly effective for the adult learner. As mentioned earlier, energizing the brain is critically important in the learning environment. A combination of thinking, moving, and a vested emotional response results in an energized brain. From their traditional schooling, students may believe that all learning occurs via spoon-fed answers and rote memorization. These learners settle into the habit of not learning, resisting learning, or feeling disengaged from the instructor and the learning experience. Students may feel isolated or unable to accomplish phases of any instruction because of prior failures earlier in their education. Other students have learned that the educator has no real effect on them; they learn in spite of the educator—a sad testimonial to their prior failed learning experiences.

The following sections discuss some ways to energize the brain and provide neural sponges for learning to occur.

Power Up the Brain

Pair and Share. Have students get on their feet and search for a partner across the room so they must move from their seat. (A pair of two is best; three people per group is the maximum.) Ask students a question and give them 30 to 60 seconds to come up with an answer, then ask a few of the groups to respond.

Ball Toss. This activity can be done indoors or outdoors. Have students stand and form a circle. Tell them that the one who has the ball is the only one who can speak. Toss the ball and ask a question. Give the students 5 seconds to respond or they must toss the ball back. This back-and-forth will allow the rest of the students to think of the answer, while waiting for the student with the ball to answer (keeps others thinking). This makes learning fun and engages all students.

Boosting Attention, Motivation, and Retention

Cooperative Learning

When students work cooperatively in a team atmosphere, they begin building confidence to foster success (**FIGURE 3.7**). **Cooperative learning** stresses teamwork, because the group only succeeds when everyone reaches the finish line.[22] Creating a brain-based learning environment is to first help students become

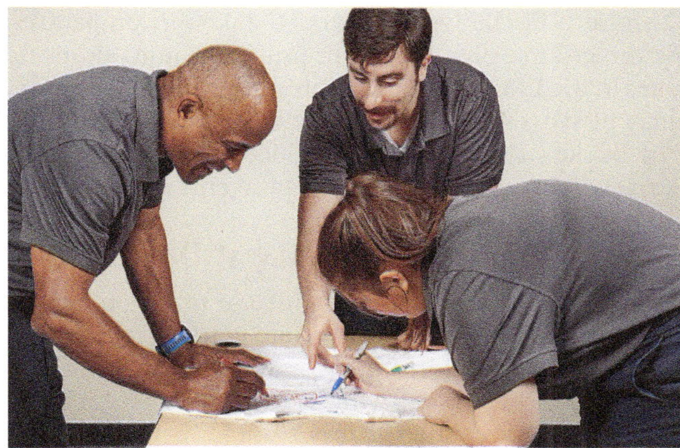

FIGURE 3.7 Cooperative learning (learning in a team setting) allows students the opportunity to develop social skills.

more confident by tapping into their interpersonal (working well with others) and intrapersonal (working well with self) domains. In the public safety and allied health classroom, the educator must stress teamwork by giving students the chance to lead, make mistakes, and refine skills in a safe setting. Students then work with each other to find common ground and create solutions through *negotiating techniques* to, as Stephen Covey noted, create a win-win scenario where everyone feels valued.[21] As students master the first two steps, they can then begin to make *personal connections* with others and respect ideas and cultural points of view that are different from their own. With each step, they become closer to understanding their own emotional intelligence (controlling personal demons), which allows them to become more socially intelligent, interacting with others more effectively. The brain is social; these strategies help foster natural leaders who are sensitive and articulate in moving others down the right path. One must be careful to not create "social chameleons"—students who attempt to do and say what others want to make a good impression.[23] These students may not stand up to the test of integrity nor develop the social skill patterns that are essential for true committed leaders. The goal of educators is to make students socially competent so that they can truly deliver great patient care.

The more we understand the brain, the more we can teach to this critical organ. To understand another, we must first begin by understanding ourselves. This may be the hardest part of teaching for educators to master—the art of reflection. Through reflection an educator can remediate their weaknesses and build on their strengths. It is only when educators can take an honest look at themselves that they can turn to students and begin to help them meet their educational and life goals.

Motivational Activities: Increasing Participation

Classroom Energizer: See It Another Way

Try to get students to think outside of the box with a strategy that gets students to think another way. The activity takes something that public safety knows and has done for years and asks that students develop another way to solve the problem. It is amazing what students can do when given the freedom to be creative and to critically think to see something another way.

Classroom Energizer: Let the Dead Speak

Have students watch a segment of shows in class, such as *Dr. G Medical Examiner*, *Forensics*, *Stories of Emergency Room*, etc. Then have them stand up and share their detailed notes with their squad. This allows those who take better notes to help those who are learning to distinguish what to write down versus what may not be as important. After 5 minutes of sharing, have them sit down and give them a 10-question test. This allows them to test their active listening skills, improve their note taking, and improve their patient assessment with actual patient care situations.

Classroom Energizer: Carousel around the Room

Orchestrating the classroom and lab the same way can reduce learning and become routine for instructors and students alike. Humans are creatures of habit—they often sit in the same chair or row, drive the same route to work, etc. Instead, have students move as a squad to a different area of the classroom each time they come to class. This simple method can improve attention, energize students, and break the monotony that may hinder learning.

Classroom Energizer: Attitude Determines Altitude in Life

Students need to be encouraged to giving each other "love" by clapping every time another student presents or participates in a positive manner. It is critical to release dopamine, vasopressin, serotonin, and the mood elevators that come with positive reinforcement. Building a collaborative culture and a safe, encouraging environment can reap huge benefits in retention and student graduation numbers.

Classroom Energizer: Medical Mind Mapping

Several strategies integrate previous knowledge with new knowledge. Interactive mind mapping is one way to accomplish this for students. Draw any shape on the board and write a disease or injury, then draw lines and bubbles extending from this center. Have students come to the board to write signs, symptoms, or any important information that is commonly seen (**FIGURE 3.8**). Have another layer of bubbles where students can write in special considerations. This activity is energizing, thought provoking, and relevant for all learning preferences.

Classroom Energizer: Flexible Focus

To create a higher learning opportunity to focus the brain, have students role-play or debate a medical issue they may encounter. An example might be the right to die (assisted suicide). For this example, the instructor could poll the class regarding who agrees and who disagrees. The instructor can then have the students with the same perspective gather in one area. Once they are in this group, give them 5 minutes to discuss how they are going to defend their issue but with one change: They must defend the opposite view. This will allow students to have a different perspective, encouraging a flexible focus.

Classroom Energizer: Dump the Bucket

Have students write down on a 3 × 5 card something they do not like about the profession or the classroom environment. Have students turn in these ideas every 2 weeks. This allows instructors to take the temperature of the group, solve classroom problems, and address issues in the EMS profession. Some of the topics addressed may be woven into lecture. See what can be dumped in the bucket, changed, and modified. This strategy gives students the idea that they can be agents of change.

Classroom Energizer: Take It Outside

It is critical to take students outside to do an activity each day. Students will appreciate getting fresh air and sunshine as they form a circle and pass the ball back and forth. The student who catches the ball must answer a question, then throw the ball back to the instructor. This is a great energizer for a brain that is built for survival rather than formal education.

Classroom Energizer: The 5-Minute Teacher

In this activity, students are assigned roles as teachers in teams of two and must deliver a 5-minute review on certain subject matter in each and every class session (**FIGURE 3.9**). For example, students are assigned the role of skills reviewer, acronym reviewer (three each class session), pharmacology reviewer (two medications each class session), patient assessment card reviewer (medical and trauma), etc. Educators can use this activity to get students active in helping keep each other current on important information.

Classroom Energizer: Mozart Effect

It has long been thought that classical music increases blood flow to the brain, leading to a higher level of

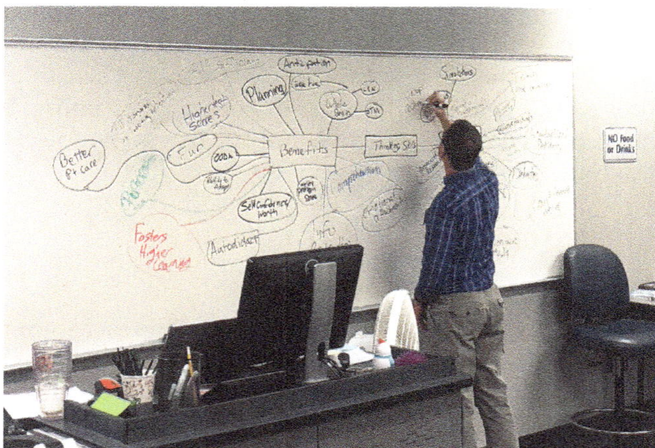

FIGURE 3.8 In a medical mind mapping activity, students reinforce their knowledge of diseases and injuries in an interactive format.

Courtesy of the National Association of EMS Educators.

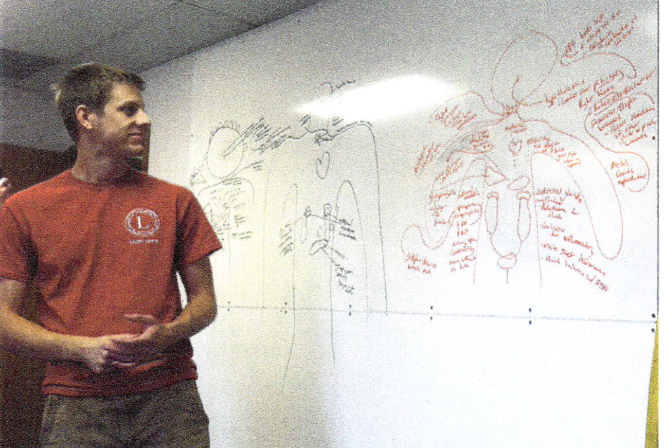

FIGURE 3.9 Having students present to the class allows them to be actively involved in their education and engages the brain.

Courtesy of St. Charles County Ambulance District.

learning and thinking. Researchers have identified that human brains are built to respond to music in powerful and productive ways.[24] Armed with this powerful tool, music gives educators an advantage to engage emotions and increase energy in the classroom. Try playing music (in a variety of genres) during breaks or when students are engaged in group activities to see how the energy in the classroom is transformed.

Passion

The instructor's passion creates an increased awareness and piques the interest of students with learned helplessness. Educators must be passionate about teaching to reach all of their students.

Learned Helplessness: Combating an Unhealthy Brain

How many educators have heard students say, "I am not a good test taker," "I am not a leader," "I cannot do this," or other negative phrases? These statements limit the brain's success. Even if these thoughts are not stated aloud, they may be reflected by a lack of student participation. These are signs of a condition called **learned helplessness**, which causes the brain to make unhealthy choices. It is the educator's job to nurture an unhealthy brain back to health. The number of students who have learned helplessness may surprise even a seasoned educator.

Eric Jensen states, "There are varying levels of learned helplessness . . . about two-thirds of students are likely candidates."[2] Learned helplessness physically changes the brain. The amount of norepinephrine, **gamma-aminobutyric acid (GABA)**, serotonin, and dopamine are decreased, while activation of the amygdala and the amount of the hormone cortisol are increased. These lower levels of biological markers do not cause learned helplessness; rather, it is the reverse: learned helplessness causes the lower levels of biological markers. As educators work to correct learned helplessness, these levels can return to normal and create a healthy brain.

All educators must work to instill confidence and build students into leaders so they can work with others to create successful patient outcomes. Many students have a burning desire to make a difference, but lack the confidence to see themselves achieving their goals. Jocko Willink and Leif Babin (two retired U.S. Team 6 Navy Seals) wrote about this in their 2015 book titled *Extreme Ownership*.[25] During training that involved racing large rubber boats, the Seals found that when they put the physically smaller recruits into a boat with a painted Smurf on the bow (this marking indicating that they could not or may not meet the standard), the men in that particular boat—class after class—worked to ensure that they would step from the shadow of uncertainty and into the light of success. Instead of setting an expectation of failure, they chose to work together as a team and became the number one boat in the class.

To begin the process of making an unhealthy brain into a healthy brain, one must realize that it will test the instructor's patience. The first step is to make these students stakeholders in the learning process and not tourists in the classroom. Integrating students into teams and giving them jobs provides the learner with a peer support system that improves their confidence, and this confidence allows them to have greater control in their learning.[26] Teamwork takes the student from passivity to activity in the classroom and begins to rewire the brain with a more can-do attitude.

Keep the classroom positive by encouraging and mentoring student success by believing in what is being taught. The seller must convince the buyer that the deal is good; similarly, educators must believe in what they are promoting. Learned optimism starts with an enthusiastic approach to learning. If the instructor is excited about the topic, students cannot help but be intrigued with the possibility of what they will learn.[27] It is important that educators maintain a positive and supportive environment that is devoid of false praise—make it genuine. Educators who fake praise or give too many external rewards can make a learned helpless brain become negatively dependent.[28]

Have students take an active role in and outside of the classroom. Nothing can refocus a brain better than socializing it to believe it can make a difference. Students can participate in decision making in the classroom, participate in projects for local fire and

Praise Reports

In a praise report, squad leaders have members of their squad stand up while they recognize each other for doing well. A squad member reads narrative reports from their clinical or field assignments or verbalizes how a student helped someone in the class. Give recognition by clapping to let them know they matter to the program, to the class, and to the profession.

Belonging

Foster a sense of belonging via activities such as community service events or projects that improve the profession or the classroom. Involve students in presenting their program and profession at community events. Ownership not only fosters pride but also activates the brain in a positive way. Even wearing a uniform and belonging to a squad can create relevance to the student and a feeling of belonging.

EMS departments, attend local or state meetings, or engage in research projects. Involvement in meaningful experiences in any area of the EMS profession can lead to retooling a brain in a positive and productive manner.

The brain is a challenging frontier. Each day, researchers learn more about how the brain works and, therefore, how educators can be more effective. It is important that students make decisions in the classroom: Indecision is a decision to be indecisive. Educators now know that the **whole brain** must be used. In fact, a new term called **relative lateralization** has been coined. Relative lateralization refers to using both sides of the brain.[29] Educators must take these concepts into account and develop new strategies to combat the disruptive effects of a disengaged brain. In the end, it takes a little effort, a lot of patience, and a commitment to creating an active and engaging classroom to get brains out of intensive care and rehabilitate them back into the wonderous world of learning.

Types of Intelligence

It has long been believed that intelligence centers around just a few variables. In ancient Greece, Plato argued that he was intelligent because he knew the limitations of his own ignorance. Aristotle, a student of Plato, claimed that humans were capable of quickly understanding situations and then could make a good moral choice—this was wisdom. Being familiar with the newer concepts of multiple intelligences, emotional intelligence, and social intelligence helps an educator set up students and the classroom for success.

Multiple Intelligences

Howard Gardner, a professor at Harvard University, was the first to add an "s" to intelligence. He believes that intelligence has been too narrowly defined and that educators only test and acknowledge particular aspects of intelligence. Dr. Gardner argues that there are **multiple intelligences**, and that existing definitions of intelligence leave out the majority of intelligent people by failing to see diverse types of intelligence and the implications of these types of intelligences.[30] To date, Gardner has outlined eight intelligences that redefine and challenge past assumptions about what is and who is intelligent (**TABLE 3.2**).[30]

TABLE 3.2 Eight Intelligences

Type of Intelligence	Description
Intrapersonal intelligence	Knowing oneself, feeling confident and comfortable in one's own shell. Having self-control, setting goals, having peace with self, and working to get the most out of life. Knowing oneself—emotional intelligence.
Interpersonal intelligence	Responding to those around oneself by identifying solutions, needs, and emotions to overcome problems. Working and playing well with others—social intelligence.
Verbal-linguistic intelligence	Writing and speaking effectively. This intelligence is tested and scored for entrance to professions and college.
Logical-mathematical intelligence	Working effectively with numbers, effectively using deductive and inductive reasoning, forming and testing hypotheses. Used in testing for entrance to professions and colleges.
Musical intelligence	Composing, analyzing, playing, and creating music.
Spatial intelligence	Seeing the big picture, having the mental imaging capability to remember details and directions, and having space recognition.
Body-kinesthetic intelligence	Controlling body movements, having flexibility, having hand–eye coordination.
Naturalistic intelligence	Survivalists, having knowledge or instincts about living things such as plants or animals, being attuned to nature.

Modified from Gardner, Howard. 1999. *Intelligence Reframed: Multiple Intelligence for the 21st Century*. New York: Basic Books.

If educators look beyond the old definition of intelligence and see students from a different perspective, they can teach to each student's unique intelligences and be more successful. Educators must break the outdated paradigm that only 10% of students are gifted. The truth is that over 90% of students may be gifted. It is up to educators to identify ways to reach them. Many educators have failed to teach to the students' intelligences and have done a disservice to so many who would have made great practitioners had their education not been based on a flawed, antiquated system. It is time to broaden the educational horizons and speak the "love language" of students, rather than continue to teach as originally taught. Theories give pause to see if it is possible to improve how education is delivered. It is through this improved practice that students will succeed because of educators, not in spite of educators.

Emotional Intelligence

Emotional intelligence centers around a self-awareness that starts with understanding one's own emotions and how these can affect student behavior either positively or negatively. The better educators understand emotions, the better students are able to read the emotions of others accurately.[23] The critical element in understanding emotions is the strength of an individual's empathy. Empathy builds self-awareness and connects people with others. Many students lack an understanding of themselves and, sadly, this transfers to those inside and outside of their social circle. It is important that educators strive to achieve the following:

- Connect with themselves (setting the tone/example)
- Create opportunities to practice empathy (community service)
- Grade student progress (behavioral evaluation)
- Encourage students when they demonstrate an awareness and empathy for others (praise reports)

Educators must teach the art of treating the entire illness—the body and the soul. When educators teach students to concentrate on the emotions of the patient, they will see something remarkable—the patient has greater trust and hope. Attitude and the affective domain matter and can make all the difference. Teaching students how to talk to patients, actively listen to them, and touch them in appropriate ways can lead to improved outcomes for patients. When healthcare professionals practice emotional intelligence, they engage their personality, smile more, and share more of themselves. As students begin the process of coming to terms with their emotions, educators can see it play out as they interact with others, showing their social intelligence.

Social Intelligence

Social intelligence is defined by Dr. Daniel Goleman in his book, *Social Intelligence,* as the ability to sense another's feelings (empathy) and thoughts (attunement) and interpret them correctly (social cognition).[23] Goleman went one step further by saying it is not enough to know how to read others; one must engage in smooth social interaction (synchrony). The key is to present oneself effectively in social situations (self-presentation), shape these outcomes (influence), care about others (concern), and act to meet others' needs.[23] Social intelligence is a skill to ensure that people can connect and cohesively "play in the sandbox together," so to speak. This is an essential intelligence for all healthcare professionals who must face difficult situations on a daily basis. Social intelligence does not happen on its own—it must be nurtured in and out of the classroom. There are many ways to teach and, most importantly, model this important intelligence, and it begins with a drive to be better people and better professionals.

Harvard University's Jerome Kagan is quoted as saying, "Although humans inherit a biological bias that permits them to feel anger, jealousy, selfishness and envy and to be rude, aggressive and violent . . . they inherit an even stronger biological bias for kindness, compassion, cooperation, love and nurture—especially toward those in need."[23] EMS students see the best of the human experience, but too often they also see the worst of human experience. Without education and strategies to cope, they may become cynical, angry, distanced from their compassion, and distant or callous to patients, family, and friends. With the public safety suicide rate climbing,[31] what are educators and the profession doing to arm students before they begin their work in the streets? Is it not the educator's responsibility to provide clinical experiences that deal with death and dying, like hospice? Should there not be clinical experiences where, for example, students see poverty up close and witness the struggle of fellow Americans in a close and personal way?

Community service is an instructional methodology that integrates community with academic instruction. It is an essential part of a student's education to see the human condition up close, and teach students how they can make a difference—not only in the medicine they will give, but by listening to patients, showing empathy, and appropriately touching patients in healing ways (**FIGURE 3.10**). Touch can have an incredible positive effect for the patient and the provider.

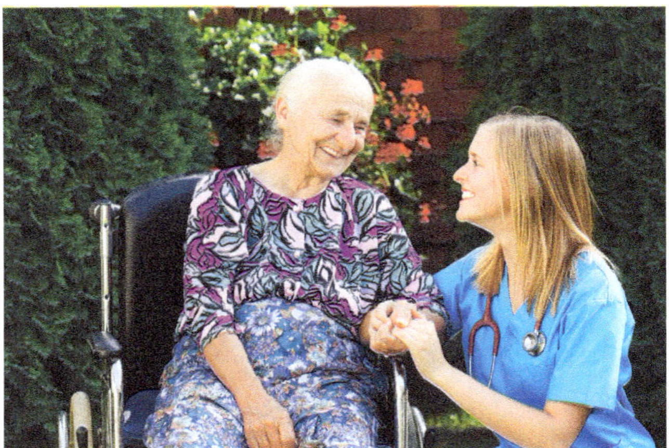

FIGURE 3.10 As part of their EMS training, students should be taught appropriate types of touch that can be used to enhance patient healing.

Building Social Intelligence through Community Service

Educators must get a sneak peek into student attitudes, problem-solving abilities, and temperament *before* students join the workforce. Researchers now state: "Personality tests are better predictors of future career success than letters of recommendation, interviews, and educational credentials."[22] Educators are pretty good at assessing the cognitive domain (thinking) and the psychomotor domain (hands on), but many have not explored the most powerful domain for learning and retention: the affective domain. The affective domain is the least understood and yet is the most powerful educational tool that many educators fail to measure. So, how can educators improve a student's personality, values, and heart? Shaping and measuring the affective domain through community service—sometimes referred to as service learning—give both the educator and student insight into what the future will bring (**TABLE 3.3**).

Community service allows students to think at a higher level, reflect on their core values, and engage themselves and their peers in civic responsibility. Such service creates opportunities for the students to participate in effective and authentic education. Educators must see their role as not just providing facts and figures, but helping to shape the core, providing experiences that allow students to compare and challenge their values with those of others. This is a small part of what community service offers—a chance to give students real-life experience while connecting with the community.

There are three areas that benefit from student engagement in community service: the students, the teaching institution, and the community as a whole.

The benefit to students beyond enhanced critical thinking skills lies in the fact that they are given an opportunity for personal growth, improved self-esteem, personal satisfaction, a sense of community, and a better grasp of the problems and concerns of the people that they hope to serve.

The educational institution benefits through delivering students who are more prepared to meet the challenges of a stressful profession. An institution that offers community service opportunities has a stronger motivational and inspirational base, enhanced learning opportunities, concentration on human needs, and a lower attrition rate due to an increased student satisfaction.

TABLE 3.3 Implementing Community Service in an EMS Education Program

1. Brainstorm community service events.	Examples of events that fulfill community needs include a toy drive, a Dr. Seuss reading program, Habitat for Humanity, Ronald McDonald House, first aid stations, assisted living residences, etc.
2. Treat community service like any other clinical/field assignment.	Document it with clinical forms. Ask students what they learned and felt about their social interactions. Build the grade into the curriculum; if it is not graded, this signals to the student that it is not important.
3. Set rules.	The attributes of professional behavior should be evaluated at all times and include the following: courteous and respectful interaction, refusal of money or services, wearing full uniform at all events, and checking in and out with preceptors at the site.
4. Encourage community involvement.	Ask organizations of interest to sit on the EMS advisory board to help shape the professional future.
5. Team up with other schools or programs.	Doing so increases cooperation and effectiveness. Show students the power of working together, and involve them in powerful and productive ways.

The community benefits from an improved relationship with and increased involvement with the teaching institution, increased community support and commitment, and a chance to preview students before they join the public safety professional workforce.

The truest form of success for an educator is what the student takes away when their time in class is done. The most powerful student experience is the opportunity to find themselves, reflect on their values, shape their passion, and be challenged to care more for others than themselves. Community service can help educators take a giant step forward in creating competent and compassionate healthcare professionals.

Summary

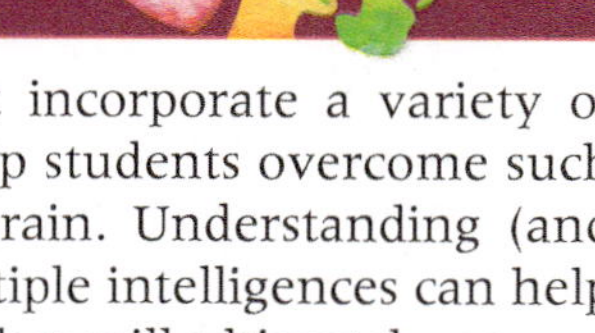

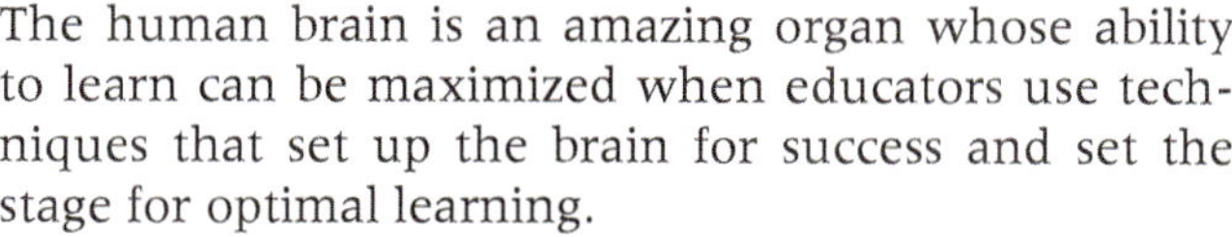

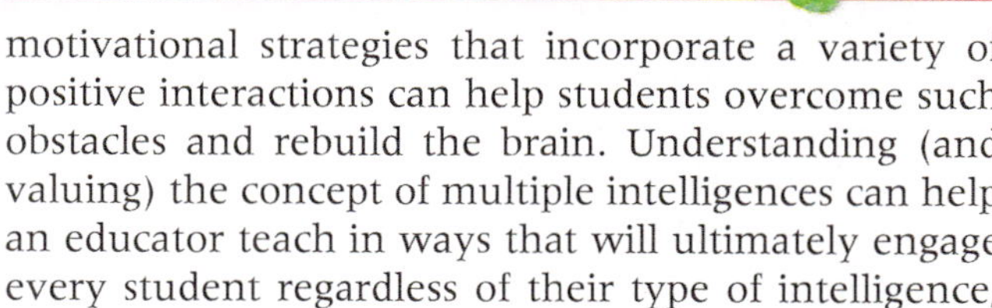

The human brain is an amazing organ whose ability to learn can be maximized when educators use techniques that set up the brain for success and set the stage for optimal learning.

Educators must effectively integrate a variety of tactics to energize the brain and engage students. Strategies range from group work, to getting students out of their seats and physically moving, to assigning students to speak in front of the class, to using music or television while students arrive. Providing a variety of formats and activities helps students build bonds with each other and support each other along their education and career paths. It is important to train and test students to perform skills exactly the way they are performed in the field so that upon graduation, they are best prepared. It is also important to get students out of the classroom to practice in a real-world environment.

Students may face challenges such as limited bandwidth and lack of confidence. Educators who use motivational strategies that incorporate a variety of positive interactions can help students overcome such obstacles and rebuild the brain. Understanding (and valuing) the concept of multiple intelligences can help an educator teach in ways that will ultimately engage every student regardless of their type of intelligence, thereby bringing out the best in each student.

Educators must also teach to the affective domain by planning and developing activities that give students the opportunity to develop and by grading students on this domain to stress its importance. Involving students in community service events is an effective way to provide this experience, if it is taken seriously through structure, documentation, and grading.

Last but not least, educators must put their egos aside, slow down, and allow themselves to recharge so they can best serve their students.

Glossary

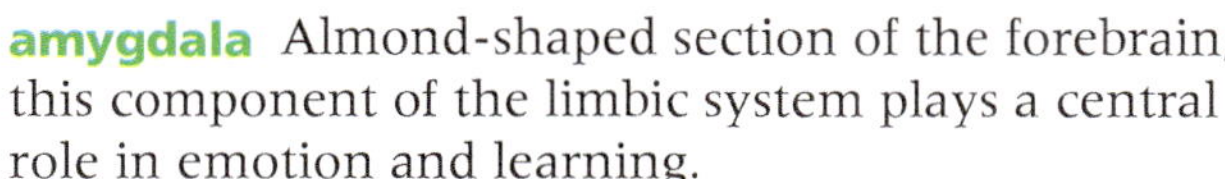

amygdala Almond-shaped section of the forebrain; this component of the limbic system plays a central role in emotion and learning.

axon Electrically sensitive fiber of a neuron responsible for the transmission of information away from the nerve cell.

bandwidth In the context of brain-based learning, refers to the available space in the brain for learning.

brain-derived neurotrophic factor (BDNF) Natural substance released by the brain to improve cognition (thinking) and boost how neurons talk with one another.

central sulcus The longitudinal fissure in the brain that lies on the outside edge of the hemisphere.

cerebellum Region of the brain that is most responsible for producing smooth, coordinated muscle movements.

cerebral cortex Outermost layer of the brain, responsible for creativity, planning, language, and perception.

cooperative learning Type of learning in which students work together in a team atmosphere.

corpus callosum Thick band of nerve fibers that connect and allow for communication between the left and right hemispheres of the brain.

declarative memories Memories of which a person is consciously aware, and which are known to be true, can be seen, and can be measured as fact.

dendrites Branching fibers of axons that act as receptors of information; they receive messages from other neurons and deliver them to the main body of the nerve cell.

emotional intelligence Type of intelligence in which people is aware of and understands their own emotions.

gamma-aminobutyric acid (GABA) Most common inhibitory neurotransmitter; it quiets neurons and can exist in up to one-third of synapses.

glial cells Most abundant cell types in the central nervous system; they provide support for and insulation between the surrounding neurons.

hippocampus Area in the limbic system that moves learning from short-term memory into long-term memory.

homeostasis State of equilibrium referring to the body's ability to remain internally stable while external environments vary.

hypothalamus Area in the limbic system that maintains homeostasis by regulating temperature, sleep, and nutrient intake through internal monitoring; also plays a role in the immune system.

intentional thinking Process of actively deciding to think about a topic, being aware of one's own thoughts, and shaping thoughts in order to drive toward a specific result.

learned helplessness Self-concept that one is not good at something or is unable to achieve something.

longitudinal fissure The anatomical separation between the right and left hemispheres of the cerebrum.

medulla oblongata Spinal cord termination about 1 inch into the lower brain.

mirror neurons Neurons that fire when a person performs or thinks of a familiar action, or when seeing another performing that action.

multiple intelligences Concept that there is more than one type of intelligence.

neurogenesis Production of new neurons.

neurons Nerve cells; central nervous system cells that generate and transmit information from nerve impulses.

nondeclarative memories Memories of which one is not consciously aware, but which are used to perform motor skills.

pons Part of the brainstem that serves as a bridge between the medulla and the midbrain and aids the medulla in respiratory regulation.

prefrontal cortex Region of the brain located in the anterior frontal lobe that is responsible for reasoning, planning, judgment, empathy, abstract ideas, and conscience.

relative lateralization Using both sides of the brain.

reticular activating system (RAS) Area of the brainstem that is responsible for keeping the brain alert by heightening awareness to respond to stimuli related to the sympathetic nervous system's "fight or flight" response.

serotonin Inhibitory neurotransmitter that plays a role in sleep, mood regulation, memory, and learning.

social intelligence Type of intelligence in which a person has the ability to sense another person's feelings and thoughts, and interpret them correctly.

soma Cell body.

somatosensory cortex Area that receives the bulk of thalamocortical projections from the sensory input fields.

sylvian fissure Groove separating the parietal lobe of the brain from the temporal lobe.

thalamus Area in the limbic system that organizes cognitive activities, including memory.

whole brain Use of all areas of the brain to process and control all aspects of human interaction.

References

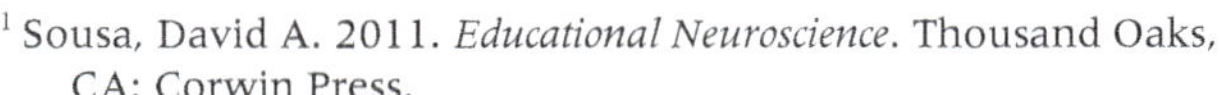
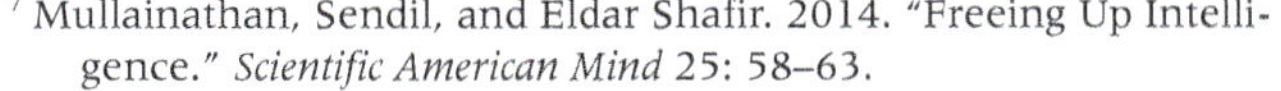

[1] Sousa, David A. 2011. *Educational Neuroscience*. Thousand Oaks, CA: Corwin Press.

[2] Jensen, Eric. 2008. *Brain Based Learning: The New Paradigm of Teaching*. Thousand Oaks, CA: Corwin Press.

[3] Chopra, Deepak, and Tanzi, Rudolph. 2012. *Super Brain*. New York: Harmony Books.

[4] Goleman, Daniel. 1995. *Emotional Intelligence: Why It Can Matter More than IQ*. New York: Bantam.

[5] Dosenbach, Nico U., Binyam Nardos, Alexander L. Cohen, Damien A. Fair, Jonathan D. Power, Jessica A. Church, Steven M. Nelson, et al. 2010. "Prediction of Individual Brain Maturity Using fMRI." *Science* 329: 1358–61. http://dx.doi.org/10.1126/science.1194144.

[6] Linde, Nancy. 2012. *399 Games, Puzzles & Trivia Challenges Specially Designed to Keep Your Brain Young*. New York: Workman Publishing.

[7] Mullainathan, Sendil, and Eldar Shafir. 2014. "Freeing Up Intelligence." *Scientific American Mind* 25: 58–63.

[8] Maxwell, John. 2003. *Thinking for a Change*. New York: Warner Business Books.

[9] Medina, John. 2008. *Brain Rules*. Seattle: Pear Press.

[10] Silva, Alcino J. 2017. "How One Memory Attaches to Another." *Scientific American*. 27, no. 3S.

[11] Gold, Sunny S. 2013. "How to Be a Better Boss." *Scientific American Mind* 24, no. 3: 18. http://dx.doi.org/10.1038/scientificamericanmind0713-18a.

[12] Rogers, S. 2013. "How the Science of Mindfulness Can Improve Attention and Lift Your Mood." *Scientific American Mind* 24, no. 1: 33.

[13] Grossman, Dave, and Christensen, Loren W. 2007. *On Combat: The Psychology and Physiology of Deadly Conflict in War and in Peace*, 2nd ed. Millestadt, IL: Warrior Science Publications.

[14] Vuontela, Virve, Pia Rama, Antti Raninen, Hannu Aronen, and Synnöve Carlson. 1999. "Selective Dissociation between Memory for Location and Color." *NeuroReport* 10: 2235–40.
[15] Walker, Morton. 1998. *The Power of Color.* Wazipur, Delhi: B. Jain Publishers.
[16] Ostrander, Sheila, and Lynn Schroeder. 1991. *Super-Memory: The Revolution.* New York: Carroll and Graf Publishers.
[17] Indoor Air Quality Scientific Findings Resource Bank. 2018. "Temperature and School Work Performance." Berkeley Lab/ LBNL Indoor Environmental Group website. Accessed December 7, 2018. https://iaqscience.lbl.gov/performance-temp-school.
[18] Ornstein, Robert E. 1991. *The Evolution of Consciousness: The Origins of the Way We Think.* New York: Simon & Shuster.
[19] Griesbach, Grace S., David A. Hovda, Raffaella Molteni, Aiguo Wu, and Fernando Gomez-Pinilla. 2004. "Voluntary Exercise Following Traumatic Brain Injury: Brain-Derived Neurotrophic Factor Upregulation and Recovery of Function." *Neuroscience* 125: 129–39. https://doi.org/10.1016/j.neuroscience.2004.01.030.
[20] Knecht, Stefan, Caterina Breitenstein, Stefan Bushuven, Stefanie Wailke, Sandra Kamping, Agnes Flöel, Pienie Zwitserlood, and E. Bernd Ringelstein. 2004. "Levodopa: Faster and Better Word Learning in Normal Humans." *Annals of Neurology* 56, no. 1: 20–6. https://doi.org/10.1002/ana.20125.
[21] Covey, Stephen R. 1989. *The 7 Habits of Highly Effective People.* New York: Simon & Shuster.
[22] Rogers, Carl R., and Jerome H. Freiberg. 1994. *Freedom to Learn*, 3rd ed. Upper Saddle River, NJ: Prentice Hall.
[23] Goleman, Daniel. 2006. *Social Intelligence: The New Science of Human Relationships.* New York: Bantam.
[24] Weinberger, Norman M. 2004. "Music and the Brain." *Scientific American* 291, no. 5: 88.
[25] Willink, Jocko, and Leif Babin. 2015. *Extreme Ownership: How US Navy Seals Lead and Win.* New York: St. Martins Press.
[26] Glasser, William. 1999. *Choice Theory: A New Psychology of Personal Freedom.* New York: Harper-Collins.
[27] Seligman, Martin E. P. 1998. *Learned Optimism: How to Change Your Mind and Your Life.* New York: Pocket Books.
[28] Kohn, Alfie F. 1993. *Punished by Rewards: The Trouble with Gold Stars, Incentive Plans, A's, Praise, and Other Bribes.* New York: Houghton Mifflin.
[29] Proverbio, Alice M., Valentina Brignome, Silvia Matarazzo, Marzia Del Zotto, and Alberto Zani. 2006. "Gender Differences in Hemispheric Asymmetry for Face Processing." *BMC Neuroscience* 7, no. 1: 44. https://doi.org/10.1186/1471-2202-7-44.
[30] Gardner, Howard. 1999. *Intelligence Reframed: Multiple Intelligence for the 21st Century.* New York: Basic Books.
[31] Vigil, Neil H., Andrew R. Grant, Octavio Perez, Robyn N. Blust, Vatsal Chikani, Tyler F. Vadeboncoeur, Daniel W. Spaite, and Bentley J. Bobrow. 2018. "Death by Suicide: The EMS Profession Compared to the General Public." *Prehospital Emergency Care* Sept: 1–6. https://doi.org/10.1080/10903127.2018.1514090.

Additional Resources

Buzan, Tony, and Barry Buzan. 1995. *The Mindmap Book*, 2nd ed. London: BBC Books.

Covey, Stephen R. 2004. *The 8th Habit: From Effectiveness to Greatness.* New York: Simon & Shuster.

Lavie, Nilli. 2005. "Distracted and Confused? Selective Attention Under Load." *Trends in Cognitive Sciences* 9, no. 2: 75–82. https://doi.org/10.1016/j.tics.2004.12.004.

Mani, Anandi, Sendhil Mullainathan, Eldar Shafir, and Jiaying Zhao. 2013. "Poverty Impedes Cognitive Function." *Science* 341, no. 6149: 976–80. http://dx.doi.org/10.1126/science.1238041.

National Aeronautics and Space Administration website. nasa.gov.

Sousa, David A. 2001. *How the Brain Learns*, 2nd ed. Thousand Oaks, CA: Corwin Press.

CHAPTER 4

Principles of Adult Learning

OBJECTIVES

At the conclusion of this chapter, the educator will be able to:

Cognitive Domain

1. Compare and contrast the adult learning theories of pedagogy and andragogy to understand how to best facilitate the learning process.
2. Identify characteristics that are unique to the adult learner that inspire creative development of learning opportunities.
3. Identify physiological variables in the learning environment that impact the learning process.
4. Identify psychosocial variables in the learning environment that impact the success of student outcomes.
5. Describe strategies that motivate students to learn that can be applied to the classroom, lab, clinical, and field experience environments.
6. Compare and contrast intrinsic and extrinsic motivational principles that contribute to student learning and professional growth.
7. Identify intrinsic and extrinsic barriers for adult learners that can inhibit positive outcomes.
8. Discuss the theory of margin in relationship to an adult learner's ability to balance personal and professional lives during the learning process.
9. Discuss the importance of the role of the educator as a facilitator during experiential learning activities.
10. Identify examples of applying the theory of context-based learning in the classroom and lab experiences.
11. Based on Maslow's hierarchy of needs, explain how intrinsic and extrinsic motivation can assist a student's professional growth.
12. Identify strategies that can minimize the effects of instructor-generated load to improve a student's motivation to learn.

Psychomotor Domain

There are no psychomotor objectives for this chapter.

Affective Domain

1. Value the understanding of adult learning theories by developing strategies to apply in classroom and lab activities to foster student success.

"To become an educator is to accept responsibility for the flame of the lamp of knowledge that was passed to you from teachers and mentors who lit your way and for you to carry forward, lighting the way for those in the future whose lives you will touch and change forever."

~ William Raynovich

CHAPTER GOAL This chapter presents the principles that form and underlie the sound practices of emergency medical services (EMS) education. These principles inform EMS educators about the best educational practices that ultimately result in the effective education of adult EMS learners.

The principles and modalities of adult education, including EMS education, are in an accelerating state of transition from traditional face-to-face lecturing and paper-based testing toward a variety of innovative modalities, such as flipped classroom models and computer, digitized, and Internet-based instruction, testing, and feedback.[1,2] The traditional fundamental principles of adult education, including those used commonly in EMS education, remain as sound and applicable as ever; however, the innovative modalities have been transformational and are expanding student access, affordability, flexibility, and personalization. Furthermore, in recent years a new trend toward expanded professional roles for EMS providers, with broader and more flexible scopes of practice, such as community paramedicine, mobile integrated health care, critical care, and aeromedical paramedicine, are becoming formally recognized with national and international registries, standardized curricula, accreditation, and certifications.[3,4] This chapter presents and updates long-standing traditional principles of adult education. It also presents an update on newly emerging principles and practices occurring in the domain of adult education and, in particular, EMS education.

Contemporary approaches to learning and classroom instruction are shown in **TABLE 4.1**. These are intended to serve as reference sources for this chapter and the remainder of the full text.

The learning styles, needs, responses, and expectations of adults differ from those of younger learners. Even when educators teach emergency medical responder (EMR) or emergency medical technician (EMT) courses to adolescents in high school, the instruction and learning that take place follow adult education principles more closely than the principles involved in teaching children. The skillful educator utilizes techniques that enhance student motivation, comprehension, and retention by incorporating the principles of adult learning.

Historical Foundations of Adult Education Principles

Several significant historical educators and events are universally recognized as making contributions to adult education. For example, Socrates (c. 470–399 BCE), the philosopher and teacher of Plato, is credited with being among the first to introduce critical thinking in teaching through reflection, systematic questioning, and examining evidence.[5] We should acknowledge Socrates, if for no other reason, for advising adult educators to "start where the students are."[6]

John Dewey was a pioneering polymath (an intellectual accomplished in multiple disciplines) and a leader in educational theory. He promoted pragmatism and reflective teaching and learning through applied experiences, doing, and interaction. These are touchstones of excellence in EMS education today.[7] According to Dewey, "If we teach today's students as we taught yesterday's, we rob them of tomorrow."[8]

One of the most influential adult educational theorists was Malcom Knowles. His contributions to the understanding of the differences between how adults and young people learn and retain information have had a profound impact on education over the past 60+ years.[9] An understanding of these differences helps educators design and present educational experiences effectively. A logical place to start such a discussion is with the concept introduced by Knowles in 1968 and which is now the most basic and universally recognized concept in adult education—*andragogy*. **Andragogy** is the art and science of teaching adults. Knowles used the term *andragogy* to differentiate the principles of adult learning from those centered on children, or **pedagogy**.[10]

Pedagogy versus Andragogy

Autonomy and Self-Direction

Adults expect and enjoy independence, or a degree of **autonomy**, in what they learn and how they learn it. They like to have control over their learning. Moreover, for adults, learning is a process of omnidirectional sharing with the instructor as well as with fellow students. While the adult learner may have a degree of discretion and self-determination in the learning process, the instructor is responsible for facilitating the learning processes, as

TABLE 4.1 Contemporary Approaches to Learning and Classroom Instruction

Approach	Brief Description	Sample Activities
Active learning	Instructor assigns challenging problems that require students to engage in activities that require exploration or discovery of fundamental elements of a problem or issue, analytic components, theoretical explanations, possible interventions or treatments, and higher-level explanations and remaining problems, or unknowns.	Students must address challenging ethical issues, such as caring empathetically for an intoxicated driver with minor injuries who, by running a stop sign, caused a motor vehicle incident that killed two schoolchildren, 6 and 8 years of age. The class is assigned to work in small groups to present a case analysis. The instructor hands out five complex, challenging clinical cases to the class, such as patients in extremis with ARDS, cardiac shock, and pulmonary embolism presenting with vague symptoms.
Student-centered learning	Instructional approach that promotes active learning, in which students are given responsibility, flexibility, and autonomy for mastery of competencies. This includes student choice in how, when, and why to study selected elements of the curriculum, making the student a stakeholder in the educational process and a shared experience.	Assignments may include group work, case studies, role-play, scenarios, writing assignments, games, and other activities that promote collaboration, communication, and problem solving.
Collaborative learning	Students are assigned to work in groups to solve problems or develop skill sets.	The instructor can create interactive classroom activities, such as debates or jigsaw or trivia games. Students can be assigned to work collaboratively on a community-based problem or a major paper, such as developing an MCI demonstration for a classroom or other community-based exposition.
Experiential learning	Students are engaged in realistic or actual learning experiences.	Clinical and field internships Patient care laboratories, such as cardiac codes, trauma labs, and medical lab sessions with manikins and model students Students learn to intubate on manikins and in the OR and ECU.
Problem-based learning	Instructors facilitate learning by having students tackle complex multifaceted problems in small groups while the instructor provides scaffolding, modeling experiences, and opportunities for self-directed learning.	Students handle a case in stages. First, they are dispatched to an MVC and discuss their preparation and "preflection" en route. When they arrive at the scene, they are presented with photographs of the incident scene. They discuss hazards, logistics, materials, and triage priorities. As they "approach" each patient, they are presented with preliminary "first look" findings, etc.

Abbreviations: ACLS, advanced cardiac life support; AMLS, advanced medical life support; ARDS, acute respiratory distress syndrome; BCLS, basic cardiac life support; ECU, emergency care unit; EVOC, emergency vehicle operator course; HIPAA, Health Insurance Portability and Accountability Act; MCI, mass-casualty incident; MVC, motor vehicle crash; OR, operating room; OSHA, Occupational Safety and Health Administration; TLS, trauma life support.

Modified from Slavich, George M., and Philip G. Zimbardo. 2012. "Transformational Teaching: Theoretical Underpinnings, Basic Principles, and Core Methods." *Educational Psychology Review* 24, no. 4: 569–608. https://doi.org/10.1007/s10648-012-9199-6.

opposed to simply providing knowledge points or facts to students. Brookfield suggests that direction and guidance from the educator are essential because many adults need help in determining their learning needs.[11]

Adults approach education with the expectation of learning new skills and knowledge, and they tend to stay focused on the final goal—successful completion of the program. Ultimately, they want to be well-prepared to practice competently and to pass state or national exams. In light of this, adults are less tolerant of wasted time and tasks that have no apparent value; they prefer to gain a return on the investment of their time and energy. In fact, educators should expect more criticism from the adult learner than from the younger learner, especially when students feel that their expectations are not being met.

Omnidirectional Learning

In the context of education, **omnidirectional learning** is based on an open dialogue in the educational environment, where the instructor serves as facilitator rather than as an expert who imparts knowledge. In an omnidirectional sharing environment, the instructor engages all students in discussions, encouraging and requiring them to contribute substantively. Responses are not just to the instructor (bidirectionally), but to everyone in the educational setting, or omnidirectionally. The role of the omnidirectional instructor is critical in that the dialogue must be carefully guided, with the goal of promoting constructive dialogue that stays topically relevant and meaningful rather than devolving into off-track casual chat sessions or worse, hostile debates.

Life Experience

By the time a person reaches adulthood, they have accumulated many life experiences. The adult learner has the advantage of being able to relate new facts and concepts to real-life experiences; this enhances and reinforces the adult learning experience. Adult EMS classes typically include students with wide-ranging levels of expertise and educational backgrounds. This means the instructor can draw upon the students' experiences and incorporate them into the instruction. In this adult learning model, all members of the class share information and experiences with one another. In fact, in some areas of the curriculum, students may have more information and experience than the instructor does. With this in mind, the educator should strive to ensure that class communication is multidirectional and is more a dialogue than a lecture.

TEACHING TIP

The degree to which a professional is recognized for having a rich depth of knowledge and understanding, and the ability to apply those professional skills, is that professional's level of expertise.

Expertise involves "seeing the invisible." Novices can see only the obvious—that which is present and occurring. Experts see what is missing and what isn't happening.[12]

Level of Experience

Experienced EMS educators appreciate that students will have widely varying background experiences and learning potentials. The range of experience about the EMS profession will typically range from rank novices who have no first-hand understanding about the profession to highly experienced and clinically advanced students, such as emergency nurses, respiratory therapists, and even emergency physicians and trauma surgeons. It is a challenge for an instructor to teach a class where one or more highly experienced clinicians are mixed with a group of students who have no EMS experience and may never have taken care of a patient. With such a wide range of backgrounds and experiences, the key is to strive to respect the motivations, backgrounds, knowledge, and skill sets of all students, value the experiences that each brings to the educational setting, and maintain an engaging pace and depth of instruction that is relevant and meaningful to the full class.

TABLE 4.2 describes novice, advanced beginner, competent practitioner, proficient, and expert learning levels. Regardless of the level of EMS experience among the students, teaching to a higher degree of performance is rewarding for both the students and the instructor, and it is, to a degree, achievable. The principle is to set the bar just beyond the students' grasp and encourage them to strive for excellence and a higher degree of professionalism. With experience, the educator develops the capacity to visualize how complex, challenging clinical situations develop and how to project, or anticipate, further developments and outcomes.

Problem-Centered Orientation

Adults are "relevancy oriented," which means they need to know *why* they are being told to learn something before they are receptive to learning it. Therefore, educators must ensure that instruction is

TABLE 4.2 Levels of Expertise

Level	Description
Novice	Initial learning is about recognition of elements or facts (situations, tools, and environmental factors) and appropriate or required individual operational tasks (or steps), and satisfactory or deficient outcomes.
Advanced beginner	Operational performance is based on repeated operational experience with an understanding of how the elements, or steps in processes, function to reach a desired outcome. While able to perform a set of tasks, or steps, according to a well-defined procedural outline, or algorithm, expert guidance is required to deviate from the standardized learned steps.
Competent practitioner	Action plans and procedures are routinely developed and executed and may be modified accordingly, as needed. However, the speed and flexibility that comes with mastery have not yet been developed.
Proficient	Situations are perceived in their entirety, rather than as distinct components, or events. Action plans are not plotted out in steps, but are viewed as a complex of integrated actions to be executed. Exceptional situations that require alternative actions or solutions are perceived and appropriate modifications to operational plans can be executed smoothly.
Expert	Situations are perceived free of rules (guidelines, maxims, algorithms, and operational plans). Experts intuitively grasp the full situation and zero in on required actions, without wasting time and energy on unnecessary or nonessential considerations or processes. Performance is fluid, flexible, and efficient.

Modified from Benner, Patricia. 1984. *From Novice to Expert: Excellence and Power in Clinical Nursing Practice*. Menlo Park, CA: Addison-Wesley.

The Progression from Novice Learner to Expert

Glaser described the progression from novice learner to expert as follows:[13]

- Novices advance from awkward and inconsistent performances to smoother, more balanced, consistent performances.
- Specific individual actions, or steps of processes, become smoother and integrated into overall operational processes, or strategies.
- Perceptions shift from being isolated actions focused on specific tasks and events, to becoming comprehensive visualizations and contextual parts of complex events.
- Self-reliance develops, along with the capacity to form effective alternate strategies, or solutions, as needed.

Expert perceptions of tasks and situations yield the visualization of problems and solutions that those less experienced cannot see.[13] Experts also perceive fine distinctions. They are able to apply higher-order rules, such as integrating and truncating complex processes that those with less experience may not yet be able to apply. An example would be a response to a mass-casualty incident in which numerous patients have been injured where immediate lifesaving interventions and rapid triage and transportation are critical. An expert may be overwhelmed yet still able to act decisively and effectively, whereas a novice may simply be overwhelmed and tend to focus on a single patient or challenge.

Finally, regarding teaching and expertise, according to Glaser, attempting to teach students to "think like an expert" has not been shown to be effective, although one of the most effective teaching modalities has been high-fidelity simulation.

The progression from novice to expert is incremental and requires extensive experience. Instructors must recognize that this is difficult to obtain within the time constraints of most EMS educational settings. It is also difficult for many instructors who have reached the stage of expertise to clearly remember the steps it took to get there.

problem-centered, rather than subject-centered. For example, paramedic students may not value instruction in the fundamentals of human anatomy and physiology until that depth of knowledge becomes relevant to specific medical conditions and how they are encountered and treated in the field. This challenge becomes more complex when the EMS educator seeks to give relevant instruction on higher-level basic science topics, such as biochemical ion gate electrophysiology or acid–base values interpretation. Future providers often lack a strong educational background in such fields. There are several ways for instructors to motivate those students, however, including the following:

- Demonstrate to students that the ion gate electrophysiology has parallels to the cardiovascular and nervous systems, so that once the fundamental principles of electrophysiology are understood, the students can then understand the assessment of the patient as well as interactions between medications the patient is taking and those being administered.
- Inform students that, in the future, they will be performing many biomedical tests in the field, as well as providing interfacility transports in which they will work with hospital patient care records containing lab results and that, by understanding those results, their patient care will be significantly enhanced, contributing to their professional competence.

Goal Orientation

Adults are pragmatic by nature. In other words, they want to be able to apply the information they learn immediately, or at least have some understanding of how their learning will be of direct benefit to them. Adults generally do not tolerate studying anything that they cannot apply to tasks they expect to perform. Moreover, adults appreciate an educational program that is organized with clearly defined course components designed to help them to achieve their goals.

Although Knowles himself,[10] along with others,[11,14–16] have at times questioned the validity of the differences between andragogy and pedagogy, the previously mentioned attributes of learners throughout the stages of their development may aid the educator in developing teaching techniques. Ultimately, the transition from childhood to adult varies from individual to individual, and there is no discrete point that suddenly occurs at a particular age.

Other Characteristics of Adult Learners

Adult learners typically display characteristics that can be divided into two broad categories: physiological and psychosocial. Although adults are much more diverse than children physiologically, sociologically, and psychologically, general characteristics and central tendencies are presented here; the educator must bear in mind, however, that individuals vary broadly.

Physiological Variables

Physiological variables in adult learners specifically relate to how changes in vision, hearing, energy levels, and overall health affect learning. These variables involve the natural process of aging and maturation.

Distractions

For nearly all younger generation students, smartphones, laptop computers, and tablet devices are a way of life. What may be completely ordinary behavior to younger students, who routinely check updates on social media and the latest news on their devices, may be intolerable distractions to some older instructors and other learners sitting in the same class. The educator may attempt to ban electronic devices in the classroom, but that will be a futile battle in most settings and often will only result in tension. An effective alternative is for the educator to skillfully integrate interactive technology, such as Web-based response systems or social media, into the learning environment (**FIGURE 4.1**) in the form of "backchannel" communications (see the box *Backchannel Communications*). Other learning distractions include televisions, background office and emergency radio chatter, and emergency apparatus entering and exiting the station. The educator must be aware of these environmental distractions and must work to minimize them as much as possible.

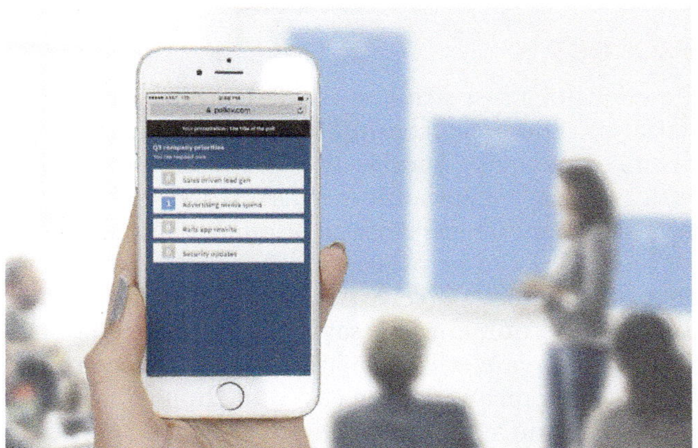

FIGURE 4.1 Web-based response systems, social media, and other technology can be used to enhance class activities.

Courtesy of Poll Everywhere.

Backchannel Communications

Backchannel communications involve utilizing classroom "polling" platforms (or clickers) and links or other ways to survey student feedback and attitudes as the class is progressing. In this way, the students may engage their electronic communication devices actively in providing input and feedback into the learning process. For example, "Was that a cardiac tamponade or a pulmonary embolus? Vote now!" "Which medication would you administer? What dosage? Ah, I see that 80% of the class knew this answer right off! Excellent. Let's consider possible alternatives."

Psychosocial Variables

The psychosocial differences of adult learners include the differences in adult versus child learning behaviors. For instance, adult learners may vary in their established attitudes, beliefs, and values, and they may be more rigid in their thinking than younger learners. Through years of living, adults have acquired set patterns of behaviors, along with set ideas and beliefs about right and wrong, and fact and fiction. These patterns may need to be "unset" or challenged for learning to take place. New ideas and ways of doing things cannot be forced on adult learners; they must be soundly demonstrated through logic and good evidence. Adult learners must understand and believe the new knowledge or technique before they will be willing to abandon their beliefs or past practices.

Success

The educator must strive to create learning situations that afford the greatest potential for learning success; this includes taking special care not to embarrass the adult learner. When adult learners are placed on the defensive, they are less likely to be open to learning and are more likely to be protective of their thoughts and feelings; they may perceive the classroom as an unsafe learning environment. The saying "praise in public and criticize in private" clearly applies to the adult learner. This does not mean that the educator should structure all learning and assessment activities so all learners can succeed on early attempts. "Failures" in a safe learning environment can be a healthy, meaningful experience when effective coaching and feedback are provided in a collegial setting. Students must accept that not every clinical call will go well. They must learn to objectively reflect on their performance to determine how it can be improved in the future.

Respect

Returning to school is often a momentous decision for an adult learner, and it often represents a considerable investment of time, energy, and money. Having made the important and commendable decision to return to school, the adult learner expects, and deserves, to be treated with respect. The resourceful educator draws upon the wealth of knowledge and experiences of the adult learners to enrich the level of instruction and overall eagerness for learning; this benefits all students in the class. It is the instructor's responsibility to model respect toward every student and to instill an environment of mutual respect among all class members.

Critical Thinking Skills

Adults learn best by adding new information to an already existing framework, and they have greater difficulty remembering isolated facts, especially those thought to be irrelevant, or trivial. The educator must seek the most effective approach to developing and presenting course material. Knowing the educational and professional backgrounds of students is important in making these determinations. With this knowledge, the educator can add new information to the students' existing frameworks, or expertise.

TEACHING TIP

The educator should get to know the students' backgrounds, so they can better integrate new ideas with those ideas students already know. Linking new information to old is a particularly effective way to aid information retention in the adult learner.

Practical Limitations and Considerations

The adult learner has competing responsibilities, and the EMS instructor who does not consider these factors risks losing good students. These limitations and considerations may involve scheduling challenges, scarce time, financial stresses, conflicts between job and family responsibilities, and transportation problems. It is important that the educator respect the challenges that each student faces (**FIGURE 4.2**).

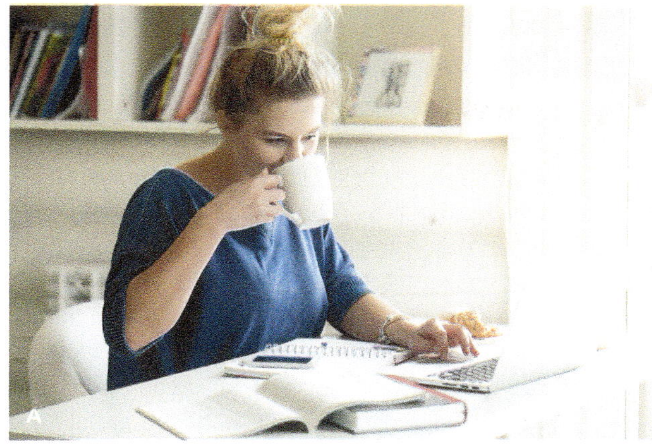

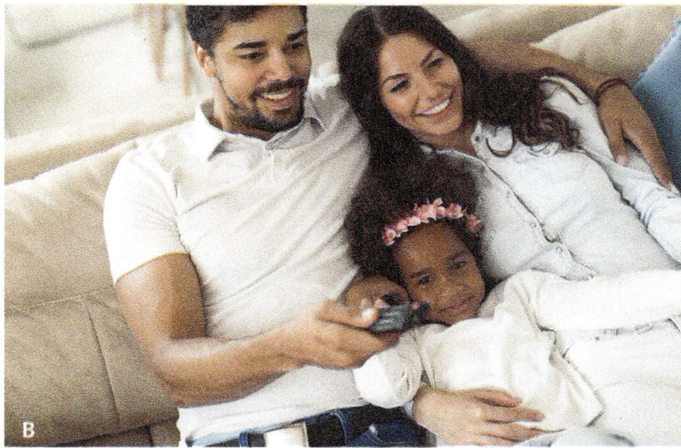

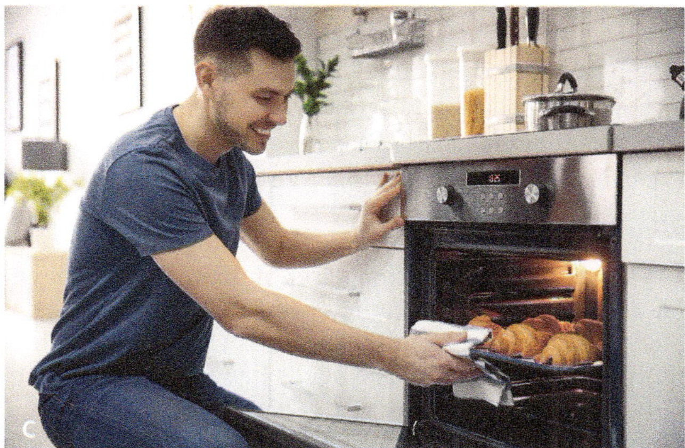

FIGURE 4.2 Teaching adults means teaching people with varied life experiences and responsibilities.

A. © Fizkes/Shutterstock; **B.** © Nd3000/Shutterstock; **C.** © Africa Studio/Shutterstock

Principles for Teaching Adult Learners

With adult learners, instructors should do the following:

- Involve students in the planning process.
- Actively engage students in the learning process.
- Incorporate a variety of teaching methods to meet the needs of students with a variety of learning styles.
- Focus on real-world situations.
- Emphasize how the learning can be applied.
- Practice information quickly after it is presented.
- Relate the material to the learner's past experience.
- Allow debate and challenge of ideas, while suppressing nonsensical or political challenges (e.g., avoiding time-consuming academic discussions on topics such as euthanasia, right-to-life, surgical skills such as C-section deliveries, or whether paramedics should be able to go into independent practice and such).
- Listen to and respect the opinions of learners.
- Encourage learners to be resources to the instructor and to one another.
- Use students to assess learning.
- Give learners control (e.g., when, where, and how they can learn—videos, extra reading, small groups, practice labs; provide specialized areas of learning, such as a focus on trauma, medical emergencies, pediatrics, or geriatrics).
- Reinforce positive behavior whenever possible.

Motivation

Adults typically have different motivators for learning than do younger students. The instructor can apply an important classroom management and performance enhancement tool by understanding what motivates students, because motivation creates the desire to learn. By learning the students' motivators, the instructor can understand student behavior and choose relevant motivational tools. For example, students who are trying to provide for their family on an EMT salary can be reminded that the top five students in the paramedic class will be guaranteed interviews for openings at one of the most highly respected regional ambulance services, and that the service has a track record of offering positions to each such student interviewed in the past. Such information may strongly motivate a student to excel in the program. For example, an educator may share with a class the results of research by Fernandez, Studnek, and Margolis that reported that paramedic licensure required for employment was one of the independent variables that predicted passing the National Registry of EMTs written examination.[17]

TEACHING TIP

Active listening is an important and effective communication skill, and requires determination and practice in order to develop proficiency. During class, it is tempting to divide attention between several students at once, but that is not always effective. Instructors should self-monitor how actively and attentively they listen to each student. Active listening can also help to identify a student's motivators.

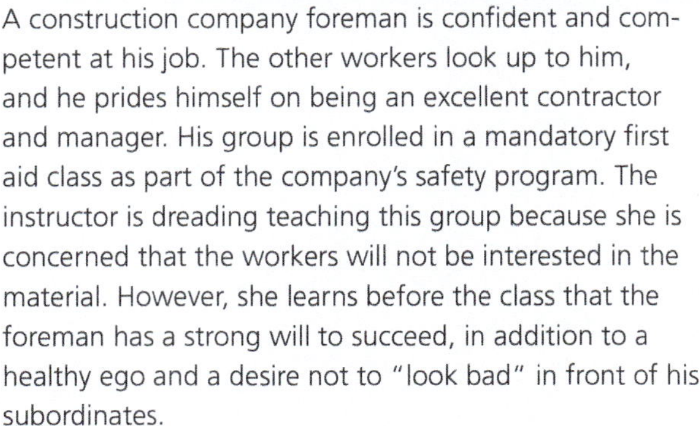

CASE in Point

A construction company foreman is confident and competent at his job. The other workers look up to him, and he prides himself on being an excellent contractor and manager. His group is enrolled in a mandatory first aid class as part of the company's safety program. The instructor is dreading teaching this group because she is concerned that the workers will not be interested in the material. However, she learns before the class that the foreman has a strong will to succeed, in addition to a healthy ego and a desire not to "look bad" in front of his subordinates.

The instructor knows that she has a useful tool with which to motivate this group—by identifying the foreman as the team leader and encouraging and supporting his learning. By helping him to succeed, she will ensure that he stays motivated to master the material, while simultaneously motivating his group to learn the information and perform well.

Additionally, the instructor uses examples that are relevant to the students' experiences. She describes accidents and injuries that could occur on a construction jobsite. When teaching spinal immobilization, she uses the example of a roofer who falls while laying shingles. When teaching hemorrhage control, she uses the example of a framer who cuts himself while using a power saw. The students see the relevance of the class to them personally, and they are more motivated to pay attention and practice the skills presented in class. In fact, several students pursue supplemental learning beyond the classroom by attending additional classes in construction site safety.

Intrinsic and Extrinsic Motivators

Motivators are divided into two groups: intrinsic (internal) and extrinsic (external).[18] *Intrinsic motivators* are internal drives for behaviors, such as a desire to help others, to achieve, or to serve the community, or a need for personal or professional growth and development, to boost one's self-esteem, or to be competent and succeed in life. Another intrinsic motivator is to make new social contacts or to maintain existing social relationships, or sometimes just to relieve boredom. Adults are usually more highly motivated by intrinsic factors than by extrinsic factors.

In contrast, *extrinsic motivators* come from outside of the individual. Examples of extrinsic motivators include the possibility of a promotion, a bonus, additional vacation time, or the need to find or maintain a job.

Once an instructor knows and understands a student's motivators, it is possible to use language, examples, and incentives relevant to the student to provide motivation to learn.

Maslow's Hierarchy

A discussion of motivation would be incomplete without including Abraham Maslow, one of the seminal pioneers in the field of human motivation. He worked on his theory over a period of many years, from 1943 through 1971, making alterations as he sought to refine understanding of the subject. The resulting theory is deemed **Maslow's hierarchy of needs**. In fact, the hierarchy has evolved over the decades and has influenced many fields, including education. Maslow's hierarchy can be helpful to educators as they seek to identify and understand student needs and motivations.[19,20]

Maslow, a humanist, believed that people strive for a higher potential and desire to reach higher levels of their calling—to become fully functioning persons—or, as he describes it, to achieve "self-actualization." Moreover, individuals can grow and actualize their potential in the right environment; but in a less-than-healthy environment, individuals do not grow to meet their potential.

Maslow's theory comprises a hierarchy of levels of *basic* needs, or deficiency needs, then progresses to *higher* needs, or growth needs, which can be attained only when the more basic needs have been met. At the lowest level of the hierarchy, basic needs are physiological, such as oxygen, food, water, and a reasonably constant body temperature. An individual who is deprived of any of these basic physiological needs would be controlled by them and would desperately seek to attain them. Until these needs are satisfied, the individual cannot move to the next level. Students who are distracted by a classroom environment that is too hot or too cold, or who fail to have sufficient breaks to meet personal needs, may be distracted from learning.

Safety and security needs, the next level in the hierarchy, describe the ability to be free from fear of physical danger and to feel secure. Safety is presumed by most adults until a serious emergency or a major disruption in some social structure occurs. Examples of events that have raised safety concerns and questions of needs in recent decades include the 9/11 attacks and the 2012 Sandy Hook Elementary School shooting in Newtown, Connecticut. Young children, on the other hand, almost constantly feel the effects of insecurity, and they need to feel safe when they are in new places and around strangers. Likewise, students must feel safe in the classroom to fully participate in learning. A classroom environment that allows bullying or sarcasm may inhibit students from speaking out or engaging in the learning experience for fear of being mocked or belittled.[21]

The next level in the hierarchy is the need for love, affection, and belonging. Maslow explains that individuals strive to overcome loneliness and separation from family, friends, and society. This level of need includes not just receiving love and affection, but also giving love and affection. If there is difficulty attaining a sense of belonging, individuals may substitute achievement. Student teams or groups can promote a sense of belonging. Likewise, a classroom of inclusion, where all students are shown that their opinions and contributions are valued, can create an atmosphere where students feel that sense of belonging.

The next level of Maslow's hierarchy of basic needs includes esteem. An individual has the strength and motivation to strive to fulfill this need only when the more basic needs have been met. Humans must have a stable, high level of respect for themselves and respect from others. Becoming competent and gaining recognition (validity from others) produce feelings of self-confidence, power, and usefulness to society. Some individuals may not always seek to fill these needs through constructive behavior; sometimes they may seek attention through disruptive or immature actions. In the classroom, everyone must be encouraged and offered the opportunity to participate in all activities. Allowing one person in a group or class to lead in every exercise or activity does little to improve the self-esteem of others. It is the instructor 's responsibility to ensure all are given equal opportunities to demonstrate their ability to excel.

Once the basic needs have been met, an individual, according to Maslow, is ready to pursue the higher level, or "growth," needs. Although Maslow initially identified self-actualization as one need, after more study he identified four specific levels: cognitive needs, aesthetic needs, self-actualization needs, and self-transcendence needs. Again, each of these levels of need is attempted only after lesser needs have been met. Cognitive needs include knowing, understanding, and exploring. Aesthetic needs include order and beauty. Self-actualization is reaching one's potential, or, as described by Maslow, "What a man can be, he must be." This is an intrinsic motivation; it is not related to what others think is important. Self-transcendence is a connection to something beyond the ego; it involves helping others to find self-fulfillment and to reach their potential. Offering nontraditional learning opportunities or activities within the curriculum allows students to experiment and to demonstrate their creative talents. This enriches the student experience and the classroom environment, allowing some students the chance to reach toward those higher needs.

Instructors must be able to talk to students to understand life events that may impact their motivation. Considering Maslow's hierarchy and determining where students stand within the hierarchy may assist instructors in understanding and addressing the specific needs of students (**FIGURE 4.3**).

Honors

Presenting honors or awards can be a two-edged sword. There is no doubt that recognition is a strong motivator for some students. However, the students who do not receive recognition may be resentful. Nevertheless, recognizing the student who completes a program with the highest grade average or one who has gained nearly universal admiration from faculty, clinical instructors, and fellow students is appropriate. Such awardees must be thoughtfully chosen and reflect achievements or qualities that are worthy of special recognition. Time and effort must be invested to make the selection fair and objective. The criteria for granting such awards should be disseminated to all students early in the program.

If done appropriately and professionally, awards can acknowledge exceptional performance or behaviors demonstrated by the students who are selected.

Programs may also find it useful to use rubrics to score students for eligibility for honors and have the faculty collectively make the selection of students to honor. This has the advantage of making the process as transparent and objective as possible.

Careful consideration should be given to presenting awards or end-of-class certificates. Certainly, accomplishments should be celebrated. Completing any one of the four levels of EMS education can be a significant achievement for an individual student. These moments should be celebrated, but not at the expense of those students who failed to progress. If there is no formal graduation ceremony, some programs reserve the last day of class to present course completion certificates. They also use this time to register students who have successfully completed their coursework for either their state or national examinations. Students who have not successfully completed the course do not need to attend the last day. This practice avoids embarrassment for students who have not met the

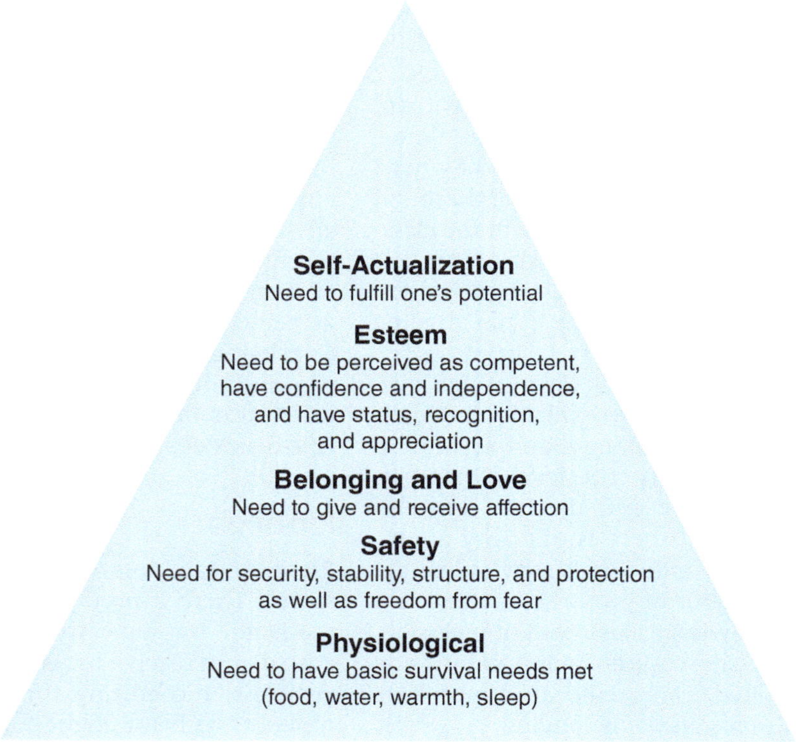

Self-Actualization
Need to fulfill one's potential

Esteem
Need to be perceived as competent, have confidence and independence, and have status, recognition, and appreciation

Belonging and Love
Need to give and receive affection

Safety
Need for security, stability, structure, and protection as well as freedom from fear

Physiological
Need to have basic survival needs met (food, water, warmth, sleep)

FIGURE 4.3 Maslow's hierarchy of needs.

requirements for certification. It is common for schools to allow students who have made satisfactory progress but lack some clinical hours or final course requirements to participate in the graduation ceremony. Their official graduation certificate is awarded when all program requirements are completed.

Positive Affirmation

Developing a positive mindset is one of the most powerful instructional strategies for giving feedback on performance. Positive-thinking techniques, visualization, and positive affirmations are highly effective methods to increase levels of performance in stressful situations. They are, however, the most generally underutilized motivational techniques used in EMS education. Most experienced master educators know that a student's attitude is the most important factor in training.

Barriers to Learning

Not all learners come to the classroom fully prepared to learn. Some may lack adequate motivation. Others may be physically exhausted due to a heavy work schedule or a demanding family situation, such as having a young child or two in the home (**FIGURE 4.4**).

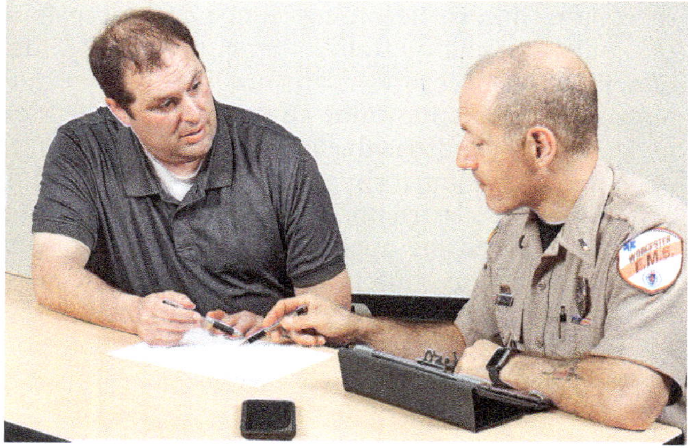

FIGURE 4.4 Scheduling problems and bureaucracy can be significant barriers to learning.

Others may have innate learning disabilities, such as dyslexia or attention deficit hyperactivity disorder (ADHD), while others may simply lack confidence.[22–25]

Educators should understand that such barriers exist and that they may be able to effect positive changes in students through their roles as mentor, guide, and advocate. The educator must strive to decrease barriers whenever possible and must encourage learners

CASE in Point

Aiko is enrolled in an advanced EMT class. She has taken several other EMS courses and is well known by all of the instructional staff. Aiko is a strong learner and has not had struggles in any of her classes. During the academic portion of the class, she has routinely announced aloud her excellent test and quiz scores to the annoyance of her classmates.

During the live intravenous (IV)-start lab, each student is given 10 attempts to start five successful IVs. Failure to accomplish this task results in a failing grade and prevents the students from progressing to the clinical portion of the class. Aiko missed her first four IV attempts. She was able to start two successful IVs on her fifth and sixth attempts, but required close coaching. On her seventh attempt she was unsuccessful. She now has only three attempts left and they must be successful IV starts. To add more pressure, she is the only student in the class who will need to use all 10 attempts to complete this portion of the lab.

Aiko resented any suggestion of remediation, viewing that as an embarrassing failure. However, with additional coaching and tactful support, her skills improved and she was able to successfully start her next two IVs. When she missed the seventh attempt, however, she became outwardly negative and was heard saying, "I can't do this."

The lead instructor knows Aiko's problem is not her psychomotor or cognitive skills. He knows that she is only lacking in confidence and manual practice. He instructs Aiko to focus on other skills for the rest of the day. At the end of the class he asks Aiko for a few minutes of her time and they discuss how she views her IV starts. She is shy and defensive, saying that she only needs to concentrate harder. He suggests to her that she wait 5 days before actually trying to perform additional starts and to spend several minutes per day visualizing successful IV starts. He instructs Aiko to stay positive and clearly envision herself successfully completing at least five IVs every day. Aiko returns the following week and successfully starts all three of the remaining IVs.

to explore ways to overcome their personal barriers. Encouraging attention to intrinsic motivators (e.g., success, helping others) may also be helpful. These barriers might otherwise limit students' ability to grow as prehospital EMS providers and to become lifelong learners.

Accommodation for Disabilities

Key points for the EMS educator with regard to accommodation of disabilities include the following. For more information, see Appendix B, *Disabilities in EMS Education*.

1. Don't make assumptions about the potential capabilities of an applicant based on perceived or diagnosed disabilities.
2. Every EMS responder and educator has their own sets of skill strengths and weaknesses—we are not all equal in all three domains (cognitive, psychomotor, and affective).
3. There are several federal laws that govern how academic programs must assess and accommodate admitted students with disabilities.
4. Specialized professional counsel and support are advised when confronting an applicant or an admitted student with a disability, whether diagnosed or not.
5. Case law is evolving, as is technology. An impairment that could not be reasonably accommodated yesterday might well be accommodated today or tomorrow!

Selected Learning Theories

This section examines several selected theories of learning and offers practical lessons that educators can gain from these theories. Although dozens of theories, preferences, and concepts are associated with learning in educational psychology, five of the more common types have been selected for discussion here. These include self-directed learning, the theory of margin, transformational learning, experiential learning, and context-based learning.

Self-Directed Learning

The theory of **self-directed learning** involves many related concepts, such as self-planned learning, self-teaching, autonomous learning, and independent study. Distributed learning and distance education are also frequently used modalities for self-directed learning.

Self-education has been described as nothing more than the manner in which information is acquired—that of learning without an instructor present.[26] However, the absence of an instructor, although an important characteristic of self-directed learning, is only *one* of several characteristics of self-directed learning. At least three additional characteristics are particular to self-directed learning:

- A longer learning time period
- A wider range of studies
- A higher level of subject mastery and critical thinking

Self-direction in learning comes from a lifelong learning perspective. Kidd supports this view in the following passage: "It has often been said that the purpose of adult education, or of any kind of education, is to make the subject [student] a continuing, 'inner-directed,' self-operating learner."[27]

Self-direction in adulthood is a process in which learners assume primary control of what they desire to learn. Moore describes self-directed learners as individuals who can identify learning needs when a problem must be solved, a skill acquired, or information obtained. They are able to articulate their needs in the form of a general goal, differentiate that goal into several specific objectives, and define fairly explicitly the criteria for successful achievement. In recognizing their needs, they gather the information desired, collect ideas, practice skills, work to resolve their problems, and achieve their goals. In evaluating, the learners judge the appropriateness of newly acquired skills, the adequacy of their solutions, and the quality of new ideas and knowledge.[28]

A related view of self-directed learning that stresses the phases of a learning process has been offered by Knowles:

> In its broadest meaning, "self-directed learning" describes a process in which individuals take the initiative, with or without the help of others, in diagnosing their learning needs, formulating learning goals, identifying human and material resources for learning, choosing and implementing appropriate learning strategies, and evaluating the learning outcomes.[10]

The EMS instructor can apply this theory by creating a classroom environment that includes two elements. First, implement an *institutional* process in which students are made responsible for identifying their learning needs and deciding on the strategies they plan to use to reach them. Then, promote self-directed learning from the point of view of an *internal* process. In other words, students are encouraged to set their own goals in terms of learning outcomes. By doing so, students take responsibility for their own learning.

For example, the instructor might plan an activity on the first day of class that requires students to immediately assume responsibility for their own learning. Another approach might be to simply suggest self-learning strategies that motivated students can utilize. For example, multitudes of free or relatively inexpensive learning resources exist. These resources can be utilized by students who prefer to learn independently or by those who require additional learning support systems. The box *Self-Study Learning Resources* provides a few examples. Instructors can also assign students to define their career choice (EMT, advanced EMT, or paramedic) by investigating a variety of resources and to write a paper with their definitions, observations, and findings. Instructors who ensure that students have initial success with their self-directed assignments can help motivate them in their studies and, in the process, can help them become lifelong learners.

Entry-level EMS education is, by its nature, driven by specific competencies and deadlines that somewhat restrict self-directed learning because of its limitations. By definition, self-directed learning allows students to decide what to learn; an entire program based on this concept would not be practical in EMS. In addition, this type of learning may take longer to achieve as students define their objectives and develop their plans for learning.

Self-directed learning does, however, offer many advantages. Knowles felt that it increases learning because it is based on individual learner initiative, it is an essential element needed to move toward maturity, it makes the learner take responsibility for their own learning, and it develops essential independent learning skills needed to stay current as knowledge evolves.[29] The ability to continue learning independently is an important skill for EMS professionals. EMS instructors should provide tools for learners to pursue self-directed learning. Guiding students to find appropriate resources and seeking opportunities to encourage independent learning within the classroom empower students to become self-directed learners after graduation.

Self-Study Learning Resources

Some examples of self-study learning resources include the following:

- Many self-study electrocardiogram (ECG) books are available; however, free self-study Internet sources are also available, such as https://ekg.academy/ and www.slideserve.com/onan/ekg-self-study-guide.
- An example of a study source on the topic of arterial blood gas analysis can be found at https://medicforyou.in/abg-interpretation-made-easy.
- An example of an anatomy and physiology study source is available at https://chancesforyouth.com/2018/08/14/human-anatomy-and-physiology-pdf-free-download/.

CASE in Point

The EMT instructor looked at the requirements of the National EMS Education Standards for the EMT course and tried to imagine how to possibly cover all of the material adequately. It appeared there was no possible way to have the students learn to be proficient in their skills, understand what they were doing, and still cover every topic during class. Yet, realizing the students are all motivated adults, he concluded that surely they could learn much of this on their own. With that in mind, he devised a self-learning plan that would help to improve his class in several ways.

First, he took the required bloodborne pathogens and Health Insurance Portability and Accountability Act (HIPAA) of 1996 materials that had been added to the curriculum and placed them into a self-directed learning module that had to be completed and passed (by a written test) before students could even register for the courses. This would be the first "commitment filter" because competition to get into the class was strong.

Second, he took the medical terminology, hazardous materials, and weapons of mass destruction (WMD) modules and, from these, created self-directed learning modules that had to be completed by students during class at specific points in the schedule. The medical terminology module was required within 1 week of the start of class. The hazardous material module was required to be completed by the fourth class. Completion of the WMD module was required by the end of the program, but it had to be submitted before students could take the certification exam.

By shifting this content to self-learning modules, the instructor increased contact hours for content related to patient care skills and materials that the students would use on most of their EMS calls. The outcome was a better-prepared, less frustrated, better-performing class.

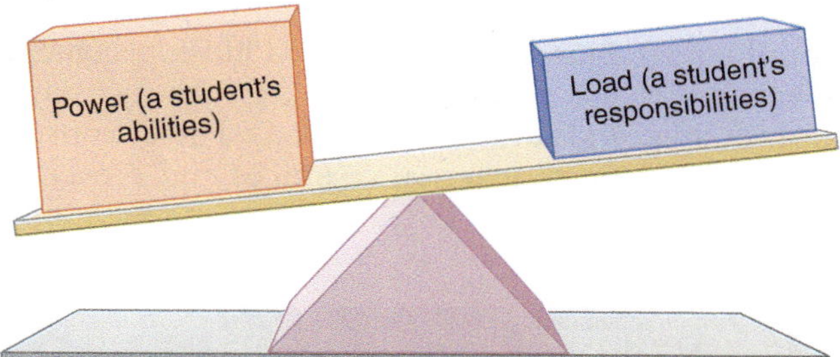

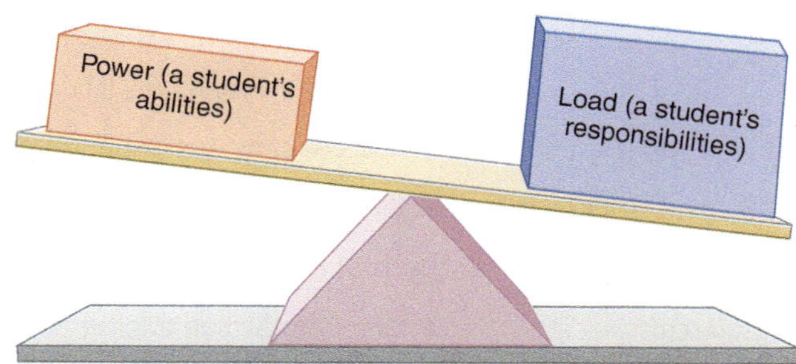

FIGURE 4.5 The theory of Power-Load-Margin.

Power-Load-Margin Theory

The theory of **Power-Load-Margin**, commonly called the theory of margin, provides a model for looking at how much ability (*power*) a student has compared with how much learning the student needs to accomplish (*load*). *Margin* is the difference between power and load. This theory is one way of describing the pressures placed on an individual during the learning process. In general, the greater the margin an individual has, the more likely the individual is to succeed. **FIGURE 4.5** depicts the theory of margin.

Research behind the Theory

Howard Y. McClusky, an experimental psychologist, examined adult learning and introduced the theory of margin in the early 1960s.[30] He believed that the theory was essential for understanding adult lives, especially as adults age and the various demands of family and career increase.

According to McClusky, the key factors of adult life are the load that the adult carries in living and the power that is available to that person to carry the load.[31] He described *load* as the demands, both self and social, that are required by a person to maintain a minimal level of autonomy. He described *power* as the individual's resources, abilities, possessions, and position on which the individual can draw to cope with the load; *margin* is the difference between the power and the load. The greater the margin a person has, the more likely it is that the person can deal with the load, because the person has greater reserve capacity. A student with an overwhelming load, caused by the need to work a full-time job and take care of children and possibly an ill parent, may have no margin for handling any additional duties or stressors, including even the most minimal educational load.

McClusky further divided load into two groups of interacting elements: external and internal. The *external load* consists of tasks involved in normal life requirements (e.g., family, work, and community responsibilities). *Internal load* consists of life expectancies developed by the people themselves, such as aspirations, desires, and future expectations. Power consists of a combination of external resources and capacities such as family support, social abilities, and economic abilities. It also includes various internally acquired or accumulated skills and experiences that contribute to effective performance, such as resilience, coping skills, and personality.

FIGURE 4.6 shows an example of two daily schedules: one with no margin versus one with margin.

A. DAILY SCHEDULE WITH NO MARGIN		
8:00–8:30 a.m.	Roll call and quiz; collect homework assignments; discuss issues from the prior day and any scheduling concerns	Lead instructor
8:30–9:00 a.m.	Quiz review and hand out teaching notes for the day; go over specific requirements for completion	Lead instructor
9:00–10:00 a.m.	Lecture: Cardiac anatomy (chambers, septa, valves, vessels)	Lead instructor
10:00–11:00 a.m.	Cardiac anatomy workshop (dissection and small group reviews)	Lead instructor
11:00 a.m.–12:00 p.m.	Lecture: Cardiac physiology (sodium–potassium ion channels)	Lead instructor
12:00-1:00 p.m.	Lunch	Cafeteria
1–3:00 p.m.	Lecture: Introduction to electrophysiology (atrial rhythms and blocks)	Lead instructor
3:00–4:30 p.m.	ECG rhythms workshop (static strips and small group reviews)	Lead instructor
4:30–5:00 p.m.	Daily review and assignments for next day; to be turned in at 8:00 a.m. ■ 25 end-of-chapter questions (SA node and atrial pathways) ■ 25 ECG rhythms (atrial waveforms and abnormalities)	Lead instructor
5:00–6:00 p.m.	Dinner	Home
6:30–9:00 p.m.	Regional EMS Council Meeting (QA discussion: review of calls)	City Hall, G-17

B. DAILY SCHEDULE WITH MARGIN		
8:00–8:30 a.m.	Roll call and quiz	TA
8:30–9:00 a.m.	Quiz review	TA
9:00–10:15 a.m.	Lecture: Cardiac anatomy and physiology	Lead instructor
10:15–10:30 a.m.	Break	
10:30 a.m.–12:00 p.m.	Cardiac anatomy and physiology workshop	Lead instructor
12:00–1:00 p.m.	Lunch	Cafeteria
1:00–2:45 p.m.	Lecture: Introduction to electrophysiology	Lead instructor
2:45–3:00 p.m.	Break	
3:00–4:30 p.m.	ECG rhythms workshop	TA
4:40–5:00 p.m.	Daily review and assignments for the next day. ■ Five end-of-chapter questions ■ 10 ECG rhythms	Lead instructor
6:30–9:00 p.m.	Regional EMS Council QA Meeting	City Hall, G-17

FIGURE 4.6 A representation of the theory of margin as it applies to life, learning, and comprehension. **A.** Daily schedule with no margin. **B.** Daily schedule with margin.

There are several thematic points that apply to the theory of margin in these examples. The schedule with no margin (Schedule A) contains more detailed information, but that additional information isn't necessary to highlight the activity. Second, in the schedule that contains margin (Schedule B), the activities have been eased, with two 15-minute breaks inserted. These breaks cost half an hour of instructional time, but the overall effect of the planned instruction for the day will be much better—and more realistic—with these breaks built in, as no actual schedule should contain two 4-hour periods without breaks. There are several areas where the student load has been eased, with the message that the student margin should also be increased. This occurs in the area of overnight assignments, which are reduced in Schedule B. Assigning homework is appropriate; however, most times, the same amount of learning can be achieved with a few good sample exercises and a reduction in excessive problems. That does not mean students should not do more exercises; in fact, they should do as many as they need in order to reach competency. However, the instructor does not need to review multiples of repeated questions, when a good sampling of a few assigned questions would be sufficient. Regardless of the approach, the overall impact of increasing the margin and reducing the load can be a great enhancement for adult education, and education in general.

TEACHING TIP

Demands on the instructor are significantly eased by the introduction of a teaching assistant (TA). Some would argue that a TA would be a prohibitive cost for most programs, and is not attainable at many institutions. In fact, TAs can be quite cost effective; for example, an outstanding student may be willing to serve in that capacity if offered discounted tuition.

Practical Application of the Theory

Instructors can affect their students' margins in both positive and negative ways. McClusky's Power-Load-Margin theory can be applied to the degree that instructors contribute to the increase or depletion of margin in the lives and capacities of adult students.[32] Day and James, at the University of Wyoming,[33] in a series of interviews with adult students, found numerous examples of instructor-generated load that they categorized into four areas: attitude, behavior, task, and environment.

One of the most surprising findings of this research was that the attitudinal and behavioral dimensions of the instructor-generated load were identified more than three times as often as the task dimension.

In other words, adults adjust their margins to deal with the expected task demands assigned to them by the instructor better than they do with interpersonal issues. Unexpected demands, such as an instructor's attitude and behaviors, create barriers to a student's ability to satisfactorily complete a learning objective.

Day and James identified several ways in which instructors can minimize the effects of instructor-generated load.[33] These techniques include the following:

1. Recognize and understand that margin exists in adult students.
2. Understand that student concerns do not center merely on the content of the course.
3. Recognize that an instructor can contribute both positively and negatively to the learner load, and that the way in which instructors do so is through behaviors, learning environment, attitudes, and the structure and content of classes.
4. Address issues of margin during the first class, and occasionally revisit the topic at appropriate times, such as a week or two before a major examination.

TABLE 4.3 lists instructor behaviors that increase student load; it also lists behaviors that instructors can emulate to avoid increasing load.

The theory of margin provides a framework for discussion of both how much work a given EMS course typically requires and how much time a student has to devote to the course. In addition, it gives both the instructor and the student a conceptual model by which to discuss how illness, personal problems, and work and family problems can add up to an unmanageable situation. Perhaps the most powerful component of this model is the way that an educator's attitude, lack of organization, or use of busywork can dramatically narrow a student's margin, thus reducing the student's performance and chance of success in a class.

Transformational Learning

The theory of **transformational learning** emerged with the work of Jack Mezirow,[34,35] and is defined as "learning that initiates and creates deep and lasting personal changes," sometimes known as a "paradigm shift."[36] In transformational learning, acquisition of specific knowledge and skills is often secondary to the deeper and lasting change in perception and thought. Although EMS educators generally are not oriented toward intentionally seeking out transformational-learning opportunities for their students, such experiences often appear unexpectedly for the students simply due

TABLE 4.3 Examples of Instructor-Generated Load-Creating Behaviors versus Load-Reducing Behaviors

Load-Creating Behaviors	Load-Reducing Behaviors
Attitude	
Instructor treats learner as an inferior person.	Instructor treats learner with respect, as an equal.
Instructor ignores learner's opinion.	Instructor solicits and listens to learner's opinion.
Instructor is too impatient.	Instructor is patient.
Instructor is too rigid.	Instructor is flexible.
Behavior	
Instructor has distracting mannerisms.	Instructor's mannerisms are not distracting.
Instructor mumbles or is difficult to understand.	Instructor speaks clearly.
Instructor is disorganized.	Instructor is organized.
Instructor avoids eye contact.	Instructor makes eye contact.
Tasks	
Instructor gives inappropriate assignments.	Instructor gives appropriate assignments.
Instructor's guidelines for assessment/grades are unclear.	Instructor's guidelines for evaluation/grades are clear.
Instructor gives busywork.	Instructor gives meaningful work.
Instructor allows too little time to complete assignments.	Instructor allows sufficient time to complete assignments.
Environment	
Learning environment is too hot or too cold.	Learning environment is not too hot or too cold.
Lighting is poor.	Lighting is adequate.
Desks and chairs are uncomfortable.	Desks and chairs are comfortable.
Noise or other distractions can be heard from neighboring classrooms.	Noise or other distractions cannot be heard from neighboring classrooms, or are minimized.

Modified from Mendler, Allen, and Randi Moody. 2001. *Motivating Students Who Don't Care: Successful Techniques for Educators*. Bloomington, IN: National Educational Service.

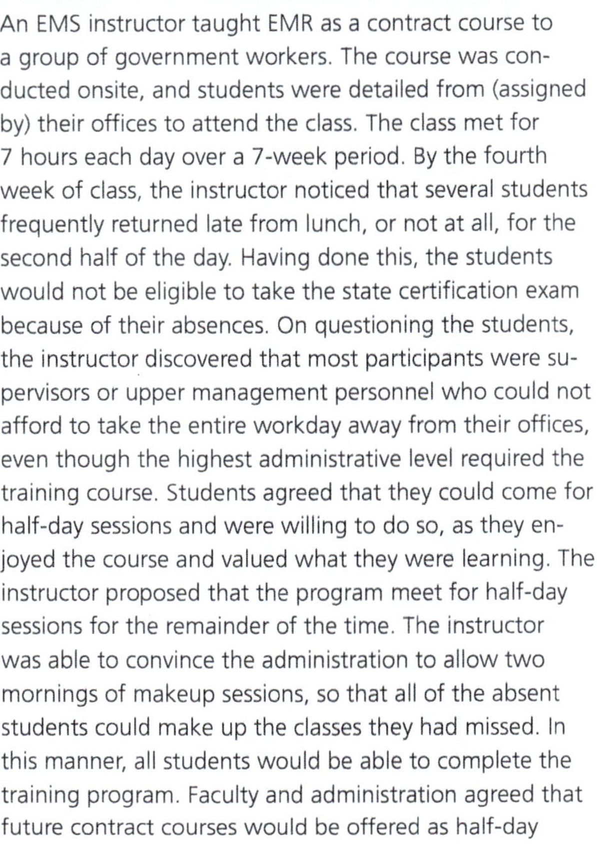

CASE in Point

An EMS instructor taught EMR as a contract course to a group of government workers. The course was conducted onsite, and students were detailed from (assigned by) their offices to attend the class. The class met for 7 hours each day over a 7-week period. By the fourth week of class, the instructor noticed that several students frequently returned late from lunch, or not at all, for the second half of the day. Having done this, the students would not be eligible to take the state certification exam because of their absences. On questioning the students, the instructor discovered that most participants were supervisors or upper management personnel who could not afford to take the entire workday away from their offices, even though the highest administrative level required the training course. Students agreed that they could come for half-day sessions and were willing to do so, as they enjoyed the course and valued what they were learning. The instructor proposed that the program meet for half-day sessions for the remainder of the time. The instructor was able to convince the administration to allow two mornings of makeup sessions, so that all of the absent students could make up the classes they had missed. In this manner, all students would be able to complete the training program. Faculty and administration agreed that future contract courses would be offered as half-day sessions.

This instructor applied the theory of margin by increasing the power the students had (by responding to their need and allowing them to help devise a solution) and decreasing their load, thus increasing their margin.

to the nature of EMS and exposure to dramatic and unexpected life and death events. Many instructors can recall times when a student approached them at some point during or after the class and said, "EMS has changed my life. Now I know what I want to do." EMS educators should be on the lookout for those seminal moments that can transform the lives of students and influence their entire careers.

Research behind the Theory

Transformational learning is based on the concepts of *meaning perspectives*, or one's overall worldview, and *meaning schemes*, or smaller components that contain specific knowledge, values, and beliefs about one's experiences.[34] A number of meaning schemes work together to generate one's meaning perspective.

CASE in Point

A student, Josef, came into the instructor's office frustrated and ready to quit. He told the instructor that he could not do the medication calculations no matter how hard he tried. The instructor, similar to every paramedic program instructor who has taught medication calculations, sat and listened attentively. Yes, medication calculations are one of the most challenging tasks for some students to learn, and some students *never* master the calculation skills that are essential to be a paramedic. However, this was a very bright student who was "blocked" in this particular learning area for some reason; he *believed* that he simply could not learn these calculation tasks.

The instructor thought about the student's background and about why Josef might not be learning the skill. The instructor realized that he was a licensed cosmetologist, a beautician who ran his own business. The instructor asked Josef, "Don't you have to calculate your business expenses every month? Project the supplies you need and order them? Calculate how much they will cost? Calculate the costs of your utilities, lease, taxes, and other business expenses? Don't you have to anticipate how many customers you will have, how long it will take you to serve each one, and schedule them?" The instructor then asked, "How is all of that any more complicated than medication calculations? Isn't it all the same, except for changing dollars to milligrams, and ounces to bottles, instead of milligrams to kilograms?"

Josef's expression changed in an instant. He smiled. His eyes lit up. He said, "I got it!" He stood up and walked out of the office, passed the pharmacology test with high scores, and today is a practicing paramedic. He is also a critical care nurse. He had a *transformational learning experience* that occurred in one brief moment—just by being asked the right questions at the right time.

Meaning perspectives are shaped during childhood and youth, and they form the basis for a person's view of the world from their own perspective. They operate as perceptual filters that determine how individuals will organize and interpret the meaning of their life experiences.

Perspectives on one's life and career change and evolve naturally as the number and depth of life experiences increase. However, there are occasions when significant events occur that induce powerful emotional responses. These life-changing events may include intensely personal negative experiences, such as divorce, death of a loved one, health crises, financial upheavals, and unexpected job changes. They may involve large-scale incidents such as the 9/11 attacks or a mass shooting. When these events occur, people process their individual perspectives and how deeply they are affected by the events. However, transformational learning does not take place if the perception of the events fits comfortably into one's worldview. If, however, the event causes an emotional upheaval and cognitive dissonance regarding what one believes, a transformative learning experience may occur as the new information shifts the meaning and perspective to a new position.[35]

Practical Application of the Theory

Although transformational learning has a powerful potential for enhancing and accelerating a student's self-actualization processes, an EMS instructor must consider some important points in attempting to bring about such processes. Baumgartner advises instructors to consider ethical questions that may arise in the planning and delivery of transformational learning.[37] He also discusses the dynamics and the balance of power in the classroom, emphasizing the necessity for a trusting and ethical relationship between students and instructors. Students who see the instructor as an authority figure may be reluctant to challenge conventional values, beliefs, and interpretations of events. Thus, Baumgartner recommends that educators adhere to a formal code of ethics and engender a safe forum for adult educators in which mutual support and exploration of transformational learning events can take place.

It is not uncommon for transformational learning to elicit strong emotional responses from both the student and the instructor, often unexpectedly. Because of their powerful potential, the instructor should take the time to deal with transformational learning moments when they occur. For example, a class discussion about medical maladies among the homeless leads to a larger discussion of the nature of homelessness. The instructor gives a research assignment to a group of interested students, instructing them to find relevant information about the topic. As the students research the topic, several of them find the information to be very powerful and alter their preexisting thoughts regarding the homeless. As a result, they feel better prepared and more empathetic to the homeless patients they contact in the field.

The wise educator avoids controversial political discussion in the EMS educational setting. Discussions about political parties, candidates, religions, gun control, the right to life, and capital punishment are wisely relegated to classes that specifically address ethics, political science, and philosophy. In the EMS setting, such discussions only result in a loss of learning time and classroom calm. As a corollary principle, it is also wise to never include questions of this nature on any written, oral, or practical test.

TABLE 4.4 outlines transformational teaching.

TABLE 4.4 Transformational Education

Theoretical Underpinnings
Promote individual and collective self-efficacy
Challenge habits of mind and points of view
Realize ideal self and vision for future
Transcend self-interests to achieve shared goals
Basic Principles
Facilitate mastery of key core concepts
Enhance strategies and skills for learning and discovery
Promote positive learning-related attitudes, values, and beliefs
Core Methods
Establish a shared vision
Provide modeling and mastery
Challenge and encourage students
Provide personal attention and feedback
Create experimental lessons
Promote preflection and reflection

Modified from Slavich, George M., and Philip G. Zimbardo. 2012. "Transformational Teaching: Theoretical Underpinnings, Basic Principles, and Core Methods." *Educational Psychology Review* 24, no. 4: 569–608. https://doi.org/10.1007/s10648-012-9199-6.

Experiential Learning

Experiential learning can be explained simply as learning by doing. Kolb developed an early experiential learning model (based on work by Dewey, Piaget, and Lewin), but many new experiential models have developed over time. At first glance, this principle appears simple, but to learn rather than just do, the learner must move through a cycle that involves (1) an experience, (2) meaningful reflection to see the experience from several perspectives, (3) abstract thought to derive concepts and key ideas from the experience, and (4) critical thinking and problem solving to try out the new ideas by actively testing them in another situation (FIGURE 4.7).[38,39]

Later theorists wrote that the Kolb model neglected the individual learners and the important role their characteristics and past experiences play in learning. In addition, the critical relationship of emotion in situational learning was emphasized. A positive experience that enhances self-esteem, peer trust, and confidence is more likely to contribute to meaningful learning.[39] Negative emotions, such as fear, must be acknowledged for the student to move forward.

The instructor plays an important role as facilitator to promote learning in experiential situations. Developing challenging scenarios using simulation with standardized patients or manikins and scheduling appropriate clinical and field experiences form the foundation for experiential learning in the EMS classroom. Instructors can assist students to reflect and manage emotions associated with experiential learning by debriefing, discussing, or having them journal. Deliberate facilitation may be needed to help the students generate meaning from the experience so that they can identify how to improve performance and use their knowledge in new or different situations. During this phase, the instructor may suggest or lead the students toward other ways to solve the

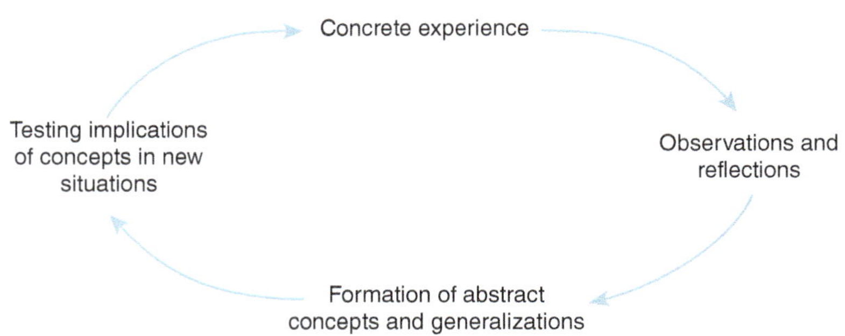

FIGURE 4.7 Experiential learning—concrete experience, meaningful reflection, abstract thought, and active testing.

CASE in Point

The EMT course covered the topic of child abuse and neglect. During the lesson, the instructor noticed that one student was withdrawn and quiet. This was out of character for the student. The instructor approached the student during the break to see if there was an illness, or if something else was an issue of concern. The student related a story from childhood and explained how a best friend had been the victim of child abuse. The student told how he had watched his friend endure several years of abuse, and that he had been sworn to secrecy. Because they were both young children at the time, he thought that he was doing the right thing by not telling. The student spoke of the feelings of loss when his friend moved away suddenly and he never heard from him again. He told the instructor how this experience had caused him to want to become an EMT, so he could help other children in similar situations. The instructor urged the student to share this story with the rest of the class, and when the break was over, he did. All of the students were riveted during his story, and another student shared a similar experience with the class. This led to a much deeper discussion of the topic than could have been possible from the instructor's lecture alone. The whole class could clearly see how this experience had transformed the life of the student involved.

problem in the future, or to identify areas in which additional skill practice or knowledge is needed. Effective coaching promotes student confidence to test their new problem-solving skills or knowledge in new situations. Good coaches also understand the progression of cognitive, psychomotor, and affective development and challenge students in incremental steps of increasing difficulty and complexity, to avoid overwhelming and intimidating students while reinforcing their increasing competency with "stair step" successes.

Context-Based Learning (Situated Cognition)

Context-based learning (situated cognition) is a type of experiential learning that assumes that information is more easily learned if it is taught within the environment where it will actually be used by the student.

Research behind the Theory

Lave and Wenger state that effective learning manifests as a function of the activity, context, and culture in which it occurs—*the situation*.[40] This contrasts with most traditional classroom learning theories where learning activities are most often presented in an abstract form and out of context. For example, in the past, students learned about starting an IV line in a lecture with screen projections and demonstration bags of solutions, administration sets, lines, sterilizing wipes, gauze, and tape. Then, the drip rate was calculated on a blackboard and on sheets of paper. In context-based learning, a realistic environment and social interaction are critical components of learning. Today, students learn about starting IV lines in realistic laboratory settings. They are presented with a series of realistic scenarios that require responses that lead to learning. For example, the student is presented with a dehydrated patient in shock. They must determine what must be done, how it must be done, and then they must do it.

Students become experientially involved in a "community of practice." The community is made up of experts and novices. Experts are identified as individuals with real-life experience that reflects the content, whereas novices are those who wish to learn the content but have minimal or no practical experience. The community, which comprises both experts and novices, creates a dynamic learning environment.

Situated learning is usually unintentional, or incidental, rather than deliberate. Lave and Wenger call the process "legitimate peripheral participation." Content is learned, and value is "assigned" to it by the students when they have the opportunity to interact in the same environment as experienced practitioners.[41]

Practical Application of the Theory

Educators should strive to make every case scenario and simulation as realistic as possible. This can be achieved through carefully crafted scripts and a realistic environment. If a lab can be made to appear like a living room or a motor vehicle collision, learning will be enhanced. As an example, many EMS programs have installed realistic patient-transport compartment labs in classrooms.

Lave and Wenger provide an analysis of situational learning in five different settings: Yucatan midwives, native tailors, Navy quartermasters, meat cutters, and alcoholics.[41] In all cases, the researchers observed a gradual acquisition of knowledge and skills as novices learned from experts in the context of everyday activities. In EMS, students who have opportunities to observe and practice their skills with real vials,

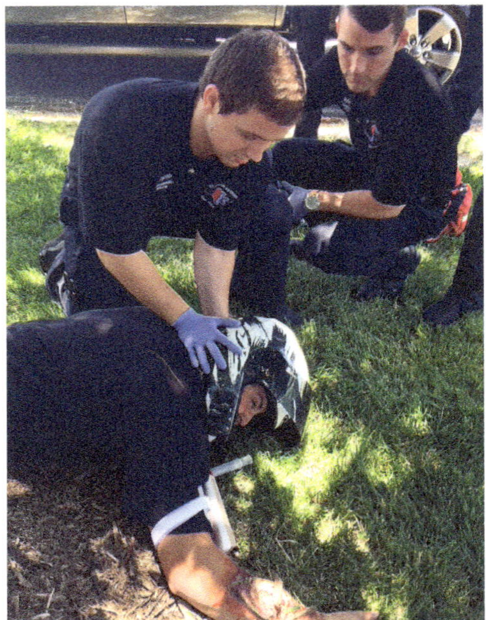

FIGURE 4.8 Students who participate in real-life environments are more likely to be successful learners.

Courtesy of St. Charles County Ambulance District.

needles, and syringes in real-life environments with interaction with field providers benefit greatly. Although formalized internships may not be practical for every EMS class at every level of training, the opportunity for students to participate in patient scenarios in well-scripted and environmentally realistic laboratory settings provides a reasonable alternative (**FIGURE 4.8**).

CASE in Point

The students were nearing the end of their didactic training and were beginning to transition into the field internship phase of the program, during which they would spend time in the field setting with preceptors from the ambulance service. The primary instructor, clinical coordinator, medical director, and field preceptors were meeting to finalize the details of their rotations. The newly hired primary instructor was nervous because he felt the students' skills were weak, and that this would reflect poorly on his teaching abilities. During the final practical skills evaluations, several students scored as "marginal" or "average," and one even failed the evaluation totally and would have to complete a remediation cycle before being allowed to attend field clinical rotations. The clinical coordinator reminded everyone that the students were novices, and that the preceptors needed to work closely with them to develop their skills in all three domains of learning: cognitive, affective, and psychomotor. After the first couple of weeks of field rotations, the primary instructor noticed the students were performing well on in-class scenarios and simulations. The instructor could not understand why they had suddenly improved so dramatically in their performance. During a mentoring session with the program medical director, the instructor began to understand how the theory of contextual learning was affecting student performance. The instructor was motivated to include more practical application exercises in future courses.

Summary

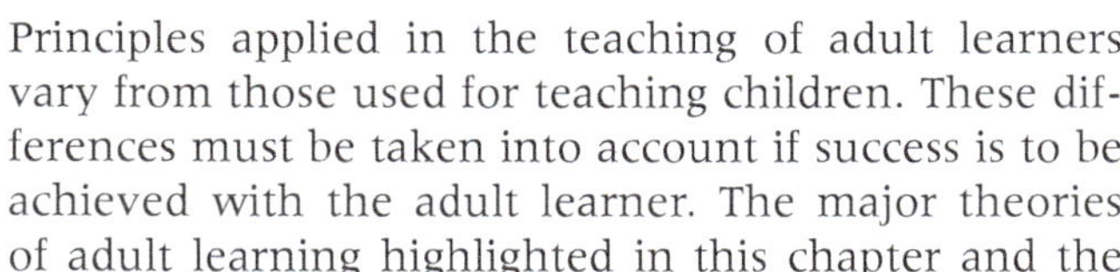

Principles applied in the teaching of adult learners vary from those used for teaching children. These differences must be taken into account if success is to be achieved with the adult learner. The major theories of adult learning highlighted in this chapter and the corresponding examples will aid educators in applying them in practical ways to help students succeed. EMS educators will have a greater capacity for tailoring classroom activities effectively and successfully when they attain a fuller understanding of how adults learn.

Glossary

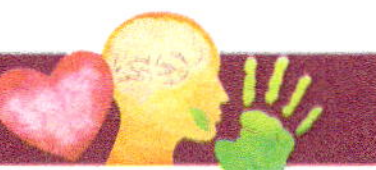

andragogy The art and science of teaching adults.

autonomy Independence.

context-based learning (situated cognition) Learning strategy that places the lesson within the actual situation in which it will be used.

experiential learning Learning by doing.

Maslow's hierarchy of needs Theory that identifies an incremental series of human needs. Individuals must satisfy the lower-level needs to achieve the higher levels.

omnidirectional learning Type of educational environment that is based on an open dialogue in which the instructor serves as facilitator rather than an expert. Discussion responses are directed to everyone in the educational setting, not just to the instructor.

pedagogy The art and science of teaching children.

Power-Load-Margin theory Model that examines the relationship between power (ability) and load (demands on learner).

problem-centered Type of learning in which the student is placed in the context of a real-life situation and must apply knowledge from many subjects in order to resolve an issue at hand.

self-directed learning Learning without instructor presence.

transformational learning Learning theory centered around creating change in perception and thought.

References

[1] Sutton, Kimberly K., and Josh DeSantis. 2017. "Beyond Change Blindness: Embracing the Technology Revolution in Higher Education." *Innovations in Education and Teaching International* 54, no. 30: 223–8. https://doi.org/10.1080/14703297.2016.1174592.

[2] Tainish, Ryan. 2016. "Thoughtfully Designed Online Courses as Effective Adult Learning Tools." *Journal of Adult Education* 45, no. 1. Accessed February 12, 2019. https://www.questia.com/library/journal/1P3-4042660331/thoughtfully-designed-online-courses-as-effective.

[3] Raynovich, Bill, Chris Nollette, Gary Wingrove, Mike Wilcox, and Connie J. Mattera. 2018. "NAEMSE Position Paper on Community Paramedicine and Mobile Integrated healthcare." *JEMS.* Accessed February 12, 2019. https://www.jems.com/ems-insider/articles/2018/january/naemse-position-paper-on-community-paramedicine-and-mobile-integrated-healthcare.html.

[4] Stuhlmiller, David F. E., John R. Clark, Sean Caffrey, Mark Betterton, Chris Nollette, and William Raynovich. 2018. "National Association of EMS Educator's Position Paper on the Critical Care Paramedic." *Prehospital Emergency Care.* https://doi.org/10.1080/10903127.2018.1536772.

[5] McPherran, Mark L. 2010. "Socrates, Plato, *Erôs* and Liberal Education." *Oxford Review of Education* 36, no. 5: 527–41. https://doi.org/10.1080/03054985.2010.514433.

[6] Swardson, H. R. 2005. "Socratic Teaching under Postmodern Conditions." *The Philosophical Forum* 36, no. 2: 161–82. https://doi.org/10.1111/j.1467-9191.2005.00198.x.

[7] Day, Michael, and Clifford P. Harbour. 2013. "The Philosopher and the Lecturer: John Dewey, Everett Dean Martin, and Reflective Thinking." *Education and Culture* 29, no. 1: 105–24. https://doi.org/10.1353/eac.2013.0008.

[8] "John Dewey Quotes" *Goodreads.* Accessed January 2, 2019. https://www.goodreads.com/author/quotes/42738.John_Dewey.

[9] Slavich, George M., and Philip G. Zimbardo. 2012. "Transformational Teaching: Theoretical Underpinnings, Basic Principles, and Core Methods." *Educational Psychology Review* 24, no. 4: 569–608. https://doi.org/10.1007/s10648-012-9199-6.

[10] Knowles, Malcom. 1988. *Andragogy Not Pedagogy!* New York: Associated Press.

[11] Brookfield, Stephen. 1988. "Developing Critically Reflective Practitioners: A Rationale for Training Educators of Adults." In *Training Education of Adults: The Theory and Practice of Graduate Adult Education*, edited by Stephen Brookfield, 99–105. New York: Routledge.

[12] Klein, Gary A., and Robert R. Hoffman. 1982. "Seeing the Invisible: Perceptual-Cognitive Aspects of Expertise." In *Cognitive Science Foundations of Instruction*, edited by Mitchell Rabinowitz, 203–26. Mahwah, NJ: Erlbaum.

[13] Glaser, Robert. 1976. "Cognition and Instructional Design." In *Cognition and Instruction*, edited by David Klahr, 303–15. Hillsdale, NJ: Lawrence Erlbaum Associates.

[14] Imel, Susan. 1988. *Guidelines for Working with Adult Learners.* Syracuse: ERIC Clearinghouse on Adult Career and Vocational Education.

[15] Imel, Susan. 1999. *New Views of Adult Learning.* Syracuse: ERIC Clearinghouse on Adult, Career and Vocational Education.

[16] Brookfield, Stephen D. 1986. *Understanding and Facilitating Adult Learning: A Comprehensive Analysis of Principles and Effective Practice.* Milton Keynes, UK: Open University Press.

[17] Fernandez, Antonio R., Jonathan R. Studnek, and Gregg S. Margolis. 2008. "Estimating the probability of passing the National Paramedic Certification Examination." *Academic Emergency Medicine* 15, no. 3: 258–64. https://doi.org/10.1111/j.1553-2712.2008.00062.x.

[18] Mendler, Allen, and Randi Moody. 2001. *Motivating Students Who Don't Care: Successful Techniques for Educators.* Bloomington, IN: National Educational Service.

[19] Maslow, Abraham H. 1971. *The Farther Reaches of Human Nature.* New York: Viking Press.

[20] Greene, Lloyd, and George Burke. 2007. "Beyond Self-Actualization." *Journal of Health and Human Services Administration* 30, no. 2: 116–28.

[21] Fullerton, Lynn, Scott Oglesbee, Steven J. Weiss, Amy A. Ernst, and Vanessa Mesic. 2018. "Assessing the Prevalence and Predictors of Bullying among Emergency Medical Service Providers." *Prehospital Emergency Care* 17: 1–6. https://doi.org/10.1080/10903127.2018.1470208.

[22] Goto, Stanford T., and Connie Martin. 2009. "Psychology of Success: Overcoming Barriers to Pursuing Further Education." *The Journal of Continuing Higher Education* 57: 10–21. https://doi.org/10.1080/07377360902810744.

[23] Darkenwald, Gordon G., and Thomas Valentine. 1985. "Factor Structure of Deterrents to Public Participation in Adult Education." *Adult Education Quarterly* 35: 177–93. https://doi.org/10.1177/0001848185035004001.

[24] Fujita-Starck, Pamela J. 1996. "Motivations and Characteristics of Adult Students: Factor Stability and Construct Validity of the Educational Participation Scale." *Adult Education Quarterly* 47: 29–40. https://doi.org/10.1177/074171369604700103.

[25] McKendry, Stephanie, Marty Wright, and Keith Stevenson. 2014. "Why Here and Why Stay? Students' Voices on the Retention Strategies of a Widening Participation University." *Nurse Education Today* 34, no. 5: 872–7. https://doi.org/10.1016/j.nedt.2013.09.009.

[26] Brockett, Ralph G., and Roger Hiemstra. 1991. *Self-Direction in Adult Learning: Perspectives on Theory, Research and Practice.* London and New York: Routledge.

[27] Kidd, J. R. 1973. *How Adults Learn.* New York: Association Press.

[28] Moore, Judith A., Stephen Cote, Stephen Vantassel, Tim Graeme, and Kevin Andrews. 2003, Spring. "EMS Stress-Training Concept

'Kobayashi Moru' Scenarios." Domain 3. National Association of EMS Educators.

[29] Langenbach, Michael. 1988. *Curriculum Models in Adult Education*. Malabar, FL: Krieger Publishing.

[30] McClusky, Howard Y. 1963. "The Course of the Adult Life Span." In *Psychology of Adults*, edited by Wilbur C. Hallenbeck, 10–20. Chicago, IL: Adult Education Association of USA.

[31] McClusky, Howard. 1974. "Education for Aging: The Scope of the Field and Perspective for the Future." In *Learning for Aging*, edited by Stanley M. Grabowski and W. Dean Mason, 324–55. Washington, DC: Adult Education Association of the USA.

[32] McClusky, Howard. 1970. "An Approach to a Differential Psychology of the Adult Potential." In *Adult Learning and Instruction*, edited by Stanley M. Grabowski, 80–95. Syracuse: ERIC Clearinghouse on Adult.

[33] Day, Michael, and James, James. 1984. "Margin and the Adult Learner." *Mountain Plains Adult Education Association Journal of Adult Education* 13: 1–5.

[34] Mezirow, Jack. 1981. "A Critical Theory of Adult Learning and Education." *Adult Education Quarterly* 32: 3–24. https://doi.org/10.1177/074171368103200101.

[35] Mezirow, Jack. 1997. "Transformative Learning: Theory to Practice." *New Directions for Adult and Continuing Education* 74: 5–12. https://doi.org/10.1002/ace.7401.

[36] Clark, M. Carolyn. 1993. "Transformational Learning." *New Directions for Adult and Continuing Education* 57: 47–56. https://doi.org/10.1002/ace.36719935707.

[37] Baumgartner, Lisa M. 2001. "An Update on Transformational Learning." *New Directions for Adult and Continuing Education* 89: 15–24. https://doi.org/10.1002/ace.4.

[38] Zull, James E. 2002. *The Art of Changing the Brain*. Sterling, VA: Stylus.

[39] Merriam, Sharan B., Roemary S. Caffarella, and Lisa M. Baumgartner. 2007. *Learning in Adulthood*, 3rd ed. San Francisco: John Wiley & Sons.

[40] Lave, Jean. 1988. *Cognition in Practice: Mind, Mathematics, and Culture in Everyday Life*. Cambridge, UK: Cambridge University Press.

[41] Lave, Jean, and Etienne Wenger. 1990. *Situated Learning: Legitimate Peripheral Participation*. Cambridge, UK: Cambridge University Press.

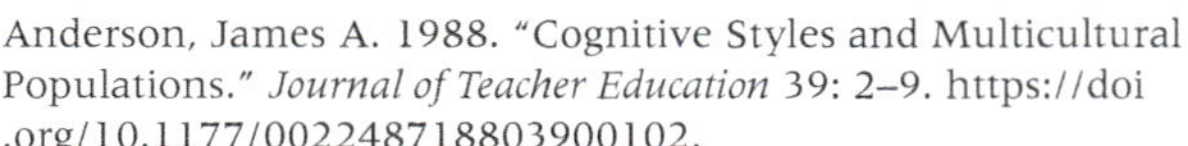
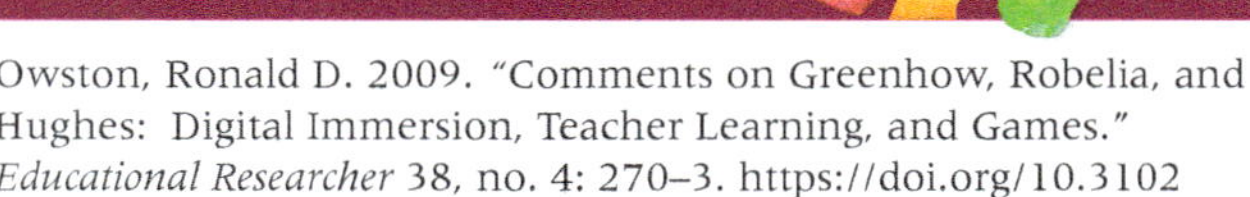

Additional Resources

Anderson, James A. 1988. "Cognitive Styles and Multicultural Populations." *Journal of Teacher Education* 39: 2–9. https://doi.org/10.1177/002248718803900102.

Boud, David, Rosemary Keogh, and David Walker (Eds.) 1985. *Reflection: Turning Experience into Learning*. London: Kogan Page.

Jarvis, Peter. 1994. "Learning." In *ICE301 Lifelong Learning* 1, no. 1. London: YMCA George Williams College.

Knowland, Victoria C. P., and Michael S. C. Thomas. 2014. "Educating the Adult Brain: How the Neuroscience of Learning Can Inform Educational Policy." *International Review of Education* 60, no. 1: 99–122.

Kolb, David A. 1984. *Experiential Learning*. Englewood Cliffs, NJ: Prentice Hall.

Kolb, David A., and Ronald Fry. 1975. "Toward an Applied Theory of Experiential Learning." In *Theories of Group Process*, edited by Cary L. Cooper, 33–57. London: John Wiley.

Krzyzewski, Mike, and Donald T. Phillips. 2000. *Leading with the Heart: Coach K's Successful Strategies for Basketball, Business, and Life*. New York: Warner Books.

LeNoue, Marvin, Tom Hall, and Myron A. Eighmy. 2011. "Adult Education and the Social Media Revolution." *Adult Learning* 22, no. 2: 4–12. https://doi.org/10.1177/104515951102200201.

Mullen, Rebecca, and Linda Wedwick. 2008. "Avoiding the Digital Abyss: Getting Started in the Classroom with YouTube, Digital Stories, and Blogs." *The Clearing House* 82, no. 2: 66–9. https://doi.org/10.3200/TCHS.82.2.66-69.

Nichols, Mark. 2003. "A Theory for eLearning." *Journal of Educational Technology & Society* 6, no. 2: 1–10.

Owston, Ronald D. 2009. "Comments on Greenhow, Robelia, and Hughes: Digital Immersion, Teacher Learning, and Games." *Educational Researcher* 38, no. 4: 270–3. https://doi.org/10.3102/0013189X09336673.

Pavlik, John V. 2015. "Fueling a Third Paradigm of Education: The Pedagogical Implications of Digital, Social and Mobile Media." *Contemporary Educational Technology* 6, no. 2: 113–25.

Schwenk, Thomas L., and Neal Whitman. 1987. *The Physician as Teacher*. Baltimore: Williams and Wilkins.

Simms, Julia, and Dave S. Knowlton. 2008. "Ideas in Practice: Instructional Design and Delivery for Adult Learners." *Journal of Developmental Education* 32, no. 1: 20–30.

Song, Yanjie, Morris S. Y. Jong, Maiga Chang, and Weiqin Chen. 2017. "Guest Editorial: 'HOW' to Design, Implement and Evaluate the Flipped Classroom? A Synthesis." *Journal of Educational Technology & Society* 20, no. 1: 180–3.

Taylor, Nancy E. and Linda Valli. 1992. "Refining the Meaning of Reflection in Education through Program Evaluation." *Teacher Education Quarterly* 19, no. 2: 33–47.

Tennant, Mark. 1997. *Psychology and Adult Learning*, 2nd ed. London: Routledge.

Weimer, Maryellen. 2002. *Learner-Centered Teaching: Five Key Changes to Practice*. San Francisco: Jossey-Bass.

Yakimowski, Mary E., and Michael P. Alfano. 2013. "Can Principles of 'Good Practice in Assessment' Work within Higher Education? A Case Study of an Interdepartmental Assessment Exchange Project." *Journal of Assessment and Institutional Effectiveness* 3, no. 2: 77–105. http://dx.doi.org/10.5325/jasseinsteffe.3.2.0077.

CHAPTER 5

Learning Styles: Concepts and Controversies

OBJECTIVES

At the conclusion of this chapter, the educator will be able to:

Cognitive Domain

1. Discuss how emotion and empathy attached to learning experiences impact memory.
2. Identify activities that involve learning for long-term memory.
3. Identify how sensory input in the classroom environment stimulates curiosity, attentiveness, and retention.
4. Compare and contrast strategies to motivate students with auditory, kinesthetic, and visual learning preferences.
5. Identify characteristics of the global versus analytical learning styles that impact the classroom and lab learning environment.
6. Identify characteristics of the social versus independent learning styles that impact the classroom and lab learning environment.
7. Compare and contrast the converger, diverger, assimilator, and accommodator experiential learning styles and how they impact the types of learning experiences in the classroom, lab, clinical, and field settings.
8. Identify various resources that assist the educator in assessing student learning preferences.
9. Discuss the importance of evaluating the educator's learning preferences and how those preferences impact student learning in the classroom and lab.
10. Identify classroom and lab strategies that balance the various student learning styles for active learning and long-term memory.

Psychomotor Domain

There are no psychomotor objectives for this chapter.

Affective Domain

1. Value diverse classroom and lab experiences to promote knowledge and skill acquisition by using a variety of methods of instruction to enhance positive student outcomes.
2. Defend research findings that support and question the relevance and impact of learning styles on student achievement.
3. Defend the importance of not stereotyping students into a singular learning style or preference.

“The whole purpose of education is to turn mirrors into windows.”

~ Sydney J. Harris

CHAPTER GOAL This chapter explores the concept of learning styles, considers controversies surrounding this concept, and explains the use of learning styles to facilitate learning and memory.

When an educator walks into a classroom, they face a group of learners—each with specific levels of intelligence, experience, aptitude, maturity, and interest. The educator's job is to convey knowledge, skills, and attitudes to each student. In doing so, one of the educator's greatest challenges is to determine the most appropriate means or process for facilitating that learning. In addition, the educator must strive to make learning a meaningful, pleasant, and rewarding experience for the learner. Learning experiences should promote knowledge acquisition, as well as retention, that results in a change in behavior.

A vast amount of research in the neurosciences has provided much information about the brain and how it perceives, processes, and stores information. Each learner has a unique means of perceiving, processing, and storing knowledge and skills. In recent years, this unique means has been called "learning" or "thinking" styles or preferences.

The Neuroscience

Neuroscience has supported the view that people learn differently and that the brain is an ever-evolving structure. This is at the root of learning style theory. Research in the neurosciences has provided educators with valuable insights into learning and how to teach to the ways people learn.[1] (See Chapter 3, *Brain-Based Learning*.)

As John Medina described in his book, *Brain Rules*, neuronal change is a dynamic process that constantly fosters neuronal growth to efficiently transfer information. However, there is a remarkable difference in growth patterns of neurons from one person to the next, despite exposure to the same stimuli or, in the case of a student, new information.[1,2] This explains why two students may come away from the same class with different impressions. It is the types and numbers of senses involved in learning experiences that determine how individuals learn and what they retain.[2]

For example, movement enhances the learning process by improving cognitive function. (See Chapter 3, *Brain-Based Learning*.) The following sections discuss additional findings in neuroscience that relate to education.

Neuroscientific Findings That Relate to Education

Multitasking

The ability to multitask depends on what concept is being referred to. In one respect, the brain multitasks daily. For instance, the brain controls the heart rate while a person reads; it coordinates chewing gum while walking; and it allows a person to read music while their fingers find the keys on a piano or guitar. However, when it comes to paying attention, humans cannot multitask attention-rich inputs simultaneously.[2] Interruptions have a price. Research suggests that a person who is interrupted takes 50% longer to accomplish a task and makes up to 50% more errors. The brain naturally focuses attention sequentially. People who think they can multitask are actually rapidly switching attention between tasks requiring their attention.[3,4]

Effect of Emotions on Learning, Memory, and Recall

Medina asserts that emotions are useful in the learning process because they make the brain pay attention.[2] One of the more interesting results of research pertaining to emotion is the finding that empathy may be one of the most important characteristics, if not *the* most important characteristic, of teaching that influences student performance.[2] The feeling that the instructor

The Teenage Brain

The teenage brain has its own challenges. During puberty, extensive changes happen throughout the body, including in the brain. According to Jensen, the changes occurring in the adolescent brain are as dramatic as those that occur in the infant brain.[5] Major changes occur in morphological and functional development, including development of neurotransmitters and synaptic plasticity.

The teenage brain is highly receptive to new information, making new connections and new dendrites. The teen is more likely to opt for immediate reward than is a mature adult, and more teens opt to engage in risky behavior for the novelty of the experience. Teens also exhibit a lack of the planning and foresight that is more characteristic of adult behavior. Teens are still learning to understand and manage emotions, and they may have trouble with self-regulation.

These changes have an effect on learning and long-term memory. The instructor may find themselves acting as a mediator—asking questions and providing safer alternatives to risk taking.

cares is a major factor in motivation and retention of learning.[2]

Circadian Rhythm

The human sleep-wake cycle is regulated by the brain. These cycles have been documented and are known as circadian rhythms. One of these rhythms, the psychological/cognitive cycle, regulates a person's ability to focus on incoming information with intent to learn.[1] The low point of this rhythm is in the mid-afternoon, the time when most people experience transient sleepiness. Sitting for as little as 15 to 20 minutes during that time period, in class or in a meeting, may result in people nodding off. This has significant implication for classes that may be scheduled during that time period. By getting students up and moving by changing the type of activity or style of presentation method during class every 20 minutes, instructors can help engage the brain and motivate students to learn.

Sleep deprivation also has a profound impact on learning and memory. It is so prevalent that there is now a recognized phenomenon called *delayed sleep-phase syndrome*, characterized by a pattern of difficulty falling asleep at night, difficulty waking up in the morning, and fatigue during the day with increased alertness at night. During sleep, the brain consolidates, organizes, and distributes information and skills for long-term storage. Sleep is critical for transfer to long-term memory.[1,2,5] Encouraging and mentoring students to maintain a school, work, and life balance will enhance their memory and learning experiences.

Memory

There are three stages of memory: (1) sensory (immediate), (2) working (short-term), and (3) long-term.[1] Some stimuli processed in temporary memories are eventually transferred to long-term memory. As mentioned previously, it is known that emotions affect memory—both positively and negatively. A student who has made an emotional investment is more likely to be attentive. Simulations, role-playing, journal writing, and real-world experiences are all examples of strategies to help students connect emotions to content.

The findings listed here are just a small number of the discoveries that can profoundly affect teaching and learning. To help understand exactly how this information can be helpful, it is important to revisit the senses.

The Senses

The senses are the main conduit through which a learner experiences and interacts with the learning environment. Neuroscience has identified specific regions of the brain that play crucial roles in visual, auditory, and kinesthetic processing.[6] The primary senses used in learning have been identified as auditory (hearing), visual (seeing), and kinesthetic or tactile (physical movement or touch). Smell is the strongest sense to access long-term memory. Most people have sensory preferences for how they receive information from their environment. Due to the sensory impact on learning, use of reality-based scenarios in the classroom is essential in developing a student's ability to utilize their senses regarding situational awareness, both at scene arrival and throughout patient care. Implementing smells, sounds, and realistic patient situations fosters critical thinking as well as a culture of safety.

Each person has a preferred method of processing or thinking. For instance, some prefer an analytical approach to organizing information while others may prefer a more global approach and need to see the end result before the pieces of information make sense. How a learner organizes and processes information is a fluid dynamic and occurs as a natural part of thinking. It is difficult to separate organizing from processing because they often occur in concert with one another. Collectively, these preferences have been termed a **learning style**.

Early on, Carol Ann Tomlinson (1999) suggested that how students learned involves more than a learning style.[7] Research in neuroscience has supported this contention.[1,2,5] Much of the current research supports Tomlinson's initial proposal that (in addition to a learning style) how the learner processes, remembers, and uses what is learned; their intelligence; culture; and gender all contribute to learning outcomes. She proposed using the term *learning profile* because it was more accurate. While that terminology has not gained widespread acceptance, current learning style models, such as Dunn and Dunn's Learning Style Model, include a variety of factors. **FIGURE 5.1** depicts categories and factors included in Dunn and Dunn's learning styles.

The Controversy

While there may continue to be controversy on the depth of impact of learning styles on knowledge and skill acquisition, research is ongoing. An understanding of learning styles can be applied in mentoring, precepting, and presentation styles in the classroom and lab setting. Flexibility and creativity in content delivery in working with students with different preferences may assist students in understanding information and acquiring skills more easily, better cementing them into long-term memory. Educators can change how

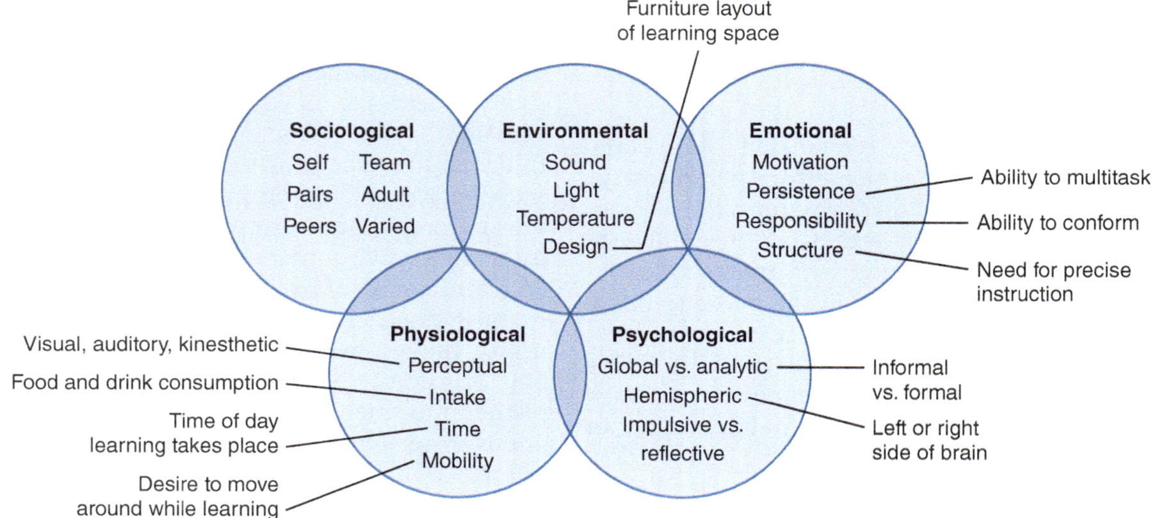

FIGURE 5.1 Dunn and Dunn Learning Style Model.

Modified from Bhat, Mehraj Ahmad. 2014. "Understanding the Learning Styles and Its Influence on Teaching/Learning Process." *International Journal of Education and Psychological Research* 3, no. 1: 9–13.

information is shared and assessed for better knowledge achievement. Educators should work toward having a variety of methods to teach within the domains of learning to obtain positive student outcomes.

Introduction to Learning Styles

Many educators adopted the learning style definition proposed by Dunn and Dunn: "A learning style is the way in which each learner begins to concentrate on, process, absorb, and retain new and difficult information."[8] This textbook uses the following modification: Learning style is a unique means of taking in, processing, and retaining knowledge and skills.

Using learning styles to help guide classroom activities can be very helpful. To begin, it helps to examine two undisputed facts: First, people do not all learn in the same way or at the same pace. Some read instructions first, and others just put things together and do not read instructions unless things do not work. Others listen to the presentation first, then read the textbook. Others need to see a skill in action before the written or spoken explanation makes sense.

Second, some topics lend themselves to a specific modality. For instance, students will not learn to apply a traction splint by hearing about it; they must handle the device and manipulate the parts before learning how to apply it. In this way, it becomes integrated into long-term memory. Similarly, students will not learn to prepare documentation by just watching someone fill out a patient care report.

Richard Felder, a teaching/learning scholar from North Carolina State University, indicates that the ideal balance among learning style categories depends on the subject, level, and learning objectives of the course and the backgrounds and skills of the students. Providing opportunity for students to be aware of their learning preferences can assist them with class preparation, with reading assignments, and with note-taking skills.

If educators follow the premise that the point of using learning styles is to achieve a balance between the preferences of the chosen model, then all students will have a degree of comfort in the modality they prefer. They also may develop important skills they might never develop if only taught in their preferred mode. Therefore, developing an understanding of learning styles can be helpful in creating a stimulating climate for learning. The goal of applying and utilizing learning style techniques is to enhance understanding through higher-level thought processes, enable application of textbook information to real-world situations, and achieve long-term retention.

Learning Styles

Learning styles are multidimensional; that is, they involve sensory input, organizing/processing, context, experience, and environment. Because of this, the learning styles of students will vary both within individual students and within the group. An educator may have to simultaneously reach learners who are visual, analytic, and independent, as well as those who are kinesthetic, global, and social—and all variations in between.

An important point to remember is that adult learners, although they have a learning preference, can adjust to other learning styles and use different styles for learning different types of material. Adults are capable of learning in almost any situation. However, the efficiency and enjoyment of the learning process for each student will vary, depending on how closely it matches their preferred learning style. For example, a visual learner may be required to listen to a podcast as part of a class assignment. Although they may not find this experience as pleasurable as seeing an illustrated lecture on the same topic and may need to listen to the audio recording repeatedly to master the material, the student can ultimately learn from the exercise.

Educators commonly remark that they have students who are "book smart" but cannot seem to grasp practical skills (these students are often assimilators or convergers, as discussed later in this chapter). Other learners can memorize a long list of facts but cannot seem to put them all together to develop a coherent plan of patient care. In these cases, the problem is not that these learners lack intelligence; rather, they learn some material more easily when it is presented in a style that matches their learning preference. Likewise, students may struggle with material that is presented in a style that is not congruent with their preferred method of learning.

In addition to learners who prefer a specific sensory input when processing new material, some will place importance on the context in which the information is presented. For example, some learners can easily grasp theoretical concepts presented verbally or in writing, whereas others can learn the material only when it is presented through concrete examples.

Sensory Preferences

When sensory stimulation involves more than one sense, learners retain information better. Many educational resources note that up to 90% of information can be retained when a learner says what they are doing while performing an activity—just saying something aloud or writing it improves retention by 70%. The combination of seeing and hearing, such as with an illustrated lecture, improves retention by 50%; seeing alone provides 30%, hearing 20%, and reading 10% toward retention.[9] While the exact origin and accuracy of these specific numbers have been called into question, this sensory involvement explains why it is a common practice to supplement instruction with visual and auditory aids, such as slides and audiotapes. The educator must reach out to learners through as many senses as possible, to attempt to address as many individual learning styles as is reasonably possible.

Keep in mind that learning style involves, first, how information is acquired by the senses, then, how the brain perceives and processes that information, and finally, how the brain recalls that information. This section describes auditory, visual, and kinesthetic learning preferences.

Auditory Learners

People who learn best by hearing information are considered to prefer **auditory learning**. They benefit from oral presentation of information, discussion, listening, and verbalizing. They are comfortable listening to a taped lecture or an audiobook and, in general, want to talk about their learning (**FIGURE 5.2**). Auditory learners can be reached using phrases such as, "I hear you," and, "Listen up, class." These learners absorb didactic material best when it is taught through lectures, oral presentations, and class discussions.

When learning new skills, auditory learners must hear the instructions and any noise or tones produced by the equipment. For instance, when learning how to apply a traction splint, the auditory learner would prefer to have the instructions read to them as they observe its application.

When electrocardiogram (ECG) recognition is introduced, the auditory learner would be best taught by speaking out the rhythms, such as, "Beat, beat, complex, beat, beat, complex" for a second-degree block. They would also be inclined to "talk their way through" analyzing the ECG strip. In practice, an auditory learner would want to turn on and listen to the cardiac monitor tone while treating a patient.

Visual Learners

Individuals who need to see what they are learning are considered to prefer **visual learning**. They benefit from the visual presentation of material and learn best when they can look things up, write things down, and watch the performance of a skill. Educators can help these learners "see" the words by using handouts, videotapes, pictures, slides, overheads, illustrations, posters, radiographs, X-rays (**FIGURE 5.3**), and moulage. These individuals may speak in terms of "seeing you around" and "try to picture this." Returning to the traction splint and ECG examples, visual learners need to look at the splint and observe its application prior to applying it themselves. In terms of the ECG example, they prefer to study an ECG strip and perhaps mark intervals to help determine the rhythm. They tend to watch the monitor whenever possible.

Kinesthetic Learners

People who learn through physical movement are considered to prefer **kinesthetic learning**. They prefer to associate movement and tactile experiences with learning. Educators can enhance learning for kinesthetic learners by providing opportunities for students to take things

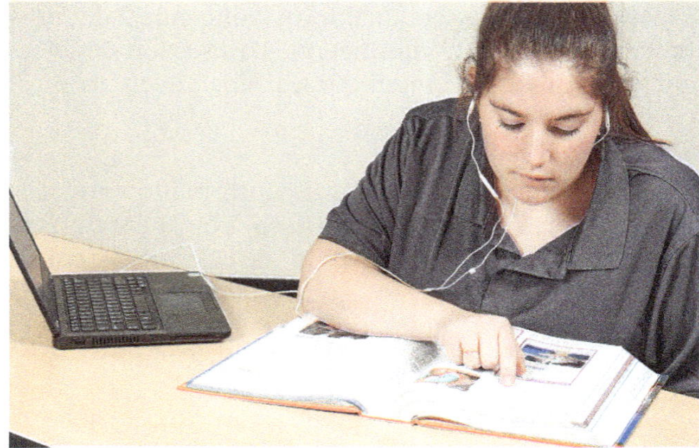

FIGURE 5.2 An example of auditory learning.

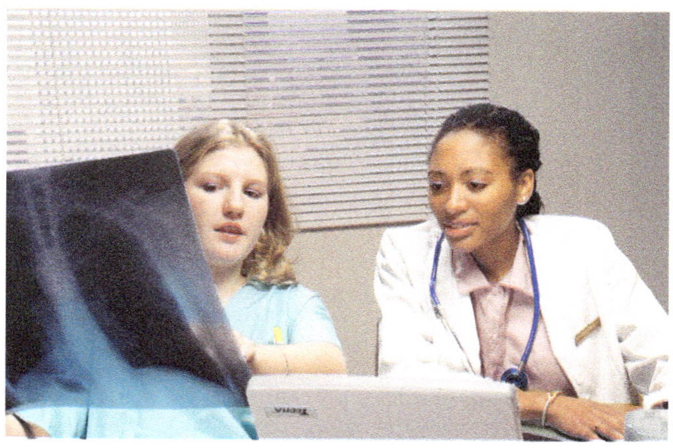

FIGURE 5.3 Visual learners may benefit from relating anatomy classes to X-rays.

apart, make things work, and use their hands for tactile stimulation (**FIGURE 5.4**). For example, when teaching the anatomy of the heart, the educator could pass around an anatomic model so students can feel the structure or dissect an animal heart, cutting it apart to identify the chambers and feel the thickness of the walls, etc. Kinesthetic learners may say "catch you around," or, "let's get going." Laboratory sessions, scenarios using manikins/programmed actors with actual equipment, and role-playing are all effective learning activities for kinesthetic learners. They can also benefit from "air writing," in which key terms, formulas, and other short statements are written in the air with the hand or finger.

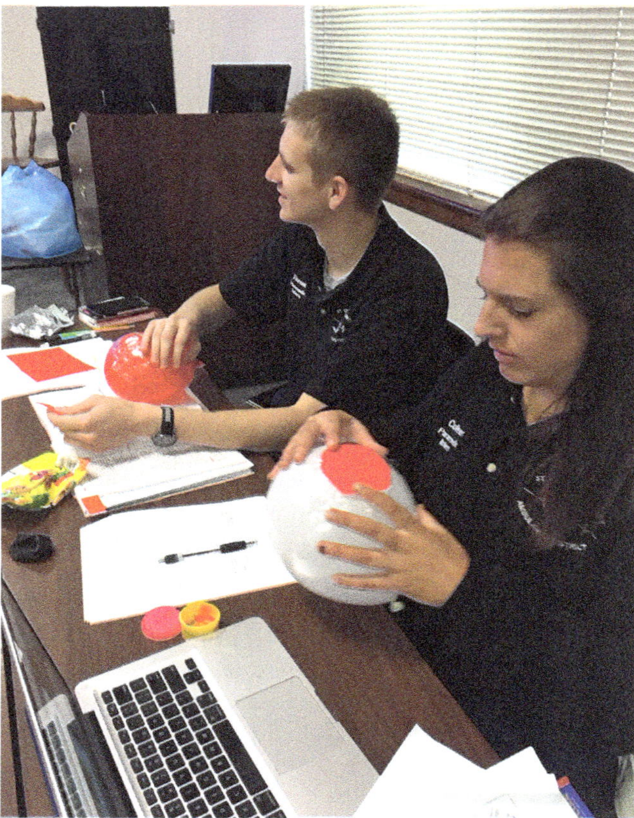

FIGURE 5.4 Touching and feeling things can help the kinesthetic learner to understand and retain information.

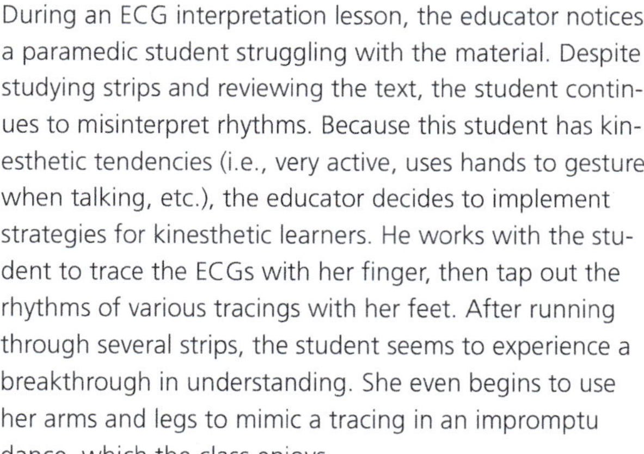

CASE in Point

During an ECG interpretation lesson, the educator notices a paramedic student struggling with the material. Despite studying strips and reviewing the text, the student continues to misinterpret rhythms. Because this student has kinesthetic tendencies (i.e., very active, uses hands to gesture when talking, etc.), the educator decides to implement strategies for kinesthetic learners. He works with the student to trace the ECGs with her finger, then tap out the rhythms of various tracings with her feet. After running through several strips, the student seems to experience a breakthrough in understanding. She even begins to use her arms and legs to mimic a tracing in an impromptu dance, which the class enjoys.

Organizing and Processing Information

Once information is gained through the senses, the brain organizes and processes it in a preferred manner. This occurs on both a cognitive level and through experience. Methods of organizing and processing information include the following characteristics:

- Analytic
- Global
- Social
- Independent

Analytic Learners

People who are logical thinkers organize and process information logically, sequentially, and in small parts that build toward a whole. These individuals are considered to prefer **analytic learning** and are often described as "left-brained." Using the analogy of a forest and the trees, the analytic learner has to separate the forest from the trees. In so doing, this learner cannot see the forest for the trees. They will look at every tree in the forest before feeling certain enough to conclude that it is a forest. For instance, when assessing a patient for difficulty breathing, this student will look for all signs of difficulty breathing before concluding that difficulty breathing is present.

Analytic learners work comfortably by following a protocol or algorithm. They are well served by lectures that follow outlines, clear reading assignments, and multiple choice questions on exams. They typically enjoy spelling, numbers, reading, analysis, and speaking. Using the ECG example, the analytic learner will look at an ECG strip and immediately begin a systematic analysis: Is it regular or irregular? Fast or slow? Is there a P wave? As another example, analytic learners may categorize signs and symptoms of respiratory diseases with each one on a separate index card. Once they have learned the diseases individually, they can then begin to compare and contrast similarities and differences in the respiratory patient presentations, which will be needed as they begin to perform scenarios with these patient complaints.

When learning a skill, analytic learners benefit from detailed steps of the procedure provided in written and visual materials. These students are most comfortable mastering steps and specific information. They need encouragement to learn judgment and global, applied concepts.

Structure, in terms of both educational process and material presented, is important to analytic learners. They may get frustrated if they discover inconsistencies between what is said in class and what their books say, or between what is taught and what they have previously learned. In addition, they may be uncomfortable with learning that is out of sequence, or when the order of learning has been changed or rearranged. For the analytic learner, order of delivery and consistency in the message are very important.

These learners may get tied up in the details, which may delay decision making. It may be of benefit if the educator can help them determine when an end point has been reached so they can make a decision.

Global Learners

People who think in terms of the big picture and who need to see the whole before the parts are considered prefer **global learning**. They are often described as "right-brained." Returning to the forest and the trees analogy, the global learner will look at several trees, quickly declare it a forest, and then begin to see individual trees. This is the student who cannot see the trees for the forest. They are the ones who, at first glance, quickly declare the patient is having a myocardial infarction and, when they are asked how they know, may say "I just know." The clues the patient exhibited (clutching chest, sweating, body position, facial expression, etc.) must be brought to their conscious attention.

These learners tend to be creative, artistic, imaginative, emotional, and intuitive. They may be less likely to follow protocol, preferring to treat patients based on outcome, rather than on process. Global learners can also process information simultaneously; thus, they may easily move back and forth between activities and tasks. A common example of the global learner is the student who can be engaged in a motor task while giving instructions to others or interacting with students who are doing other tasks.

When teaching global learners, it is important for the educator to start with an overview of the lesson, so the students know where they are going. These students are most comfortable focusing on the global concepts and intuition, and they need encouragement to learn specific steps and the theory behind applications. They also need to be encouraged to think of "what else could this be" to avoid tunnel vision.

Global learners may enjoy working in teams. If the pace of instruction lags or is too tedious, they may become bored or distracted because they have already moved ahead to the conclusion. Techniques appropriate for these learners include mental imagery, drawing, maps, metaphors, and experiential learning.

These learners run the risk of jumping to conclusions that may or may not be accurate. They need to be encouraged to think of likely possibilities to avoid tunnel vision. These learners benefit from going back to look at the parts to justify their conclusions.

Social Learners

People who process information best when engaged in multiple tasks in busy environments with other learners are considered to prefer **social learning**

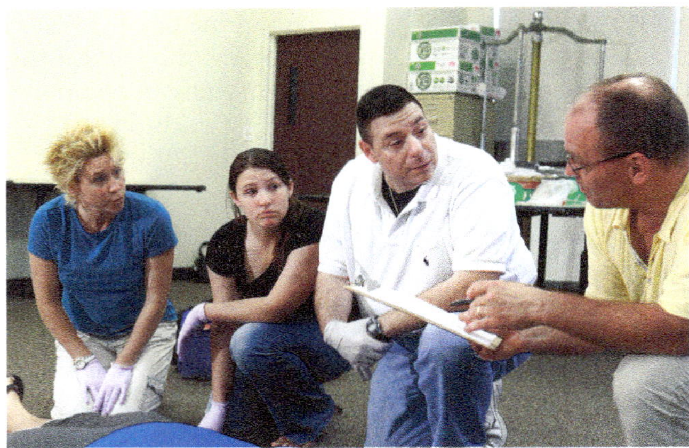

FIGURE 5.5 Social learners usually enjoy group projects and teamwork activities.

(**FIGURE 5.5**). They tend to enjoy study sessions, group projects, and cooperative learning. Educators should provide opportunities for group work in class, classroom discussions, study groups, and skills groups. For social learners, background noise in the classroom or practice area, such as music or a radio, is not necessarily distracting and can even be helpful to a point. Social networking media can be used to facilitate learning for these individuals. An example of an activity for learners who prefer peer interaction is to provide a small group of students with a case study to discuss and determine the diagnosis and treatment interventions. Such collaboration encourages effective communication skills, teamwork, and the process of critically thinking through the emergence of several possibilities identified to achieve the goal.

Independent Learners

People who prefer to process and organize information independently, isolated from other learners, are considered to prefer **independent learning**. They tend to seek quiet, undisturbed study environments, and react well to reading assignments, written exams, and reports. They may be uncomfortable in "touchy-feely" classroom situations led by an educator who encourages social interaction through group exercises and projects. The response and demeanor of independent learners should not be mistaken by the social educator as lack of enthusiasm or disdain for the content; rather, the student may be uncomfortable with the presentation style. When asked to participate in a group, independent learners do better when they receive an assignment, have time to work by themselves, and then return to the group with the results.

Experiential Learning Styles

In addition to cognitive learning styles, educators need to be aware of their students' **experiential learning** styles.[9] This is especially true when considering practical experiences both in the field and in the classroom.

Experiential learning provides the benefit of involving all of the senses in an active learning process. Edelman and Tononi state it simply as "doing precedes understanding."[10] Additionally, experience can involve an emotional reaction, which results in a change of body state (COBS).[10,11] COBS helps by focusing attention. This involves the hippocampus (a part of the reticular activating system) in quickly creating a durable memory store of the experience that includes all of the individual's senses. Research suggests that experience dictates future decision making (more than classroom teaching) in a real-world environment.[2] The impact of experiential learning can be enhanced by well-run debriefings when experiences are discussed in a nonpunitive environment.

Experiential learning styles are broken into four components:

- Convergers
- Divergers
- Assimilators
- Accommodators

Convergers

The **converger** has dominant abilities in abstract conceptualization and active experimentation. A converger favors the practical application of ideas. When teaching convergers, they will strive to find the reasoning behind why a new concept or skill matters before they are willing to try something new. Ideas without obvious practical applications, such as microbiology, may be difficult for them to grasp unless the connection to practice is made.

Divergers

The **diverger** brings together concrete experimentation and reflective observation. Divergers are reflective and like to think through their experiences. They are skilled observers and often would prefer to watch something done first before they have an experience.

Often, they reflect on an experience long after it occurred, even if they were not directly involved.

Assimilators

A combination of abstract conceptualization and reflective observation defines the **assimilator**, who is apt to create theoretical models. Assimilators like to understand the theory before they put something into practice. Assimilators tend to believe that, without understanding the theory completely, they cannot treat a patient. For example, they need to understand why a medicine or procedure works before they try it.

Accommodators

An **accommodator** is a doer and is often the first to volunteer for a new experience. This person adapts to the circumstances at hand, usually through plans and experimentation. This characteristic represents the union of concrete experience and active experimentation. Accommodators often jump into a new experience, even if they have not learned the new concept, just to "try it out." Accommodators do not see the reason for learning theory when they can just do it.

Assessing Students' Learning Styles

Before developing an instructional plan that addresses variations in student learning styles, the educator may want to assess the learning styles of the people in the group. Because those who pursue a given profession often have similar learning styles, an assessment can allow the educator to focus on the predominant learning style of the group of students.

An educator can assess students' learning styles informally in various ways, including talking with students and getting to know them; observing their behavior individually and in groups when different teaching strategies are employed; and analyzing their success in learning and retention, given different teaching strategies. For example, when an educator is talking with a student, if the student uses gestures or moves about, the educator observes that the student may be a kinesthetic learner. If the educator notices that a student speaks the words to himself while reading, then the student most likely is an auditory learner. If, after material is presented by lecture, the student does not do as well on a quiz than they did with previous material presented via video, the student is probably a visual learner. Educators can also assess students using a formal assessment process or a standardized test; this can occur as part of a program entrance-exam process or at the beginning of an individual course.

The educator is cautioned against using test results to "prejudge" learners. Many factors beyond learning style preference, such as innate intelligence, motivation, previous learning success, and culture, contribute to learning and student success. Finally, even if the class appears to have a dominant learning style, the educator must continue to vary the instructional approach to stimulate as many senses as possible.

Although many standardized tests for learning styles exist, those that are most commonly used in health professions education include the Dunn and Dunn[8] Learning Style Inventory, the Health Occupations Basic Entrance Test, and the Myers–Briggs Type Indicator.

Learning Style Inventories

The concept of determining an individual's learning style was pioneered by Kolb, with the introduction of Kolb's Learning Style Inventory.[11] The inventory is completed by answering a series of questions that identify a person's preference for learning in four areas: concrete experience, reflective observation, active conceptualization, and active experimentation. Kolb refers to these four areas as "learning cycles." By adding together scores for the various learning cycles, four types of learners are identified, as discussed earlier: converger, diverger, assimilator, and accommodator (**FIGURE 5.6**).

In addition to Kolb's inventory, other measures of assessing learning style have been developed. The learning style model of Rita Dunn and Kenneth Dunn, mentioned earlier and depicted in Figure 5.1, is one of the most researched and tested learning style inventories.[12] This model breaks learning styles down into five stimuli, each with its own group of elements (**TABLE 5.1**). The learner completes an inventory, which asks questions related to the five stimuli and their elements. From the information gleaned about the elements, a learner can categorize their preference for learning in terms of the five main stimuli. This inventory gives the learner more information about how they like to learn than is provided by the cognitive information–processing model of Kolb, which tells the learner how they learn. The Dunn and Dunn model also provides more information on learning preferences that is of value to the educator.

The Myers–Briggs Type Indicator (MBTI) is another popular and well-researched model. The MBTI

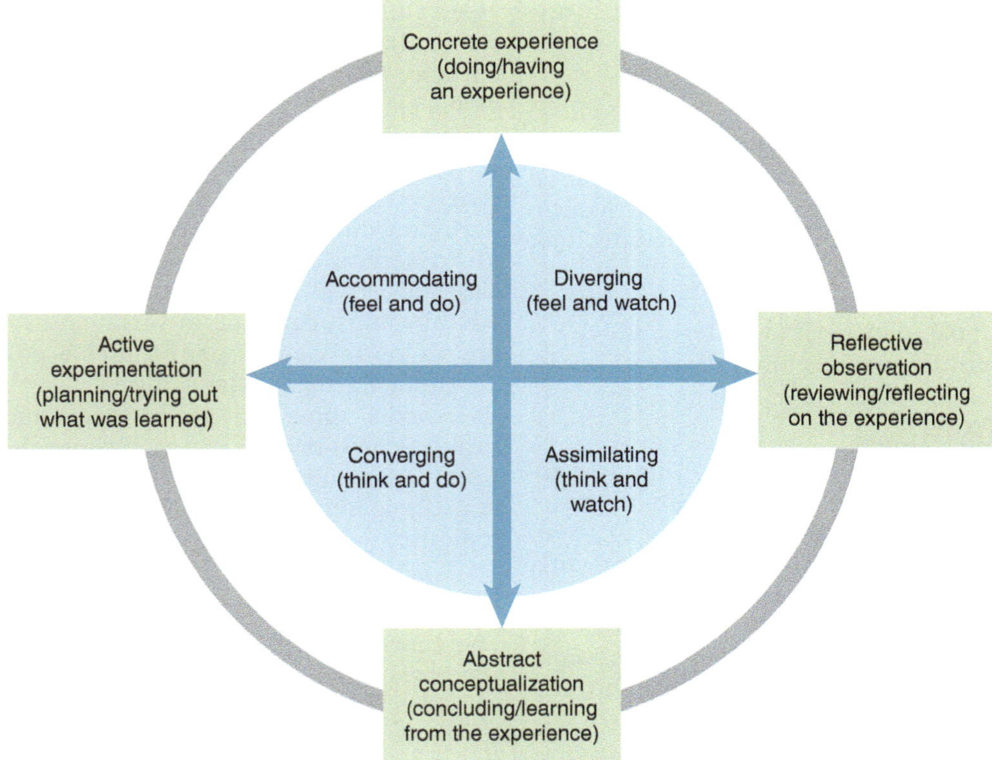

FIGURE 5.6 Experiential learning styles; Kolb's learning style model.

Modified from Bhat, Mehraj Ahmad. 2014. "Understanding the Learning Styles and Its Influence on Teaching/Learning Process." *International Journal of Education and Psychological Research* 3, no. 1: 9–13.

TABLE 5.1 The Learning Style Model

Stimuli	Elements
Environmental	Lighting Sound Temperature Seating arrangement
Emotional	Motivation Persistence Responsibility Structure
Sociologic (i.e., how people learn)	Alone or with peers Authoritative adult or collegial colleague Variety in learning or routine pattern
Physiological	Perceptual skills Time-of-day energy levels Intake (eating) Mobility
Psychological	Hemispheric Impulsive or reflective Global or analytic

Modified from Damasio, Antonio. 2000. *The Feeling of What Happens: Body and Emotion in the Making of Consciousness*. New York: Harcourt Brace.

is designed to determine a person's personality type.[13] It is based on the theory of personality characteristics and types originally developed by the psychoanalyst Carl Jung in the early 1900s. Isabel Myers and Katharine Briggs expanded on Jung's theory to the extent it is today.[13] The MBTI determines preferences on four dichotomies:

1. **Extraversion–Introversion**. Describes where people prefer to focus their attention and get their energy—from the outer world of people and activity, or their inner world of ideas and experiences
2. **Sensing–Intuition**. Describes how people prefer to take in information—focused on what is real and actual, or on patterns and meanings in data
3. **Thinking–Feeling**. Describes how people prefer to make decisions—based on logical analysis, or guided by concern for the impact on others
4. **Judging–Perceiving**. Describes how people prefer to deal with the outer world—in a planned, orderly way, or in a flexible, spontaneous way

Multiple Intelligences Toolbox[15]

Logical/Mathematical

- Abstract symbols/formulas
- Calculation
- Deciphering codes
- Forcing relationships (connecting ideas)
- Graphic/cognitive organizers
- Logic/pattern games
- Number sequences/patterns
- Outlining
- Problem solving
- **Syllogisms**

Musical/Rhythmic

- Environmental sounds
- Instrumental sounds
- Music composition/creation
- Music performance
- Percussion vibrations
- Rapping
- Rhythmic patterns
- Singing/humming
- Tonal patterns
- Vocal sounds/tones

Bodily/Kinesthetic

- Body language/physical gestures
- Body sculpture/tableaus
- Dramatic enactment
- Folk/creative dance
- Gymnastic routines
- Human graph
- Inventing
- Physical exercise/martial arts
- Role-playing/mime
- Sports games

Verbal/Linguistic

- Creative writing
- Formal speaking
- Humor/jokes
- Impromptu speaking
- Journal/diary keeping
- Poetry
- Reading
- Storytelling/story creation
- Verbal debate
- Vocabulary

Interpersonal

- Collaborative skills teaching
- Cooperative learning strategies
- Empathy practices
- Giving feedback
- Group projects
- Intuiting others' feelings
- Jigsaw
- Person-to-person communication
- Receiving feedback
- Sensing others' motives

Intrapersonal

- Altered states of consciousness practices
- Emotional processing
- Focusing/concentration skills
- Higher-order reasoning
- Independent studies/projects
- Know thyself procedures
- Metacognition techniques
- Mindfulness practices
- Silent reflection methods
- Thinking strategies

Visual/Spatial

- Active imagination
- Color/texture schemes
- Drawing
- Guided imagery/visualizing
- Mind mapping
- Montage/collage
- Painting
- Patterns/designs
- Pretending/fantasy
- Sculpting

Naturalist

- Archetypal pattern recognition
- Caring for plants/animals
- Conservation practices
- Environmental feedback
- Hands-on labs
- Nature encounters/field trips
- Nature observation
- Natural world simulations
- Species classification (organic/inorganic)
- Sensory stimulation exercises

Instructor's Lesson Guide Sample[16]

Course: Paramedic

Session Reference: 6–5

Topic: Heart blocks

Level of Instruction: Cognitive

Time Required: 3 hours

References: Paramedic ECG textbook based on education standards

Preparation

Attention: Instructor provided

Motivation: Instructor provided

Objective: At the conclusion of this lesson, the student will be able to identify the three degrees of cardiac conduction blocks, given a real or simulated ECG tracing, without assistance, to a written test accuracy of 75%.

Overview:

- Anatomy and physiology of the heart
- Supraventricular conduction system
- 1st-degree block
- 2nd-degree block
- 3rd-degree block

Learning Activities

Verbal/Linguistic

In pairs, students read, discuss, and question textbook information.

Visual/Spatial

Students identify on a heart model the location of the sinoatrial (SA) and the atrioventricular (AV) nodes, the internodal pathways, and the nodal blood supply.

Musical/Rhythmic

Students compose a percussion piece that mimics the flow of the electrical pulse through a heart with the blocks.

Intrapersonal

Individually, students identify life events that involved a delay or blockage of communications with another person.

Logical/Mathematical

In small groups, students develop flow charts of the conduction pulse moving through the heart.

Bodily/Kinesthetic

Using paper and soda straws, as well as glue and scissors, students construct models of the heart's conduction system.

Interpersonal

Students role-play patients with each degree of heart block and share symptoms with each other.

Naturalist

Students create lists of events in nature that are similar to the underlying pathophysiology of the heart.

Summary

Review

- Anatomy and physiology of the heart
- Supraventricular conduction system
- 1st-degree block
- 2nd-degree block
- 3rd-degree block

Summary

Each learner brings to the classroom a preference for the ways they perceive, process, and store information. To maximize learning, the educator must be aware of these differences, must employ a variety of teaching strategies, and must provide a variety of learning activities that will reach all students. Similarly, educators must be sensitive to the fact that they, too, have a preference for learning that influences their teaching style and their interaction with students.

The traditional approach to learning styles has been to describe them in terms of sensory perception and social interaction. Theories such as Gardner's multiple intelligences have expanded the view of learning styles and challenged educators and curriculum developers to introduce new and varying ways of presenting material.

Glossary

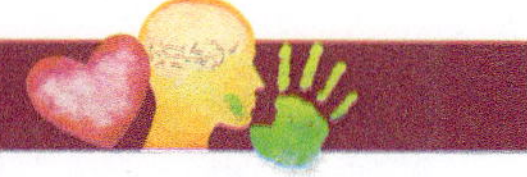

accommodator Experiential learning style in which concrete experience and active experimentation are preferred; favors doing.

analytic learning Preference for processing information in a logical, sequential manner.

assimilator Experiential learning style in which a combination of abstract conceptualization and reflective observation are preferred; favors creating theoretical models.

auditory learning Preference for learning through sound.

converger Experiential learning style in which abstract conceptualization and active experimentation are the dominant preferences; favors practical application of ideas.

diverger Experiential learning style in which concrete experimentation and reflective observation are preferred; favors observing before experiencing.

experiential learning Active learning process that engages all senses.

global learning Preference for processing information by seeing the whole before the parts.

independent learning Preference for processing information alone rather than in a group setting.

kinesthetic learning Preference for learning through touch.

learning style Preferred method of learning.

social learning Preference for processing information effectively while multitasking in a group setting.

syllogism Type of argument in logic that contains a major and minor premise and a conclusion.

visual learning Preference for learning through imagery.

References

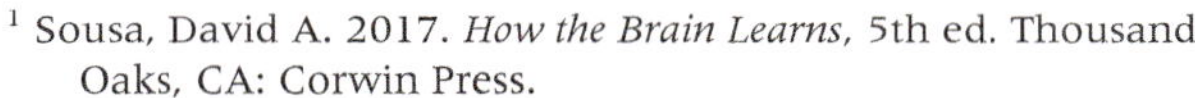

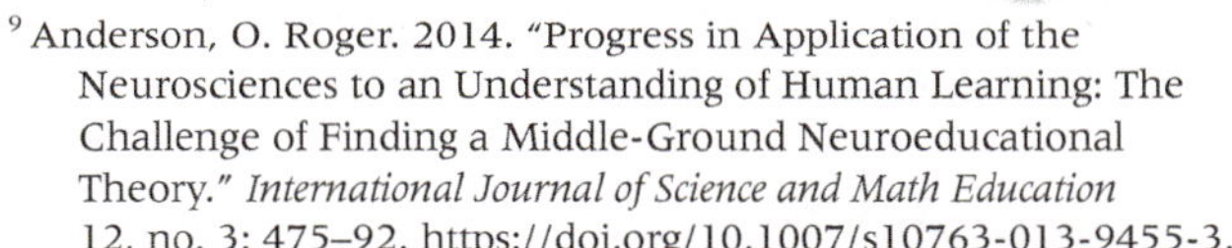

[1] Sousa, David A. 2017. *How the Brain Learns*, 5th ed. Thousand Oaks, CA: Corwin Press.

[2] Medina, John. 2008. *Brain Rules: 12 Principles for Surviving and Thriving at Work, Home and School*. Seattle: Pear Press.

[3] Yeung, Nick, Leigh E. Nystrom, Jessica A. Aronson, and Jonathan D. Cohen. 2006. "Between-Task Competition and Cognitive Control in Task Switching." *Journal of Neuroscience* 26, no. 5: 1429–38. https://doi.org/10.1523/JNEUROSCI.3109-05.2006.

[4] Spink, Amanda, Charles Cole, and Mary Waller. 2008. "Multitasking Behavior." *Annual Review of Information Science and Technology* 42, no. 1: 96–8. https://doi.org/10.1002/aris.2008.1440420110.

[5] Jensen, Eric. 2006. *Enriching the Brain*. San Francisco: Jossey-Bass.

[6] Howard-Jones, Paul A. 2014. "Neuroscience and Education: Myths and Messages." *Nature Reviews Neuroscience* 15: 817–24. https://doi.org/10.1038/nrn3817.

[7] Tomlinson, Carol A. 1999. *The Differentiated Classroom: Responding to the Needs of All Learners*. Alexandria, VA: Association for Supervision and Curriculum Development.

[8] Dunn, Rita S., and Kenneth J. Dunn. 1978. *Teaching Students through Their Individual Learning Styles: A Practical Approach*. Reston, VA: Reston Publishing.

[9] Anderson, O. Roger. 2014. "Progress in Application of the Neurosciences to an Understanding of Human Learning: The Challenge of Finding a Middle-Ground Neuroeducational Theory." *International Journal of Science and Math Education* 12, no. 3: 475–92. https://doi.org/10.1007/s10763-013-9455-3.

[10] Edelman, Gerald, and Giulio Tononi. 2000. *A Universe of Consciousness: How Matter Becomes Imagination*. New York: Basic Books.

[11] Damasio, Antonio. 2000. *The Feeling of What Happens: Body and Emotion in the Making of Consciousness*. New York: Harcourt Brace.

[12] Jensen, Eric. 2008. *Brain-Based Learning: The New Paradigm of Teaching*, 2nd ed. Thousand Oaks, CA: Corwin Press.

[13] Myers, Isabel, and Peter B. Myers. 1995. *Gifts Differing*. Palo Alto, CA: Consulting Psychologists Press, Inc.

[14] Keirsey. n.d. "What Is Your Temperament?" Accessed March 30, 2019. http://www.keirsey.com.

[15] Lazear, David. 1999. *Eight Ways of Knowing: Teaching for Multiple Intelligences*, 3rd ed. Arlington Heights, IL: Skylight Professional Development.

[16] Campbell, Linda, Bruce Campbell, and Dee Dickinson. 1999. *Teaching and Learning through Multiple Intelligences*. Needham Heights, MA: Allyn & Bacon.

Additional Resources

Lalley, James P., and Robert H. Miller. 2007. "The Learning Pyramid: Does It Point Teachers in the Right Direction?" *Education* 128, no. 1: 64–79.

Pashler, Harold, Mark McDaniel, Doug Rohrer, and Robert Bjork. 2008. "Learning Styles: Concepts and Evidence." *Science in the Public Interest* 9, no. 3: 106–16. https://doi.org/10.1111/j.1539-6053.2009.01038.x.

Riener, Cedar, and Daniel Willingham. 2010. "The Myth of Learning Styles." *Change: The Magazine of Higher Learning* 42, no. 5: 32–5. https://doi.org/10.1080/00091383.2010.503139.

Willingham, Daniel T., Elizabeth M. Hughes, and David G. Dobolyi. 2015. "The Scientific Status of Learning Styles Theories." *Teaching of Psychology* 42, no. 3: 266–71. https://doi.org/10.1177/0098628315589505.

CHAPTER 6

Culture in the EMS Classroom

OBJECTIVES

At the conclusion of this chapter, the educator will be able to:

Cognitive Domain

1. Recognize the dimensions of culture.
2. Define *cultural competency* and *cultural humility*.
3. Describe how instructor biases can impact student outcomes.
4. Outline the many ways in which students can be different from one another.
5. Distinguish between equity and equality.
6. List ways to incorporate classroom strategies that embrace student differences.
7. Describe how to develop a culturally sound curriculum.

Psychomotor Domain

There are no psychomotor objectives for this chapter.

Affective Domain

1. Commit to the need to teach through a cultural lens.
2. Create a learning environment that honors the values, beliefs, and characteristics of each student.

"We are all different, which is great because we are all unique. Without diversity life would be very boring."

~ Catherine Pulsifer

CHAPTER GOAL The goal of this chapter is for the educator to explore strategies to teach effectively in a culturally diverse classroom.

Individuals view life through a unique set of perspectives, shaped by years of accumulated experiences and interactions with the world. They absorb and reject the thoughts, opinions, and ideas of others based on the lives they have lived. Within the emergency medical services (EMS) classroom, educators should allow and encourage the presentation of dissimilar, and sometimes conflicting, viewpoints. Instructors have the ability and power to provide the information and setting necessary to promote better awareness and understanding of diversity among students, both within the classroom and later outside of the classroom, when students enter the field as interns and finally as practitioners. The United States has one of the most diverse populations of people, ideas, and cultures in the world. Most people have heard the United States referred to as a "melting pot." Population data bear that out, reflecting great diversity in age, race, and religion throughout the country.[1] Many EMS instructors and providers understand the complexities involved in caring for patients and working in a diverse society. However, the EMS profession could improve the elements of diversity seen in its curricula, its education processes, and its practitioners. The Longitudinal Emergency Medical Technician Attribute and Demographic Study (LEADS) indicated that approximately 85% of those registered with the National Registry of EMTs are male, and 85% are white.[2] Because there appears to be a disparity between the diversity of the general population of the nation and that of EMS providers, it is crucial that the instructor work toward including elements of culture and diversity throughout the curriculum.

This chapter cannot and should not serve as the only guide in that effort. It will, however, identify key concepts (1) to better prepare EMS providers to treat patients within a diverse population, and (2) to improve diversity within the profession, beginning with a culturally aware educational environment (**FIGURE 6.1**).

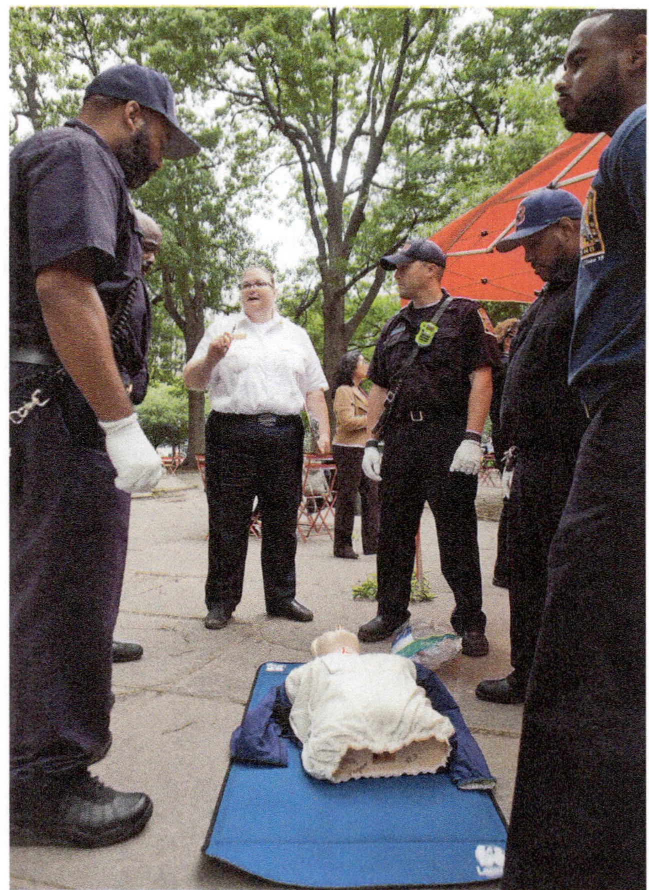

FIGURE 6.1 Instructors have the ability to promote understanding of diversity among students and patients.

Teaching through a Cultural Lens

Much of what informs people about the world around them is in the culture that surrounds them, often in unseen ways. Within this context, **culture** is defined as the attitude, values, and behaviors of a particular group of individuals. All people belong to more than one culture; within the EMS classroom there may be a multiracial gay Christian male sitting next to a Caucasian heterosexual agnostic female who grew up in poverty. Both are in class to learn about the same topic and may have several shared values that attracted them to the profession. However, it is unlikely that they view the world around them in the same way. It is also unlikely that these students learn in identical ways. Multiply the differences in culture by the number of students in the classroom and it quickly becomes apparent that a one-size-fits-all approach to teaching will not be successful for all.

There has been ongoing debate and discourse over whether an individual from outside a culture can, through intent and study, become "competent" in the belief system of a particular culture (**cultural competency**). Early efforts to develop culturally competent curricula were often limited in scope and effect, focusing on overt behaviors such as dress, language, and customs. By its very nature, such curricula can only skim the surface of a multifaceted and complex set of parameters that define a culture.

Rather than try to become completely *competent* with all forms of culture that might exist within the classroom, it may be more effective for the instructor to develop a perspective of **cultural humility**—acknowledging that the understanding of culture is a never-ending process of exploration. Hook and colleagues defined cultural humility as the "ability to maintain an interpersonal stance that is other-oriented (or open to the other) in relation to aspects of cultural identity that are most important to the [person]."[3] In developing a sense of "other," the educator commits to developing a sense of self (self-critique and reflection), has a desire to correct power imbalances that exist within classrooms, and is willing to advocate for student success.[4]

In developing cultural humility, instructors must commit to several values, including the following:

- The concept that one's own ethnocentrism and background shape how they interact with students whose background is different from theirs
- That teaching and learning occurs against the broad backdrop of society and all of its dominant and subordinate values
- A willingness and ability to use culturally aware strategies to promote learning for all[5]

Becoming aware of culture and how it impacts learning is a challenge for any educator. It begins by learning about one's own sense of being.

CASE in Point

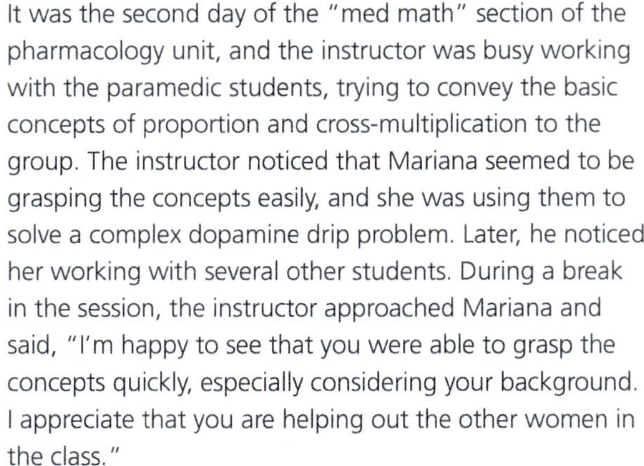

It was the second day of the "med math" section of the pharmacology unit, and the instructor was busy working with the paramedic students, trying to convey the basic concepts of proportion and cross-multiplication to the group. The instructor noticed that Mariana seemed to be grasping the concepts easily, and she was using them to solve a complex dopamine drip problem. Later, he noticed her working with several other students. During a break in the session, the instructor approached Mariana and said, "I'm happy to see that you were able to grasp the concepts quickly, especially considering your background. I appreciate that you are helping out the other women in the class."

There was a momentary pause in the classroom conversation, as the students closest to the instructor overheard the comment.

Mariana appeared puzzled. "Why are you surprised?" The instructor responded, a bit awkwardly, "I assumed that you probably were not well prepared in your high school math classes."

Silent for a moment, Mariana replied with a tinge of frustration, "I'm not sure why you would think that. Actually, I excelled in math. Furthermore, I resent the idea that I could only help other women, especially because I helped three male students as well!"

Instructor, Know Thyself

All humans are susceptible to having biases. This is not a value statement; it is simply fact. The Merriam Webster Dictionary defines **bias** as "an inclination of temperament or outlook; *especially* a personal and sometimes unreasoned judgment."[6] For example, an instructor may unreasonably believe that most people for whom English is a second language are unable to communicate as a healthcare provider. That instructor might feel obligated to use simpler words rather than the medical terms in order to "accommodate" these students. This instructor's judgment is not based on any reasoned discourse.

Bias can take many forms. Examples include bias against particular ethnicities, gender, ages, socioeconomic classes, religions, political persuasions, and sexual orientations. The Case in Point gives an example of a person who held multiple biases, which created a negative synergistic effect on his attitude and behavior toward others. In this case, the instructor has a bias against a Latina's ability to understand and excel in math.

Biases become dangerous when they are manifested as behaviors. An instructor's behavior in the classroom can and will affect the probability of success for many students. An instructor who believes students can succeed makes that prospect more likely than one who believes they will fail. Students' sense of self-efficacy (i.e., their sense of "I can do it!") is directly related to the classroom environment and the instructor's expectations of those students.[7] EMS instructors must be aware of the impact their attitudes may have on students, and they should remain diligent to prevent their own biases from negatively affecting the perceptions of those students.

To deal with or reduce bias, one must first acknowledge its existence. Performing a critical self-reflection and recognizing one's own personal biases are ways to begin a process of self-discovery and a greater awareness of one's own potential biases. Instructors should try to see lessons and other course materials through the perceptions of others and should consider enrolling in cultural diversity classes offered through a local college or university. For example, the U.S. Department of Health and Human Services Office of Minority Health has a free, online cultural competency curriculum for disaster preparedness and crisis response for educators to enroll and use in their classroom.[8] For instructors who have already critically examined and dealt with these issues, it remains incumbent upon them to challenge students to do the same.

TEACHING TIP

Ask a colleague to review exams and lesson plans for possible cultural bias.

Diversity in the Classroom

A tremendous amount has been written about cultural competency within a variety of environments, including the worksite and the classroom. Early efforts in EMS education focused on identification of the unique traits of specific groups, based on gender, ethnic, and religious lines.[9] Although those who made these attempts meant well, the truth is that the very act of defining group characteristics can reinforce stereotypes that such efforts are designed to minimize. Instructors who try to modify their teaching practices based on "laundry lists" of characteristics will quickly run into issues associated with any one-size-fits-all approach, namely, that not all members of a specific group of individuals are completely alike.

Stereotyping assumptions will likely cause discomfort for the student and the instructor. This discomfort may rise to a level of anger and open frustration that disrupts the class. Students within the classroom may include representatives from a wide variety of groups. Alternatively, instructors may be faced with a group of culturally similar students and may find themselves in the minority. How many ways can a single group of students be dissimilar?

- Age (younger versus older, nontraditional students)
- Appearance (e.g., hair length, hygiene, tattoos, piercings)
- Disorders (e.g., physical, emotional, and psychological/psychiatric disabilities)
- Gender identification (e.g., female, male, transgender)
- Generational (e.g., baby boomers, Gen-Xers, Gen-Yers, millennials)
- Learning ability (e.g., attention deficit disorder, dyslexia, underprepared educational background)

Generational Learning: Is There Really a Difference?

Much has been said, discussed, and debated about the role of generations and the ways people learn. There are many labels that the general media has used over the years to describe certain age groups; a simplified way to describe these differences is as follows:

- **Baby boomers**. Individuals born between the mid-1940s and mid-1960s; born in the era that included the post-World War II boom period in the United States and prior to the general mistrust of U.S. government involvement in Vietnam.
- **Gen-Xers**. Short for Generation X, a term first used by Douglas Coupland in a novel describing teenage lifestyles in the 1980s,[10] the birth dates of this generation span roughly from the mid-1960s to the early 1980s.
- **Millennials**. Sometimes termed "Generation Y," "Net-Gen," or the Digital Generation, their birth dates span from the 1980s to the late 1990s.
- **Post-millennials**. Also called Gen-Z or iGen, these individuals have birthdates spanning the mid-1990s to the mid-2010s. This is the generation that is currently entering the EMS workforce.
- **Gen-Alphas**. Those born between the mid-2010s and 2025.

A Web search will produce literally millions of popular articles, blogs, and opinions on the similarities and differences of perception, values, and judgments among the different generations. Yet there is little scientific data that supports specific educational methods, geared toward apparent generational traits, to actually improve learning outcomes.[11] For example, it would be a mistake to believe that a millennial student would learn better with technology-based tools, simply because they use social media sites easily, or possesses a smartphone, or sends text messages without a second thought. Rather, it has been suggested that the "Net-Gen" individual, while adept at being an end user of Internet technology, has a shallower base of knowledge about how the technologies work than previous generations,[12] and the instructor cannot assume that such students know how to use the technology in support of their learning.

Generational stereotypes, like any stereotypes, are poor criteria to use to select teaching tools or methods. *Keeping the information relevant, interesting, and appealing to the student's intrinsic values* is the educator's best tool for excellent teaching.

- Language ability (e.g., first language other than English, using poor grammar, depending heavily on slang)
- Marital status (e.g., cohabitating, divorced, married, single, widowed)
- Parenting (e.g., no children, older or younger children, stepchildren, adopted children, or older, dependent parents)
- Political views (e.g., conservatism, liberalism, libertarianism)
- Race/ethnicity (categories listed here are from the U.S. Census Bureau[1] and are used on most federal and state forms: American Indian, Alaska Native, Asian, Native Hawaiian or other Pacific Islander, Black or African American, Hispanic or Latino, White, and multiracial)
- Religion (e.g., Buddhism, Christianity, Islam, Romany, Wicca)
- Sexual orientation (e.g., bisexual, heterosexual, homosexual, asexual)
- Socioeconomic status (e.g., indigent, poor, middle class, wealthy)

Careful review of this list should lead to the realization that even apparently homogeneous students can be different in many ways. This should not be surprising, as it reinforces what is commonly known: *Each student is an individual* and does not deserve to be limited to being viewed as a "representative" of any one group. Students should be considered complex beings with much to offer the class. Each possesses experience and knowledge that can add to the richness of the classroom experience for other students and for the instructor.

Power in the Teaching Relationship

The relationship between student and instructor can be a powerful one, although not in the sense of power meaning "strength." In this case power refers to the control that an instructor exerts over the relationship with the student. For example, the instructor sets the teaching schedule, grades the tests, assigns the clinical rotations, and designs the curriculum, just to name a few obvious tasks. The student usually has little or no control over these areas. Another aspect of that control is the ability to decide what is taught in the classroom. The instructor may, knowingly or not, taint the material that is being taught by injecting elements of bias into lessons. Effects of bias can be seen in individual lessons and even throughout an entire curriculum. For example, although many major publishers have worked to minimize it, not all EMS textbooks equally portray individuals from ethnic minority groups and women in positions of authority.[13] In fact, the lack of diversity in a profession makes it difficult for publishers to obtain photos of a wide range of diverse providers. The images and the feel of a textbook can influence an entire course. This is not to say that diversity is the only element to consider when one is choosing a text; however, it is something that should be closely evaluated.

TEACHING TIP

When selecting a textbook, the instructor must be fully aware of the level of diversity (and equity) demonstrated in that text. It can be as straightforward as examining the number of images showing diversity of patients and EMS personnel, or the use of gender-specific pronouns such as "he" or "she."

Instructors should not be afraid of embracing diversity. Some instructors may be tempted to ignore student diversity when it could in fact contribute to the learning environment, not only of those individuals but also of the whole group. For example, an instructor may have students from a rural, agricultural community who could directly speak to the hazards of farm machinery. Students with medical military experience could speak to the provision of care in austere environments. Their unique cultural experiences could help to make the material more relevant for the entire class.[14] It would be tragic to ignore this wealth of information and to rely solely on textbooks.

TEACHING TIP

Learning about students' cultural differences occurs throughout the program. One strategy to begin the process is to ask students to pair up on the first day of class and tell each other something that few people know about. Then ask each member of the pair to incorporate that information as they introduce their partner to the rest of the class. This exercise can tease out clues about student experiences that are not necessarily caught in the formal application process.

Equity versus Equality

Equity is not equality. Equality implies that every student receives the same level of attention and support. Equity disputes the underlying notion that every student is equally prepared to succeed. Establishing equity within the classroom paves the way for success for every student. By recognizing that each student's academic ability is impacted by issues related to culture, the instructor can implement approaches that deliberately foster excellence in learning.

Fostering equity extends beyond the EMS classroom. The learning inequities associated with primary (K–12) education and poverty present a barrier to a profession that emphasizes reading as a primary method of learning information.[15] Students may need additional resources such as tutors and learning communities to overcome systemic barriers to academic success.

Opportunities to Integrate Classroom Diversity

There are many ways for an educator to create an environment that takes advantage of a classroom's diversity, rather than minimizes it. Not all approaches will work with every instructor. Instructors should decide which of the following suggestions might work for them, based on their background and comfort level. Then, they should try these suggestions or develop their own ideas; they may find these efforts to be surprisingly interesting and effective.

Instructional Materials

Attention to details influences the tone of the classroom. A small effort to include diversity in the names and characteristics of patient models, scenarios, printed materials, and visual aids goes a long way toward making students feel comfortable and valued in their learning situations.

Ethnicity and Gender

Spoken and written language should be racially/ethnically and gender nonspecific, or genders should be used with equal frequency. Contrived or forced neutrality (e.g., using "he/she") should be avoided. The instructor can use "he" or "she" in alternating scenarios and test questions or can use generic phrases such as "the patient" and "the EMT." Scenarios can be used to challenge misperceptions and to strengthen positive role models. For example, a scenario might be written in which the nurse is male and the EMS supervisor is female. By challenging traditional perceptions, these scenarios help to expose students to greater possibilities, so they can develop an openness to incorporating those possibilities into their practice.

Identifying the race, ethnicity, or gender of patients in written scenarios is not always necessary. In general, this information can be legitimately omitted, allowing students to focus on the clinical issues at hand. However, there are times when these characteristics are significant elements of a person's medical history (e.g., when genetic disorders such as sickle cell or Tay–Sachs disease are considered). When clinically indicated, ethnic and gender identifiers should be used. Care should be taken, however, to avoid reinforcing negative—and unfounded—stereotypes. Cite accurate statistics, and frame these relevant concepts against the broad background of medicine for the entire class.

It can be helpful to discuss the contributions of different ethnic groups to the field of medicine as part of the curriculum and not spotlight it as a side topic. A reference librarian can serve as an excellent resource.

Printed Material and Visual Aids

The educator should ensure that models and simulated situations reflect a wide variety of cultural backgrounds. For example, computer images of people of different genders and from various ethnic, cultural, and/or religious backgrounds can be used. Scripted scenarios should also incorporate a wide range of socioeconomic factors. Frequent reviews of textbooks by instructors for issues of equity and diversity will help to ensure the quality of the text and the degree to which it encourages diversity. Feedback from students is also helpful.

Instructional Strategies

Instructors who provide variations in teaching and learning strategies in their classrooms help ensure that they will meet the needs of a diverse group of students. For example, an instructor may allow students to submit a video, PowerPoint, or podcast in lieu of a written paper. However, educators must ensure fair assessment of student learning and avoid the risk of instructor bias when creating situations where an assessment is not fair for everyone.

Presentation

Rather than using only one type of presentation format (e.g., lecture), the educator should use a variety of teaching strategies. The student body within any given classroom community is likely to represent a wide range of learning styles. The use of multiple methods of instruction will help to enhance the learning of the class. Examples of teaching methods include small group exercises, take-home case studies, debates, large group discussions, Web-based lessons, and role-playing.

As information-sharing technology and social media continue to be integrated into everyday tasks, instructors can take advantage of the different platforms and provide even greater access to their educational material. For the generation of students who grew up with the Internet, the 24/7 availability of learning resources is not only useful, but expected. These developments do come with a caveat; what is posted by students and instructors in the public space may be easily misinterpreted, or worse, may be seen as insensitive and offensive. Educators must develop strong, consistent guidelines to ensure what is shown is a fair representation of the program and its participants.

Assessment

Instructors must be aware of their own biases when they are assessing a student's performance. It may be helpful to have students identify written assignments with a code name, or an institution-assigned identifier, so their identities are shielded during grading. Two or more instructors may videotape or observe practical scenarios and role-playing to establish an "average" score. These safeguards work in two ways: They help students by ensuring that they are not unfairly penalized, and they help instructors to avoid favoritism.

Student-Educator Relations

Learning is more likely to occur when an instructor creates a safe classroom climate. It is an important aspect of an instructor's role to take concrete steps to create that climate.

Awareness

Students come from diverse and complex backgrounds. *Nothing about them should be assumed.* For example, comments about social activities that assume all students are heterosexual, middle class, or Christian should be avoided. One must not assume that the most obvious perception of a student's ethnicity (or even gender) is correct (e.g., a person who might be thought of as Hispanic American may self-identify as white American). As the nation becomes increasingly diverse, the percentage of people who identify with a multiplicity of heritages (and races) also increases. Students must be permitted to explain who and what they are and how they want to be identified.

Terminology

The educator must be sensitive to changing terminology. For example, Asian Americans may not want to be referred to as Oriental, Hispanic Americans may prefer to be called "Chicano" or "Latino," and persons from diverse families may wish to be referred to as "multiracial." If it is necessary to categorize, *ask which labels are comfortable or preferable.*

Spotlighting

One must not force a student to be the spokesperson for any group. For example, when describing the higher frequency of alcoholism or diabetes within a particular group, the instructor must not single out a member of that group to be its spokesperson. An educator could simply pose a question about the disease to the entire class and allow anyone (including students who are members of the group disproportionately affected) to offer a response or personal anecdote, of their own accord.

Knowledge

Instructors should get to know their students (**FIGURE 6.2**). Office hours, class "down time," and any other lull in activity can be used to find out about personal background and learning styles. The educator can become better informed about different cultures by researching, reading, and participating in culture-specific activities. One method of learning about someone else's culture is to find expert informants. These are people who live in and are respected within their communities. Examples are as disparate as local store owners, religious leaders, schoolteachers, and parents. Students should be encouraged to write scenarios for the class that are based on personal experiences. This approach helps to validate students' lives for the group, and it shows that the instructor values what is shared.

Behavior

One must lead by example. Instructors should exhibit the actions desired in their students. If comments are made in the classroom that focus on negative stereotypes, the instructor should take time to discuss and counter them

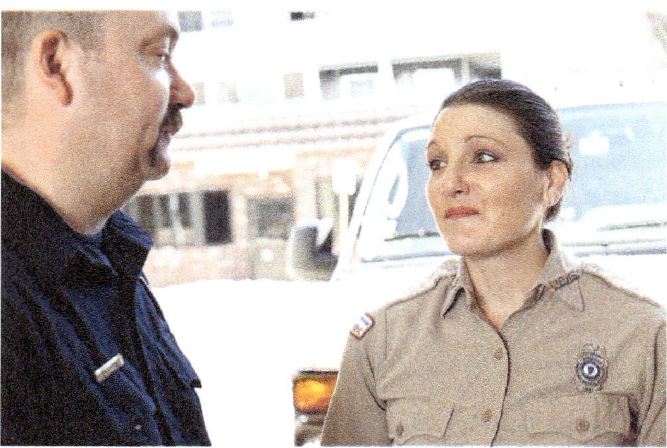

FIGURE 6.2 Getting to know students as individuals enables the instructor to better understand their backgrounds and values.

with accurate information. If the instructor does not have the information available at the time, they should reach out to key informants in the community for help. Typically, these people are well known and highly respected members of a community who are eager to help share information about their community.

Environment

The educator must create a classroom environment that is a safe haven for discussion and exploration. Distasteful or abusive remarks, even if spoken in jest, must not be tolerated. It is important to remember that what is humorous to some may be hurtful to others. An instructor must develop and enforce classroom rules that prohibit language and behavior that is racist, misogynistic, or otherwise discriminatory.

Acceptance

Many elements of everyday behaviors are influenced by cultural rules. For example, in some cultures, people consider it disrespectful for a child (the student, regardless of age) to make eye contact with an elder (the instructor), whereas many in our society value such eye contact, considering it a sign of respectful attentiveness. Other students may not want to shake hands, as it conflicts with cultural or religious upbringing. The instructor who is aware that such cultural disconnects exist can avoid embarrassing and even infuriating moments.

Preparing Students to Incorporate Diversity Awareness into Their Practice

Open communication is an essential element to any successful group endeavor. Instructors must foster clear dialogue within their learning setting to promote learning and develop a collegial group experience.

Culture

When the word "culture" is mentioned, images of racially or ethnically based differences often come to mind. Many social scientists, however, define culture as an amalgamation of customs, experiences, languages, and beliefs common to a defined group. For example, various regions of the nation are described as having uniquely identifiable cultures with predominant characteristics for that area (e.g., Southeastern states, Appalachia, inner-city urban areas). The same can be said for regions of the world (e.g., Central America, South Pacific, Middle East).

Social scientists define culture as a group of people who share experiences, language, and values that permit them to communicate knowledge not shared by those outside the culture. An example of a culture is EMS itself. How many providers have used the jargon of the profession ("10-8," "Code 3," "ALS") in a conversation with people outside the industry, only to have someone look quizzically at them. When EMS providers get together and begin talking, they should take pity on the non-EMS person who tries to keep up with the discussion. Any person who is looking from the outside in would likely be confused about what is being said and meant.

This lack of "getting it" by the non-EMS person is an example of low cultural competency. It is possible that students in the EMS classroom come with culturally specific elements in their communication. The EMS instructor must be aware of this potential challenge and should build tools to overcome it. One strategy would be to invite students to write down a list (with definitions) of words and phrases they commonly use, that a person outside the culture may not be familiar with. Another strategy would be to simply ask students what they mean any time an unknown word is noted in the classroom.

Transcultural communication can open doors to greater understanding, but it can also lead to misunderstanding. Misunderstanding, often caused by ignorance, can make or break the medical management of an event. The following section provides some suggestions on how to reduce the occurrences of misunderstanding; ways to implement a culturally aware medical curriculum are discussed.

Developing a Culturally Sound Teaching Curriculum

Instructors expect to follow specific steps for students to learn skills such as airway management. It is equally important to design purposeful strategies to promote their skills related to cultural awareness.

Needs Assessment

Not all areas of the United States are similar in terms of the cultures that exist. For example, the incidence of homelessness may be greater in an urban, inner-city area than in a sparsely populated rural area. A needs assessment, or evaluation, should be conducted by the EMS instructor for the purpose of ascertaining which

CASE in Point

It was early Monday morning, and an EMT instructor was just about to begin her class. About half of the students were in the classroom; some were reviewing their textbooks, while others were texting or otherwise engaged with their phones. As the instructor came into the room, she noticed that a few students were congregated toward the back of the room. Devin was relating to a group of students the details of an EMS call he had observed the previous day. The instructor overheard a few laughs but did not really pay attention to the conversation. Soon, the class came to order, and the day's lesson on cardiac emergencies began.

During lunch, April came to see the instructor in her office. This student was visibly angry and obviously needed to talk. Concerned, the instructor closed the office door and listened carefully to her. Apparently, the conversation that Devin was leading earlier involved a patient who had end-stage AIDS, necessitating an urgent call for EMS. The student had been riding along as an EMT observer with the crew. April had overheard the other student making comments such as, "Homosexuality is a sin" and "AIDS is what you get when you're gay." Even though she was not part of the discussion, she was angered by the comments, especially because her sister had died of AIDS only 6 months earlier.

The instructor asked the student if she said anything to the other student about his comments. She shook her head—no; she felt very uncomfortable talking to him directly. Angrily, April said, "I just want him to know that not all AIDS patients are gay, and even those who are do not deserve to suffer like that!"

Follow-Up

After the upset student left the instructor's office, the instructor spent the remainder of her break finishing her lunch and thinking about how she could manage the situation. Despite her own discomfort and anger about what Devin had said to his classmates, she knew she had to intervene to try to turn a tense situation into a learning experience for all involved. In her conversation with the instructor, April had indicated that she was not seeking an apology from the other student, nor did she want to get him "into any trouble."

The instructor decided to implement the following plan:

1. At the next break, she would pull Devin aside and determine what he had actually said during the discussion. She would advise him that, if stated as reported, the comments would be seen as poor affect based on the class rubric for professional behavior. The instructor would also provide Devin an opportunity to express his feelings about what was said and about how another person perceived his comments. However, she would make sure that he understood that the comments he had made were inappropriate, and that he must not make similar ones in the future. Later that day, she would document her conversations with both students, possibly having each student sign a copy of the respective incident reports.
2. At the next class, she would engage the class in a short discussion about verbal behavior in the classroom, as well as in the clinical setting. She felt it would be important to reinforce to the entire class how critical it is to be mindful of other people's feelings and perceptions, in case a conversation is accidentally overheard. She would be careful to avoid "shutting down" the student who had made the comments and would make sure that he continues to feel valued as a member of the classroom community.
3. Later in the semester, she would provide additional information about HIV and AIDS through handouts, Web links, and class discussions.
4. She would schedule clinical rotations with a local AIDS hospice. Each student would be required to submit a written summary of the experience and to share it with the entire class in a discussion or presentation.

terms, customs, and other cultural elements should be introduced into the curriculum to best serve local, regional, and national needs.

Sometimes what is needed is evident. For example, the rapid influx of an ethnically based population, for whom English is not the primary language, may necessitate a specific training effort to educate the EMS system about basic practices and traditions within that population. Many texts are available to learn more about the theory of evaluation techniques. (For more information, see the works of Hunter, Guskey, Tyler, and Scriven in the Additional Resources section of this chapter.)

Research

Research can often be the most labor intensive step of developing a culturally sound curriculum. What information is needed during preparation of the lesson plan that will deliver the concepts? Often, the information cannot be found in traditional EMS textbooks. However, it can be found in many places, including libraries, the Internet, journals, and textbooks. (For more information, see Sue and Sue in the Additional Resources section of this chapter.) Other sources may provide more accurate and relevant information to EMS than can be found in published writings. One such source consists of those persons identified as community leaders or key informants within the population in question.

Issues of culture arise in all areas of education. The educator can also look to other medical disciplines for position papers, culturally aware curriculum development, and other tools that can be used in the EMS classroom.

Other Resources

Local service agencies often focus on specific groups within a community and can offer a wealth of information about their clientele. Many such agencies are more than happy to share their expertise with anyone who wishes to become more enlightened. For example, a local council on aging might offer an entire presentation on the psychosocial issues the elderly face when living alone, or they might help to arrange for elderly persons to serve as patients during presentation of a unit on geriatrics.

In addition to local resources, many helpful sources of information are available at the federal and national levels. Organizations such as the American Medical Association (AMA) and the American Association of Medical Colleges (AAMC) have released compendiums of references on the needs and resources of specific populations. The American Association of Universities and Colleges (AAUC) has compiled resource information on culturally aware teaching practices. (Some of these sources can be found in the Additional Resources section of this chapter.)

Instructional Strategies

Many cultural concepts can be integrated directly into the medical curriculum that is being taught. In doing so, the instructor must take the time needed to develop and establish the "ground rules for a safe environment." These rules must include statements assuring all students that they will have the opportunity to speak and to be heard. Students must know, however, that there are limits to this free speech. This limit in the classroom, as in society, means that one person's right to expression stops at the next person's nose. That means students may speak, they may be honest, and they may disagree; they may not, however, attack one another. So, although ideas may be torn apart (i.e., with the use of reasoned arguments or discourse), people may not be. The instructor must present these rules to the class and must ensure that all participants understand and agree to abide by them. Students should be given an opportunity to read and add to or argue against the specifics of the list of rules, but in the end, they must all sign a contract of agreement with the final document.

Instructors can incorporate diversity into a classroom community by employing a variety of educational methods, including some of those discussed in the following paragraphs.

Case Studies

These scenario-based lessons describe for students an event, the actions taken, and the outcomes. For example, students may be given a written exercise that contains a short scenario about an elderly woman who was found "down" in her apartment by neighbors. The case proceeds to detail what the responding crew found, how they treated the patient, and how the patient responded. These types of scenarios may be created to include a wide variety of diverse elements, such as gender identification, race, or religious backgrounds. If these elements are included, it would be worthwhile to have individuals who are culturally competent in these areas review the case for unintentional bias or stereotyping.

Guest Presentation

Invite members of various cultures to present information. If the community of interest is a particular religious group, a member of the local house of faith could be invited to present a lecture to the class. This lecture might include a brief history of the group, an explanation of its core beliefs, and any special information that would be particularly useful during an emergency (e.g., perhaps members of this faith do not accept blood products or medications, or perhaps they permit female patients to be touched only by female caregivers). Students should be encouraged to ask questions, and the presenter must be made to feel welcome, even when the presenter's beliefs seem strange or extreme. Other examples might include the LGBTQI community, ethnic populations, and age groups.

Community Outreach

Students often engage in community-minded projects, such as staffing first aid stations, providing blood pressure checks, and giving bicycle safety lectures (**FIGURE 6.3**). It could be helpful for the instructor (or the program) to sponsor such efforts in targeted communities. Students could set up a health education booth at a community center in an ethnic minority neighborhood, or they may provide free cardiopulmonary resuscitation (CPR) classes for a low-income, single-parents group. The communities that receive these services may, in turn, share intimate knowledge about the group. Students may be invited to attend local festivals or events, an opportunity that would further their understanding and appreciation of that culture.

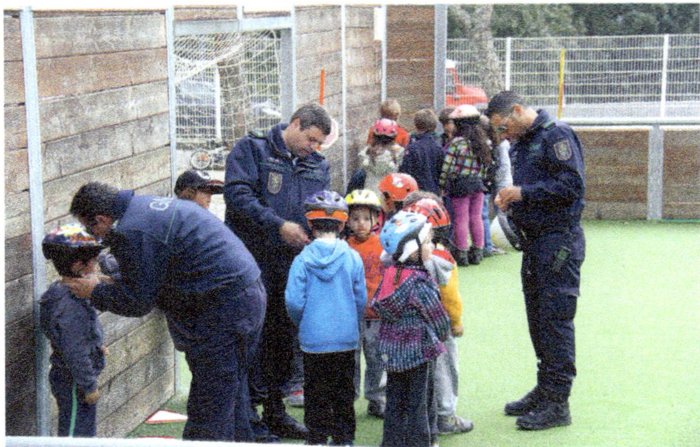

FIGURE 6.3 Injury-prevention activities sponsored by the educational program can be educational for the community, as well as for school-age students.

Group Discussions

Open forums are best supported by clear guidelines and goals. If some students in the class identify themselves as members of the community of interest, they should be invited (not compelled) to share their thoughts and experiences. Other sources of information are local community leaders (e.g., ministers, business owners, and instructors). The instructor must begin such discussions with a brief outline of the rules for the event. These rules must establish that ideas are welcome but attacks are not. Each student must feel safe if open and frank discussions are to occur. The instructor should function as the facilitator, guiding the discussion but not controlling it. The instructor will be the guide on the side—not the sage on the stage.[16]

CASE in Point

"Uh oh. What did I do now?" the instructor thought to himself as he walked into his supervisor's office. Everyone knows just how unpleasant visits like these can be. No notice, no warning—he was getting dressed for shift in the locker room when the overhead page requested his presence on the second floor.

He was a bit surprised when he entered the office. In addition to his supervisor, an elderly man was sitting in the room. Smiling, the supervisor introduced the instructor to the director of the senior citizen assistance office of the county health department.

"Remember when you were talking about the number of hip fractures you were handling at the elder care high-rises downtown?" the supervisor asked.

"Uh huh," the instructor replied. (He was actually ranting and about how ambulance resources were being used to handle these cases. It seemed like a unit went to a report of a "person found down" several times a week!)

"Well," the supervisor said, "by chance, I was talking to the director here about another issue, when I mentioned this might be a problem. He has offered to listen to your complaint and offer some assistance." The three began a discussion about identifying the nature of the problem.

Follow-Up

First, the instructor established a common ground with all interested parties—everyone involved in this case understands the serious effects of a fractured hip in an elderly patient. Next, the three discussed the possibility of performing a risk analysis to determine what factors increase or decrease the likelihood of a fall. The county's public health office probably has a tool for gathering such information. Those data could be used in the design of a safety program that eliminates hazards (e.g., loose carpeting replaced with a nonslip version, handrails added to all rooms) and teaches residents how to monitor their personal risk index. Last, the instructor decided to establish a train-the-trainer model by which he would prepare his staff to go out into the community and educate the staff at the elder care centers.

CASE in Point

During a recent class discussion, the instructor presented information about scene assessment (the global survey). She stated that some EMS agencies provide bullet-resistant vests for their personnel. One local agency does this, and they allow the employees to wear the "over the shirt" type of vest whenever the employees believe it is justified. Roann asked why most of the EMS personnel she knows wear the vests only when they get a call to go to areas of town that are primarily populated by ethnic minorities. The class immediately began a debate about the "facts" that these parts of town have more calls that are violent and that EMS is more likely to be threatened in these areas. Some members of the class describe this as a reasonable precaution. Others describe it as racial profiling. They turn to the instructor and look for guidance. What does she do?

Follow-Up

First, the instructor distills the arguments on both sides to their most salient points (e.g., crime rates, number of past EMS assaults, overall violence in the areas). Then, she gets each side to do some research to back up their beliefs. They could examine publicly available statistics and invite local community leaders to discuss the issue. She asks that each side bring their results back into class and present them to one another. This case is based on local practices, so it would be appropriate to bring in a representative of the local EMS agency to explain the reasoning that went into the policy's creation and implementation.

Practical Skills

Ideally, an actor is brought into the skills laboratory for each practical scenario. The actor must be prepared to play the patient role. Care should be taken to create scenarios that inform students and even challenge perceptions. For example, a scenario about a pregnant teenager should not always include a person of one particular racial/ethnic or socioeconomic group. If actors are not available, students can be coached to take on the patient roles and to conduct the research necessary to perform the role accurately. Although they may be labor intensive, such exercises can stimulate alternative learning opportunities for all students involved.

Clinical Rotations

Clinically oriented rotations can be supplemented by limited observations in nontraditional settings. For example, if the community of interest includes severely intellectually disabled patients, students may be assigned clinical rotations with a center that specializes in the care of these patients. Such rotations could provide students with expert opinions and a chance to put a face on the disorder, thereby making it more meaningful to them.

Identity

Instructors and students make assumptions about others. These assumptions include labels of ethnicity, religion, disability, and more. One strategy that is useful for challenging such potentially erroneous assumptions is known as the "identity game." During this type of exercise, students might be asked to elaborate (by writing on an index card) on how they see themselves (e.g., "heterosexual, Christian, male"). Each student could label the card using a code name known only to the instructor. These completed cards would be turned in to the instructor, who would then randomly assign the cards to other members of the class. The students' assignment would be to try to identify the classmate whose card they were given. The class would be polled to see how many students were able to identify the author of their card.

Facilitating any identity activity requires that the instructor model sensitivity and skill. The class must be monitored to ensure that a climate of respect is maintained throughout the activity. Many other examples of identity and cultural awareness exercises can be found online. See the Additional Resources at the end of this chapter for some suggested sites.

Role-Playing

Students are asked to identify a group (e.g., ethnic, gender, religion) that is different from their own. They are then assigned to play parts in a patient care scenario based on their new identity. For example, a Christian female student may play the part of an elderly Jehovah's Witness male patient, or an ethnic minority male student might play the part of a nonminority male fire fighter. This exercise has been used in EMS classrooms with great success. However, a degree of caution must be issued. These portrayals can be full of stereotypes and clichés. Some will break down walls and use humor to demonstrate the ridiculousness of such beliefs. Others may cause hurt feelings and have the potential to create disharmony within the classroom community. It is recommended that this exercise be used in classrooms in which there is a tradition of open dialogue, and one in which the instructor feels comfortable that a safe environment will be maintained.

Communication Games

Through games, students can learn the importance of communication and ways that it can be affected. One example of this type of game would be to split students into two groups. Group A would be asked to leave the classroom and go into the skills laboratory to prepare equipment for extremity splinting. Once in the lab, this group would be told to reverse the meanings of their words (e.g., they will say "more" when they mean "less," or "right" when they mean "left"). When Group B enters the lab, they would be told to partner with the people already there. The ensuing confusion can be humorous. It can also demonstrate how communication, usually taken for granted, can lead to misunderstanding and even be counterproductive.

Using the Critical Incident Questionnaire in Diverse Classrooms

Stephen Brookfield feels that the Critical Incident Questionnaire (CIQ) classroom assessment technique is particularly helpful to use in diverse classrooms.[17] The tool is simple. Students are asked to anonymously jot down the answers to the following questions at the end of a class period:

1. At what moment in class this week did you feel most engaged with what was happening?
2. At what moment in class this week were you most distanced from what was happening?
3. What action that anyone (instructor or student) took this week did you find most affirming or helpful?
4. What action that anyone took this week did you find most puzzling or confusing?
5. What about this class surprised you the most? (This could be about your own reactions to what went on, something that someone did, or anything else that occurred.)[17]

The instructor informally summarizes the results and shares common areas of concern with the class. There are many uses and benefits of the CIQ. In diverse classrooms, the CIQ may alert the instructor to teaching strategies that are meeting the diverse learning needs of the class, or to classroom activities that are seen by some students as unfair or alienating. This tool contributes to a sense of inclusivity within the classroom and permits students to express sensitive concerns in a nonthreatening manner so they can be addressed.[17]

Summary

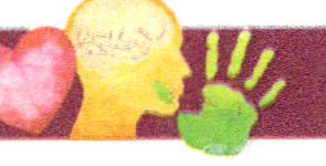

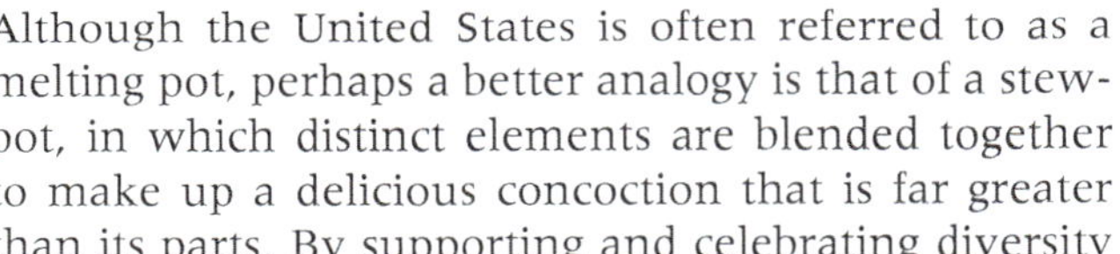

Although the United States is often referred to as a melting pot, perhaps a better analogy is that of a stewpot, in which distinct elements are blended together to make up a delicious concoction that is far greater than its parts. By supporting and celebrating diversity in the EMS classroom, students can become better prepared to deliver care with greater empathy for and understanding of the many cultures and groups they will encounter. These future healthcare providers may become more attuned to the diversity of the EMS profession itself and, where needed, they may even improve it.

Glossary

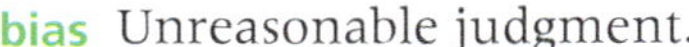

bias Unreasonable judgment.

cultural competency Awareness of beliefs and customs of cultures.

cultural humility Understanding of culture in which a person is open to another person's cultural identity and is open to exploring and learning about it.

culture Amalgamation of customs, experiences, languages, attitudes, values, and beliefs common to a defined group.

equity In the context of education, practices and approaches that set up every student for success and deliberately foster excellence in learning.

References

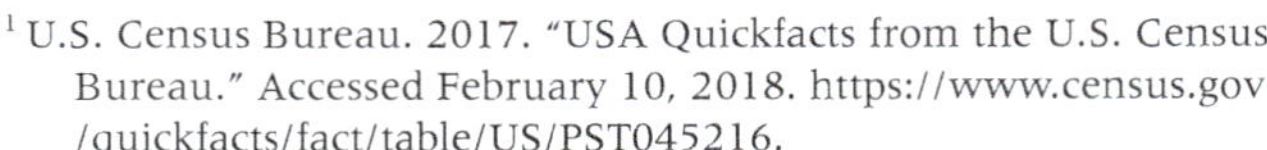

[1] U.S. Census Bureau. 2017. "USA Quickfacts from the U.S. Census Bureau." Accessed February 10, 2018. https://www.census.gov/quickfacts/fact/table/US/PST045216.

[2] Crowe, Remle P., Roger Levine, Jennifer Eggerichs, and Melissa A. Bentley. 2016. "A Longitudinal Description of Emergency Medical Services Professionals by Race/Ethnicity." *Prehospital and Disaster Medicine* 31, S1: S30–69. https://doi.org/10.1017/S1049023X16001072.

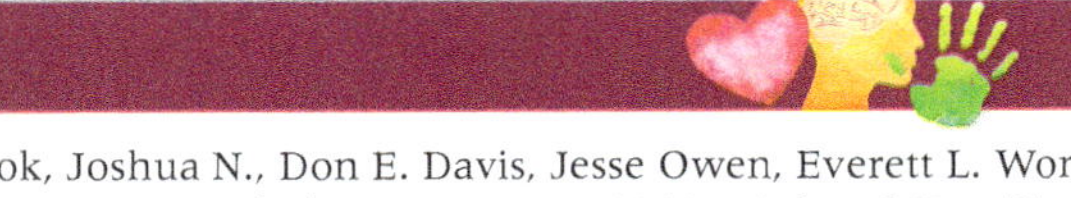

[3] Hook, Joshua N., Don E. Davis, Jesse Owen, Everett L. Worthington, Jr., and Shawn O. Utsey. 2013. "Cultural Humility: Measuring Openness to Culturally Diverse Clients." *Journal of Counseling Psychology* 60, no. 3: 353–66. http://dx.doi.org/10.1037/a0032595.

[4] Tervalon, Melanie, and Jann Murray-Garcia. 1998. "Cultural Humility versus Cultural Competence: A Critical Distinction in Defining Physician Training Outcomes in Multicultural Education." *Journal of Health Care for the Poor and Underserved* 9: 117–25. http://dx.doi.org/10.1353/hpu.2010.0233.

[5] Weinstein, Carol S., Saundra Tomlinson-Clarke, and Mary Curran. 2004. "Toward a Conception of Culturally Responsive Classroom Management." *Journal of Teacher Education* 55, no. 1: 25–38. https://doi.org/10.1177/0022487103259812.

[6] "Bias." 2018. In *Merriam-Webster.com*. Accessed July 1, 2018. https://www.merriam-webster.com/dictionary/bias.

[7] Bandura, Albert. 1997. *Self-Efficacy: The Exercise of Control*. New York: W.H. Freeman.

[8] U.S. Department of Health and Human Services, Office of Minority Health. "Why Use Culturally and Linguistically Appropriate Services (CLAS) throughout a Disaster?" Accessed December 10, 2018. https://cccdpcr.thinkculturalhealth.hhs.gov/.

[9] Honeycutt, Linda. 1997. "Cultural Diversity: Essential Education." *Journal of Emergency Medical Services* 22, no. 8: 39.

[10] Coupland, Douglas. 1991. *Generation X: Tales for an Accelerated Culture*. New York: St. Martin's Press.

[11] Reeves, Thomas C. 2007. *Do Generational Differences Matter in Instructional Design?* Athens, GA: University of Georgia.

[12] Oblinger, Diana G., and James L. Oblinger (Eds.). 2005. *Educating the Net Gen*. Washington, DC: EDUCAUSE.

[13] Hunter, Sandy L. 2003. "Defining and Valuing Diversity in EMS." *Journal of Emergency Care and Transportation* 32: 88–9.

[14] Cole, Henry P. 1997. "Stories to Live By: A Narrative Approach to Health Behavior Research and Injury Prevention." In *Handbook of Health Behavior Research IV: Relevance for Professionals and Issues for the Future*, edited by David S. Gochman, 325–49. Louisville, KY: University of Louisville.

[15] García, Emma, and Elaine Weiss. 2017, September 27. "Education Inequalities at the School Starting Gate." *Economic Policy Institute*. Accessed January 18, 2019. https://www.epi.org/publication/education-inequalities-at-the-school-starting-gate/.

[16] Collison, George, Bonnie Elbaum, Sarah Haavind, and Robert Tinker. 2000. *Facilitating Online Learning*. Madison, WI: Atwood Press.

[17] Brookfield, Stephen D. 2006. *The Skillful Teacher: On Technique, Trust, and Responsiveness in the Classroom*. 2nd ed. San Francisco: Jossey-Bass.

Additional Resources

Agency for Healthcare Research and Quality. 2012. "Improving Patient Safety Systems for Patients with Limited English Proficiency. Appendix A: Recommendations for Staff Training." http://www.ahrq.gov/professionals/systems/hospital/lepguide/lepguideapa.html.

Canadian Centre for Diversity and Inclusion. 2017. "Getting Started: Diversity and Identity Toolkit." https://ccdi.ca/media/1587/toolkit-1-getting-started-diversity-and-identity.pdf.

Gonchar, Michael. 2017, March 15. "Film Club: 25 Mini-Films for Exploring Race, Bias and Identity with Students." *The New York Times*. https://www.nytimes.com/2017/03/15/learning/lesson-plans/25-mini-films-for-exploring-race-bias-and-identity-with-students.html.

Goto, Standord T., and Connie Martin. 2009. "Psychology of Success: Overcoming Barriers to Pursuing Further Education." *The Journal of Continuing Higher Education* 57: 10–21. https://doi.org/10.1080/07377360902810744.

Guskey, Thomas R. 1958. "Does It Make a Difference?" *Educational Leadership* 59, no. 6: 45–51.

Guskey, Thomas R. 1998. "The Age of Accountability." *Journal of Staff Development* 19, no. 4: 36–44.

Hunter, Sandy L. 2005. *The Role of Gender, Race and Self-Efficacy in Career Choice for Primarily Male-Oriented, Primarily Female-Oriented and Minority Under-Represented Professions* [PhD Thesis]. Lexington, KY: University of Kentucky.

Hurtado, Sylvia, June C. Han, Victor B. Sáenz, Lorelle L. Espinsoa, Nolan L. Cabrera, and Oscar S. Cerna. 2007. "Predicting Transition and Adjustment to College: Biomedical and Behavioral Science Aspirants' and Minority Students' First Year of College." *Research in Higher Education* 48: 841–86. https://doi.org/10.1007/s11162-007-9051-x.

Jeffreys, Marianne R. 2007. "Tracking Students through Program Entry, Progression, Graduation, and Licensure: Assessing Undergraduate Nursing Student Retention and Success." *Nurse Education Today* 27: 406–19. https://doi.org/10.1016/j.nedt.2006.07.003.

Lie, Désirée A., Elizabeth Lee-Rey, Art Gomez, Sylvia Bereknyei, and Clarence H. Braddock, III. 2011. "Does Cultural Competency Training of Health Professionals Improve Patient Outcomes? A Systematic Review and Proposed Algorithm for Future Research." *Journal of General Internal Medicine* 26, no. 3: 317–25. https://doi.org/10.1007/s11606-010-1529-0.

National Highway Traffic Safety Administration. 2008. "EMS Workforce for the 21st Century: A National Assessment." https://www.ems.gov/pdf/research/Studies-and-Reports/National_Workforce_Assessment.pdf.

Reason, Robert D. 2009. "An Examination of Persistence Research through the Lens of a Comprehensive Conceptual Framework." *Journal of College Student Development* 50, no. 6: 659–82. http://dx.doi.org/10.1353/csd.0.0098.

Reason, Robert D., Patrick Terenzini, and Robert J. Domingo. 2006. "First Things First: Developing Academic Competence in the First Year of College." *Research in Higher Education* 47, no. 2: 149–75. https://doi.org/10.1007/s11162-005-8884-4.

Scriven, Michael. 1967. "The Methodology of Evaluation." In *Perspectives of Curriculum Evaluation*, edited by Ralph W. Tyler, Robert M. Gagné, and Michael Scriven, 39–83. Washington, DC: American Educational Research Association.

Sue, Derald W., and David Sue. 2002. *Counseling the Culturally Diverse: Theory and Practice*. 5th ed. New York: John Wiley & Sons.

Tyler, Ralph W. 1949. *Basic Principles of Curriculum and Instruction*. Chicago: University of Chicago Press.

University of Houston, Division of Student Affairs and Enrollment Services, Center for Diversity and Inclusion. Diversity Education. "Activities." https://www.uh.edu/cdi/diversity_education/resources/activities/.

PART III

Education Essentials

Like a building whose integrity is only as strong as the foundation it rests upon, an educator's teaching is strengthened and supported by a clear understanding of core concepts in education. This part of the text explains the learning domains, incorporating the revisions to Bloom's taxonomy in the cognitive domain. Specific details within these chapters outline strategies to develop solid goals and objectives that will provide clear guidance for educators and learners regarding what they should know and be able to do at the end of the lesson. Then, it describes how to create effective lesson plans and provides useful information about the nuts and bolts that are essential to planning teaching to maximize student learning.

Although it may not be as glamorous or attention-getting as the architectural details found on its facade, the foundation of a building provides the stable platform from which those details shine. This concept easily applies to teaching. An educator's ability to convey ideas and concepts in a brilliant way depends first on the ability to integrate the domains of learning into\ a comprehensive, deliberate lesson plan—one that is tailored specifically to the learning needs the educator has identified. Strong implementation of that plan in a supportive learning environment is the rich architectural detail that students will notice and appreciate.

Educators should return to these chapters from time to time to reacquaint themselves with this material. With additional experience, an educator may be able to more readily apply the information and reevaluate what they are doing—and why.

CHAPTER 7

The Learning Environment

OBJECTIVES

At the conclusion of this chapter, the educator will be able to:

Cognitive Domain

1. Define the characteristics of a student-centered learning environment.
2. Describe how the learning environment affects learning outcomes.
3. Explain the importance of establishing academic and professional expectations.
4. Explain safety concerns in the learning environment.
5. Describe three physical environment considerations that contribute to a conducive learning experience.
6. Describe three psychological environment considerations that contribute to a conducive learning environment.
7. Describe three virtual environment variables that are different than those of the traditional classroom.
8. Explain three considerations of the lab and clinical environments that are not concerns in the lecture classroom.

Psychomotor Domain

There are no psychomotor objectives for this chapter.

Affective Domain

1. Value how a safe, student-centered learning environment affects learning outcomes.
2. Defend how a positive learning environment promotes student engagement for lifelong learning.

> **"A student-learned class is a place where students of all sorts of labels come together as equals to form a new type of learning environment."**
>
> ~ Thomas Armstrong

CHAPTER GOAL This chapter explores how emergency medical services (EMS) educators can effectively set and maintain an appropriate physical and psychological learning environment in order to achieve student learning.

Being an educator involves much more than simply imparting knowledge and anecdotes. An effective educator is responsible for ensuring student success by providing an appropriate learning environment.[1]

According to *The American Heritage Dictionary of the English Language*, the term *environment* is defined as: "The combination of external or extrinsic physical conditions that affect and influence the growth and development of organisms" and "The complex of social and cultural conditions affecting the nature of an individual or community."[2] A learning environment is an environment designed with student learning in mind.[3,4] When used to describe an educational setting, the term *environment* can be associated with positive or negative perceptions for the student or the instructor. A positive learning environment is one that allows for a free exchange of ideas and information, one in which students feel safe asking questions and the educator has or acquires the necessary tools to answer those questions. It is one in which the atmosphere is supportive and students are encouraged to concentrate on academic success. Additionally, a positive learning environment is one that consistently demonstrates respect for students, as well as for the educator. A negative environment prohibits or interferes with learning, and students may feel inadequate or may believe that their ideas do not matter or cannot be expressed.

In 1943, Abraham Maslow published his theory regarding human motivation and developed a hierarchy of needs.[5] (This theory is discussed further in Chapter 4, *Principles of Adult Learning*.) According to this theory, all individuals have needs that must be met, from basic survival needs, to the need for self-actualization, to transcendence, that is, helping others to self-actualize. Once these needs are met in systematic order, individuals are motivated to realize their true potential, and self-fulfillment can occur. This is a crucial step, because motivation affects engagement, and engagement is required for learning.[6]

In 1970, Malcolm Knowles reintroduced the concept that the environmental climate surrounding learning could affect learning, an idea that had been explored for many years by early educational theorists. Since that time, research has shown that a multitude of physical, psychological, and social factors can affect learning.[7–11] Physically, the environment needs to be comfortable and conducive to learning (**FIGURE 7.1**). Psychologically, students need to feel safe and respected in the classroom, free from ridicule or bullying, and able to ask questions. Socially, positive relationships and teamwork established in the classroom can enhance the learning experience and prepare students for the workforce. Additional considerations for the virtual environment, and other environments outside of the traditional classroom, are also important responsibilities of the EMS educator (**FIGURE 7.2**).

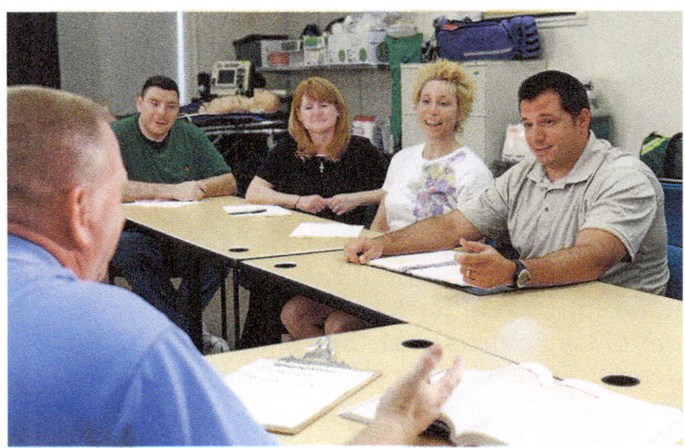

FIGURE 7.1 A student-centered physical environment must have adequate and functional resources such as proper lighting and furniture.

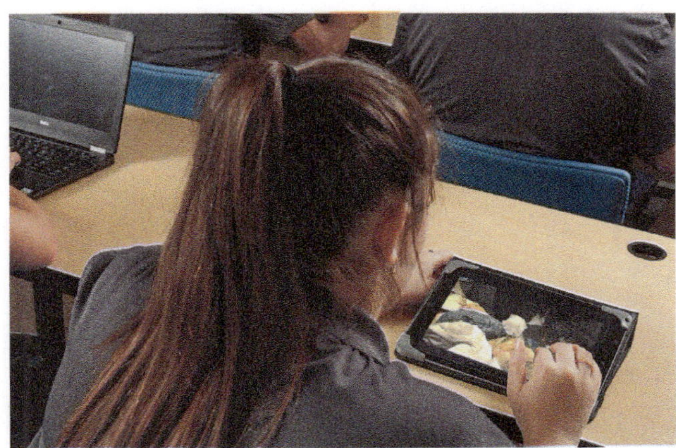

FIGURE 7.2 The virtual environment must also be student-centered.

Classroom Introductions

The Welcome

Introductions can greatly affect the learning that takes place thereafter.[1] Sights, sounds, smells, atmosphere, and rapport with the instructor established early on can potentially establish the culture for the remainder of the class or course. Each classroom, each school, develops its own culture—a blending of external and internal experiences. The culture developed gives meaning to the learning process that occurs in the class. Thus, even before class begins, the educator needs to give special attention to ensure a positive learning experience can occur (**FIGURE 7.3**).

Prior to the first day of class, an online welcome or orientation can be an effective means for setting the tone, easing some of the anticipation the students may have, and showing the instructor's immediacy and dedication. There are many tools available to instructors for asynchronous introductions, even if the class is a traditional face-to-face delivery.

When the class does meet for the first time, something as simple as the instructor learning the names of students and helping them to learn one another's names can quickly break the ice, as a first step in creating a positive learning environment. Furthermore, it reinforces that the educator values the students as individuals and expects that they value one another.[12–14]

Student Introductions

Providing an opportunity for students to introduce themselves can also have a significant impact on their motivation to work as a team. It provides the instructor an opportunity to gain an impression of the student's personality, comfort level in a group environment, and any previous experience that the student might bring to the cohort. Student introductions also put the students on notice that the learning environment will consist of collaboration and dialogue, and that they will be a part of the learning process, not simply a passive spectator.

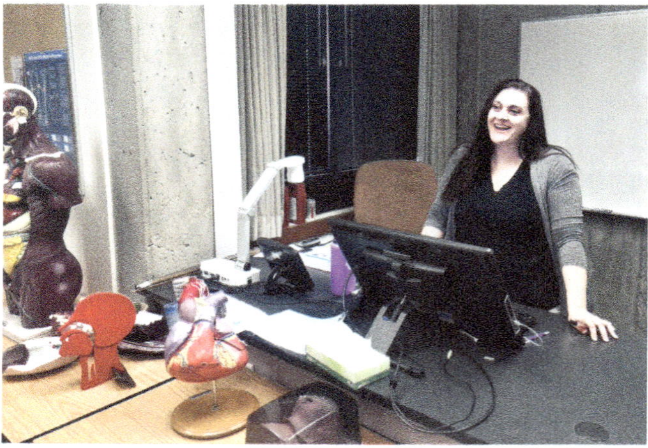

FIGURE 7.3 A warm and friendly smile from the instructor can go a long way toward setting a positive learning environment.

Courtesy of Bill Robertson.

TEACHING TIP

On the first day of class, an educator can play an icebreaker game, which can take many different forms. One method is to place all the students' keys in a basket. Each student then draws out a set of keys (other than their own) and attempts to tell the class the characteristics of the person who owns the keys. The owner of the keys then stands and states their name, why they are attending the class, and something unique about themselves.

Another suggestion is the "Two Truths and a Lie" game. For this icebreaker, students says three things about themselves—two truthful statements and one lie. The other students then vote on which is the lie and give their reasons for their vote. This game usually results in some interesting discoveries about students, proving that often, truth is stranger than fiction.

Housekeeping

A fundamental part of creating a comfortable learning and teaching environment is ensuring that the basic needs of both the student and the educator are met. This includes giving directions about where the restrooms and refreshments can be found and providing adequate break times. A general rule is to schedule a break approximately every 60 to 90 minutes. Breaks should be regular, so students know when to expect them. The class may include students with disabilities that may require special consideration for time or assistance. Instructors must ensure students have the opportunity to discuss needed accommodations with a disability resource so that the instructor makes appropriate accommodations.[12] (See Appendix B, *Learning Disabilities in the EMS Classroom*, and Americans with Disability Act for further information.)

Setting Expectations

Students enter the classroom from a variety of cultures and backgrounds and with a variety of preconceptions about learning.[14] The educator should recognize this and immediately set the standard of expected behavior and achievement. By setting a standard, the educator maximizes each student's chances for learning success.

The Syllabus

The syllabus or student handbook represents a written contract of sorts that outlines the expectations of many aspects of the program. This document clearly outlines the learning expectations of the course and evaluation of coursework. It contains information about appropriate behaviors and consequences of unacceptable behaviors. The syllabus protects the educator and the student and provides a consistent place for students to review class expectations. The syllabus should be reviewed with all students early on. Doing so helps clarify the intent of the policies within the document, clarifying misconceptions or misinterpretations of its content.

Adult education focuses on a student-centered environment; thus, the syllabus should be student-centered as well.[15] A student-centered syllabus provides more than just an outline; it provides guidance. All syllabi should have objectives, but a student-centered syllabus includes the rationale for the objectives. It provides recommendations and advice on what areas of the course require extra time and resources and points out content with which students typically struggle. Student-centered syllabi can also be designed to give students flexibility in some assignments. Such an approach suggests to the students that they have some autonomy in the process. Careful development of a syllabus that demonstrates that students are valued has been shown to improve student views toward faculty and the program.[15]

Instructor Expectations

Students should know their instructor's expectations early. Establishing expectations on the first day of class allows students to focus on the coursework.

Instructors should explain the expectations for student participation in the learning process. An adult education environment is most effective when students learn as much from one another as they do from the instructor. This only occurs when student participation is required within the EMS educational environment. The nature of the EMS occupation prohibits its providers from being passive in the learning process or in the delivery of patient care. Providers must be confident and assertive in their actions.

TEACHING TIP

It is important for instructors to follow the timeliness policy. Instructors must start and finish on time, or students won't believe the instructor values that policy.

Passing cognitive and psychomotor assessments is not the only evaluation of a candidate's ability to work in the demanding world of EMS. Assessing affective behavior is also important.[16] Instructors have an obligation to inform students of their expectations in the domains of appropriate affective or professional behavior.

Required attendance is not always assumed by students. Mandatory attendance requirements as dictated by the program, school, agency, state, or accrediting bodies should be clearly defined and published. Students should be made fully aware of attendance expectations, as well as the consequences of failing to meet those expectations. An established policy on tardiness and absences related to class, lab, clinicals, and field experiences will help both the student and the instructor plan accordingly in the event of unforeseeable circumstances that will require a student to be absent.

It is safe to say that personal electronic devices such as smartphones, tablets, and laptops are an entrenched part of our culture.[17] The use of such devices is no longer considered a luxury, but a necessity. Although there is a developing trend toward using personal electronic devices as a means of delivering, assessing, and sharing knowledge in the educational environment, they can still cause significant distraction when their use is not facilitator controlled.[18] Students should clearly understand the policy regarding the use of personal electronics and designated forms of social media in the classroom, lab, clinicals, and field. Educators should formally share this policy at the beginning of a course and have students acknowledge it.

Student Expectations

Instructors should try to learn what students expect of them. Remember that the adult educational environment is a collaboration, but it is also an agreement of sorts. The instructor agrees to provide all the tools and strategies to facilitate the learning process, and the student agrees to learn.

Students come to the classroom with certain expectations.[19] Allowing the student the opportunity to share their expectations early in the course gives the instructor a chance to reflect on whether their curriculum and educational methods are going to accurately meet those expectations.

The Physical Environment

The physical component of the learning environment can vary greatly depending on the nature of the course. Principles discussed here certainly apply to the physical classroom, but with the expansion of technology, a physical classroom is no longer a requirement. The physical environment can include a classroom, library, laboratory, informal space, and virtual space.[20] Regardless of where a class takes place (as discussed in Chapter 3, *Brain-Based Learning*) the educator needs to ensure that the environment contributes to a positive learning experience.

Students expect certain components within the physical classroom—adequately functional furniture and lighting, instructor-smart podiums, available student computers in libraries, and wireless Internet access. The physical facilities are the visual component of the learning environment. As a result, students consider the physical environment to be an important factor in their selection of a school.[21,22] It is the responsibility of the educator to ensure that all physical resources within the environment are working well and fit the needs of the students.

Room Temperature

The temperature in the classroom should be at a comfortable setting for the task at hand, as mentioned in Chapter 3, *Brain-Based Learning*. This may mean having the heat turned down slightly on skills days when the students are actively moving around. Students should also be advised that they might wish to bring a sweater to class if they are normally cold, as the environment will be controlled to ensure the comfort of the majority.

Lighting

The lighting should be adjustable so that it can be dimmed to make best use of audiovisuals, but light enough for demonstrations or taking notes, or perhaps completely off when simulating a nighttime environment for a scenario.

Distractions

Distractions such as noise, bright sunlight, and interruptions can also affect the learning environment.[6] Whereas some sources of distraction are out of the educator's immediate control, anything that can be done to minimize distractions improves the learning environment. For example, the educator should ask that students shut off mobile phones or turn them to vibrate and accept only emergency calls. Instructors should set an example by putting their electronic devices to vibrate also. When conducting outside simulations, the instructor should hold the class in a discrete area that prevents pedestrian traffic from coming through.

Safety in the Classroom

Rules for classroom safety should be explicitly stated by the educator and listed in the course syllabus. Students should demonstrate behaviors that ensure safety around special equipment and with other class members to prevent harm to anyone in the classroom. Universal precautions should be followed at all times in an effort to minimize the risk of exposure.

The educator plays the role of the recognized leader in the classroom. As the leader, the educator is responsible for setting, enforcing, and modeling the norms of conduct. This means that the instructor must clearly identify the expectations of the students throughout the course. Situational awareness and safety precautions should be included in the syllabus and discussed during the first day of class. If inappropriate behavior occurs, it is important that the matter be discussed with the student in a timely, consistent, and fair manner.[23,24]

Seating Arrangements

Ideally, an educator should be able to configure and reconfigure a classroom in a variety of ways to accommodate the instructional strategy for that session. Furniture that can be rearranged is preferable. Furniture should be comfortable and should fit students and the classroom well. If 8-hour class sessions are planned, padded seats are essential. If class will not last longer than 2 hours, padded seats may be optional.

A variety of classroom set-up strategies are possible, depending on the learning objectives and class size. A few examples are as follows:

- **Traditional**. The traditional classroom set-up is ideal for a large number of students. It is instructor focused and often used by expert faculty to deliver information to large groups. This style is not recommended for small group work or for psychomotor skill development. This structure may allow students to "hide" behind others, and it can be difficult for some students to see over others. The educator at the front of the room may also have difficulty seeing all the students in the room and may focus only on the first row, inhibiting interaction with other students.
- **Theater**. The theater classroom set-up is optimal for a large number of students. In this type of configuration, the seats rise from the front to the back, allowing better visibility of the educator and any instructional media or demonstrations. In addition,

this arrangement allows the educator to have better eye contact with the group as a whole, but is usually still instructor centered. This style is not recommended for small group work.

- **Circle, square, and rectangle—open**. This style places the educator in the center of a U-like shape and works well for both instructor- and student-centered activity. The educator may sit with the group or may enter the center area. This can be an ideal set-up when all students are expected to participate in a discussion, as it allows them to see one another. It can also work well for a psychomotor demonstration. In a lecture scenario, the instructor should be cognizant that depending on where they stand, their back may be to some students.
- **Circle, square, and rectangle—closed**. This classroom set-up places the educator either sitting or standing off to the side after instructions are provided. It can be an ideal set-up for a discussion group when all students are expected to participate, as it allows students to see one another. This design is very student-centered. Similar to the open version, this type of set-up is not recommended for lectures or presentations.
- **Grouped**. With this classroom set-up, small groups are arranged around different round tables or workstations. The focus of instruction is within the space of each individual table or station and is student-centered. It is important with this style that the educator circulates around the room, or that additional educator facilitators assist in monitoring the work at the individual stations. This set-up allows some privacy between workstations. Visualization of each station may not be an issue, but it can be controlled with partitions or room dividers. It is important to maintain adequate room between stations or tables to allow for movement and to reduce the noise level. Groups can be working on the same activity simultaneously (but independently), or they can be working on different activities. With this set-up, the educator balances between monitoring and allowing students to direct their own learning. This set-up is less effective for lectures or presentations, as inevitably some of the students' backs will face the presenter (**FIGURE 7.4**).

Audiovisual Equipment

As part of the physical environment of the classroom, the educator must ensure that audiovisual equipment is in working order and that a back-up is planned and available. (See Chapter 16, *Using Technology to Enhance Classroom Learning*, for more information on audiovisual equipment.)

Extra Considerations

To create a positive, student-centered learning environment, the instructor should be able to evaluate the classroom and answer questions such as the following:[1,6,11,13,25,26]

- Is the room of adequate size?
- Is there adequate space for each student to sit, take notes, and view the reference materials?
- Can each student see and hear the instructor and any audiovisual presentations, role-plays, or scenarios?
- How can the lighting be changed so that there is adequate light for skills, lecture presentations, or discussion activities?
- If the classroom has windows, how can natural light be adjusted to achieve optimal lighting for audiovisual presentations?
- How can environmental controls be adjusted if it gets too hot or too cold?
- Where is the space for breaks that allows for eating and drinking?
- Where are the emergency exits and automated external defibrillator (AED)?
- Where are the restrooms?
- Where is the equipment stored? Is it accessible to students?
- Is the classroom space accessible to students with a variety of physical disabilities, such as the need to use a wheelchair?
- How can distractions from the outside environment be minimized (e.g., closing doors or windows to minimize interfering noise)?
- Is lighting/security for the parking area adequate?

The Virtual Learning Environment

Alternative means of educational delivery are no longer the exception. Hybrid and fully online delivery have become common in EMS education.[13,27,28] Delivering education using an online environment does not excuse the instructor from following the tenets of good educational design and delivery. In fact, additional preparation must be considered that is generally not a concern in the traditional face-to-face classroom.

The hallmark of effective educational delivery as we know it today consists of, at a minimum, the knowledge, skills, and attitudes as described in Bloom's

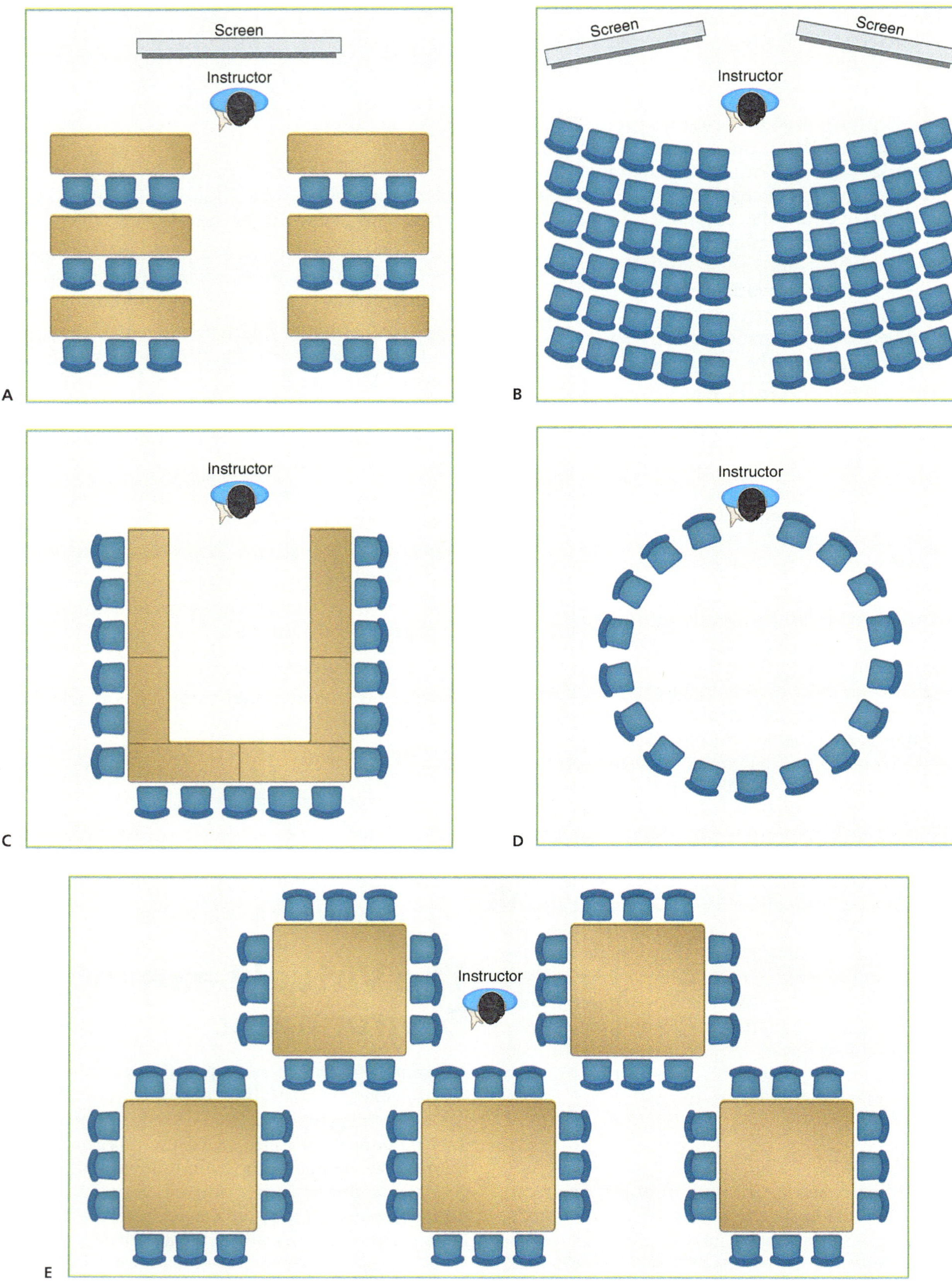

FIGURE 7.4 **A.** Traditional. **B.** Theater. **C.** Open. **D.** Closed. **E.** Grouped.

Taxonomy.[29] Although skills are difficult to teach and assess in the virtual classroom environment, knowledge and attitudes are not.

Many of the best practices of adult education that are effective in the traditional classroom can also be implemented in the virtual classroom. Tools such as discussion forums, asynchronous video lectures, group projects, interactive e-books, and more, have all been shown to enforce the transfer of pertinent knowledge as well as, if not better than, the face-to-face classroom.[30] (See Chapter 17, *Tools for Distance Learning*, for further information on virtual classroom creation and delivery.)

CASE in Point

At the conclusion of her first year of teaching for a university-based paramedic program, Christie noticed on her course evaluations that some of her students expressed discontent regarding the length of her lectures. At 8 hours per day, many students had difficulty staying focused, especially after lunch. Having recently read about new research on flipped classrooms, Christie wondered how she might use this method as a means to effectively deliver the same amount of content, while reducing the number of hours students spend in her classroom.

After consulting with a colleague, Christie learned of many resources available to help "flip" the classroom, such as online asynchronous video lectures, interactive e-books, and engaging classroom activities. By allowing students to acquire much of the necessary knowledge online, prior to coming to class, she can now use the shortened face-to-face classroom time to apply and reinforce their new knowledge with engaging group activities and dialogue.

The Psychological Environment

The effective educator sets the psychological tone of the learning environment by establishing the psychological parameters of behavior. It is essential that the expectations of the course be thoroughly discussed on the first day and be a component of the syllabus. It is the educator's responsibility to create a psychologically safe environment, in which students can make and learn from their mistakes. Psychologically safe environments exist in an atmosphere of mutual respect, shared responsibility, and safety. The relationship between student and educator is extremely important, and it has been directly related to student academic satisfaction.[31] The following sections describe strategies that can be used to establish and maintain an effective learning environment.[7,23,31,32]

Mutual Respect

One should strive to establish positive adult-to-adult rapport with students. The educator should treat students as adults whose life experiences can contribute to their learning and the learning of the entire class. The rapport between student and faculty is a powerful component of the learning environment, impacting the level of student engagement, quality of student learning, and behavioral issues. In positive environments, educators express enthusiasm for learning, are respectful, use appropriate humor, and voice expectations that all students can learn.

Shared Responsibility

A participatory environment should be fostered, where students share responsibility for their own learning. The educator role provides guidance and facilitation in the pursuit of knowledge. The learning environment should encourage intellectual freedom and creativity. It should promote trial and error with constructive feedback and represent an interactive learning agreement between students and educators. Students value a supportive environment, one in which they perceive that the educator is making sincere efforts to assist them in the learning process.[33] Student-centered learning activities are important to encourage shared responsibility for learning. (See Chapter 11, *Introduction to Teaching Strategies*, for additional information on student-centered learning.)

Safety in Learning

Abraham Maslow found that growth requires change, and change results from a sense of inner safety.[25] While physical safety is also important (see *Safety in the Classroom*), inner safety refers to student emotions, and this is a crucial consideration for the EMS educator to facilitate a welcoming and conducive environment for learning. Creating a safe place for students to learn without fear of ridicule is extremely important in the creation of a positive learning environment.[34] To motivate students to value the learning process, it must be safe and free of intimidation by fellow students, the instructor, or the administration. (See Chapter 25, *Legal Issues for EMS Educators*, and more information on the safe learning environment laws.)

Learning requires an environment in which the student is at ease and is able to experiment and learn from making mistakes. As a general rule, in a safe and positive learning environment, the following can be expected:[7,10,13,23,35,36]

- Students are free from harm.
- Students are free from discrimination.
- Students are free from sexual harassment.
- Students are free from teasing and hazing.
- Students and educators exhibit tolerance and acceptance.
- Students and educators encourage new ideas.

CASE in Point

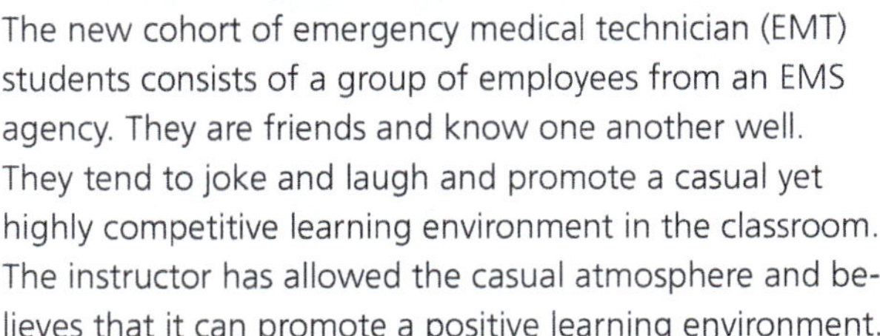

The new cohort of emergency medical technician (EMT) students consists of a group of employees from an EMS agency. They are friends and know one another well. They tend to joke and laugh and promote a casual yet highly competitive learning environment in the classroom. The instructor has allowed the casual atmosphere and believes that it can promote a positive learning environment.

However, there are two students who are not doing well in class. The instructor suspects that these two students may be intimidated by the other students. They do not ask questions, and when they do, the instructor notices nonverbal cues from the other students that appear to be condescending. These two students are reluctant to practice during skills sessions and seem to lack confidence.

The instructor talks to the class about the class environment and the importance of respect for all students in the class. The educator plans, if improvement is not noted, to consider pairing the two students with more assertive students in the class who have good leadership skills and could serve as mentors. Or, the offending students could be spoken to individually, the root cause of the behavior determined, and disciplinary procedures implemented if necessary. Whatever the best solution, the plan requires an improvement in the psychological environment of the class. Both individuals and groups of individuals must be held accountable for expected behavior and encouraged to contribute to a safe and positive learning environment for everyone involved.

TEACHING TIP

It is easier for an instructor to lighten up on class control, as trust and respect develop over time, than to start with less control and attempt to tighten up.

It is important for an educator to establish a classroom culture that accepts mistakes as a normal part of learning. Trial and error should be encouraged, and students should not feel that they will be punished for errors.[37] It is important for educators to realize that their response to student mistakes is critical in motivating students to try again and meet with success. How the instructor deals with the mistake can result in the student engaging or disengaging from the learning process. The instructor can acknowledge that the incorrect answer may seem plausible under the circumstances, and then discuss the correct answer with an explanation about why it is correct. The instructor should find something positive to say about the answer before explaining why it is incorrect. Every attempt should be made to provide an opportunity to learn from mistakes.

Discussion of a student's poor performance and collaborative strategies for improvement should be conducted in private when possible. The student must feel comfortable enough to "get it wrong" if the student is to progress to a point where they can "get it right."[1,23,38] In certain situations, such as high-technology simulations, performance as a team is addressed in the debriefing process.

Intellectual Challenge

Research shows that students are more motivated to learn when challenged to think and connect previous knowledge to new knowledge.[7,13] Setting a challenging pace, sometimes to the point of discomfort, is an important aspect of creating a dynamic learning environment. This pace must stimulate curiosity without overwhelming students and causing them to give up. It also should not be so easy that nothing is accomplished or learned by the experience.

CASE in Point

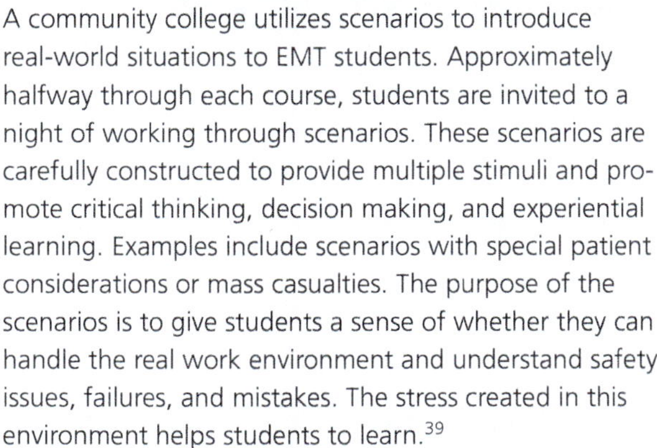

A community college utilizes scenarios to introduce real-world situations to EMT students. Approximately halfway through each course, students are invited to a night of working through scenarios. These scenarios are carefully constructed to provide multiple stimuli and promote critical thinking, decision making, and experiential learning. Examples include scenarios with special patient considerations or mass casualties. The purpose of the scenarios is to give students a sense of whether they can handle the real work environment and understand safety issues, failures, and mistakes. The stress created in this environment helps students to learn.[39]

Conflict

Conflict is a fact of life in higher education classrooms and can be dealt with constructively. Effective educators are not afraid of conflict—they realize the moment presents an opportunity for them to manage the situation and for students to enhance their level of understanding. The best educators understand this and learn how to manage conflict in an effort to bring positive and fair outcomes for all involved. Positive conflict is constructive and can help keep the class energized and creative. It is the educator's responsibility to build and maintain an environment that encourages all students to become equal participants in the learning process.[23]

In an effort to keep the conflict positive, the educator is faced with the challenge of managing the behavior appropriately.[6] The student grapevine moves quickly, and the manner in which the instructor manages the conflict will be remembered and will set the tone for future discussions in the classroom. Attention should be focused on how to make the conflict a constructive learning experience for the students.

There are three steps to effective classroom conflict management:[40]

1. **Clarify the problem**. Ask questions in an effort to clearly understand the issue at hand. After receiving feedback from students, the educator should restate the problem. This step identifies the students involved and clarifies the issue so that everyone has the same understanding.
2. **Identify a workable solution**. Have students offer suggestions for solutions, and work together to identify an agreeable solution. All parties should work together with positive attitudes and identify ground rules and criteria for the solution.
3. **Apply the solution**. Have students work together to develop a plan of action and ensure the implementation of the agreed-upon solution.

Negative behaviors such as foul language, loud voices, angry tones, and disrespect are disruptive and should not be permitted in the classroom. Students should understand that while differences of opinion are acceptable in the classroom culture, everyone in the room must still be treated with respect.

Behavioral Problems

Students enrolled in classes have the right to expect a safe environment and appropriate behavior from fellow classmates, as well as from professional educators in the classroom, lab, and clinical setting. Immature and disruptive behavior on the part of students deters serious academic students from enrolling in future courses. Moreover, such disruptive behavior adversely affects the learning environment of all students enrolled in the course, and it distracts the educator from their role as instructor and facilitator.

Most behavioral problems can be avoided by publishing behavioral expectations at the beginning of the course. These expectations can be listed in the syllabus, but should also be emphasized on day one by listing them on the whiteboard or during the introduction if the course is online. By posting them at the start of the course, the instructor has a clearly defined reference to which they can refer when there is a need to address a behavioral issue with a particular student or students. This reduces the chances of a contentious student disputing whether their behavior was permissible.

The Social Environment

It is important for the educator to remember that the learning environment is dynamic. As the individuals in a group get to know one another, the social interactions between them may change. This can create an evolving learning environment, which can be positive. For example, if everyone is speaking up, asking questions, and learning from one another because they feel safe to do so within the group, that is obviously a positive change. The key is to establish mutual respect and classroom expectations, so that the classroom relationships are not disruptive to the other members of the class.

At a fundamental level, the classroom experience can be thought of as a social arrangement. At the center of the social participation is the educator, who may possess a high degree of expertise in an academic discipline but may not be as skilled at promoting the positive social environment needed for effective learning.[23] It is important that the educator set the tone and maintain the tone even as class dynamics change. Studies have shown that learning increases when there is a positive rapport between students and educator.[41]

The instructor is the primary role model in the classroom. To act appropriately as a role model, the educator should clearly demonstrate the behaviors that students should exhibit. By modeling appropriate conduct, the instructor stands the best chance of developing the desired behaviors in students. Being on time to class, dressing in a professional manner, treating other instructors with respect, and refraining from inappropriate language are all examples of how an instructor can set positive impressions for students.

Using New Technologies

Virtual classrooms are not the only examples of how expanding technology has affected educational delivery. The use of technology to create a simulated "real environment" for students may result in successful practice as well. In addition to simulations, examples of using technology in the classroom include online library databases, virtual reality simulations, and computer-generated games. The use of diverse types of technology can create a dynamic environment that facilitates learning. This also allows the instructor to assess learning and student responsiveness in an engaging and less stressful environment. Student- or instructor-designed use of technology can create a fun place for learning. However, educators should be cautious about implementing new technologies simply because it is the latest shiny object on the market. The same considerations of adult learning methodology and effectiveness should be practiced for all new teaching tools.

Encouraging Teamwork

A career in EMS will involve many team activities; therefore, teamwork skills are essential. Group projects are an effective way to teach students about working in a team, improving accountability, and sharing ideas through discussion. The optimal group consists of less than five students; this size allows for individual student contribution and at the same time prevents the more industrious student from doing the majority of the work. Although instructors may encounter students who have already developed excellent team skills, they are more likely to find students who need coaching on teamwork and group dynamics.[23] For educators, a basic knowledge of how groups form and function is important for promoting positive team activities.

As groups form, there is a predictable dynamic to the growth of the team. Different stages may take varying amounts of time to evolve. Awareness of team stages seems to shorten their duration, as team members have an awareness of what will occur and know the language to describe group dynamic problems that they encounter.

Four stages of group growth are shown in **TABLE 7.1**. The first step is the **forming stage**, wherein team members encounter one another for the first time. The dominant theme of this stage is that members attempt to define the task assigned to them. Because the group has not worked together before, there are no set ground rules or expectations. Expectations must be clarified before the team can progress. Instructors should develop specific responsibilities for each team member, including the role of Team Leader. Assigning job responsibilities similar to those that students will encounter in the workforce helps identify the value of each team member in contributing to tasks or goals.

TABLE 7.1 Stages of Group Growth

Stage	Name	Student's Role	Instructor's Role
1	Forming	Define tasks	Clarify expectations
2	Storming	Determine hierarchy	Guide conflict
3	Norming	Establish cohesiveness	Maintain rules
4	Performing	Find balance	Affirmation

Modified from Tuckman, Bruce W. 1965. "Developmental Sequence in Small Groups." *Psychological Bulletin* 63, no. 6: 384–99. http://dx.doi.org/10.1037/h0022100.

As the group begins to establish goals and expectations, invariably, conflicts arise. This leads to the second stage—the **storming stage**. The dominant theme of this stage is the jockeying for position by team members as they struggle to define the team's leadership. This struggle can cause arguments and conflicts among team members, even when there is agreement on the real issue. In some cases, this conflict is externalized to the educator.

As conflicts are settled and a leadership system for the team emerges, the team progresses to a point at which interpersonal relationships grow more important than the team goal. This is the third stage—the **norming stage**. The dominant theme of this stage is emphasis on getting along, even when disagreements and open discussions are necessary. A sense of cohesion develops, and the team has now established and is maintaining ground rules.

This gives rise to the fourth stage—the **performing stage**. During the performing stage, the team balances interpersonal relationships with the team's needs, and results begin to occur. By the time this stage is reached, the team has developed the ability to work through group problems.[42]

Although it is difficult to observe teams going through this process, it is important for the educator to realize that the process itself is what allows students to learn teamwork skills. The role of the educator in team development is to guide students through these phases, pointing out landmarks and assisting them in working through obstacles.

Special Considerations

Because of the dynamic and sometimes unique nature of EMS education, educators should pay careful attention to detail when planning activities in the various settings to maximize the ability of the students to learn.

Nonlecture Environments

Increasing the reality of the learning environment may promote critical thinking, improve student confidence, and enhance performance. As learning settings become more complex, students integrate higher levels of thinking skills and psychomotor skills. No longer is simple knowledge adequate for performing a task; students must function at the application level or problem-solving level to perform in the clinical and field environment. (See Chapter 8, *Domains of Learning*.) When psychomotor skills are taught, students in clinical settings must apply these skills to a patient situation. For example, it is one thing to recite the sequence for cardiopulmonary resuscitation (CPR) in class, but quite another to recognize that a patient lying on the ground in a parking lot is not breathing and has no pulse. Utilization of safe outdoor areas, kitchens, bathrooms, or other in situ settings as learning environments can be an effective approach for improving performance.[11,26]

The learning environment can also be specific to location. For example, a student who has come from a rural area may be comfortable transporting patients for 30 to 60 minutes but fail to perform all treatments in a timely fashion in the urban setting, where transport times are generally less than 10 minutes. The problem in this case is likely the change in the environment, and not the student's knowledge base. Skill training around efficiency, multitasking, and delegation may provide keys to this student's success. An EMT student who has worked for a rural ambulance provider for 3 years may have a level of discomfort during an internship at a large, urban fire department. Emotions and stress may interfere with the ability to recall information and perform skills adequately. Acclimating to the fire service may do more in this situation to improve performance than any amount of studying. The plan for improvement should include activities to increase the student's comfort level at the station and with station personnel. An option for helping the student acclimate to an unfamiliar environment may include providing additional observation time before patient care tasks are added to the student's assignments.

Students entering a clinical environment for the first time, in which they are introduced to staff members and oriented to the facility, feel more comfortable and are set up for more successful learning.[38] However, as new variables are introduced within that environment, such as a difficult patient or unfamiliar equipment, the student's comfort and safety may become challenged.[9,24]

The Laboratory

Prior to working with live patients, students should become familiar with their skills and interventions so they can perform them safely and effectively under direct supervision. The instructor needs to consider numerous variables to ensure that student time in skills labs is safe and effective.

- **Safety**. As mentioned previously, safety should be considered in terms of physical practice by learners and educators (**FIGURE 7.5**) and in terms of a psychological environment free from ridicule. The educator must also consider any inherent danger associated with skills or any potential danger to the simulated patient. For example, caution is needed when defibrillation is demonstrated. Electrical shocks can be dangerous when performed on manikins and should never be performed on standardized patients. The educator should clearly define what is safe and should enforce it. Additionally, the educator must ensure safety with appropriate knowledge and use of universal precautions, proper disposal of sharps, proper body mechanics, and all aspects of a safe physical environment. Special precautions may be necessary when students are introduced to certain exercises.
- **Visibility**. For learners to model and imitate a skill, they must be able to see all aspects of the process. It

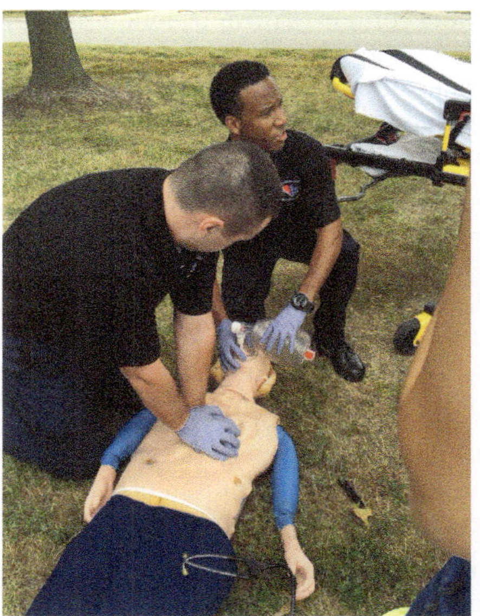

FIGURE 7.5 Physical safety when practicing clinical skills includes use of standard precautions.

is important that the educator place tables, chairs, and the equipment set-up so that it is easily viewed by all students. This includes instructor demonstrations and observation of a student practicing a skill or task. Other students should not have barriers that would inhibit vision or discussion.

- **Equipment**. The necessary equipment, supplies, and teaching aids should be identified and secured. An instructor should never assume that the equipment and materials needed to conduct the skills lab will be available in the classroom. This is especially true in multiuse facilities, where different instructors and different classes meet. Equipment should be checked for damage and that all parts are in working order. Documentation of who checked the equipment, including the date and time, should remain easily accessible in the lab. Often students are assigned this responsibility, with a team leader double checking for accuracy.
- **Cognitive load.** Human brains have a limited capacity to process new material.[43] Once that capacity is reached, additional content that is presented will go unlearned. Therefore, it is important that educators attempt to eliminate or minimize content that is not related to the material to be learned (such content is also known as extraneous load). The lab environment is bursting with extraneous load. This includes everything from trying to figure out how to check a pulse on a high-fidelity manikin, to trying to guess the expectations of different lab instructors. These can tie up valuable processing space in the student's brain, which is then not available to learn new content. The appropriate operations and use of all instructional technologies, as well as specific expectations of the task at hand, are variables that the educator is responsible for explaining before learning takes place.
- **Rehearsal**. Regardless of how many times or how well an educator can perform a skill, it is always prudent to practice the skill before class. This is especially true when a special model or equipment is used that is different from what the educator routinely uses. Demonstration accuracy by faculty is key to the student learning process.
- **Practice space.** The educator must ensure that sufficient space and equipment are provided for learners to practice a skill.
- **Encourage self-learning**. Set the expectation that learning new skills depends on student motivation to learn and valuing the importance of the skill. After instructors demonstrate a particular skill, they should expect that students will watch one another, go through a detailed skills checklist, and work through their mistakes before asking the instructor to watch them perform the skill. This type of peer mentoring and self-learning practice encourages lifelong learning.

CASE in Point

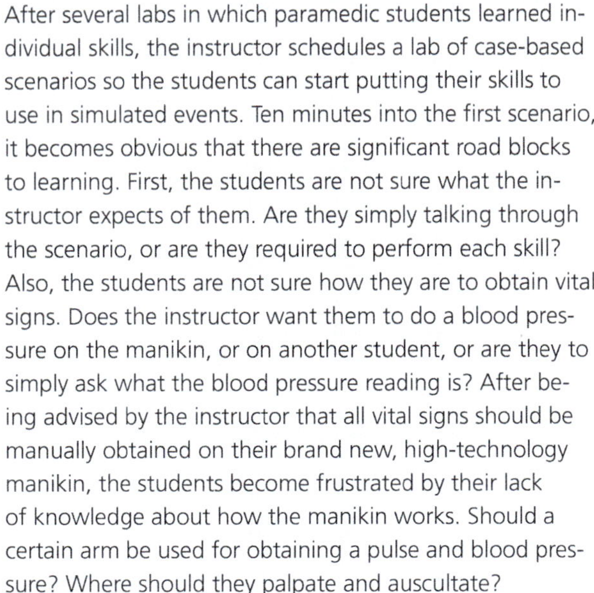

After several labs in which paramedic students learned individual skills, the instructor schedules a lab of case-based scenarios so the students can start putting their skills to use in simulated events. Ten minutes into the first scenario, it becomes obvious that there are significant road blocks to learning. First, the students are not sure what the instructor expects of them. Are they simply talking through the scenario, or are they required to perform each skill? Also, the students are not sure how they are to obtain vital signs. Does the instructor want them to do a blood pressure on the manikin, or on another student, or are they to simply ask what the blood pressure reading is? After being advised by the instructor that all vital signs should be manually obtained on their brand new, high-technology manikin, the students become frustrated by their lack of knowledge about how the manikin works. Should a certain arm be used for obtaining a pulse and blood pressure? Where should they palpate and auscultate?

The students have used a considerable amount of cognitive energy trying to learn the logistics of this scenario, none of which had anything to do with assessing and treating a patient. Ideally, this lab, as with any lab with new equipment, would have started with an orientation and time to practice using the equipment to ensure safety and competency. The instructor has an obligation to inform students of what is expected of them in the scenario and how the simulated equipment is to be used. By doing so, the students can focus their attention on the scenario, becoming more comfortable with the dynamics of patient care rather than becoming frustrated by the logistics.

- **Simulate real environments**. Where possible, an educator should use real props to simulate an actual working environment. For example, moving a patient from a sofa is different from moving someone off a classroom chair.
- **Attire**. Students should be advised when they will be performing psychomotor tasks so that they may wear appropriate clothing—for protection and to prevent embarrassment. This also applies to the instructor. Dress codes should be clearly stated for students and faculty. Be sure students are aware of any policies that require different attire in lab than what is acceptable in lecture.

Clinical and Field Environment

The clinical and field environments are very different from the lecture and lab environments with which the student is familiar. Clinical can be quite intimidating to the student, especially for those with little or no experience. It is important that the instructor address all components of the clinical environment, especially because they are not always there to troubleshoot when the students are in need.

- **Patient consent**. Be sure students understand the process of obtaining consent from patients prior to performing any interventions. Often, patients are not comfortable having students care for them. The student should always be identified as a student so that there is full disclosure to the patient about who is caring for them.
- **Preceptor orientation**. Students should never be left under the direction of a preceptor who does not know the student's objectives. Leaving preceptors in the dark can result in the student not receiving the exposure for which they are there, or worse, performing interventions for which they have not been properly prepared. Charge nurses in each clinical area should be given a packet of information regarding student objectives while attending clinicals. This information should be discussed to ensure understanding. Charge nurses should share this information with their assigned preceptors.
- **Adequate space and exposure**. The instructor is obligated to ensure that students are placed in a clinical environment that is appropriate to meet their objectives. Clinical environments that have too many students for the space or patient volume can be both ineffective and burdensome for the clinical site and the preceptors.
- **Safety**. Just as safety is crucial in the classroom, so too should it be a priority in clinical. It is important that the student be apprised of all safety policies set forth by the clinical site and that the extra burden of the student does not put the students, staff, or patients at additional risk. Students should have access to all of the same safety precautions that are available to the staff, such as infection control equipment. Additionally, students should be oriented as to where to find such equipment and how to use it.
- **Attire**. Clinical sites may require different uniform or attire than that of lecture or lab. Some clinical sites have specific policies regarding hair, jewelry, and visible tattoos. The instructor is responsible to be aware of these policies and to orient the student regarding those expectations prior to their first rotation.

Student Characteristics

Although a caring classroom and a positive instructor foster a better learning environment and decrease disruptive behaviors, the fact is, there are students who will challenge the instructor. The syllabus should clearly define professional behavior expectations and the consequence of failing to meet those professional attributes. The following are a few of the behaviors that every instructor will face.

The Late Comer

This is the student who regularly comes to class or lab late. Fellow students watch the offending student arrive late week after week, and silent frustration begins to build in the classroom setting.

- The educator can start the class with a quiz or other classroom assignment that encourages everyone to show up on time. A missed quiz could negatively affect the student's grade and is a strong deterrent to coming in late.
- The educator can pull the student aside and counsel them regarding the tardiness. Have specific problems kept the student from coming to class on time? Most EMS students are holding down a job while attending class or may have long travel times to get to class. Have the student put together and sign a plan that will solve this problem, now and for the future.

The Bored Student

This is the student who appears to be bored by the class. Their boredom may be observable through body language or lack of participation. The lack of interest could be related to the pace of the class or the lack of group activity; or, the student may not understand the material or may be preoccupied with work or family responsibilities.

- The instructor can create an opportunity for the student to participate by allowing the student to present a portion of the material. Actively engaging students makes them stakeholders in the learning process and creates active learners.
- The educator could visit with the student in an effort to identify the underlying issue. The problem may be a personal issue that has nothing to do with the instructor or the material that is being presented. The pace of the class may be too slow or too fast, a fact that can be discovered in talks between the educator and the student. Once the issue is identified, the instructor and student can write a corrective plan of action together.

The Social Butterfly

Social butterflies tend to spend more time visiting with everyone as opposed to learning. They tend to hold side conversations and seem more interested in socializing. This behavior interrupts the instructor's presentation. Some students may even use the classroom as a dating pool. Although the class should be a friendly and interactive environment, clear rules and guidelines must be in place to create boundaries to which both the instructors and the students have agreed.

- These students may require a job assignment in class that will allow them to put their people skills to work. The instructor can channel these students in a positive manner that can add to rather than detract from the classroom experience.
- A brief discussion with the student focusing on the effects of their behavior on the class may be in order.

The Introvert

Every classroom has a few introverts, who are more comfortable avoiding discussion. These students may not seem like active participants. They remain distant, keeping themselves invisible in the group.

- These students need to become involved in the learning process. Traditionally, instructors were taught to bring these students out by putting them on the spot through Socratic questioning in the classroom. However, this may cause further isolation and may lead the student to drop the class, feeling that they are being singled out.

  A better strategy is to have the student lead a small group discussion or group activity. This scales down classroom interaction to a few members and allows the student to take a more active role. In addition, it allows the instructor to promote a sense of belonging and ownership.
- Encouraging these students to take chances is another strategy that can work to their advantage. Rewarding small wins when they take small risks can lead to bigger risks that are safe and allows these students to become more social. The instructor must be careful not to put these students in a position that they cannot handle.

The Domineering Student

As future healthcare providers, allied health students are encouraged to be assertive in their communication. However, a dominant student can disrupt the learning environment. Typically this type of behavior is learned and offers a reward or payoff for the student. Discussion with the student to understand the root cause and consequences of this behavior will help with a behavioral or disciplinary action plan.

- Small groups with other students serving as the leaders can help to direct energy in other areas. Students in the group will, if carefully selected, be able to manage this personality type.
- Assign a project to the student if they are asking too many questions and causing the class to get off-track. The educator can compliment the student on being inquisitive and ask the student to research the topic and report to the class during the next meeting.
- If the behavior is consistently disruptive, the educator should confront the student and explain how the student can participate positively in the classroom. Explaining how their behavior affects the learning of other students can help the domineering student realize the outcomes of such behavior.

The Sleeper

EMS students usually work a job or have family responsibilities in addition to taking classes. The responsibilities of a student can result in little sleep or personal time.

- Calling on various students verbally to answer questions is a good way to encourage involvement and keep all students on their toes.
- Ensure that students have a break every 30 to 60 minutes.
- Involve students in learning activities other than the traditional lecture format. Group activities can work wonders in keeping students engaged in the learning process. Changing the presentation style every 20 minutes can keep students interested and is a necessary part of teaching the adult learner.

The Confused Student

Confused students have problems grasping the material. In addition to their poor grades, they may exhibit this by not engaging with the instructor or other students or by asking excessive irrelevant questions. The latter can slow down the instructor's presentation style and may lead to palpable frustration among student peers.

- The educator should provide students with clear expectations and a detailed plan on how to accomplish the goals of the class. The instructor can begin by outlining the classroom lecture for the day or for the week, so that the student can have a picture of how instruction will proceed.

- Group projects, like small groups comparing class notes before class dismissal, can help reinforce theory to this student, and establish a social network upon which academic assistance can occur. Peer support can be a powerful, nonthreatening, and reassuring strategy.
- Tutoring can also be arranged by faculty at prearranged times to help clear up any confusion.

The Hostage

Those who teach in agencies or companies who require their employees to attain a mandatory EMS certification or require monthly continuing education deal with this student type. These students shuffle into the classroom and strike an almost defiant pose. For the new instructor, this is one of the most difficult groups to teach. Even seasoned instructors may develop a sense of dread knowing they have to motivate these students.

To manage this type of student, instructors must recognize that motivation results from an interrelationship between internal student factors. Their motivation is based on the value they put on the learning goals and their belief that they are capable of achieving those goals (called *expectancy*). These intrinsic factors determine student behavior and how they see the environment, whether supportive or unsupportive. So, a disorganized classroom or one the learner feels is unfair will quickly dissolve positive attitudes.[44] Establishing a positive classroom environment from the first day of class is critical. Educators must clearly articulate the importance of each step of the learning process to help students achieve their individual learning goals to focus on their success. Educators must also make the content meaningful to student practice by incorporating relevant cases or examples. Instructors should integrate quality improvement data to show why the training is needed.

The educator can take clues for dealing with this type of student from the Motivational Framework for Culturally Responsive Teaching developed by Wlodkowski and Ginsberg.[45,46] The framework identifies four components (**TABLE 7.2**):

1. **Establishing inclusion**. This element includes developing a safe classroom community where each student's opinion is valued and in which others in the group have the community's best interests in mind. Involving students in meaningful group activities can enhance their feelings of self-worth and their engagement in the learning process. The Socratic questioning method, case studies, and role-play are examples of providing an interactive group dynamic.
2. **Developing attitude**. Students desire to learn because they believe the material is relevant. This fosters curiosity and interest that is necessary to establish intrinsic motivation to learn. Instructors should harness the fact that these students must achieve licensure or maintain their credentials to continue employment by coaching them in a positive manner toward that goal. Educators should incorporate quality improvement data when available to demonstrate the need for the training. Fernandez, Studnek, and Margolis found that the need to pass the licensure exam to retain employment is associated with increased success on the exam.[47]
3. **Enhancing meaning**. Learning experiences engage and challenge the students and include the learner's perspectives and values. Instructors should

TABLE 7.2 Strategies for Motivating Students

Component	Name	Instructor's Role	Example
1	Establish inclusion	Create safe learning environment	Group activities
2	Develop attitude	Foster immediacy	Focus on the importance of licensure by examination
3	Enhance meaning	Provide opportunities for context	Use real-life examples
4	Engender competence	Provide sufficient opportunities for mastery	Provide continuous feedback and affirmation

Modified from Wlodkowski, Raymond J. 2008. *Enhancing Adult Motivation to Learn,* 3rd ed. San Francisco: Jossey-Bass; Wlodkowski, Raymond J. 2004. "Creating Motivating Learning Environments." In *Adult Learning Methods: A Guide for Effective Instruction,* 3rd ed., edited by Michael W. Galbraith, 141–64. Malabar, FL: Krieger Publishing.

allow students to apply information in contexts that simulate real life so they see how the pieces of their education fit together to permit them to succeed in real-life patient situations. Instructors should provide real-life case examples when possible to illustrate the value of the material.

4. **Engendering competence**. Most students are capable of learning material they believe is valuable, and they also want to be proficient at relevant tasks. Providing the opportunity to demonstrate mastery of tasks and providing frequent positive feedback promote feelings of success that further motivate the learner.

It is important that all disruptions and breaches of classroom behavior be documented, so that if and when disruptions become persistent, a record of noncompliance is available to support the instructor's actions regarding a disciplinary process or, when appropriate, dismissal. A concise written statement of the behavior, including its impact on others and the intervention provided, is important. These behaviors should be documented on the affective (professional behavior) assessment.

Additionally, the educator may ask the student to formulate a learning contract or corrective action plan. The aim is to stop the disruptive behavior by suggesting alternatives. Students may need help to determine appropriate alternatives to disruptive behaviors. The plan for improvement should be short and concise, and should be designed for success. This plan should be written and signed by the student, the instructor, and a witness. Behavioral contracts or plans should be negotiated in a neutral, nonjudgmental tone. The educator should assist the student to move forward and plan for a better approach to classroom citizenship that will help the student succeed.

Although most classroom issues can be dealt with in conversation with the student, it is sometimes necessary for the instructor to deal with the issue in accordance with a formal disciplinary system. Instructors should check their organization's policies for the specific requirements. Formal disciplinary processes should be explained in the student handbook and during the first class session.

Summary

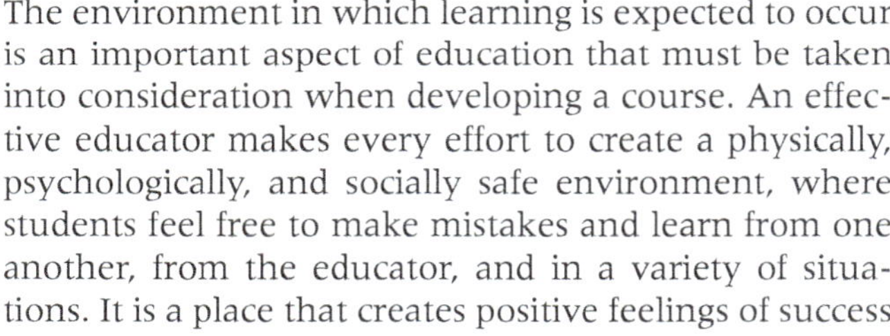

The environment in which learning is expected to occur is an important aspect of education that must be taken into consideration when developing a course. An effective educator makes every effort to create a physically, psychologically, and socially safe environment, where students feel free to make mistakes and learn from one another, from the educator, and in a variety of situations. It is a place that creates positive feelings of success and in which the educator and students are free to focus on academic success. The tactics and resources needed to foster an environment that promotes positive learning may change with each new class of students. Instructors should continually evaluate each situation and each new group of students and should review all acquired information, then devise a plan that will promote a positive learning environment for the given situation.

Glossary

forming stage Group growth stage in which team members encounter one another for the first time, attempt to define the task assigned to them, and start to determine the future course.

norming stage Group growth stage in which the team establishes and maintains ground rules.

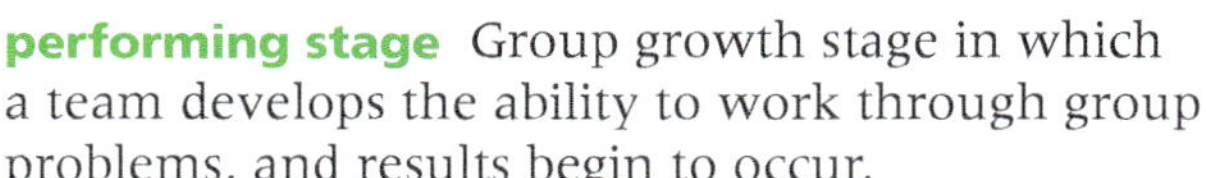

performing stage Group growth stage in which a team develops the ability to work through group problems, and results begin to occur.

storming stage Group growth stage in which team members jockey for position as they struggle to define the team's leadership.

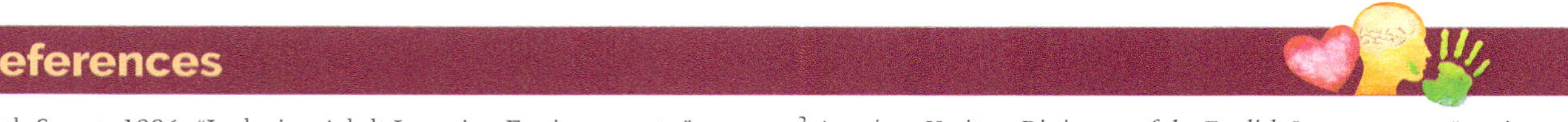

References

[1] Imel, Susan. 1996. "Inclusive Adult Learning Environments." *ERIC Digest No. 162*. Accessed February 13, 2019. http://www.ericdigests.org/1996-2/adult.html.

[2] *American Heritage Dictionary of the English Language, s.v.* "environment." Accessed May 4, 2018. https://ahdictionary.com/word/search.html?q=environment.

[3] Jackson, Gregory A., and Terrence E. Deal. 1985. "Technology, Learning Environments, and Tomorrow's Schools." *Peabody Journal of Education* 62, no. 2: 93–113. https://doi.org/10.1080/01619568509538477.

[4] Bruno, Andreina, and Giuseppina Dell'Aversana. 2018. "Reflective Practicum in Higher Education: The Influence of the Learning Environment on the Quality of Learning." *Assessment and Evaluation in Higher Education* 43, no. 3: 345–58. https://doi.org/10.1080/02602938.2017.1344823.

[5] Maslow, Abraham H. 1943. "A Theory of Human Motivation." *Psychological Review* 50, no. 4: 370.

[6] Hutchinson, Linda, Peter Cantillon, and Diane F. Wood. 2003. "Educational Environment." *British Medical Journal*, 326, no. 7393: 810–2. https://doi.org/10.1136/bmj.326.7393.810.

[7] Billington, Dorothy D. 2002. "Seven Characteristics of Highly Effective Adult Learning Programs." *New Horizons for Learning*. Accessed February 13, 2019. http://archive.education.jhu.edu/PD/newhorizons/lifelonglearning/workplace/articles/characteristics/index.html.

[8] Biswalo, Peles. 2001. "The Systems Approach as a Catalyst for Creating an Effective Learning Environment." *Convergence* 34, no. 1: 53–67.

[9] Cleave-Hogg, Doreen, and Arthur I. Rothman. 1991. "Discerning Views: Medical Students' Perceptions of Their Learning Environment." *Evaluation and the Health Professions* 14, no. 4: 456–74. https://doi.org/10.1177/016327879101400406.

[10] Diamantes, Thomas. 2002. "Improving Instruction in Multicultural Classes by Using Classroom Learning Environment." *Journal of Instructional Psychology* 29, no. 4: 277–83.

[11] Magolda, Marcia B. B. 2000. "Teaching to Promote Holistic Learning and Development." *New Directions for Teaching and Learning* 82: 88–99. https://doi.org/10.1002/tl.8209.

[12] Davis, Barbara G. 2001. *Tools for Teaching*. San Francisco: Jossey-Bass.

[13] Simplicio, Joseph S. C. 1999. "Some Simple and Yet Overlooked Common Sense Tips for a More Effective Classroom Environment." *Journal of Instructional Psychology* 26, no, 2: 111–6.

[14] Lee, Eunbae, and Michael J. Hannafin. 2016. "A Design Framework for Enhancing Engagement in Student-Centered Learning: Own It, Learn It, and Share It." *Educational Technology Research and Development* 64, no. 4: 707–34. https://doi.org/10.1007/s11423-015-9422-5.

[15] Richmond, Aaron S., Jeanne M. Slattery, Nathanael Mitchell, Robin K. Morgan, and Jared Becknell. 2016. "Can a Learner-Centered Syllabus Change Students' Perceptions of Student–Professor Rapport and Master Teacher Behaviors?" *Scholarship of Teaching and Learning in Psychology* 2, no. 3: 159–68. http://dx.doi.org/10.1037/stl0000066

[16] Brown, William E., Gregg Margolis, and Roger. Levine. 2005. "Peer Evaluation of the Professional Behaviors of Emergency Medical Technicians." *Prehospital and Disaster Medicine* 20, no. 2: 107–14. https://doi.org/10.1017/S1049023X00002284.

[17] Grinols, Anne B., and Rishi Rajesh. 2014. "Multitasking with Smartphones in the College Classroom." *Business and Professional Communication Quarterly* 77, no. 1: 89–95. https://doi.org/10.1177/2329490613515300.

[18] Norris, Cathleen, Akhlaq Hossain, and Elliot Soloway. 2011. "Using Smartphones as Essential Tools for Learning: A Call to Place Schools on the Right Side of the 21st Century." *Educational Technology* 51, no. 3: 18–25.

[19] Voss, Roediger, Thorsten Gruber, and Isabelle Szmigin. 2007. "Service Quality in Higher Education: The Role of Student Expectations." *Journal of Business Research* 60, no. 9: 949–59. https://doi.org/10.1016/j.jbusres.2007.01.020.

[20] Lippincott, Joan K. 2009. "Learning Spaces: Involving Faculty to Improve Pedagogy." *EDUCAUSE Review* 44, no. 2: 16–25.

[21] CDW Government. 2008. *The 21st Century Campus: Are We There Yet?* Accessed February 13, 2019. https://www.slideshare.net/joshmkim/the-21st-century-campus-are-we-there-yet-challenges-and-opportunities-for-campus-technologies-presentation.

[22] Han, Heesup, Kiattipoom Kiatkawsin, Wansoo Kim, Ju H. Hong. 2018. "Physical Classroom Environment and Student Satisfaction with Courses." *Assessment and Evaluation in Higher Education* 43; no. 1: 110–25. https://doi.org/10.1080/02602938.2017.1299855.

[23] Anderson, James A. 1999. "Faculty Responsibility for Promoting Conflict-Free College Classrooms." *New Directions for Teaching and Learning* 77: 69–76.

[24] Morris, William (Ed.). 1976. *The American Heritage Dictionary of the English Language*, 438. Boston: Houghton Mifflin.

[25] Mann, Karen V. 2002. "Thinking about Learning: Implications for Principle-Based Professional Education." *Journal of Continuing Education in the Health Professions* 22, no. 2: 69–77. http://dx.doi.org/10.1002/chp.1340220202.

[26] Niemeyer, Daniel C. 2003. *Hard Facts on Smart Classroom Design: Ideas, Guidelines, and Layouts*. Lanham, MD: Scarecrow Press.

[27] Firebaugh, Francille M., and David O. Watkins. 1997. "The College Embraces Technology for Education." *Human Ecology Forum* 25, no. 4: 1.

[28] Dwyer, Carol A. 1999. "Using Emerging Technologies to Construct Effective Learning Environments." *Educational Media International* 36, no. 4: 300–10. https://doi.org/10.1080/0952398990360409.

[29] Kraiger, Kurt, J. Kevin Ford, and Eduardo Salas. 1993. "Application of Cognitive, Skill-Based, and Affective Theories of Learning Outcomes to New Methods of Training Evaluation." *Journal of Applied Psychology* 78, no. 2: 311. http://dx.doi.org/10.1037/0021-9010.78.2.311.

[30] Brinson, James R. 2015. "Learning Outcome Achievement in Non-traditional (Virtual and Remote) versus Traditional (Hands-on) Laboratories: A Review of the Empirical Research." *Computers and Education* 87: 218–37. https://doi.org/10.1016/j.compedu.2015.07.003.

[31] Imel, Susan. 1988. "Guidelines for Working with Adult Learners." *ERIC Digest No. 77*. Accessed February 13, 2019. http://www.ericdigests.org/pre-929/working.htm.

[32] Imel, Susan. 1989. "Teaching Adults: Is It different?" *ERIC Digest No. 82*. Accessed February 13, 2019. http://www.ericdigests.org/pre-9211/teaching.htm.

[33] Winteler, A. 1981. "The Academic Department as Environment for Teaching and Learning." *Higher Education* 10: 25–35. https://doi.org/10.1007/BF00154889.

[34] Clapper, Timothy C. 2010. "Creating the Safe Learning Environment." *Pailal Newsletter* 3: 1–6.

[35] Backes, Charles E. 1997. "The Do's and Don'ts of Working with Adult Learners." *Adult Learning* 8, no. 3: 29–32. https://doi.org/10.1177/104515959700800314.

[36] Robins, Lynne S., Larry D. Gruppen, Gwen Alexander, Joseph C. Fantone, and Wayne K. Davis. 1997. "A Predictive Model of Student Satisfaction with the Medical School Learning Environment." *Academic Medicine* 72, no. 2: 134–9.

[37] Bierema, Laura L. 2018. "Adult Learning in Health Professions Education." *New Directions for Adult and Continuing Education* 2018, no. 157: 27–40. https://doi.org/10.1002/ace.20266.

[38] Newble, David I., and Eugene J. Hejka. 1991. "Approaches to Learning of Medical Students and Practising Physicians: Some Empirical Evidence and Its Implications for Medical

Education." *Educational Psychology* 11: 333–43. https://doi.org/10.1080/0144341910110309.

[39] Moore, Judith A., Stephen Cote, Stephen Vantassel, Tim Graeme, and Kevin Andrews. 2003. "EMS Stress-Training Concept 'Kobayashi Moru' Scenarios." *Domain 3*. National Association of EMS Educators.

[40] Holton, Susan A. 1999. "After the Eruption: Managing Conflict in the Classroom." *New Directions for Teaching and Learning* 77: 59–68. https://doi.org/10.1002/tl.7706.

[41] Sutliff, Michael, Janelle Higginson, and Sean Allstot. 2008. "Building a Positive Learning Environment for Students: Advice to Beginning Teachers." *Strategies* 22, no. 1: 31–3. https://doi.org/10.1080/08924562.2008.10590806

[42] Tuckman, Bruce W. 1965. "Developmental Sequence in Small Groups." *Psychological Bulletin* 63, no. 6: 384–99. http://dx.doi.org/10.1037/h0022100.

[43] Westby, Carol. 2018. "Cognitive Load and Learning." *Word of Mouth* 29, no. 4: 8–12. https://doi.org/10.1177/1048395018759556b.

[44] Ambrose, Susan A., Michael W. Bridges, Marsha C. Lovett, Michele DiPietro, and Marie K. Norman. 2010. *How Learning Works: Seven Research-Based Principles for Smart Teaching*. San Francisco: Jossey-Bass.

[45] Wlodkowski, Raymond J. 2008. *Enhancing Adult Motivation to Learn*, 3rd ed. San Francisco: Jossey-Bass.

[46] Wlodkowski, Raymond J. 2004. "Creating Motivating Learning Environments." In *Adult Learning Methods: A Guide for Effective Instruction*, 3rd ed., edited by Michael W. Galbraith, 141–64. Malabar, FL: Krieger Publishing.

[47] Fernandez, Antonio R., Jonathan R. Studnek, and Gregg S. Margolis. 2008. "Estimating the Probability of Passing the National Paramedic Certification Examination." *Academic Emergency Medicine* 15, no. 3: 258–64. https://doi.org/10.1111/j.1553-2712.2008.00062.x.

Additional Resources

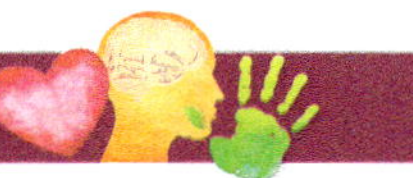

Park, Elisa L., and Bo Keum Choi. 2014. "Transformation of Classroom Spaces: Traditional versus Active Learning Classroom in Colleges." *Higher Education* 68, no. 5: 749–71. https://doi.org/10.1007/s10734-014-9742-0.

Segrist, Dan, Lynn K. Bartels, and Cynthia R. Nordstrom. 2018. "'But Everyone Else Is Doing It': A Social Norms Perspective on Classroom Incivility." *College Teaching* 66, no. 4: 181–6. https://doi.org/10.1080/87567555.2018.1482858.

CHAPTER 8

Domains of Learning

OBJECTIVES

At the conclusion of this chapter, the educator will be able to:

Cognitive Domain

1. Differentiate between the three domains of learning.
2. Understand the revisions within the cognitive domain of learning.
3. Describe the levels of mastery within each domain of learning.
4. Compare and contrast objective assessment tools appropriate for each domain of learning.

Psychomotor Domain

There are no psychomotor objectives for this chapter.

Affective Domain

1. Value the importance of developing strategies to ensure student progression of knowledge, skill, and behavior in all the domains of learning.
2. Defend the importance of teaching and assessing all domains of learning throughout a class or program.
3. Value that the assessment of progressive learning in each domain is based on objectives.

"Meaning making involves thinking, feeling, and acting, and all three of these aspects must be integrated for significant new learning, and especially in new knowledge creation."

~ Dr. Joseph. D. Novak

CHAPTER GOAL This chapter will provide the traditional perspective of the three predominant domains of learning.

For many years, researchers have identified different domains, or categories, of learning that educators use in several ways in their practice of teaching. An increased understanding of objectives will assist an educator in devising strategies for learning, teaching, and assessment. In the instructional design process, the **domains of learning** are always considered when goals and objectives are established and written. Educators also identify student knowledge and behaviors that exemplify the domains of learning. In the context of medical education, these domains are targeted in the lesson plans and in the choices regarding the teaching strategies that will be used. Finally, educators consider each domain when formulating assessment criteria and methods. The domains of learning lie behind every stage of the learning, teaching, and assessment processes.

This chapter will assist instructors to recognize how to integrate each domain of learning into their teaching practice. Adopting these strategies will promote student acquisition of the knowledge, skills, and professional behaviors essential for practice in emergency medical services (EMS).

Categorizing the Domains

Dr. Benjamin Bloom and a team of researchers first categorized the domains of learning in 1956.[1] Bloom and colleagues described three distinct domains of learning: cognitive, affective, and psychomotor.

Bloom chose the term *domain* to describe the major divisions of his concepts, because a domain is a related collection of things or items. Collectively, this work is known as **Bloom's taxonomy**. The term *taxonomy* is used to explain a hierarchy or progression of achieving competency or mastery of content, skill, or behavior. Although the taxonomy of all domains is attributed to Bloom because he was the first author of the 1956 paper, Krathwohl and Dave were the primary authors on the affective and the psychomotor divisions. Bloom's strategy is commonly used in medical education and is described in this textbook. The cognitive section of this chapter reflects the most recent revised work within the domain.

Cognitive Domain

Simply put, the **cognitive domain** describes learning that takes place through the process of thinking; it deals with facts and knowledge. For example, a student who reads a textbook and learns the contraindications of administering a certain medication is operating in the cognitive domain. Much of what medical professionals accomplish is based on the ability to acquire knowledge and use it for the greater good of patient care.

Since the time of Bloom's original cognitive domain work, other researchers have built upon his concepts and have developed other strategies of classification and additional categories of learning domains. In 2001, some of Bloom's original cohorts made revisions to the cognitive domain.[2] Anderson and Krathwohl gathered a group of educational psychologists and educators for the revision. Anderson was a student of Bloom, while Krathwohl was one of Bloom's original partners in the 1956 taxonomy.

Psychomotor Domain

The **psychomotor domain** describes learning that takes place through the attainment of skills and bodily, or kinesthetic, movements. For example, a student who physically practices in a skills station is taking steps toward competency in how to properly perform the skill and thus meet the needs associated in the psychomotor domain.

Affective Domain

The **affective domain** describes learning in terms of feelings, emotions, attitudes, and values. For example, a student who participates in case scenarios and learns to appreciate how vulnerable patients can feel when they are sick or injured is operating in the affective domain. Additionally, the affective domain covers many "soft skills" or professional behaviors, and its development is vital for career success. Specific examples include integrity, engagement, motivation, empathy, and self-discipline. This domain is essential to all of education, but in the education of healthcare professionals specifically, it is of utmost importance that aspects from the affective domain be embedded into the instructional process.

Interplay between the Domains

It is important for educators to understand that, although Bloom and his colleagues described learning processes that take place within three distinct categories, learning seldom takes place solely within one category without at least some aspect of the other two. As such, making distinctions between the three domains is artificial at best. When learning occurs, at least two domains are being used by a learner. The affective domain has been identified as the gateway to learning. When well-developed, it opens the door for the cognitive and psychomotor domain expansion. As discussed previously, if a student is closed to learning, learning will not occur. (See Chapter 3, *Brain-Based Learning*). For example, for a student to properly perform a psychomotor skill, the student must possess cognitive, affective, and psychomotor knowledge. An emergency medical technician (EMT) who performs cardiopulmonary resuscitation (CPR) effectively must first know the correct sequence of the steps for CPR (cognitive domain), must then make a decision regarding whether or not to begin resuscitation efforts through the application of ethical and moral values dictated by protocol or standing orders (affective domain), and, once the decision to treat has been made, must correctly and efficiently perform the skills (psychomotor domain). All of this is based on motivation to learn and willingness to engage in learning (affective domain).

TABLE 8.1 Taxonomy of the Domains of Learning

Levels	Cognitive Domain	Psychomotor Domain	Affective Domain
1	Remember	Imitation	Receive
2	Understand	Manipulation	Respond
3	Apply	Precision	Value
4	Analyze	Articulation	Organize
5	Evaluate*	Naturalization	Characterize
6	Create*		

*Note that the levels of evaluating and creating (formerly synthesizing) have been reversed from the original taxonomy.

Domain Levels and Dimensions

Each domain is structured into distinct divisions, or levels, that reflect the increasing depth and breadth of understanding or skill an individual achieves when progressing through the domain. Several systems of categorizing these levels are applied within each domain, and these systems are classified as either formal or informal. Of the two types, formal systems provide a greater amount of structure. Therefore, formal systems are typically used by the instructor for greater precision in determining how much content to cover on a given topic, and in identifying the appropriate depth and breadth of content for assessment purposes.

Bloom's Taxonomy for the Cognitive Domain

Bloom and colleagues originally identified and described five levels within each of the three domains of learning. In 2001, Anderson and Krathwohl led a team that revised the levels within the cognitive domain (**TABLE 8.1**). Their motivation considered many of Bloom's original concerns and criticisms that he identified with reflection and reexamination after his original 1956 publication.[2] It should be noted that specific action verbs can be used to describe behavioral characteristics required within each level. A partial listing of some of the action verbs appropriate for each level is found in Chapter 9, *Goals and Objectives*.

Cognitive Domain Dimensions and Levels

The cognitive domain contains two dimensions: the cognitive process dimension and the knowledge dimension. The taxonomy is two-dimensional as a result of the 2001 revisions.[2]

The Cognitive Process Dimension. The **cognitive process dimension** contains the actions in which a learner engages when learning in the cognitive domain.[3] These actions include remembering, understanding, applying, analyzing, evaluating, and creating. Each of these actions is assigned a level number. The levels, per the 2001 revisions, are as follows.[2]

Level 1: Remember. Remembering occurs when a learner recognizes or recalls previous knowledge from memory.

Level 2: Understand. Understanding occurs when a learner constructs meaning from differing types of functions such as interpretations, summaries, and/or written messages.

Level 3: Apply. Applying is shown by a student when learned material is used in new or differing situations, or the application of knowledge is demonstrated.

CASE in Point

Cognitive Process Dimension

A paramedic student first learns the contraindications of administering a specific medication and is able to list them (Level 1: Remember). Next, the student comprehends the adverse effects of the medication on a patient for whom it is contraindicated (Level 2: Understand). In Level 3: Apply, the student can explain the physiologic principles behind why and how the adverse effects occur with minimal assistance from the instructor. Next, given a specific patient scenario, the student is able to determine whether or not the medication would be contraindicated (Level 4: Analyze). In Level 5: Evaluate, the student accurately and efficiently performs in a patient scenario in a skills practicum and determines when to use and not use a medication. The paramedic student performs with no assistance from the instructor. In the final level, Create (Level 6), the student is able to synthesize thoughts about using a given medication (that has multiple uses) for conditions that have not yet been taught.

Level 4: Analyze. Analyzing requires that the student be able to break down whole concepts into individual, smaller parts to analyze their meaning, assess their relationships to each other and the larger concept, and understand their importance. Words that describe this level of action are differentiating, distinguishing, organizing, and attributing.

Level 5: Evaluate. Evaluating occurs when a learner can make judgments based on previous learning of standards or other criteria. In the 1956 domain, evaluation was the top level of thinking. Krathwohl and Anderson argue that evaluating precedes creating because evaluation is often a required step before one can create something.

Level 6: Create. Creating occurs when a learner puts the elements together to form a new logical pattern, structure, or concept. The reorganization of the simpler elements into a new creation or product is seen. This is the most difficult mental function. As a result, it is at the top of the cognitive domain level described by Krathwohl and Anderson.

The Knowledge Dimension. The **knowledge dimension** is a new feature within the cognitive domain and is designed to be used in addition to the action, or behavioral, components. This dimension describes the types of knowledge an educator must consider for the cognitive domain. The types of knowledge include factual, conceptual, procedural, and metacognitive[2] and are described here.

Factual knowledge is the basic elements a learner must know to be familiar with and understand a subject discipline. It entails facts, terminology, or other discrete details of knowledge related to a body of knowledge within a subject area. In EMS education, medical terminology is a great example of factual knowledge. In this example, a learner must understand terms and these terms build a foundational understanding for a subject matter such as emergency medicine.

Conceptual knowledge is learned information regarding the relationships among basic elements within the larger subject and how these concepts function together. Examples include classifications, principles, generalizations, theories, or models. An EMS education example may include concepts related to ventilation, oxygenation, and perfusion (VOP). General principles of VOP help a clinical provider understand the most essential aspects of emergency care.

Procedural knowledge is learned information of how to do something based on algorithms, techniques, or accepted methodology. In EMS, procedural knowledge can be demonstrated in very specific skills such as intubation, spinal immobilization, and cardiopulmonary arrest or resuscitation. Evidence-based medical algorithms are another example of procedural knowledge used in EMS patient care.

Metacognitive knowledge is an understanding of one's cognition. Simply stated, it is thinking about thinking in a purposeful manner. When metacognitive knowledge is utilized, learners know about their cognition, regulate learning activities, use strategic actions (such as self-assessment), and intentionally reflect; in all, these make for decisive learning improvement. Developing metacognitive knowledge allows learners to constantly grow in expertise because their existing knowledge is examined, refined, and self-directed. Purposeful actions are used to grow and further develop intelligence.

Using the levels in the cognitive process dimension and the types of knowledge in the knowledge dimension, an educator can understand interrelationships between the types of knowledge and actions required to learn them. The advantage of understanding these dimensions is that one can chart on a table the intersection of the cognitive levels and the type of knowledge (**TABLE 8.2**). With this insight, an educator can plan teaching and assessment so that they are better aligned.

TABLE 8.2 Charting the Cognitive Process and Knowledge Dimensions

		Cognitive Process Dimension					
		1 Remember	2 Understand	3 Apply	4 Analyze	5 Evaluate	6 Create
Knowledge Dimension	Factual						
	Conceptual						
	Procedural						
	Metacognitive						

Modified from Anderson, Lorin W., and David R. Krathwohl (Eds.). 2001. *A Taxonomy for Learning, Teaching, and Assessing: A Revision of Bloom's Taxonomy of Educational Objectives*. New York: Pearson.

CASE in Point

Knowledge Dimension and Cognitive Process Dimension

To illustrate use of the cognitive process and knowledge dimensions, the following example uses five objectives for learning concepts and for demonstrating gained knowledge of cardiac arrest management—specifically, the care of an adult patient in asystole.

The lesson objectives are as follows:

1. Students should be able to recall the proper rate and depth of chest compressions for adult CPR.
2. Students should be able to contrast the results (cause/effect) of proper and improper CPR.
3. Students should be able to carry out an advanced cardiac life support (ACLS) algorithm for the treatment of asystole.
4. Students should be able to distinguish important and unimportant history/findings (5Hs and 5Ts) when determining patient history.
5. Students should be able to critique personal strengths and weaknesses of one's knowledge level of the treatment of asystole.

Using the taxonomy table with both dimensions plotted, an instructor would chart the objectives as shown in **TABLE 8.3**.

The following analysis breaks down how the objectives relate to the dimensions:

- Objective 1 is simply the recall of factual details or elements (chest compression rate and depth) for good CPR. It is categorized as factual information that is remembered.
- Objective 2 is the understanding or the meaning of two ideas. The objective requires students to detect the conceptual consequences of proper CPR and improper CPR. It is therefore categorized as conceptual information to understand.
- Objective 3 requires students to carry out or apply a procedure that is based on an accepted ACLS algorithm, in this case the care of asystole. It is categorized as procedural/apply.
- When utilizing Objective 4, students have to discriminate between essential information and nonessential information when gathering a patient history to determine which "H" or "T" is relevant in the care of a patient experiencing asystole. This can be taught and assessed in the context of a megacode setting. This objective is categorized as procedural/analyze.
- Objective 5 uses metacognitive knowledge to evaluate, assess, and critique one's weaknesses, strengths, or knowledge level in regard to asystole management. Objective 5 is categorized as metacognitive/evaluate.
- Finally, rarely is an entry-level EMS student required to create new knowledge on a subject, so in this example, there is no objective associated with this category.

The benefit of simultaneously plotting the knowledge and cognitive process dimensions is to gain a more complete understanding of the nouns and verbs associated with the objectives.[3] This will lead to better decision making about teaching, assessment, and curriculum alignment. Some of these objectives would be well-suited for a written examination, while others would be best accomplished in a megacode setting; finally, personal reflection (metacognition) would be best assessed through reflection.

TABLE 8.3 Example of Charting the Cognitive Domain Using Both Dimensions

		Cognitive Process Dimension					
		1 Remember	2 Understand	3 Apply	4 Analyze	5 Evaluate	6 Create
Knowledge Dimension	Factual	Objective 1					
	Conceptual		Objective 2				
	Procedural			Objective 3	Objective 4		
	Metacognitive					Objective 5	

Key	Description
Objective 1	Students should be able to recall the proper rate and depth of chest compressions for adult CPR.
Objective 2	Students should be able to contrast the results (cause/effect) of proper and improper CPR.
Objective 3	Students should be able to carry out an ACLS algorithm for the treatment of asystole.
Objective 4	Students should be able to distinguish important and unimportant history/findings (5Hs and 5Ts) when determining patient history.
Objective 5	Students should be able to critique personal strengths and weaknesses of one's knowledge level of the treatment of asystole.

Psychomotor Domain Levels

The levels in the psychomotor domain are as follows.[2,4]

Level 1: Imitation occurs as students repeat and mimic demonstrations given by an instructor.

Level 2: Manipulation occurs as students practice the skill and begin to create their own styles of performance. Because students lack sophistication at this point, experimentation and trial-and-error are expected and should be encouraged by the educator.

Level 3: Precision is the point at which the skill should be performed without mistakes. Students should also begin to transfer its use to other situations or circumstances. However, this will be done with a high degree of error in performance, necessitating resumption of the trial-and-error process (but with a new emphasis on exploring "what if" concepts).

Level 4: Articulation occurs when students become adept, demonstrate competence, and add their own style or finesse when they perform the skill. At this level, students are able to modify their skill performance as needed and defend their choices and decisions.

Level 5: Naturalization is the mastery level of skill performance. In contrast to the cognitive and affective domains, this level is attained when the student performs the skill seemingly without any cognition required. This level is sometimes referred to as "muscle memory" or "automatic memory." True naturalization occurs when skill performance is correct despite the environment or circumstance in which the skill is performed.

Affective Domain Levels

The affective domain levels were first described by Krathwohl in his work with Bloom and Masia.[5] The affective domain levels are as follows.

Level 1: Receive. Receiving occurs as the student acquires awareness of the value or importance of learning information and expresses a willingness to learn. At this level, students may not agree with or value the actual concepts, but they are open to listening.

Level 2: Respond. Responding expands on Level 1 as the student actively participates in the learning process and begins to consider the concept further.

Level 3: Value. Valuing is the level in which the student individually perceives that the behavior has worth or value. In some cases, this is a foundational level if the concept or idea was already incorporated within a student's value system.

Level 4: Organize. Organizing integrates new, refined, or different beliefs into the student's existing value system and reconciles differences between old and new beliefs. Students should also begin to replace preexisting values that conflict with the newer ones being adopted.

CASE in Point

Psychomotor Domain

When students learn the skill of bag-valve-mask (BVM) ventilation, there is a process of building through the five psychomotor domain levels. The first time these concepts are presented, the instructor acts out the steps needed to properly use the BVM. Students are first encouraged to watch and do what the instructor demonstrates on a manikin, for example, how to seal the mask correctly over the nose and mouth and properly squeeze the bag (Level 1: Imitation). The students practice with the BVM, demonstrating various techniques such as squeezing the bag and securing the mask on the nose and mouth of the manikin (Level 2: Manipulation). As the students gain confidence in performing the proper methods of ventilating a manikin with a BVM, the instructor begins to introduce "what if" scenarios into the airway management simulation, causing the students to react and make appropriate adjustments in their treatment plans (Level 3: Precision). The students react appropriately in most scenarios and, when questioned, can defend their treatment choices with logical reasoning. This includes the ability to select different types of BVM devices (bags as well as masks) and still achieve success in securing and properly ventilating the manikin and live patients (Level 4: Articulation). When the students are presented with various scenarios in a variety of situations, the students automatically demonstrate their competence, regardless of the type of bag or mask, and achieve success in the proper ventilation of most patients (Level 5: Naturalization).

CASE in Point

Affective Domain

Isabella, an experienced EMT, is enrolled in paramedic school after numerous years in the field. Her EMS faculty member is conducting a lesson about professional and ethical pain management therapy. Isabella is attentive to the lesson regarding EMS management of pain (Level 1: Receive). The lesson continues and she becomes active in the discussion (Level 2: Respond). Eventually, Isabella begins to make a personal commitment to treat patients in a professional and ethical manner (Level 3: Value).

Next, she begins to sort through past experiences and encounters with patients who have suffered from pain. Isabella begins to establish her own professional and ethical perspective on the therapy (Level 4: Organize). No longer will she consider all patients potential "drug seekers"; rather, she will assess the patient's legitimate need for pain management.

The final domain is Characterize, Level 5. When Isabella becomes a paramedic, she begins her clinical practice and attitude for treating all patients with pain in an informed and thorough manner. She demonstrates an ethical and professional demeanor for this patient population and overcomes uninformed and critical attitudes when caring for her patients. Isabella's actions become a part of who she is as a clinical provider.

Level 5: Characterize. Characterizing is the most sophisticated level in the affective domain. It requires the development of one's own value system that governs behavior. Like Level 6: Creating in the cognitive domain, it involves a degree of metacognition as the student scrutinizes the processes used in deriving their values, beliefs, and opinions.

Addressing the Domains in Goals and Objectives

The domains of learning are used in the instructional design process for planning curriculum and writing goals and objectives. Program administrators have limited time for classroom, laboratory, and clinical/field activities, so desired learning must be defined and planned. Time must be allocated for content, psychomotor skills, and clinical experiences based on the importance of one subject over another. Educators must understand the language of an objective or goal and must discern specific meaning from the verbs used to write them. (See Chapter 9, *Goals and Objectives*.) This enables the educator to plan instructional and assessment processes that assist students in meeting the objectives and provide a means of measuring their achievement. Understanding the interrelationship between the goals and objectives and their role in clarifying strategies for learning, instruction, and evaluation will help program administrators to align teaching methodologies, student assessment, and teacher evaluation.

In the cognitive domain, terms such as *list, name, match, memorize, order, recall, recite,* and *repeat* are useful for Level 1: Remember. Level 4: Analyze of the cognitive domain uses terms such as *analyze, calculate, compare and contrast, differentiate,* and *examine*. Appreciating the differing cognitive level of these objectives contributes to better learning, instruction, assessment, and alignment. In the psychomotor domain, Level 1: Imitation employs terms such as *repeat, mimic,* and *follow,* whereas Level 4: Articulation uses terms like *demonstrate proficiency* and *perform without assistance*. In the affective domain, terms such as *accept, attempt,* and *willing* are appropriate for Level 1: Receiving, and *join* and *participate* are found in Level 5: Characterizing. Goals and objectives are more explicitly addressed in Chapter 9, *Goals and Objectives*.

FIGURE 8.1 shows a Bloom's wheel, which is used to depict the domains, levels, and sample verbs in a visual way. A complete list of examples of verbs and their corresponding domains and levels is presented in Chapter 9, *Goals and Objectives*.

Addressing the Domains in Teaching Strategies

Learning within one domain is often interdependent on learning in another domain. For example, cognitive knowledge and concepts are required for hands-on practice of psychomotor skills to be most effective. Students will achieve mastery of endotracheal intubation more quickly if they can identify the necessary equipment, understand the indications for the skill, and recite the sequence of events required for completion of the skill before they ever attempt to perform it.

At the same time, mastery of knowledge in one domain does not imply mastery in the other domains. For example, a student who can answer multiple choice exam questions about the procedure for nebulizing a medication, such as albuterol, may not necessarily be able to select the proper respiratory treatment for congestive heart failure (CHF) and asthma. The learner may be able to fully master nebulizer set-up and albuterol administration, but uses the nebulizer inappropriately to treat CHF.

As educators plan learning, they should consider the level of learning that has taken place within each domain and how it relates to their instructional objectives. This process of building new learning upon previous learning is called **scaffolding**. In the building trade, scaffolds allow an individual to move from one floor, or level, to another. They are often fragile structures that

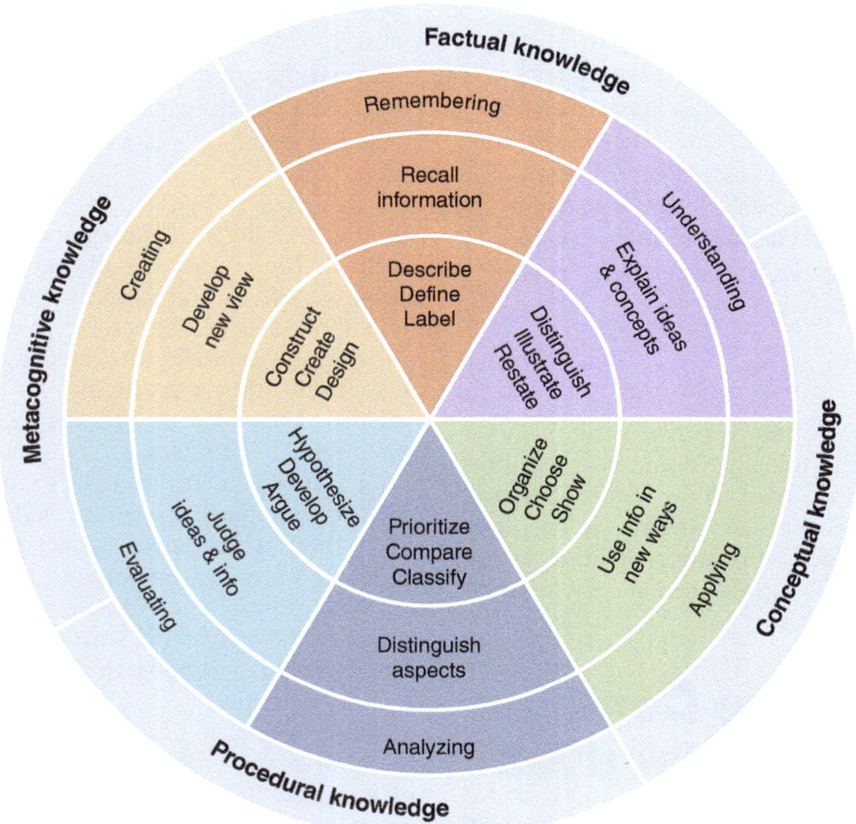

FIGURE 8.1 Bloom's wheel.

Adapted from Edutechalogy. Accessed May 6, 2019. http://eductechalogy.org/swfapp/blooms/wheel/engage.swf.

depend on firm attachment to multiple points below them. Learning scaffolds are also highly dependent upon successful performance at lower levels (FIGURE 8.2).

To properly scaffold learning, teaching strategies and assessment methods must target the top of the level in which students are learning. To do this, the instructor should review objectives from the course, unit, or lesson to determine the appropriate depth and breadth at which to teach the material.

To determine the depth and breadth, one of the two formal strategies should be used to identify the level of the objectives. The **depth** of content in a topic refers to the amount of detail the student would need to learn or perform within their scope of practice. The determination is made based on whether the student needs to know the information at a simple, fundamental, or complex level. As an example, an emergency medical responder (EMR) may learn to ask basic questions

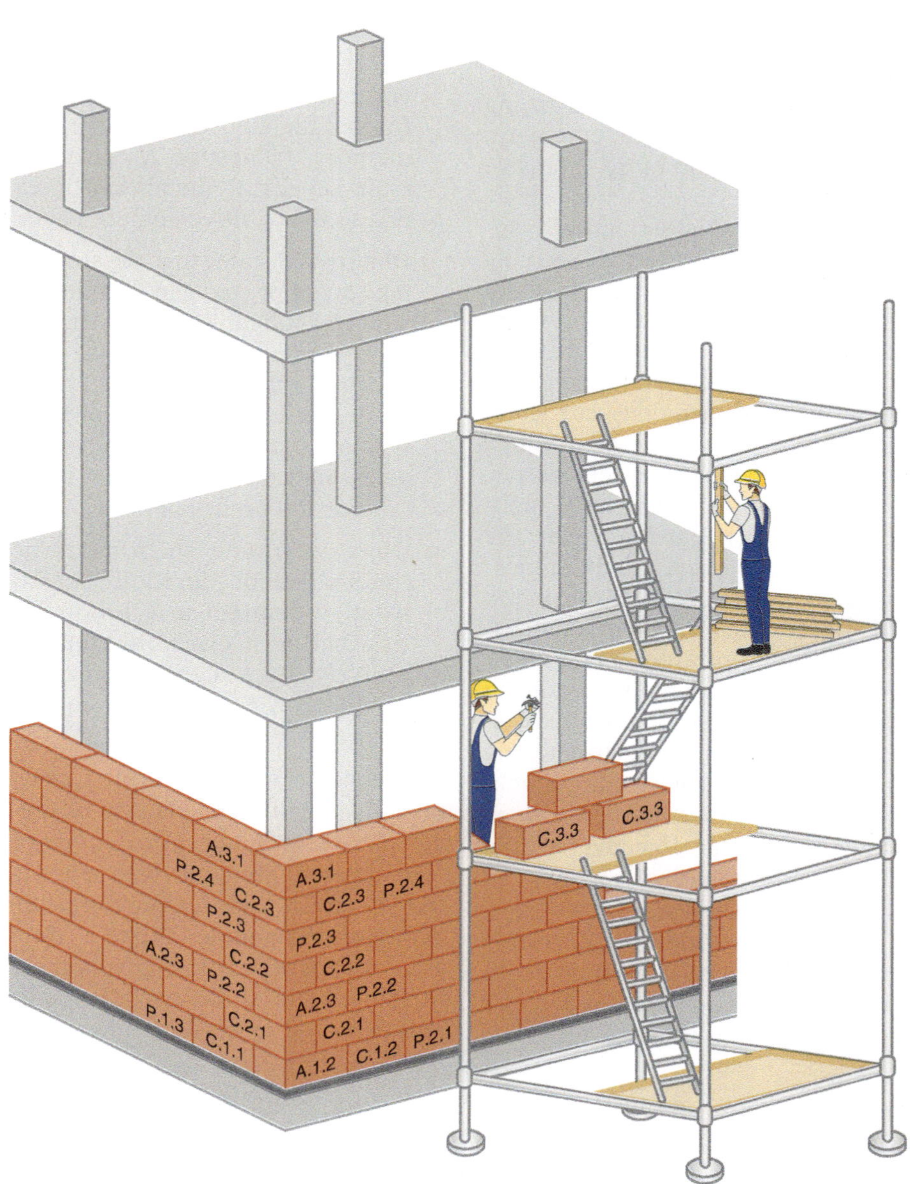

FIGURE 8.2 The process of building new learning upon previous learning is called *scaffolding*. This concept, borrowed from the building trade, structures how an individual moves up through the levels. The numbers shown here represent objective numbers in the cognitive, psychomotor, and affective domains.

to obtain a present illness history, while a paramedic may ask a more comprehensive list of questions. The EMR may obtain the patient's list of medications, but the paramedic asks about over-the-counter medications and determines the conditions for which the medications are being taken, whether they are being taken as prescribed, and the last time the patient has seen a physician. The **breadth** of information to be learned refers to the volume of topics that the student would need to learn to achieve competency in the subject. For example, the EMT may learn fundamental information regarding the anatomy and physiology of the respiratory system and a limited amount of critical respiratory diagnoses and treatments. The paramedic would build on that knowledge by learning respiratory pathophysiology; nonemergent, emergent, and critical respiratory diagnoses; and more extensive treatments.

Objectives allow an educator to systematically approach the desired learning outcomes. Classifying objectives helps teachers systematically plan ways of facilitating learning to achieve the particular objective. Differing types of objectives require differing instructional approaches. For different objectives, the instructional approaches, learning activities, curricular materials, and roles need to adjust. Using the example of respiratory emergencies, a respiratory emergency "compare/contrast" lecture could instruct and highlight the differences between CHF and asthma. The focus of this lecture would be to teach the differences in anatomy, physiology, pathophysiology, assessment, and management of the two differing emergencies. When moving to the psychomotor aspects of a respiratory emergency therapy, the students would go to the laboratory or clinical site to learn in a hands-on fashion. The cognitive objectives for this lecture would cover the knowledge associated with selecting a nebulizer and albuterol versus continuous positive airway pressure (CPAP). The psychomotor objectives would cover bodily-kinesthetic performance of the skill, in this case, using the nebulizer or CPAP.

Clever educators can devise methods for integrating learning across several domains to enhance both depth and breadth of knowledge. This is accomplished by engaging as many senses as possible to enhance retention. For example, use of multimedia, class discussion, and role-playing are all ways of successfully engaging the students' senses. Studies on retention suggest that the more the student is actively participating in the learning process and the more senses are stimulated in the learning process, the more learning takes place. Additional studies show that greater retention occurs as concepts are revisited and reviewed.[1,6]

The following are some examples of objectives pertaining to depth and breadth:

- Objective A states that the student, using a supplied list of names of seven organs, should label those organs on a manikin.
- Objective B states that the student should create a human skeleton and label all the major bones from memory. (Objective A correlates to cognitive domain Level 1: Remember, whereas Objective B correlates to cognitive domain Level 5: Create.)
- Objective C states that the student should be able to take an empty oxygen cylinder and switch the regulator to a full tank. If an instructor demonstrates this skill, but only some (not all) of the students mimic her, it is unlikely that the entire class will be successful during assessment of this skill. Skill demonstration and practice are Level 1 activities, whereas performance of a skill for testing purposes with confidence and proficiency is a Level 3 or 4 activity.
- Objective D states the student should be able to list the Six Patient Medication Rights. If, in reviewing what was taught in a lesson, the instructor realizes that he stressed only four of the "rights," it is unlikely the students will be able to perform successfully on a test of this objective based on their classroom lessons alone.

Individual student learning styles and preferences magnify the interdependence of the different learning domains. (See Chapter 5, *Learning Styles: Concepts and Controversies*.) Students who are strongly kinesthetic (hands-on) in their learning preference may have difficulty understanding cognitive concepts until they are able to experience their psychomotor application. On the other hand, students who are more attuned to feelings may require less attention to the affective domain.

TEACHING TIP

A common strategy used to assist students in attaining mastery of depth and breadth is to account for memory degradation by teaching one level beyond that required by the objective. However, if time is at a premium (which it often is), this may not be possible.

TEACHING TIP

The instructor should always consider learning styles and preferences, and how this information influences the domains of learning. (See Chapter 5, *Learning Styles: Concepts and Controversies*).

The application of learning domains to teaching strategies is more explicitly discussed in Chapter 12, *Teaching in All Domains*, and Chapter 19, *Tools for Field and Clinical Learning*.

Addressing the Domains in Assessment Methods

Educators must devise assessment strategies that determine the progressive mastery of each level in every domain. The achievement of domain objectives must be evaluated against previously established objectives. The instrument used to measure learning must be connected to the level at which the objectives were written. Different levels of objectives require different levels of assessment. For example, if the objective is to remember a stroke assessment tool rather than the larger and more important concept of stroke facility selection (primary stroke facility versus comprehensive stroke facility), a fill-in-the-blank question may be a desired tool for assessment. In this case, a learner is simply being asked to remember and regurgitate factual knowledge. A different assessment tool is needed to determine the understanding of the larger concept of stroke recognition and destination selection. A scenario-based multiple choice question(s) or essay may be desired. In this case, a learner must understand the deeper concepts to recognize differing types of stroke and the differing capabilities of hospitals.

TEACHING TIP

An instructor can take a quick look at the course grading policy to ensure that a program places equal emphasis on each domain of learning.

Educators who assume competency and fail to accurately assess students will quickly learn it becomes difficult to track students' progressive learning and competency over time. In addition, assessment should occur to ensure that students retain concepts from the previous level(s).

Written and oral exams are useful for assessing the cognitive domain. Class participation, teamwork, demonstrated leadership, and peer supervision are useful for assessing the affective domain. Skill competency exams and evaluation within the clinical setting are useful for assessing the psychomotor domain. The application of learning domains to assessment methods is more explicitly covered in Chapter 20, *Assessing Learning*, and Chapter 22, *Other Assessment Tools*.

Summary

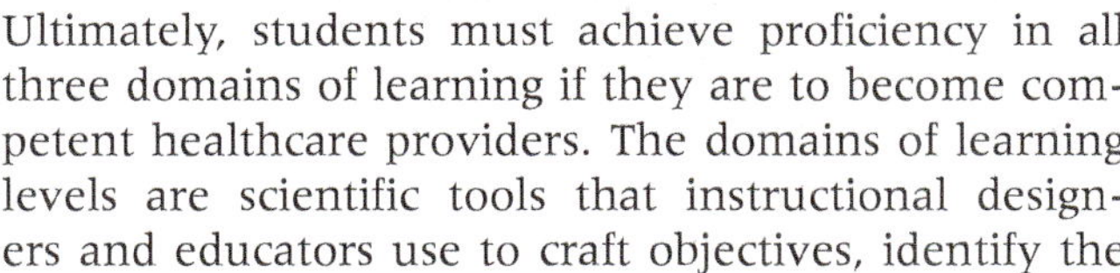

Ultimately, students must achieve proficiency in all three domains of learning if they are to become competent healthcare providers. The domains of learning levels are scientific tools that instructional designers and educators use to craft objectives, identify the appropriate depth and breadth of content to plan lessons and teaching strategies, and effectively assess learning and retention. Savvy educators recognize their importance and know how to use them in practicing and honing the art of teaching.

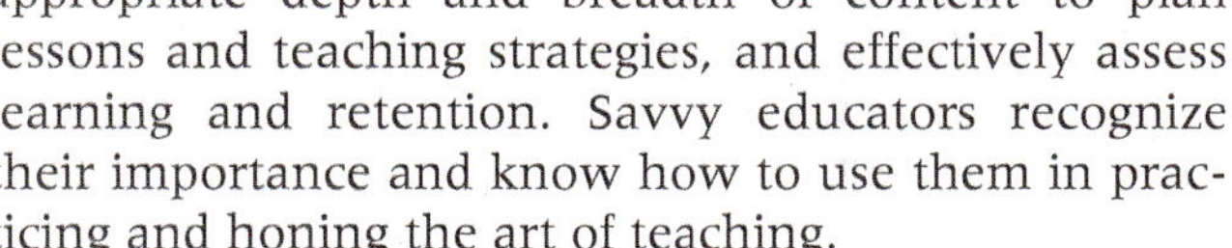

Glossary

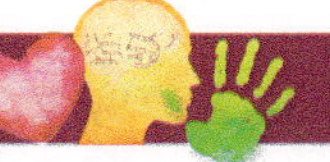

affective domain Learning in terms of feelings, emotions, attitudes, and values.

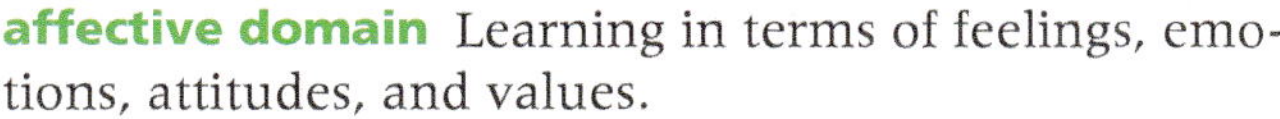

analyze Cognitive domain level that requires separation of whole concepts into individual, smaller parts to determine how the parts interrelate and understand their importance; called Analysis in the 1956 taxonomy.

apply Cognitive domain level that relates classroom information to real-life situations; called Application in the 1956 taxonomy.

articulation Psychomotor domain level that occurs when proficient and competent performance of the skill, with personal style or flair, occurs.

Bloom's taxonomy Description of the domains of learning developed by Dr. Benjamin Bloom.

breadth Volume of topics that a student needs to learn to achieve competency in the subject.

characterize Affective domain level that requires development of one's own value system that governs behavior.

cognitive domain Learning that takes place through the process of thinking; it deals with facts and knowledge.

cognitive process dimension Dimension that covers the actions in which a learner engages when learning in the cognitive domain.

conceptual knowledge Knowledge type that contains information and an understanding of a subject's principles, generalizations, or theories that are pertinent to a body of knowledge.

create Cognitive domain level in which elements are put together in a new way, to form a logical and functional whole. This is the highest mental function in the new taxonomy; called Synthesis in the 1956 taxonomy.

depth Amount of detail a student needs to learn or perform within their scope of practice.

domains of learning Categories of learning that include cognitive, affective, and psychomotor.

evaluate Cognitive domain level in which judgments are made based on existing standards and checking and critiquing content. This is now the fifth level and a precursor to creating; called Evaluation in the 1956 taxonomy.

factual knowledge Knowledge type that contains information that is essential to a subject discipline. It includes basic information, terminology, and other elements that are required for a learner to understand the discipline.

imitation Psychomotor domain level that occurs as students repeat and mimic demonstrations.

knowledge dimension Types of knowledge an educator must consider including within the cognitive domain; includes factual, conceptual, procedural, and metacognitive knowledge.

manipulation Psychomotor domain level that occurs as students practice a skill and begin to create their own styles of performance.

metacognitive knowledge Knowledge type that is an understanding of one's thinking. It uses reflective thinking to strategically improve cognition, solve problems, and think critically.

naturalization Psychomotor domain level that represents skill performance mastery.

organize Affective domain level where the learner integrates new, refined, or different beliefs into their existing value system.

precision Psychomotor domain level when the skill is performed without mistakes and transfer to other situations or circumstances begins.

procedural knowledge Knowledge type that refers to information that assists a student to do something specific within the discipline. This knowledge will typically use algorithms or protocols.

psychomotor domain Learning that takes place through the attainment of skills and bodily, or kinesthetic, movements.

receive Affective domain level that occurs as the student acquires awareness of the value or importance of learning information and expresses a willingness to learn.

remember Cognitive domain level that focuses on memorization and recall; called Knowledge in the 1956 taxonomy.

respond Affective domain level where the student actively participates in the learning process and begins to derive satisfaction from it.

scaffolding Process of building new learning upon previous learning.

understand Cognitive domain level that focuses on construction of meaning from types of functions such as written messages; called Comprehension in the 1956 taxonomy.

value Affective domain level in which the student perceives that a behavior has worth or importance.

References

[1] Bloom, Benjamin S. (Ed.). 1956. *Taxonomy of Educational Objectives, Book 1: Cognitive Domain*. New York: Longman.

[2] Anderson, Lorin W., and David R. Krathwohl (Eds.). 2001. *A Taxonomy for Learning, Teaching, and Assessing: A Revision of Bloom's Taxonomy of Educational Objectives*. New York: Pearson.

[3] Krathwohl, David R. 2002. "A Revision of Bloom's Taxonomy: An Overview." *Theory into Practice* 41, no. 4: 214. Accessed November 14, 2018. https://www.depauw.edu/files/resources/krathwohl.pdf.

[4] Dave, R. H. 1970. "Psychomotor Levels." In *Developing and Writing Behavioral Objectives*, edited by Robert J. Armstrong, 33–4. Tucson, AZ: Educational Innovators Press.

[5] Krathwohl, David R., Benjamin S. Bloom, and Bertram B. Masia. 1964. *Taxonomy of Educational Objectives. Book II. Affective Domain*. New York: David McKay Company.

[6] Cicchetti, George. 1990. *Cognitive Modeling and Reciprocal Teaching of Reading and Study Strategies*. Watertown, CT: Cicchetti Associates.

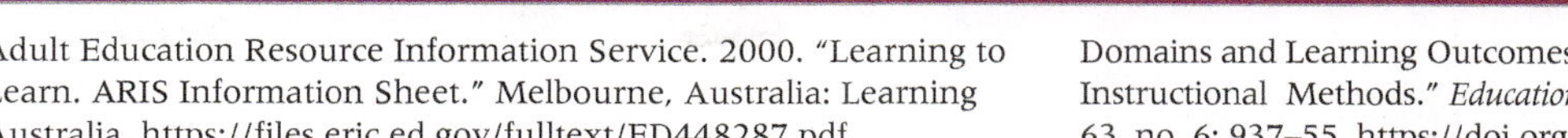

Additional Resources

Adult Education Resource Information Service. 2000. "Learning to Learn. ARIS Information Sheet." Melbourne, Australia: Learning Australia. https://files.eric.ed.gov/fulltext/ED448287.pdf.

Hodell, Chuck. 1997. "Basics of Instructional Systems Development." The American Society for Training and Development (ASTD) Infoline, Issue 9706. https://www.oreilly.com/library/view/basics-of-instructional/759706/759706_ch01.html.

Honebein, Peter C., and Cass H. Honebein. 2015. "Effectiveness, Efficiency, and Appeal: Pick Any Two? The Influence of Learning Domains and Learning Outcomes on Designer Judgments of Useful Instructional Methods." *Educational Technology Research & Development* 63, no. 6: 937–55. https://doi.org/10.1007/s11423-015-9396-3.

Mayer, Richard E. 1998. "Cognitive, Metacognitive, and Motivational Aspects of Problem Solving." *Instructional Science 26*, 49–63. https://doi.org/10.1023/A:1003088013286.

CHAPTER 9

Goals and Objectives

OBJECTIVES

At the conclusion of this chapter, the educator will be able to:

Cognitive Domain

1. Differentiate between goals and objectives.
2. Discuss the components of goals and of objectives.
3. Explain the importance of developing goals and objectives.
4. Discuss the relevance of Bloom's taxonomy in education.
5. Apply the taxonomy table when writing learning objectives.
6. Identify the components of performance alignment.

Psychomotor Domain

1. Develop objectives using Anderson and Krathwohl's revised Bloom's taxonomy.
2. Demonstrate how to write an instructional objective for each learning domain.
3. Translate the assessment of student learning into assessment rubrics.

Affective Domain

There are no affective objectives for this chapter.

"Objectives are not fate; they are direction."

~ Peter F. Drucker

CHAPTER GOAL This chapter describes how instructors can use levels within the domains of learning, as described by Bloom's taxonomy, to guide their process of writing goals and objectives.

Both emergency medical services (EMS) educators who provide initial education and training officers who provide continuing education likely have heard of educational objectives and perhaps wondered how they relate to the educational spectrum, from initial training through continuing education. Goals and objectives are considered the backbone of the instructional process. Objectives provide the educational framework for instruction by identifying what educators should teach and what students are expected to learn. They are a roadmap for the process of learning. This chapter discusses Bloom's taxonomy and its 2001 revision, the various domains of learning, performance alignment between learning and assessment, and the categorization of learning into discrete levels. This chapter then builds upon that concept by using those levels and the taxonomy table in the process of writing goals and objectives.

One approach to a systematic method of instruction is proposed in nursing and physician education. This concept utilizes the Three Cs model, which incorporates context, content, and conduct, where goals and objectives reside under content and are connected to outcomes.[1] The three Cs are as follows:

- **Context**. Consider your student population and the context. Is this initial education or continuing education?
- **Content**. Consider content when writing goals and objectives. Identify what content you are attempting to provide. Determine the most effective method for achieving student learning and what resources are needed.
- **Conduct**. Consider how to implement and evaluate whether the outcomes were met.

The Three Cs model can be employed in a broad manner to facilitate program outcomes or in a more focused manner to develop and support curriculum development and evaluation.[1]

During instructional planning, educators use goals and objectives to determine the appropriate depth and breadth of content required to teach a given topic, including differentiating between "must-know" and "nice-to-know" content. This planning helps to ensure that instruction is targeted to specific goals. Goals and objectives are also used in the test-item writing and assessment processes to effectively evaluate student learning. Finally, these tools are useful for measuring the effectiveness of the educator's teaching activities.[2]

Instructors have likely had students ask, "What do we need to know for the test?" Through goals and objectives, students are positioned to focus their learning. Students should be able to track their individual progress in a course of instruction by evaluating their ability to perform actions that relate to course objectives, for example, by answering questions, exhibiting professional behaviors, or by demonstrating skills required by class objectives to meet the course goals. Instructors should ensure that students have the course goals and objectives, understand their purpose, and use them to ensure they focus their time on relevant content and, therefore, recognize what they are expected to know for the test!

There are numerous strategies for writing objectives. Several strategies are presented here to allow instructors to determine the most appropriate strategy for their needs. The chapter focuses on a technique that uses two tiers: goals followed by objectives. Educators should determine whether their specific department uses a different strategy. If that is the case, this chapter will still be helpful, as the concepts explained here are similar to those associated with other objective- and goal-writing methods.

TEACHING TIP

Although an entry-level educator may not be required to write objectives, it is important that the educator understand how goals and objectives relate to the planning and evaluation of instruction.

Goals and Objectives

Educators can make the best use of goals and objectives when they have acquired a deep understanding of these instructional tools and can identify the differences between them. The words **goal** and **objective** are often used interchangeably and without regard for their actual meaning, which can lead to confusion. Goals and objectives are often presented in two distinct levels; objectives should always be subordinate to goals. In this textbook, a two-tiered system is described wherein the term *goal* is used only to describe the uppermost broad level of instruction and the term *objective* is used to describe the subordinate, or more detailed, level. A course may have a few goals, while a daily lesson may contain numerous detailed objectives; these objectives will ultimately lead to achievement of course goals. For example, a class may list several objectives, such as applying a tourniquet properly or identifying when a tourniquet should be applied. These detailed objectives align with the course goal of appropriately managing a trauma patient.

The first level, generally identified as the goal, recognizes the overall intent of instruction and intended outcomes. Confusion arises when this tier is called a *terminal objective* instead of the *primary goal of instruction.*[3] *Enabling objective* is another term that has been used to refer to detail-oriented objectives that progress learning toward the primary goal of instruction.[2] In completing each objective, a student makes progress toward meeting the overall goal.

Every goal statement should have at least one objective that relates to it, and usually more; every objective should relate to at least one goal. The content of the lesson, sometimes called the **declarative material**, should relate to the goals and objectives, and should not contain information that does not relate to the goals and objectives (see the section *Performance Alignment* later in this chapter for further details). Declarative information encompasses the depth and breadth of the content to be taught in the lesson plan.

TEACHING TIP

Another strategy for writing goals and objectives applies three tiers of distinct goals and objectives. In this strategy, the goal is the upper tier. The second tier is often called the primary goal of instruction, and the last tier is called the enabling objective. In this strategy, various enabling objectives are grouped together under a single primary goal of instruction that directly relates to the goal. Completion of the enabling objectives leads to completion of the primary goal of instruction. Completion of several primary goals of instruction leads to completion of the goal. This strategy of classification is useful when one is describing a program with multiple class sessions that are offered over a certain length of time. It can also be used to break down each block of instruction for a semester-long course.

Goals

Goals are philosophical statements about the intended product of learning. They are often broad, generalized, and overarching with no specific information on how learning is to be accomplished or measured. Goals are similar in nature to mission or vision statements. An educator may establish goals for an entire course, a learning module, a 1-hour skills practice, or a single case scenario. Goals are written with the end in mind.

Examples of goal statements include the following:

- The goal of this chapter is to explain the concepts of basic airway management.
- Students who attend this cardiopulmonary resuscitation (CPR) course will perform all required CPR techniques correctly on a manikin.
- Upon completion of the emergency medical technician (EMT) course, the student will be able to perform as a competent entry-level EMT.
- Upon completion of this module, students will be able to appropriately manage a trauma patient.

Objectives

For a goal to be accomplished, specific and measurable objectives must be identified. The word *objective* literally means "observable." Objectives are expressed statements of expected learning outcomes, which include results or behaviors that students are required to exhibit. As with goals, an educator should establish objectives for a course, a lesson, a skills practice, or a single classroom exercise. As objectives indicate the learning that is expected to take place, they necessitate that instructors at all levels determine what students are expected to learn, prior to lesson plan development. To establish what learning is expected, the instructor needs to decide what the student is expected to know or perform, or how the student is expected to behave as a team member or team leader.[2]

When considering objectives in EMS education and training, it is important to recognize the three domains of learning. These domains are cognitive, psychomotor, and affective. Writing objectives requires that the educator identify which domain they plan to address and then write the objectives appropriately. It is beneficial to write objectives at various levels of difficulty as well as across all three domains of learning. Later, this chapter discusses writing objectives.

Domains of Learning

It is fundamental to EMS education, both initial and continuing, that the instructor include objectives that reflect each of the domains identified in Bloom's taxonomy to ensure learning occurs across all domains: cognitive, psychomotor, and affective.[4] (See Chapter 8, *Domains of Learning*, for a detailed discussion of the domains of learning.) In order to write objectives for the course, lecture, or lesson, the educator should identify the domain in which the objectives reside. For example, if the student is to discuss shock, this should be covered in a cognitive objective; if the student is to ventilate a patient appropriately,

Student-Centered Learning in the Cognitive Domain

The cognitive domain encompasses knowledge and the development of intellectual skills and abilities. (See Chapter 8, *Domains of Learning*.) Because teachers tend to teach the way they have been taught, most defer to an instructor-centered focus, such as the traditional lecture format. Over the last decade, education has taken a definite turn toward student-centered learning and away from exposition, or the lecture format. Listening to a lecture is an example of a passive, lower level of learning.[2] However, if in the classroom the instructor provides activities that require student collaboration on applying the knowledge read in the assignment, active learning is promoted, resulting in higher levels of thinking. The instructor serves as a facilitator rather than the subject matter expert responsible for imparting all knowledge. In such a model, students learn from both the instructor and other class participants as well as through self-reflection and awareness.

The movement toward student-centered learning can be difficult to embrace. While it comes with advantages and disadvantages, it asks that educators assess the foundation of how they teach and align it with how people learn. Most people have heard the cliché, "See one, do one, teach one," and, as with all clichés, there is some value to the statement. One thing missing from the statement is "listen to how to do," emphasizing the minimal impact that listening, in this case lecture, has on learning. Most educators have worked hard to hone their lecture skills and change can be difficult. One way to embrace student perspective is for the instructor to ask two questions, "How do I wish I had been taught?" and "Is there an activity I can have students perform to achieve this objective?" The following are some ideas for presenting cognitive domain information in a student-centered form:

- Rather than lecturing on how a drop of blood travels through the body, have students act as red blood cells (RBCs) walking through a chalk-drawn model in the parking lot.
- Engage in Socratic questioning, assisting students to answer their own questions based on elemental information they already have.[5]
- Break students into groups to work on case studies.
- Have students present a topic while others ask questions.

this should be covered in a psychomotor objective; if the student is to treat patients respectfully, this should be covered in an affective objective. Once the educator establishes the domain, Bloom's taxonomy can assist in furnishing relevant verbs.

EMS is heavily dependent on skills, which fall within the psychomotor domain. EMS instructors need to ensure adequate time for skill demonstration and practice while minimizing lecture.

In EMS, it is essential that students gain competency in skills, as there may be situations where employers expect graduates to be prepared to function in the workforce from their first day of employment. A **performance gap** is the difference between actual performance and required performance.[2] For example, how are students performing compared to what is required by the program? The models for skill acquisition discussed in this chapter originate from Dreyfus and Dreyfus.[6] Dreyfus and Dreyfus assert a theory for skill acquisition.

It is important to note that students learn information and acquire skills at varying levels of acquisition. Instructors teaching students in the classroom or lab will need to know the varying levels in the sessions they teach to ensure all students are provided instruction to obtain the desired outcome level. As an example, students in initial education may reach the level of precision and are usually assessed at this level; it is unlikely that students will reach articulation or naturalization during initial education. However, training officers may expect practitioners with more experience to practice at the articulation or naturalization level for skills that are commonly performed in the field (**FIGURE 9.1**).

Dreyfus and Dreyfus identified five levels associated with skill acquisition in various occupations;[6] Benner related this information to nursing education.[7] This model is often followed by EMS.[8,9] The Dreyfus levels and associated teaching strategies are shown in **TABLE 9.1**.

In order to become expert, students must be provided with the opportunity to gain deliberate experience at increasing levels of difficulty.[9] Initial training requires a higher level of attention to recall information and for the achievement of complex tasks. The necessity for high levels of attention decreases with practice as students are able to retrieve information with less effort. **Cognitive load** refers to an effect that results from an overload of information that renders learning ineffective.[9] Beginners require a straightforward approach that reduces extraneous interference.

Training officers should understand that experience alone is not necessarily indicative of expertise. Students can progress toward expertise during continuing education opportunities if instructors are aware of existing performance gaps. Expert instructors may struggle with the ability to teach beginners if they fail to remember what it was like to learn the skill initially.[10] In such a case, it may be beneficial to utilize peers to assist learning. Levels of

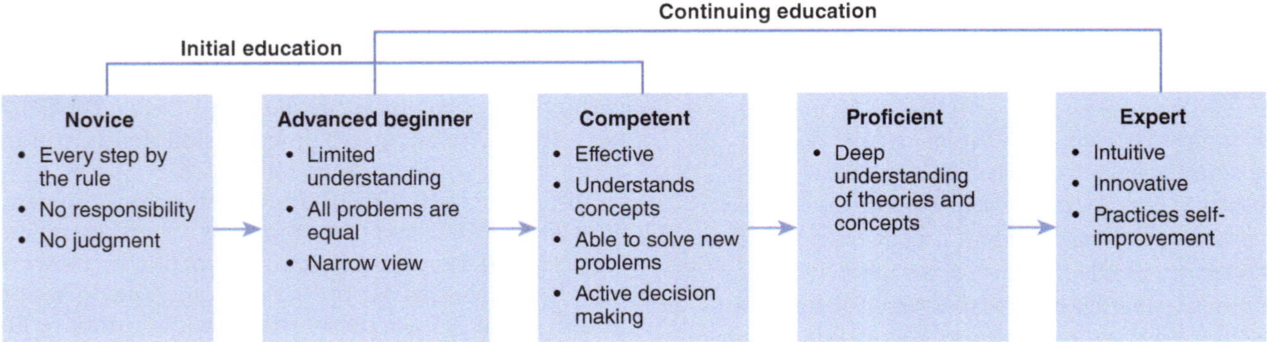

FIGURE 9.1 Dreyfus and Dreyfus model of skill acquisition illustrating levels of skill competency and characteristics of each.

Modified from Dreyfus, Stuart E., and Hubert L. Dreyfus. 1980. *A Five-Stage Model of the Mental Activities Involved in Directed Skill Acquisition*. Berkeley, CA: University of California, Operations Research Center. Accessed April 22, 2019. https://apps.dtic.mil/docs/citations/ADA084551.

TABLE 9.1 Dreyfus Levels and Associated Teaching Strategies

Dreyfus Level	Definition	Teaching Strategies
Novice	Those with no experience should practice in a straightforward manner in a precise and accurate manner.	Require the use of a peer mentor and skill sheets for *each* attempt, with immediate correction. Place the task trainer on the table; ensure easy access. Focus on technique and accuracy, not speed.
Advanced beginner	Marginally acceptable performance. Instructors should assist learners to identify patterns and make connections to improve performance.	Require the use of a peer mentor and skill sheets for *each* attempt, with immediate correction. Move the task trainer to the ground or in other more realistic and challenging locations. Include skill in simple, formative scenarios.
Competent	Moderate, specific experience. As students advance, instructors should provide progressively more challenging scenarios and encourage self-reflection.	Utilize peer mentors for skill check-offs. Provide feedback after performance. Integrate skills into challenging environments; i.e., in a difficult airway lab, place manikins under tables, in confined areas, in vehicles, or in other areas that are difficult to access, requiring the use of basic problem solving. Integrate skills into more complex scenarios to ready student for clinical and field experiences.
Proficient	Moderate, broad experience. Instructors should focus on continuous improvement and increasingly complex situations.	Integrate knowledge and skills in complex scenarios, to provide opportunity to solve complex problems to support higher levels of critical thinking.
Expert	Extensive experience, intuitive, exhibiting advanced problem-solving ability.	Utilize these practitioners to assist with instructing novice, advanced beginner, and competent-level students. Provide challenging simulations that allow self-reflection and self-awareness.

expertise may vary in different areas; for example, being an expert clinician may not reflect expertise in a supervisory or educational role.[10] Also, significant changes in circumstance could require new learning, For example, moving from a rural to an urban environment or from a transfer truck to a 9-1-1 role both require time for the individual to adapt to a changing role.

It is up to the instructor to determine which strategies are the most appropriate to support progressive learning in all domains. Some learners may respond to one strategy more favorably than another. Educators should obtain additional tools whenever possible to enhance their ability to respond to a wide variety of learners.

The Importance of the Affective Domain

More recently, the affective domain has been appreciated as an integral component of EMS education and practice. This refers to a person's values, beliefs, and attitudes and is reflected through behaviors and feelings.[2,11] Educators generally find this to be the most difficult domain to teach and assess, as it relates directly to a person's image of self. Most, if not all, employers recognize the importance of professional, appropriate, and safe behaviors in the workforce; therefore, it is imperative that educators teach, assess, and value the affective domain despite its potential challenges.

The affective domain can be observed in a multitude of venues including the classroom, lab, clinicals, and field work. Different venues provide unique areas for educators to obtain information from many different perspectives regarding a student's behaviors and attitudes. The difficulty often lies in providing clear expectations and tools for assessment for students and evaluators.

Bloom's Taxonomy

Bloom's taxonomy consists of three domains (cognitive, psychomotor, and affective), which serve as categories for objectives. (See Chapter 8, *Domains of Learning*.) Bloom's taxonomy provides clear identification of objectives within a hierarchy that evolves from simple to complex. Complex objectives build on simpler, lower-level objectives. Taxonomy is relevant in all aspects of teaching and instruction from curriculum development, to educating, and finally, assessment. Instructors must ask, what knowledge, skills, and abilities are students expected to acquire from this instruction? Incorporated within this, instructors must do the following:

1. Identify what they want students to learn.
2. Identify how they intend to provide instruction to ensure objectives are met.
3. Identify how to assess learning.
4. Identify the need for remediation.

Critical thinking and problem solving have gained recognition in the EMS world as a necessity to prepare future personnel to provide patient care within a multidisciplinary healthcare system. Critical thinking and problem solving are realized in the last three categories of Analyze, Evaluate, and Create within the cognitive domain.[12] These levels of thinking can also be taught and assessed within scenarios. EMS providers will use each of these levels when responding to calls.

A working knowledge of Bloom's taxonomy is extremely helpful when considering goals and objectives. Bloom's taxonomy provides a hierarchical framework to classify the complexity of objectives and identify at what level assessment should take place. The framework also provides a method for instructors to align goals, learning objectives, activities, and evaluation for a class, course, or entire program curriculum.[2] Revisions to Bloom's taxonomy were adopted in 2001 and reflect the emphasis on learning outcome.[13] (See Chapter 8, *Domains of Learning*.) The updated version includes action verbs, integrating a hierarchical framework from simple to complex (**FIGURE 9.2**).[14] Classifications for the revised

Lower-order thinking skills → **Higher-order thinking skills**

Remembering	Understanding	Applying	Analyzing	Evaluating	Creating
• Arrange	• Classify	• Apply	• Analyze	• Appraise	• Assemble
• Define	• Compare	• Build	• Assume	• Assess	• Build
• Identify	• Contrast	• Carry out	• Calculate	• Award	• Change
• Label	• Demonstrate	• Choose	• Categorize	• Choose	• Choose
• List	• Discuss	• Compute	• Classify	• Conclude	• Combine
• Match	• Explain	• Determine	• Compare	• Criticize	• Compose
• Memorize	• Extend	• Develop	• Conclude	• Defend	• Create
• Name	• Illustrate	• Direct	• Contrast	• Disprove	• Design
• Order	• Infer	• Execute	• Diagram	• Estimate	• Elaborate
• Quote	• Interpret	• Implement	• Differentiate	• Evaluate	• Formulate
• Recall	• Locate	• Model	• Discover	• Hypothesize	• Generate
• Recite	• Outline	• Operate	• Dissect	• Interpret	• Improve
• Recognize	• Relate	• Organize	• Distinguish	• Judge	• Invent
• Select	• Restate	• Provide	• Examine	• Justify	• Modify
• Tell	• Review	• Respond	• Inspect	• Rate	• Plan
	• Show	• Select	• Prioritize	• Support	• Predict
	• Summarize	• Solve	• Separate		
	• Translate	• Use			
		• Utilize			

FIGURE 9.2 Examples of action verbs for use in Bloom's hierarchy, showing increasing complexity within the cognitive domain.

Data from University of North Carolina at Charlotte. n.d. "Writing Measurable Course Objectives." Center for Teaching and Learning. Accessed May 18, 2018. https://teaching.uncc.edu/services-programs/learning-resources/course-design/writing-measurable-course-objectives.

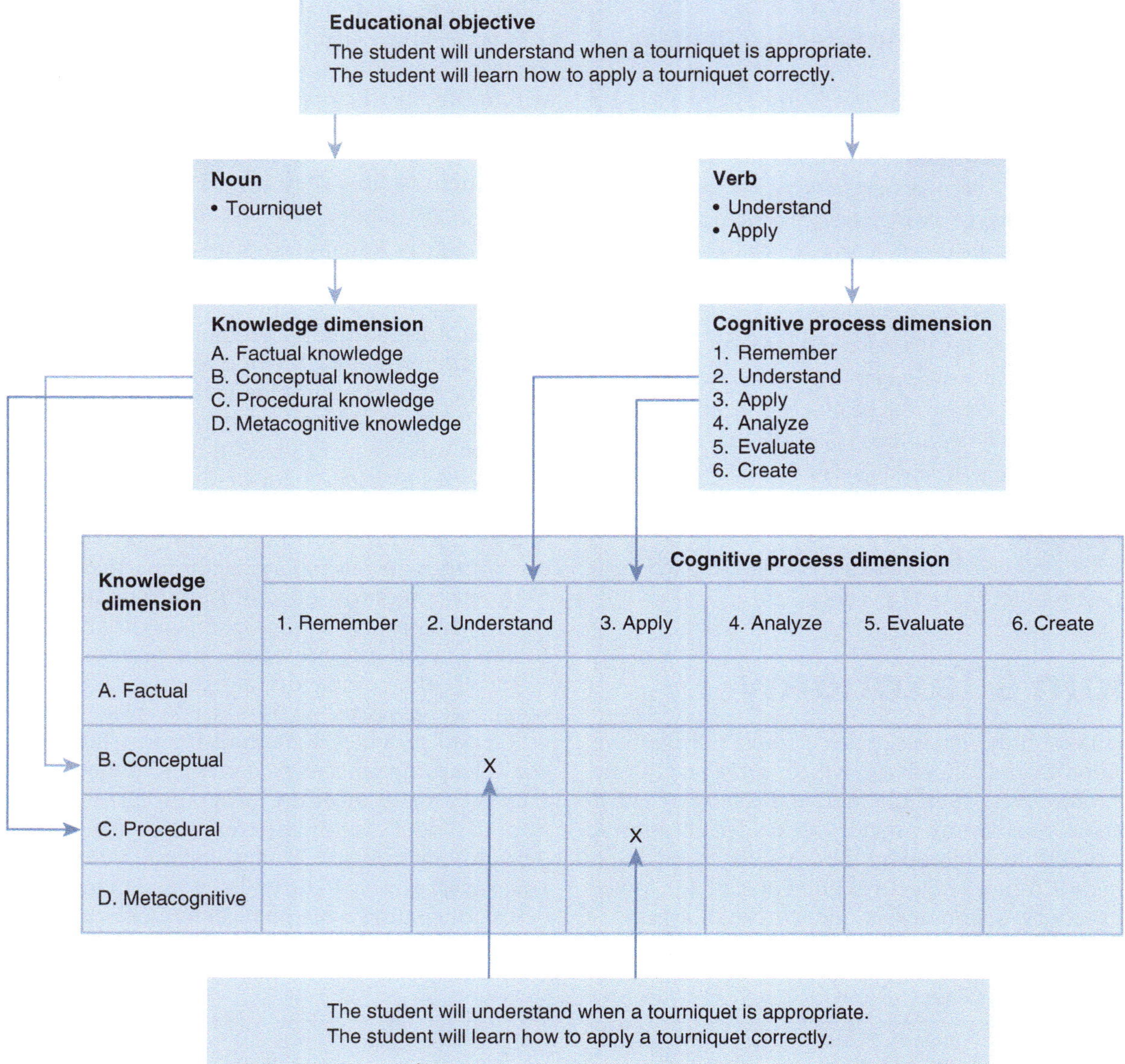

FIGURE 9.3 Example of how an objective is classified in a taxonomy table.

Reproduced from Anderson, Lorin W., and David R. Krathwohl (Eds.). 2001. *A Taxonomy for Learning, Teaching, and Assessing: A Revision of Bloom's Taxonomy of Educational Objectives*. New York: Pearson.

taxonomy in the cognitive domain include Remembering, Understanding, Applying, Analyzing, Evaluating, and Creating.[12,14]

Anderson, who led the revision, also provides a taxonomy table to assist in organization of objectives (**FIGURE 9.3**). Note that the revised Bloom's taxonomy considers four categories:[14]

1. **Factual knowledge**. Foundational components students must have (i.e., terminology)
2. **Conceptual knowledge**. The relationship between the basic elements (i.e., principles and theories)
3. **Procedural knowledge**. When and how to employ procedures or skills
4. **Metacognitive knowledge**. Comprehension of the context of information and self-awareness of strengths and limitations

Performance Alignment

The link between goals and objectives is established through an evaluation process previously referred to as *performance agreement* and currently called **performance alignment**. Performance alignment is the process of critically evaluating the goals, objectives, and declarative content for the purpose of validating their logical relationships to one another and to ensure that they adequately support one another. For alignment to exist within a body of planned instruction, each goal statement must be supported by one or more objectives that link directly to it. At the same time, each objective should link to at least one goal. The declarative content should provide the depth and breadth described by the verbs written in the objectives.

The *breadth* of the declarative content refers to the number of topics that must be taught in a particular session or module. (See Chapter 8, *Domains of Learning*, for more detail.) This information can range from simple to complex depending on the scope of practice of the provider being taught. For example, at the EMT level in the respiratory module, there may be seven disease processes discussed, while at the paramedic level there may be 12. The *depth* refers to the amount of detail within each of the topics to be discussed. The content would span from fundamental to comprehensive for each topic. Using the example of the respiratory module, at the EMT level the anatomy and physiology may be discussed for the seven diseases, while at the paramedic level the anatomy, physiology, and pathophysiology may be taught.

Any goal or objective within the block of instruction that does not have a clear link should be evaluated further for appropriateness. These "unlinked" or *misaligned* goals or objectives may represent omissions of the content required for the lesson. They may also highlight unnecessary material that should perhaps be moved into another lesson or deleted from the section altogether (**FIGURE 9.4**). For the educator,

A. PERFORMANCE ALIGNMENT

Topic: Understand circulation through the heart.

Objectives: On a written exam, with 80% accuracy, students will be able to:

1. Accurately label a diagram of the structures of the heart, vena cava, and aorta in correct anatomical terms.
2. Discuss the path of a red blood cell through the anatomical structures of the heart.
3. Correctly trace the circulation of a drop of blood through the heart (vena cava to aorta).

Class Presentation and Activities

1. Lecture: Identify the anatomical structures of the heart.
2. Activity:
   a. Instruct students to draw a large heart with chalk on the ground. The students should label the following major anatomical structures:
      i. Inferior and superior venae cavae
      ii. Right atrium
      iii. Tricuspid valve
      iv. Right ventricle
      v. Pulmonary semilunar valve
      vi. Pulmonary arteries
      vii. Lungs
      viii. Pulmonary veins
      ix. Left atrium
      x. Bicuspid valve (mitral valve)
      xi. Left ventricle
      xii. Aortic semilunar valve
      xiii. Aorta
   b. Line students up in the vena cava.
   c. Starting with the right atrium, have students walk through each structure as an RBC, naming each structure as they walk through it until they can accurately recite the correct anatomy.
3. Provide students with a diagram of the heart. Have students label the structures, then trace an RBC through the heart starting at the inferior and superior venae cavae and ending at the aorta.

The topic, objectives, and classroom presentations all align. Each objective is tied to an activity and there are no activities that are not associated with an objective.

FIGURE 9.4 An example of performance alignment (**A**) versus no performance alignment (**B**).

(*continues*)

B. NO PERFORMANCE ALIGNMENT

Topic: Understand circulation through the heart.
Objectives: On a written exam, with 80% accuracy, students will be able to:

1. Accurately label a diagram of the structures of the heart, vena cava, and aorta in correct anatomical terms.
2. Discuss the anatomical structures of the heart.
3. Correctly trace the circulation of a drop of blood through the heart (vena cava to aorta).

Class Presentation and Activities:

1. Activity:
    a. Instruct students to draw a large heart with chalk on the ground.
    b. Line students up and have students walk through the heart.
2. Demonstrate the pathophysiology of congestive heart failure by having students meet resistance as they attempt to exit the left ventricle.
    a. As the instructor provides resistance, students should back into the lungs, followed by the right side of the heart, vena cava, and liver.
    b. Discuss the difference between right and left-sided heart failure.
        i. As students are pressed backwards, have them identify signs and symptoms associated with first left-sided then right-sided failure.

The topic and objectives do not align with the classroom presentation.

- The instructor has introduced a topic not listed in the objectives, congestive heart failure, the differentiation of right-sided and left-sided heart failure, signs and symptoms associated with heart failure, as well as circulation associated with the liver.
- The instructor did not provide any information related to Objective 1 or 2.

FIGURE 9.4 *(Continued)*

TEACHING TIP

When performance alignment is assessed before instruction is provided, adjustments can be made before mistakes are made in the classroom. When alignment is assessed after instruction has been provided, content omissions or areas requiring remediation or reteaching can be identified.

the exercise of looking for and validating alignment is useful for identifying unnecessary instruction, nice-to-know information, any areas that may have been overlooked, or gaps in the lesson plan. It helps to ensure that the content found within the lesson plan and the content presented in the classroom match the goals stated for the lesson in the curricula. In general, educators can focus on teaching only the necessary and appropriate content when they evaluate alignment.

Whenever possible, an educator should conduct a postpresentation evaluation for alignment. This should occur immediately after instruction has been provided for the purpose of reviewing what was taught and identifying whether any omissions, sidetracks (superfluous content), or other deviations from the lesson plan occurred. One method for conducting this type of performance alignment is to ask students to summarize the lesson or to provide their impressions of the key points covered. Another method of conducting this assessment is through the use of post-tests. Omissions identified during the performance alignment assessment can be made up during future teaching sessions or through alternative learning opportunities outside of face-to-face instruction.

Writing an Objective

Once the goal or goals for the program or course have been identified, the work of developing objectives for a course, module, or class begins. As with goals, it is suggested that the instructor begin with the end in mind. What are students expected to learn today? An objective should be detailed enough to encompass the

CASE in Point

An educator is reviewing the lesson plan for his next presentation on the topic of interpreting 12-lead electrocardiograms (ECGs). He begins by reviewing the goals and objectives for the session. It is noted that all four of the goals listed are covered by at least one of the objectives, and each objective is linked to at least one goal. He then reviews the content for the presentation and discovers two places that lack alignment because there is a disconnection between the goals, objectives, and declarative content.

The first error he discovers is that two of the objectives listed do not seem to be covered in the declarative section of the lesson plan, so he adds the necessary material to make certain that he has covered all of the objectives. The second problem he notes is that a section of the material is not described in either the goals or the objectives for the lesson plan. As he reviews this material, he decides it is not really appropriate for this lesson but should be covered in the next one. He moves this information to the next lesson after discussing the findings with his mentor. He updates the lesson plan with these changes so that the next time this plan is used, it will be more complete. His mentor compliments him on finding the problems before attempting to teach the material.

TEACHING TIP

The postpresentation evaluation for alignment provides an excellent time for the educator to draft exam questions or select questions from a test-item bank. Once an instructor has determined that performance alignment exists and this review is fresh in their mind, then the instructor can select test items that most closely reflect the content delivered.

aspects of who, what, when, where, and how of the behaviors appropriate for accomplishing that goal. Additionally, as is recommended for goals, as the level increases, such as an entire course versus a specific module or lesson, the specificity and number of objectives decrease. At the modular, course, or lesson level, there are more objectives that relay greater detail in expectations.

Typically, the overall statement begins with, "By the end of this class, students will be able to . . . ." This is followed by a list of objectives. It is essential to keep in mind that objectives should be designed from the student's viewpoint and they should be measurable. The objective starts with an action verb that is measurable and represents what the instructor wants the student to demonstrate.[15] Finally, you may include the expectation for mastery; this occurs primarily in the realm of psychomotor skills. Mastery includes the number of points and level of competency the student is expected to obtain. For example, rarely is a student expected to achieve all the points obtainable for every skill, every time. Instead, an instructor identifies critical criteria and the minimum points required to pass a specific skill assessment, quiz, or exam.

ABCD Method

Many methods, models, and templates are available for teaching an educator how to write objectives. The generic **ABCD model**, which is commonly used, lists the parts of a behavioral objective, where ABCD indicates the required elements of information. In this model, A = Audience, B = Behavior, C = Condition, and D = Degree.[16] Objectives need not be written in the ABCD order, but should contain each of these four elements. Two simple models to follow in constructing the order for an objective include:

1. The (Audience) will (Behavior) under (Condition) to (Degree).
2. Given (Condition), the (Audience) will (Behavior) to (Degree).

The second format is more often followed and referred to as the CABD format for writing objectives.

Audience

The *audience* describes the receiver (student) of the instructional activity (**FIGURE 9.5**). When reviewing objectives before providing instruction, the educator should ensure that the intended audience matches the actual audience for the instruction. If, for example, the intended audience for the lesson is identified in the objective as advanced life support (ALS) providers, but the educator is using it for basic life support (BLS) providers, the educator will need to compensate for the disparity. In this case, the educator could supplement the lesson with additional material or, if appropriate, expand the presentation over a longer time period to account for deficits in the BLS provider's depth of knowledge.

In another situation, the audience identified in the objective may have significantly different prerequisites from the audience the instructor is about to teach or may have a different scope of practice. In this circumstance, the educator should plan additional learning opportunities, make adjustments in timing, or rearrange the lesson entirely to suit the new

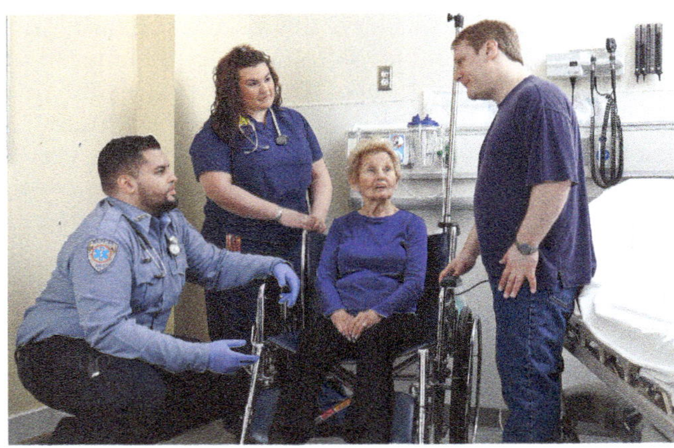

A

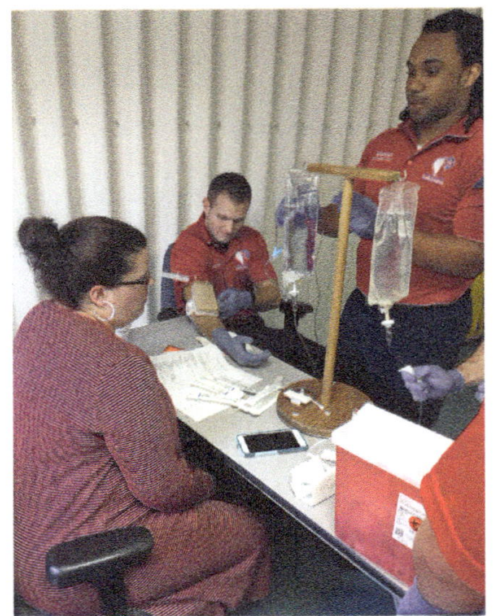

B

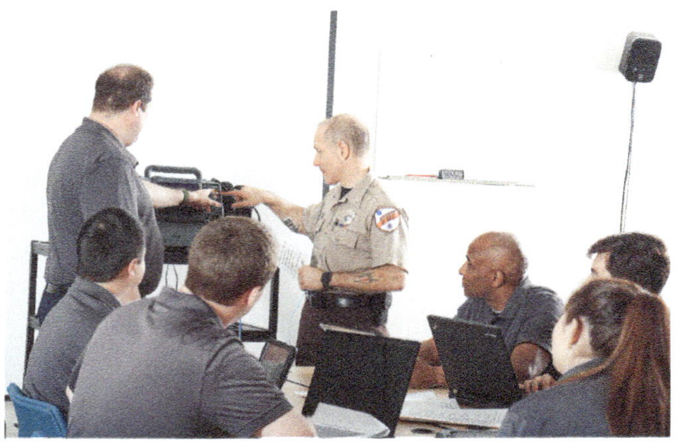

C

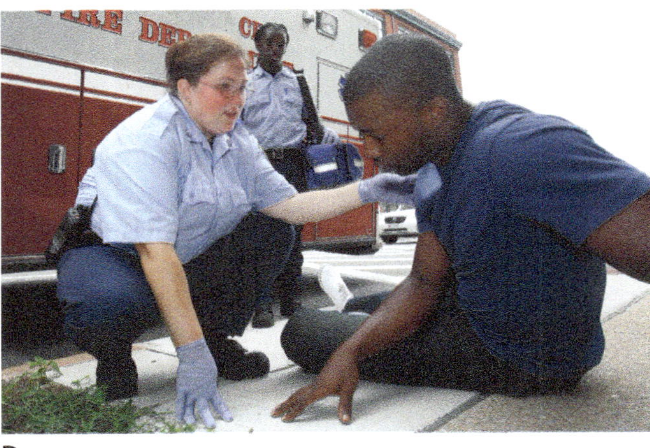

D

FIGURE 9.5 The audience (students) may be in (**A**) the hospital, (**B**) the skills lab, (**C**) the classroom, or (**D**) the field.

target audience. Because the audience remains constant throughout a series of objectives in, for example, the same lesson plan, textbook chapter, or block of instruction, the audience statement is often limited to the goal or first objective found in that series. In this case, the educator can assume the stated audience carries through for the remainder of the objectives in that section. Examples of audience statements include:

- The EMT or paramedic student
- The paramedic continuing education participant
- The cadets attending a seminar

Behavior

The *behavior* statement describes the expected outcome or capability the learner should exhibit after the instructional event has occurred. Robert Mager, a behavioral theorist, is credited with the concept that goals and objectives should be tied to measurable outcomes. The term he used to describe this relationship was *concrete*.[17] That is, any statement, or objective, tied to measurable behavioral outcomes is concrete. Objectives that are not measurable are termed *fuzzy* statements. Mager believed objectives should always be written in terms of performance so that learning can be measured. This concept is the foundation for the process of writing objectives. If an objective is written so it can be measured or observed, it becomes concrete enough to form the basis of assessment. The relationship between goals, objectives, and assessment is explored at the end of this chapter.

Review the following two objectives. According to the criteria established by Mager, objective 1 is not measurable, and objective 2 is measurable.

- **Objective 1**. The student will identify equipment used to immobilize a patient to a long backboard.
- **Objective 2**. Given a BLS ambulance stocked with all the required equipment and supplies identified by the state protocol, the student will identify every piece of equipment used to immobilize a patient to a long backboard.

Objective 1 states the audience and behavior but does not articulate any conditions or degree. It does not state how or what equipment will be used in the test, nor does it state the required score for successfully satisfying this objective. Thus, it would be difficult for an instructor to perform an assessment of this objective. Objective 2 tells both the instructor and the student that they will be required to identify all required equipment and supplies, and that they will be working with an ambulance stocked according to an established standard. Therefore, objective 2 leaves little room for subjectivity in interpretation.

If objectives are observable and measurable, a tangible product or outcome that can be scrutinized and evaluated should be the result. This product or outcome can take the form of demonstrated knowledge, performance of a skill, or expressed or modeled feeling or emotion. It can come from any of the domains of learning (cognitive, affective, or psychomotor) and can be written to correspond to any of the levels within a domain. It should be a realistic behavior related to the real-life scope of practice for the student.

Examples of behavior statements include:

- Describe the steps used to initiate a peripheral IV.
- Demonstrate how to put on sterile gloves.
- Challenge statements that do not support professional behavior and conduct.

In some educational settings, the terminology used to construct the behavioral statement carries legal connotations. In this case, there is a significant difference between phrases such as "should be able to" and "will be able to." It is important for the instructor to determine whether such a circumstance exists, and if it does, to follow the requirements accordingly when developing goals and objectives.

Condition

The *condition* portion of the ABCD objective describes any circumstance that influences the performance of behavior. It may include a list of tools or equipment that may or may not be used in completion of the behavior; it may describe environmental or weather conditions or identify specific locations or situations, such as time of day or season of the year. Time limits may also be imposed as a condition of the performance of a skill. Examples of condition statements include:

- . . . in swift-running river water with class II rapids . . .
- Given a table of assorted splinting equipment, . . .
- . . . within 1 minute . . .

Consider this example of a measurable objective for a trauma lesson: The EMT student will perform a trauma patient assessment on a simulated patient placed in a difficult-to-access location, without committing any critical errors. In this case, critical errors should be defined on the performance checklist or rubric (See the box *What Are Rubrics?*). (See also Chapter 22, *Other Assessment Tools*, for further information on rubrics.) The conditions affecting the performance (in this case, the skill of trauma patient assessment) of this objective are the use of a simulated patient (necessitating the finding of predetermined signs or symptoms) and a challenging environment. Because the condition is well articulated, both the instructor and the student can determine what behavior is expected and how it should be tested. This leaves little room for surprises during testing and helps create realistic expectations for both students and instructors.

Degree

The *degree* portion of the objective provides the standard of accuracy required for acceptable performance. It describes the actual measurement tool used to assess the student's performance and clearly identifies the point at which the student will be successful in that performance. Objectives can be measured by both **quantitative** and **qualitative** criteria. Quantitative criteria identify behaviors through conditions that impose or describe limitations (e.g., the lowest acceptable passing score, time limits, or limits on number of attempts) and provide this information as a percentage or point value. Qualitative criteria include nonnumerical observations that show underlying dimensions or patterns of relationships (e.g., expressing the value or acceptance of a concept or idea, defending a decision or action, or adopting a new behavior pattern).

Qualitative standards are often more difficult to assign numeric scores, but they can be observed for performance. The use of rubrics as evaluation tools can be helpful in qualitative measurements.

Additional factors to consider in measuring performance according to an objective are whether steps required to perform a skill are ordered (and if this order is important) and whether any factors or steps are critical to the performance. Examples of critical factors include the wearing of gloves when one approaches an appropriate patient situation and the performing of an assessment before one begins CPR. Such factors are often labeled "critical criteria," "mandatory actions," or "critical fail points" (the psychomotor examination scoring sheets of the National Registry of EMTs refer to these fail points as "critical criteria"). Failure to satisfy or perform them may result in immediate failure in the performance of an objective. Critical fail points are generally absolute, which means that failure is imposed despite an otherwise acceptable performance. Critical failure criteria should be identified in all domains of learning. For this reason, critical fail status should be reserved for extremely important steps or considerations. Some examples of degree statements include:

- . . . seven out of ten times . . .
- . . . to 80% accuracy . . .
- . . . for every patient care encounter . . .

It is important that the performance level be specifically stated; otherwise, an educator may assume that 100% accuracy is required. (Note that a performance level of 100% accuracy for quantitative or qualitative measures is not required for every objective.) Educators should scrutinize objectives carefully to determine the acceptable level of performance and should plan instructional time and emphasis accordingly. For certain items, 100% accuracy may be appropriate, such as certain airway management techniques, or calculating medication dosages. On the other hand, establishing 100% accuracy for an objective that requires team leading 12 field cardiac arrests during the program would be unattainable in most systems. In general, 100% accuracy correlates to critical criteria.

Often, it is difficult to distinguish between some of the ABCD components of an objective, as there seems to be crossover between them. Take, for example, the following objective: "Upon completion of this lesson on trauma, the student will be able to correctly demonstrate the application of a rigid splint to a simulated open fracture of the upper extremity within 7 minutes, without committing any critical errors."

Instructors may debate whether the statement "within 7 minutes" represents a condition or a degree. They may also debate whether the words "correctly demonstrate" indicate that a score of 100% accuracy is required to satisfy this objective. This objective leaves little doubt about what behavior is expected of the student (apply a rigid splint to an open upper extremity fracture) and about how the student will be assessed (it must be done correctly within 7 minutes, and the student cannot commit any critical criteria errors). The word "correctly" may cause minor confusion, but most instructors would overlook this wording because the phrase about committing critical errors sets a clear boundary.

This example draws attention to the fact that the writing of objectives is not a simple task. In this case, it is important for the educator to identify the behavior portion of the objective and to place that behavior in the proper context within the domains of learning. In so doing, the instructor can identify the depth and breadth required to teach the content so that the objective is satisfied. This objective requires problem-solving behavior via Cognitive Level 3: Applying, Level 4: Analyzing, and Level 5: Evaluating, as well as performance at Psychomotor Level 3: Precision.

TEACHING TIP

When working from goals and objectives that have been supplied to an instructor, it is critical that the educator review the objectives to ensure completeness and relevance to the audience and situation.

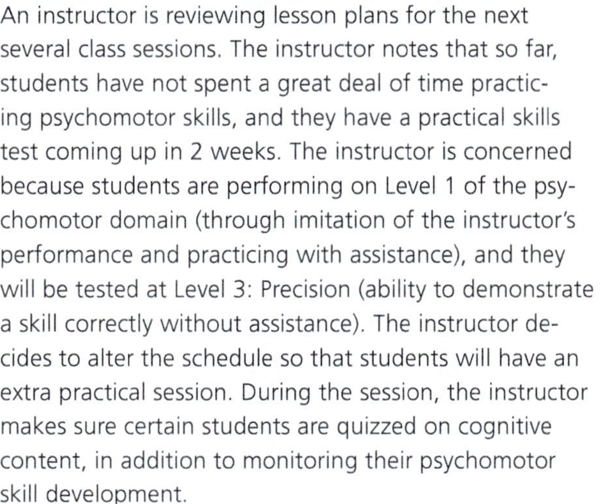

CASE in Point

An instructor is reviewing lesson plans for the next several class sessions. The instructor notes that so far, students have not spent a great deal of time practicing psychomotor skills, and they have a practical skills test coming up in 2 weeks. The instructor is concerned because students are performing on Level 1 of the psychomotor domain (through imitation of the instructor's performance and practicing with assistance), and they will be tested at Level 3: Precision (ability to demonstrate a skill correctly without assistance). The instructor decides to alter the schedule so that students will have an extra practical session. During the session, the instructor makes sure certain students are quizzed on cognitive content, in addition to monitoring their psychomotor skill development.

Checklist for Writing Objectives

- All four parts of the *ABCD* behavioral objective are present:
  - Audience
  - Behavior
  - Condition
  - Degree
- Accurate terminology is used to reflect the domain of learning level.
- Expected outcome is clearly articulated and measurable.
- Expected outcome is written in terms of behaviors to perform or observe.
- The scoring method for pass/fail is clearly articulated.
- A measurement tool is discussed or described.
- Objective supports overarching goal (performance alignment).

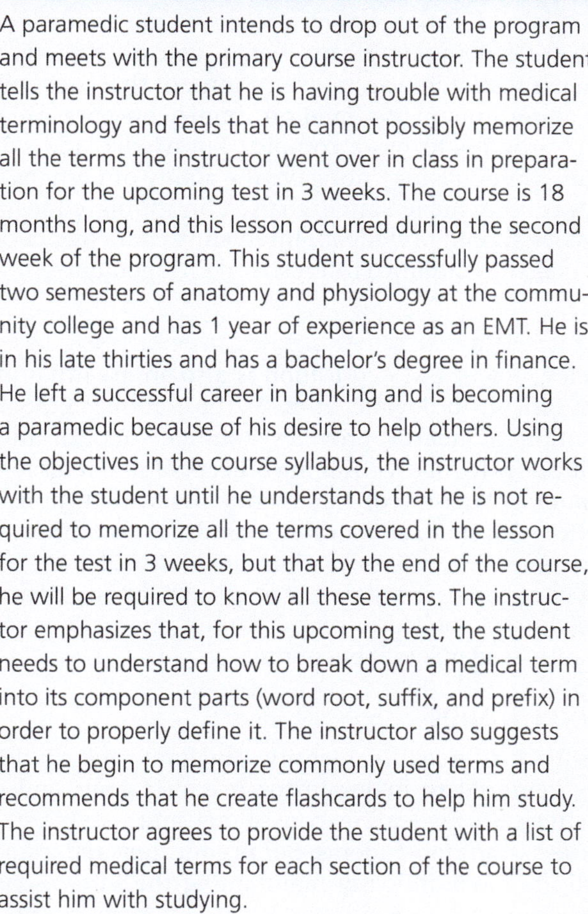

CASE in Point

A paramedic student intends to drop out of the program and meets with the primary course instructor. The student tells the instructor that he is having trouble with medical terminology and feels that he cannot possibly memorize all the terms the instructor went over in class in preparation for the upcoming test in 3 weeks. The course is 18 months long, and this lesson occurred during the second week of the program. This student successfully passed two semesters of anatomy and physiology at the community college and has 1 year of experience as an EMT. He is in his late thirties and has a bachelor's degree in finance. He left a successful career in banking and is becoming a paramedic because of his desire to help others. Using the objectives in the course syllabus, the instructor works with the student until he understands that he is not required to memorize all the terms covered in the lesson for the test in 3 weeks, but that by the end of the course, he will be required to know all these terms. The instructor emphasizes that, for this upcoming test, the student needs to understand how to break down a medical term into its component parts (word root, suffix, and prefix) in order to properly define it. The instructor also suggests that he begin to memorize commonly used terms and recommends that he create flashcards to help him study. The instructor agrees to provide the student with a list of required medical terms for each section of the course to assist him with studying.

Three Es Method

Another strategy instructors may utilize to develop objectives is the **3 Es method**, which focuses on emphasis, expectations, and evaluation.[18] The 3 Es framework allows instructors to develop objectives that reflect appropriate scope, depth, and complexity employing Bloom's taxonomy as a foundation.

Emphasis

Whether a training officer or initial instructor, an educator must identify essential information that students need to learn. *Emphasis* determines what information is the focus of student development. Inclusion of all learning domains at various levels allows prioritization of learning goals and objectives by both instructors and students. As discussed, an educator should identify broader topic goals, then narrow them down to manageable objectives. For example, an instructor may identify and prioritize airway management as a topic area. The instructor will need to decide how much time to allot to this broad topic based on the amount of time available and what areas are essential. For example, if an instructor plans to spend a week on airway management, the instructor must determine what they will cover that week, each day, and even each hour of the instructional period.

Expectations

Expectations provide students with information regarding what the instructor expects them to know and be able to do at the end of a specific course, class, or period of time. It is essential that instructors build a foundation of simple knowledge and develop more complex concepts. Instructors involved in initial training may work with a more homogenous group of students and may expect to cover all content outlined in the National EMS Education Standards and the National EMS Scope of Practice Model, whereas training officers may have a diverse group of students with varying levels of competence. The training officers can identify knowledge or psychomotor insufficiencies, then focus on specific content areas. For example, a training officer may be aware that providers struggle with correct bag-valve-mask ventilations, as well as with awareness and practice of evidence-based guidelines for oxygen application. Training officers may be able to start at a higher level of Bloom's taxonomy and expect students to engage in critical thinking and problem solving, while an initial instructor will start out at a simple recall level, incrementally increasing difficulty. It is imperative to include the affective domain in the form of attitudes and behaviors.

Evaluation

The *evaluation* process, more commonly called assessment in this text and in the field of education, is where learning outcomes are actualized. Assessments will be discussed in greater detail later in Part V, *Student Assessment and Remediation*. Objectives must be written so that they are observable and measurable and, therefore, student learning can be assessed. Often teachers write objectives that seem to meet these criteria; however, upon further examination they may be difficult to assess. Suffice to say that assessment can include a variety of activities from written and practical exams to case studies, papers, essays, reflective journals, simulations, building models, and scenarios, so educators should not limit their creativity.

One exercise that may assist students and less experienced faculty or instructional staff is to ask what the student expects to accomplish that day in the classroom, lab, or clinical setting. For example, an instructor could ask students to name the areas in which they are exhibiting competency versus sections in which they need additional attention for the attainment of proficiency. Discussing students' current status compared to expected learning can bridge the gap and make the exercise more salient.

SMART Objective Development

Another approach to developing and evaluating objectives is the **SMART method**. SMART objectives can be written for each of the domains, as well as to set personal goals. This approach focuses on objectives being specific, measurable, attainable, relevant, and time-bound (**FIGURE 9.6**).[19]

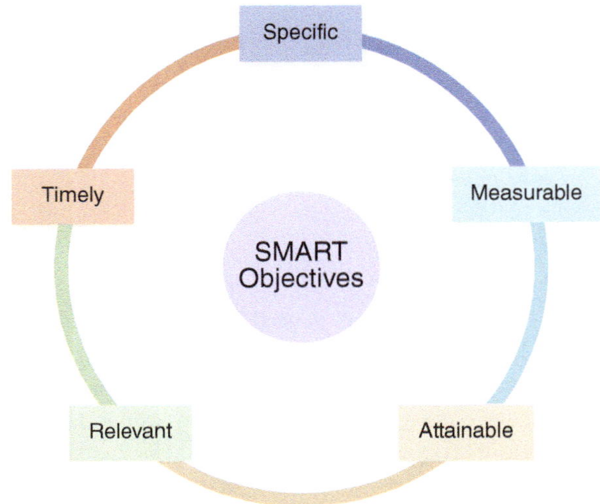

FIGURE 9.6 The components of SMART objectives.

Specific

Objectives are specific and employ action verbs that can be found in the Bloom's taxonomy table to determine the complexity and domain that the instructor is attempting to teach and ensure. Refer to the program, course, or module goals to ensure alignment. If a simple or foundational level of knowledge, as in the EMT program, is to be learned, then a verb from the lower level of the taxonomy table would be used. If the information or skill is to be learned at a complex or comprehensive level, as in the paramedic program, then a verb from a higher level of the taxonomy table would be used.

Measurable

Objectives need to be measurable so that both instructor and students can assess how well they are progressing toward achieving identified learning. Refer back to Bloom's taxonomy to choose appropriate verbs from the appropriate learning domain that can be measured by the form of assessment chosen.

Attainable

In EMS education, many objectives are necessary to ensure patient safety; however, instructors should consider a scaffolding approach to content that is complex to allow students to build on simple concepts initially and progress to more complex knowledge and skills. Some students may not have the ability or perhaps the desire to achieve stated goals. Continuing education classes should provide an interesting challenge to participants to enhance interest and engagement.

Relevant

Relevancy in EMS education is also an area that may be difficult to deviate from, as the National EMS Education Standards provides a framework for initial educators to follow. Training officers should refer to the National Registry of Emergency Medical Technicians (NREMT), state, and local standards for recertification. The must-know information and skills related to the level of competency that is measured, in any domain, need to be applied to real situations and patient complaints students will encounter.

Time-Bound

Instructors need to identify timelines that students are required to maintain for reaching goals and objectives. This will allow consistency and provide stable expectations for students. Some educators and training officers have difficulty maintaining the initial schedule provided to students, which in turn results in confusion and a dilution of standards.

Terminology and Precision

Objectives must be written with clear, unambiguous terminology that is free of jargon. All acronyms and potentially confusing terms should be clearly defined. Statements must be written in observable and measurable terms, with careful attention to ensure that action verbs used to describe the required behavior and expected outcome reflect the desired level. **TABLE 9.2** provides a listing of appropriate verbs that correspond to the various levels within the updated Bloom's taxonomy.[4]

Objectives should always be results-oriented. Unlike broader goal statements, objectives describe specific expectations. When they read an objective, there should be no doubt in the student's and instructor's minds about exactly what behavior is expected. Returning to a previous example (The EMT will perform a trauma patient assessment on a simulated patient placed in a difficult-to-access location, without committing any critical errors), imagine the difficulty this student would face if, every time the student practiced a trauma patient assessment, it was on a manikin lying supine on a blanket in the middle of the classroom floor, yet, on the night of the test, the simulated live patient was placed head down on the side of a dark hill outdoors. This example illustrates the importance of writing well-designed, relevant objectives, instructing and assessing competency to those objectives, and thereby setting up the student for success.

TABLE 9.2 Action Verbs Corresponding to Bloom's Taxonomy

Domain	Level	Appropriate Verbs
Cognitive	1. Remember	Arrange, define, identify, label, list, match, memorize, name, order, quote, recall, recite, recognize, repeat, select
	2. Understand	Discuss, explain, illustrate, indicate, infer, interpret, locate, outline, relate, restate, review, rewrite, summarize, translate
	3. Apply	Apply, choose, compute, determine, direct, develop, execute, implement, model, operate, organize, practice, prepare, provide, select, solve, use, utilize
	4. Analyze	Analyze, calculate, classify, compare, contrast, diagram, differentiate, distinguish, experiment, prioritize, separate
	5. Evaluate	Appraise, argue, assess, conclude, criticize, diagnose, evaluate, forecast, hypothesize, justify, score
	6. Create	Assemble, compose, construct, create, design, develop, formulate, generate, invent, plan, predict, prescribe, transform
Psychomotor	1. Imitation	Copy, duplicate, follow, mimic, repeat with assistance, reproduce
	2. Manipulation	Complete, demonstrate, dissemble, examine, manipulate, operate, practice with minimal assistance, put together, replicate
	3. Precision	Arrange, conduct, demonstrate to others, integrate, perform without assistance, perform without error independently
	4. Articulation	Coordinate, demonstrate proficiency, develop personal technique, modify/adjust to conditions, perform with confidence
	5. Naturalization	Build, construct, design, make, perform automatically or instinctually
Affective	1. Receive	Accept, attempt, engage, listen, notice, be open, tolerate, be willing
	2. Respond	Challenge, comply, cooperate, enjoy, examine, observe, select, support, visit
	3. Value	Accept, believe, carry out, choose, defend, devote, display, express, offer, pursue
	4. Organize	Consider, debate, dispute, favor, judge, prefer, share, theorize, volunteer, weigh
	5. Characterize	Act on, advocate, embrace, exemplify, incorporate into clinical practice, internalize, join, participate

Data from Bloom, Benjamin S. (Ed.). 1956. *Taxonomy of Educational Objectives, Book 1: Cognitive Domain*. New York: Longman.

Goals and Objectives and the Assessment Process

Once the level has been identified for the goal or objective, the instructor can determine which level the assessment tool should address. As educators consider assessment, it is important to refer to the objectives to ensure congruence. For example, if an instructor asks a student to create something, it is not possible to assess that through a multiple choice exam. The difficulty level of the verb in the objective must align with the level of difficulty expected on the assessment tool. Instead, if the objective is written at the knowledge level, the assessment should be simple recall.

Assessment tools may be formative or summative in nature. Formative assessment tools can target any level: knowledge, application, or problem solving. Summative tools should focus on the higher levels of application and problem solving. They should include some assessment to verify competency in the knowledge level, as well as at higher levels. This condition will be important in the event that the student does poorly on the assessment, as this information can help focus the remediation process by identifying where the deficit occurred. (Chapter 20, *Assessing Learning*, takes an in-depth look at formative and summative assessment tools.)

Use each of the following objectives to determine at what depth the instructor should assess and to stimulate discussion of possible assessment tools:

1. The EMT students will use their own words to correctly define, at least five of the following six terms pertaining to respiratory emergencies: *dyspnea, apnea, eupnea, hyperpnea, tachypnea*, and *bradypnea*.
2. Upon completion of this module, the students in this Advanced EMT program will be able to demonstrate insertion of a supraglottic airway, using the indicated checklist, with 80% accuracy and no critical errors.
3. Given a series of photographs of skin rashes, with 80% accuracy, the student will identify photographs that show a vesicular skin rash.

Objective 1 asks the student to provide definitions. The revised Bloom's taxonomy places this type of cognition in Level 1: Remembering. Thus, a fill-in-the-blank worksheet would be an appropriate assessment tool.

What Are Rubrics?

A **rubric** is a grading tool that uses rating scales that often incorporate examples to provide a framework to score a student's performance. Rubrics are used for both qualitative and quantitative evaluations. Rubrics work well with qualitative criteria because they provide concrete examples of the expected level of behavior or content, along with the scores or grades that will be awarded if the student meets the specifications within each category. Rubrics are also useful for more subjective assessments because they quantify the expected outcomes. Grading of essay questions is generally considered subjective but is made less so when graded with rubric tools that identify the desired level of performance within specified categories. These categories typically include content, organization, and process. Instructors determine criteria for each level ahead of time so both students and faculty have clear guidelines to define performance. For example, the rubric may state that the student will receive 5 points for each key concept that the student explains in the essay, up to a total of 50 points. It may also include a deduction of 5 points for every unrelated concept or incorrect item that the student includes in the answer. Another rubric may score the essay by creating a scale for punctuation and spelling errors, awarding up to 10 points for 0 to 5 errors, 9 points for 6 to 10 errors, 8 points for 11 to 15 errors, and so forth. Scoring within the rubric should allow for assessment of each of the dimensions of the project. Students can even be provided examples of answers for each grade range. Tools for developing rubrics can be found on various websites on the Internet.

Objective 2 asks the student to apply advanced airway skills, so they must possess knowledge and understanding (Levels 1 and 2, Remembering and Understanding), but must also apply techniques of airway management (Level 3, Applying). The objective states that the student must insert a supraglottic airway (a psychomotor activity), so a demonstration of those skills is the appropriate requirement for assessment. The evaluator should also ask questions to ensure that Levels 1 and 2 have been mastered. It would not be appropriate for the evaluator to deliberately introduce problems into the examination, as the objective does not state that such a high level of performance is expected. In the event of a problem, it may be appropriate for the evaluator to assist the student. If this happens early in the course, the student may not possess many problem-solving skills. However, because this is an advanced course, the student may be expected to have already mastered a certain number of problem-solving skills. If troubleshooting or problem solving is the expectation, it should be clearly stated in the objective, which would be at Level 4 or 5, Analyzing and Evaluating.

Objective 3 may appear to be of a higher level upon first glance, but it is operating primarily at Level 3, Applying. In this objective, the student will be shown a series of photographs, and must apply the rules and knowledge obtained in Levels 1 and 2 to decide which images meet the criteria. Students are not asked to defend their choices, compare or contrast choices, or determine whether the rash presented represents a specific disease. Because the objective states that students will be given a finite grouping of photographs to review, all the student is asked to do is to sort the images into one of two categories: those that meet the criteria and those that do not. This involves mainly knowledge Levels 1 and 2, Remembering and Understanding, along with some Level 3 skills (Applying), in that they are applying their knowledge of the rules. An assessment approach that would be appropriate for this situation would be to show students a series of slides and ask them to write "yes" or "no" on an answer sheet. Another way to assess this objective is to give students a pile of cards with the images, and ask students to sort the cards into two piles: one showing vesicular rashes and one with images that are not.

Summary

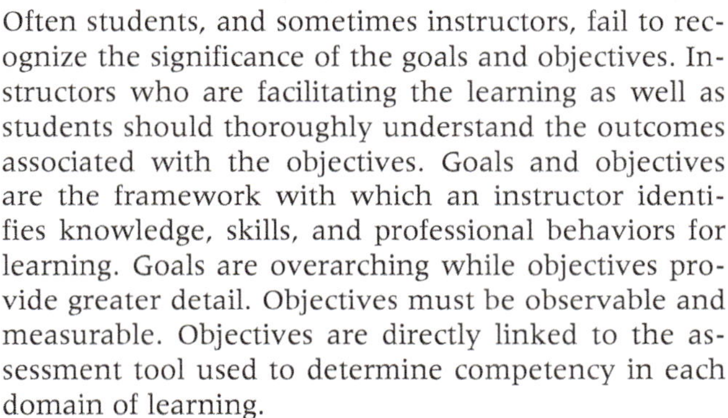

Often students, and sometimes instructors, fail to recognize the significance of the goals and objectives. Instructors who are facilitating the learning as well as students should thoroughly understand the outcomes associated with the objectives. Goals and objectives are the framework with which an instructor identifies knowledge, skills, and professional behaviors for learning. Goals are overarching while objectives provide greater detail. Objectives must be observable and measurable. Objectives are directly linked to the assessment tool used to determine competency in each domain of learning.

Educators should utilize Bloom's taxonomy and a model with which they are comfortable to write objectives that meet established criteria and the correct level of complexity. This process ensures objectives are written appropriately for the level of student being instructed and the content that is being taught. Objectives should align with the learning plan and assessment. When appropriate, the instructor should consider employing a rubric for assessing student work. Appropriate objectives aligned with content and student assessment provide a clear map for students and instructors to move toward the parallel goals of program success and, ultimately, safe patient care.

Glossary

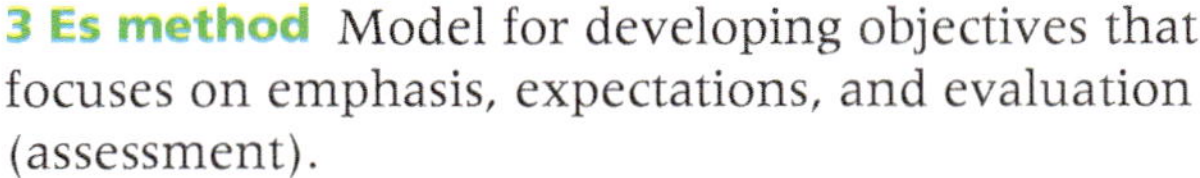

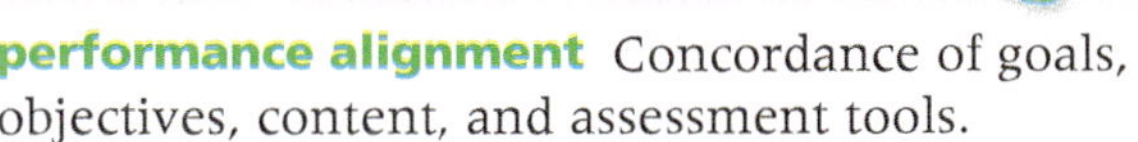

3 Es method Model for developing objectives that focuses on emphasis, expectations, and evaluation (assessment).

ABCD model Model to write objectives in which the audience, behaviors, conditions, and degree required to achieve the objective are clearly defined.

cognitive load Effect that results from an overload of information that renders learning ineffective.

declarative material Depth and breadth of the content of a lesson; the component of a lesson plan in which objectives and content are arranged and grouped in the order in which they will be taught.

goal Broad statement of instructional intent.

objective Specific, measurable learning outcome.

performance alignment Concordance of goals, objectives, content, and assessment tools.

performance gap Difference between actual performance and required performance.

qualitative Nonnumerical observations that show underlying dimensions or patterns of relationships.

quantitative Criteria that identify behaviors through conditions that impose or describe limitations.

rubric Measurement tool that establishes a framework for assessment.

SMART method Approach to writing objectives that focuses on objectives being specific, measurable, attainable, relevant, and time-bound.

References

[1] Kalb, Kathleen A. 2009. "The THREE Cs Model: The Context, Content, and Conduct of Nursing Education." *Nursing Education Perspectives* 30, no. 3: 176–80.

[2] Clark, Don. 1995. "Performance and Learning Objectives in Instructional Design." *Performance Juxtaposition*. Updated September 22, 2015. Accessed May 18, 2018. http://www.nwlink.com/~donclark/hrd/isd/develop_objective.html.

[3] Hardt, Ulrich H. 1977. "Determining Goals, Objectives, and Strategies for the Domains of Learning and Instructional Intents." *A Guide to Lesson and Unit Planning. ERIC.* ED146150.

[4] Bloom, Benjamin S. (Ed.). 1956. *Taxonomy of Educational Objectives, Book 1: Cognitive Domain*. New York: Longman.

[5] Garlikov, Rick. "The Socratic Method: Teaching by Asking Instead of by Telling." Accessed October 11, 2018. http://www.garlikov.com/Soc_Meth.html.

[6] Dreyfus, Stuart E., and Hubert L. Dreyfus. 1980. *A Five-Stage Model of the Mental Activities Involved in Directed Skill Acquisition*. Berkeley, CA: University of California, Operations Research Center. Accessed April 22, 2019. https://apps.dtic.mil/docs/citations/ADA084551.

[7] Benner, Patricia. 1984. "From Novice to Expert: Excellence and Power in Clinical Nursing Practice." *American Journal of Nursing* 84, no. 12: 147.

[8] Batalden, Paul, David Leach, Susan Swing, Hubert Dreyfus, and Stuart Dreyfus. 2002. "General Competencies and Accreditation in Graduate Medical Education." *Health Affairs* 21, no. 5: 103–11. https://doi.org/10.1377/hlthaff.21.5.103.

[9] Ramsburg, Lisa, and Ron Childress. 2012. "An Initial Investigation of the Applicability of the Dryfus Skill Acquisition Model." *Nursing Education Perspectives* 33, no. 5: 312–6.

[10] Persky, Adam M., and Jennifer D. Robinson. 2017. "Moving from Novice to Expertise and Its Implications for Instruction." *American Journal of Pharmaceutical Education* 81, no. 9: 72–80. https://doi.org/10.5688/ajpe6065.

[11] Maier-Lorentz, Madeline. 1999. "Writing Objectives and Evaluating Learning in the Affective Domain." *Journal for Nurses in Professional Development* 15, no. 4: 167–71. http://dx.doi.org/10.1097/00124645-199907000-00008.

[12] Brouchard, Gary J. 2011. "In Full Bloom: Helping Students Grow." *The Journal of Physician Assistant Education* 22, no. 4: 44–6.

[13] Adams, Nancy E. 2015. "Bloom's Taxonomy of Cognitive Learning Objectives." *Journal of the Medical Library Association* 103, no. 3: 152–3. http://dx.doi.org/10.3163/1536-5050.103.3.010.

[14] Anderson, Lorin W., and David R. Krathwohl (Eds.). 2001. *A Taxonomy for Learning, Teaching, and Assessing: A Revision of Bloom's Taxonomy of Educational Objectives*. New York: Pearson.

[15] University of North Carolina at Charlotte. n.d. "Writing Measurable Course Objectives." *Center for Teaching and Learning.* Accessed April 2, 2019. https://teaching.uncc.edu/teaching-guides/course-design/writing-measurable-course-objectives.

[16] Hodell, Chuck. 1997. "Basics of Instructional Systems Development." The American Society for Training and Development. *ASTD Infoline*, no. 9706.

[17] Mager, Robert F. 1972. *Goal Analysis*. Belmont, CA: Fearon Publishers.

[18] Medina, Melissa S. 2010. "Using the Three E's (Emphasis, Expectations, and Evaluation) to Structure Writing Objectives." *American Journal of Health-System Pharmacy* 67, no. 7: 516–21. https://doi.org/10.2146/ajhp090227.

[19] Cognology. 2017. "How to Write SMART Goals and Objectives." Accessed May 18, 2018. https://www.cognology.com.au/learning_center/howtowritesmartobj/.

Additional Resources

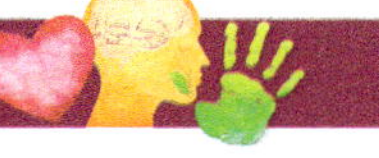

Faulconer, Emily K. 2017. "Increasing Student Interactions with Learning Objectives." *Journal of College Science Teaching* 46, no. 5: 32–8. http://dx.doi.org/10.2505/4/jcst17_046_05_32.

Gronlund, Norman D., and Susan M. Brookhart. 2009. *Gronlund's Writing Instructional Objectives*, 8th ed. Upper Saddle River, NJ: Pearson Merrill Prentice Hall.

Nooman, Zohair M., Henk G. Schmidt, and Esmat S. Ezzat (Eds.). 1990. *Innovation in Medical Education*. New York: Springer Publishing.

Smilkstein, Rita. 1993. "Acquiring Knowledge and Using It." *Gamut* 16: 41–3.

CHAPTER 10

Lesson Plans

OBJECTIVES

At the conclusion of this chapter, the educator will be able to:

Cognitive Domain

1. Describe how a well-constructed lesson plan contributes to student goal achievement.
2. Discuss the variety of resources that are available to assist with lesson plan development.
3. Identify the components of a well-constructed lesson plan.
4. Discuss the importance of identifying the equipment list and supplies in the lesson plan.
5. Identify the information that will be considered prior to the development of a lesson plan.
6. Compare and contrast the depth and breadth of content in a lesson plan between an emergency medical technician (EMT) versus a paramedic.
7. Describe the relevance of delivery of the declarative content in a logical, sequential format.
8. Discuss the relevance of inclusion of cognitive, psychomotor, and affective domain objectives in every lesson plan.
9. Discuss the versatility of lesson plans that will support online learning management systems.
10. Understand the importance of lesson plans for all training sessions led by emergency medical services (EMS) lead and lab instructors, field training officers, and continuing education instructors.

Psychomotor Domain

There are no psychomotor objectives for this chapter.

Affective Domain

1. Defend the value of inclusion of a motivational activity that promotes student curiosity to learn.
2. Value collaboration with faculty and the medical director in the development of a lesson plan.
3. Value reflection of the effectiveness of a lesson plan after each session.
4. Defend student outcomes based on the relevance of the components of a lesson plan.

> **“The whole art of teaching is only the art of awakening the natural curiosity of young minds for the purpose of satisfying it afterwards.”**
>
> ~ Anatole France

CHAPTER GOAL To understand the importance of the components in the development of an effective lesson plan as they relate to student outcomes.

The process of education can be described as a journey. As with any journey, the traveler, or student, must know where they are going and the path they will take. Along the way, various waypoints will indicate the progress that is being made. In an educational journey, the final destination is indicated by the course, or terminal objective. Waypoints along the way correspond to the student performance objectives; the roadmap that keeps the learner and the instructor on track and heading toward the final destination is the lesson plan. Thus, it can be seen that the lesson plan plays a key role in the educational process. This role is even more important as instructors move away from traditional lectures and classroom structures. An effective lesson plan incorporates various teaching techniques such as a "flipped classroom" and simulation, defining the complete roadmap for the journey.

Overview of Lesson Plans

The lesson plan is a valuable teaching tool on many levels. In addition to keeping the instructional process on track, it serves a variety of other important functions. For the instructor, whether a field training officer or continuing education instructor, it provides the basic information needed to teach as well as to prepare the lesson. A properly formatted lesson plan includes not only the materials needed to meet the lesson objectives, but also the introductory material needed to prepare the lesson. It provides information and guidance on the development and use of instructional aids. And, because it is tied to the lesson objectives, it serves as a basis for student assessment.

Lesson plans assist the instructional process and directly help the instructor. Lesson plans explain the depth and breadth of the lesson and tie together the student objectives. And, perhaps as important as the assistance they lend to the instructor, lesson plans ensure continuity and consistency in instruction.

When multiple instructors are involved in an educational program, the lesson plan serves as the "common map" that guides the course instruction. For the new instructor, or even a seasoned instructor who is moving into a new content area, the lesson plan takes on increased importance. In such cases, the contract, ancillary, or lab instructor will most likely not be the one developing the lesson plan. The primary instructor such as the lead instructor or program director typically develops, customizes, and revises the lesson plan. Those who develop and revise lesson plans need to share the lesson plan objectives with all instructors who are teaching the lesson, including the lab or continuing education instructors. Standardized courses, such as advanced cardiac life support (ACLS), typically provide lesson plans created by the sponsoring agency. Institutions or publishers that provide EMS education may produce standardized lesson plans for instructor use. The availability of prepared lesson plans can provide a generic template. Such lesson plans still require review to ensure they are relevant to the type of session being taught. For example, the topic of respiratory diseases will have differences in the depth and breadth of various content components when taught in an EMT, paramedic, or continuing education setting. Local or state content may also need to be included, which may be beyond what the national education standards require. Although advanced instructor training programs teach ways to develop lesson plans, the knowledge and process awareness needed to develop plans may be beyond the scope of the typical EMS instructor. However, even the novice instructor should be familiar with the required components of a lesson plan, able to evaluate a plan for completeness and appropriateness, and make modifications when necessary.

Purpose of a Lesson Plan

The lesson plan is truly a multipurpose tool. It serves a number of functions in the educational process, including the following:

- Ties all lesson objectives into a coherent plan of instruction
- Provides a structure or framework from which the lesson is presented
- Ensures that important material is covered, and learning objectives are met
- Plans classroom time management to determine content that students should read outside of class, content that should be reviewed in class, and how to reach application and synthesis cognitive domain levels
- Helps the instructor prepare to teach the lesson

- Matches declarative material with each objective
- Provides a basis for the development of student assessment activities
- Serves as a means by which instructor performance can be evaluated
- Helps to keep the instruction on track and on schedule
- Assists substitute or secondary instructors and instructional assistants
- Provides consistency across multiple sections of a course
- Ensures adherence to institutional goals, objectives, and standards

To ensure that the lesson achieves the learning outcomes desired, the developer should direct the design of the lesson plan.

ADDIE Instructional Design Model[1]

The ADDIE instructional design model is a common framework used to plan and implement education. It is a cyclical process that includes five elements:

1. **Analysis**: Determine learner needs, program resources, and overall goals and objectives.
2. **Design**: Construct learning objectives; determine instructional methods, learning activities, and evaluation plan.
3. **Development**: Develop content and course materials; review and pilot test.
4. **Implementation**: Conduct the training (online, direct to learners, or train-the-trainer).
5. **Evaluation**: Measure knowledge gains and learning transfer based on overall goals.

Sources of Lesson Plans

Lesson plan templates are available from a variety of sources, ranging from the course instructor, to outside agencies, to textbook publishers. Some common sources of lesson plans include the following:

- **State EMS offices**. State agencies may develop lesson plans for EMS courses in their state.
- **Primary or senior instructors**. Instructors who have been teaching a course for some time most likely will have modified existing lesson plans or developed their own. These instructors may be adept at writing lesson plans, thus serving as a lesson development mentor for new instructors. However, instructor-modified lesson plans should be tailored to a particular cohort's learning needs and should complement the instructor's preferences in teaching. Therefore, each instructor should carefully review and modify a lesson plan before it is used.
- **Publishers**. Lesson plans for nationally recognized courses are frequently obtained from publishers. Publishers of textbooks often provide not only lesson plans, but also complete instructional support packages to supplement their texts. One must remember that these lesson plans and accompanying materials are designed for a wide audience and may be biased toward a particular product or approach. They often need modification and must frequently be tailored if they are to address local system issues. Instructors should avoid relying totally on these instructional packages; they must be sure to invest sufficient time in their own lesson preparation and delivery.

  Often, packaged lesson plans are prepared to meet minimal objectives. They may not incorporate higher learning objectives or include activities designed to synthesize information and encourage problem solving and critical thinking.

  The instructor should not assume that a packaged lesson plan addresses all of the educational standards at the appropriate level. Instructors should conduct an analysis to determine whether the lesson includes the competencies, behaviors, and judgments essential to the standard. Instructors should consider customizing objectives by cross referencing with required standards and also list the standard number with the relevant objective. This may involve including activities that integrate information from earlier lessons or previous knowledge of a group of students to reinforce and build on earlier learning at each step of the program.
- **National organizations**. Several national organizations and groups produce specialty courses that cover a specific topic in detail. Examples of these "alphabet soup" or "boutique" courses include ACLS, pediatric advanced life support (PALS), and International Trauma Life Support (ITLS). Lesson plans provided for these courses vary in complexity. However, most are very basic and are designed to closely follow an accompanying video or PowerPoint presentation. Lessons are planned around a specific time frame and assessment process. Because of the administrative control associated with many of these courses, instructor variation through tailoring of lesson plans is limited. Instructors must follow the lesson plans and schedule closely because they are often one of a cadre of instructors who have been assembled to teach such a course.

- **Institutions and agencies**. Institutions and agencies such as fire departments and EMS services may produce their own lesson plans to ensure consistency and uniformity in instruction. This is usually the case with in-house and procedural training courses, especially when instruction is scheduled to occur at various geographically separated locations. A trainer or central office staff may prepare lesson plans for distribution to instructors at various locations.

TEACHING TIP

An instructor who is selecting lesson plans must make sure that the source is appropriate for the students. For example, a lesson plan on the cardiovascular system at the paramedic level would not be appropriate for use in a cardiopulmonary resuscitation (CPR) course for laypeople. Note that some commercial lesson plans have costs or restrictions associated with them. Proper permission to use a lesson plan must be obtained.

The Needs Assessment

The needs assessment encompasses the intended audience, previous knowledge, student learning preferences, academic backgrounds, barriers that may impede the learning process, and environment. This assessment should be identified prior to the development of a lesson plan and in conjunction with the objectives of the lesson.

Tools to obtain this information can be purchased from vendors or asset tests from local community colleges, or may be self-constructed. Pre-entrance applications or surveys sent to registrants with relevant questions related to the needs of the audience are assessment tools that provide information the educator will need in order to begin construction of the lesson plan. As an example, the EMT educator constructing the lesson plan will need to know the reading level of the students in an upcoming class. Understanding the reading levels of the class, as well as individual students, will help guide how the instructor addresses reading assignments in the textbooks and related handouts. A session schedule may need to be adapted to allow more classroom time to be devoted to explanation or assessment of reading assignments to promote motivation to read the materials and ensure student understanding.

TEACHING TIP

Class time is precious! Consider assigning students to read the appropriate text chapter before class time and use class time more strategically to apply learned concepts. The instructor can spend time clarifying any complex content and then applying the content to patient situations.

Parts of the Lesson Plan

As has been stated, lesson plans can come from numerous sources and may be written in a variety of formats. The adjunct or lab instructor may have little control over how a lesson plan is constructed. However, most standard lesson plans consist of the following:

- Audience description (needs assessment should be completed first)
- Lesson goal(s)
- Cognitive objectives
- Psychomotor objectives
- Affective objectives
- Recommended list of equipment and supplies
- Recommended schedule (including breaks)
- Suggested motivational activity or anticipatory set
- Declarative content (local, state, national)
- Student independent and collaborative activities (guided practice)
- Formative assessments
- Next assignment/lesson
- References
- Comment section

The format of lesson plans varies greatly according to the source. The lesson plan format may be revised depending on the purpose of the session. Variance may occur if the educator is teaching an EMT, paramedic, or continuing education session. As an example, a continuing education session may incorporate new research based on previous knowledge that may result in a change in current local practice. However, as a rule, most lesson plans include these listed parts in some form. If the selected lesson plan does not comprise all of these parts, missing sections should be added. If the instructor is inexperienced with curriculum development, the instructor should seek help in preparing the more complicated parts of the lesson plan. A list of the specific details the students will learn on a particular topic can be maintained separately in a document of declarative information, similar to an outline format.

Front End

The first few parts of the lesson plan comprise what can be called the "front end," which contains administrative details and information. This section should contain a title for the lesson or some other scheme by which the lesson can be identified and sequenced. Specific parts of the front end are as follows.

Audience Description

The audience description is just what the name implies. It is a statement describing who is the intended audience for the lesson. In a certification course, this description may be the same for all lesson plans. An example would be "entry-level EMT students." For a more advanced course, the description might be "senior paramedics with command responsibility."

TEACHING TIP

Demographics of a student population include the students' age, educational background, years of experience working in a healthcare profession, and ethnic background. This information is helpful in knowing a particular group's previous knowledge of a topic and, therefore, the extent of coverage needed in class. In addition, demographics are useful when creating squads or teams; this information can be used to ensure a variety of backgrounds is represented in each group.

Lesson Goal

Lead instructors or program directors typically develop an instructional goal for the entire course, as well as a goal or goals for each particular lesson. For example, "At the conclusion of this lesson, the student will be able to identify and describe the functions of the endocrine system." The lesson goal identifies the desired outcome of the session or program.

The lesson objective describes how the goal will be achieved. It is supported by the listed cognitive, psychomotor, and affective objectives that follow. The action verb used in the lesson goal determines, to a large extent, the instructional approach. (See Chapter 8, *Domains of Learning*, and Chapter 9, *Goals and Objectives*.) A goal that uses verbs such as "identify," "describe," and "discuss" will most likely be pursued through a lecture or presentation format. A goal that identifies "demonstrate" as the desired outcome behavior will be addressed in a practical session. The same applies to the design of the assessment method. Lesson goals that are predominantly cognitive will be assessed through summative evaluations, such as multiple choice and short-answer tests. Psychomotor goals will be assessed by methods such as observation or a skills checklist. Affective domain goals can be assessed by the student's team member or team leader behaviors during the psychomotor practical evaluation.

Lesson Objectives

The lesson objectives portion of the lesson plan is a listing of student performance objectives that support the lesson goal. Objectives are categorized according to the three domains of learning: cognitive, psychomotor, and affective. Depending on the lesson plan format or the institutional preference, objectives may be assigned a numeric sequencing. This allows the objective to be referenced on tests and other course materials. Similar to the lesson goal, lesson objectives should be reviewed with students, so they know in greater detail what will be covered in the lesson. This is especially important for concrete and field-dependent learners.

TEACHING TIP

Students should be given a complete list of objectives for each lesson of a course. That way, they know what material will be covered. Objectives also make a good study guide.

Recommended List of Equipment and Supplies

Classroom success for the instructor is most often ensured by careful preparation. This preparation process includes reviewing the material, refreshing knowledge and skills, preparing the learning environment, and preparing instructional materials. The lesson plan contains a list of equipment and supplies needed for the lesson to be taught effectively (**FIGURE 10.1**). This list may include such items as instructional models, audiovisual materials and equipment, handouts, student practice materials, and practical training equipment. Simulation-based instruction is equipment intensive, thus this list can be quite extensive and complex. The

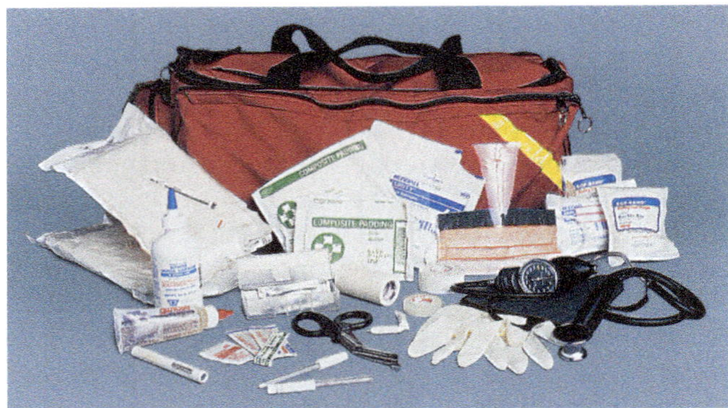

FIGURE 10.1 An equipment list is an important part of the lesson plan that should not be overlooked. Equipment should be kept updated and in working order.

TEACHING TIP

Instructors should not forget to prepare the basic "tools of instruction," such as whiteboard markers, erasers, a laser pointer, and a podium.

supply list is also useful at the completion of the lesson as a checklist to ensure that materials are accounted for and returned to their proper storage locations.

If any part of a lesson is going to fail, it most likely will be the part that is related to or dependent on equipment or technology. For this reason, the instructor should begin by becoming familiar with all material and aids to be used. Instructors should not assume that they know how something works. Instruction manuals are an excellent source of information and usually contain additional facts worth presenting to learners. Because of this, instructors should arrive well in advance of the class start time and should check and review all equipment. The instructor should not assume that because a particular audiovisual device or piece of equipment was in the classroom during the last session, it still is available. Also, instructors should know whom to contact if assistance is needed with technology. The complexity and costs of current educational technology preclude replacement or repair by the average instructor.

The instructor must have a back-up plan in the event of equipment failure or other such problems that can occur with technology-dependent lessons. The back-up plan may involve alternative aids to accomplish the lesson, material to be presented, or an entirely different lesson to replace the intended one.

TEACHING TIP

If a planned lesson cannot be presented as intended and no back-up lesson is available, the instructor can facilitate a variety of guided practice activities, such as case studies, or have students perform patient scenarios on the related content. If a face-to-face session cannot occur, conference calls or sessions such as GoToMeeting could be used. At the beginning of a course, the instructor can review prerequisite skills and knowledge. An instructor should never waste a lesson by canceling class. Practice and review are always needed.

The effective instructor always has one or two lessons "in the can" in the event of an unforeseen problem.

One area of concern in EMS education is the quality and amount of equipment available for training. Too often, outdated or broken equipment is relegated to training, or the amount of equipment is insufficient for active student participation. This sends a negative message about the service and its appreciation of training to the learner. It also violates basic educational principles in that learners are not receiving the most realistic experience during the learning process. Behavioral modeling may have as great an impact on learner development as what students are taught by the instructor. Also, a lack of equipment identical to that used in the student's practice makes it necessary for the provider to train again before they can begin functioning in the field setting. If they participate in field calls as part of their training, providers may become confused and frustrated because of differences in equipment and procedures between the classroom and the field site. Because differences in equipment may be inevitable, the instructor should encourage students to let the clinical and field preceptors know when they need orientation to a new piece of equipment, such as a different electrocardiogram (ECG) monitor.

The use of realistic simulators has become common in EMS education. Although a valuable teaching tool, the use of simulators requires specialized training on the part of the instructor as well as proper set-up. Often, a dedicated simulation lab with assigned staff is used, requiring the instructor to arrange lab time in advance and to work with the lab staff to ensure the proper objectives and skills are covered. Again, preplanning for instruction becomes a critical concern for the instructor, as does a back-up plan in the event of equipment failure or other unforeseen problems. (For more information on the use of simulation, see Chapter 18, *Tools for Simulation*.)

TEACHING TIP

A lesson plan may be designed to "teach" a particular model or type of equipment. This is especially true of lesson plans provided by equipment manufacturers. The instructor must make sure that the teaching matches the equipment the students will be using for in the field and for testing. Providing a variety of similar equipment, such as different types of traction splints, can ensure students are aware there are several types of tools to manage large bone fractures. Students must be encouraged to investigate what equipment is included on the ambulances where they will perform field experiences.

If the instructor is teaching students who provide varied services, the instructor can ask students to provide an inventory of the equipment that is available to them. In this way, the instructor can determine whether students will be using different or unusual equipment in the field. If the instructor does not have a specific piece of equipment in their training cache but students may benefit from instruction on it, they can make arrangements to borrow equipment from the service for a single class session.

Recommended Schedule

The lesson plan should identify time frames for each component of the session. This should include breaks and review time. For a practical session, it may include a schedule for practice activities. If the number of learners in a class is variable, this section may list time frames in terms of a set number of participants. For example, each group of five students could require a minimum of 40 minutes for each practical station. Of note when creating skills practical labs and testing schedules, in 2018, the National Registry of EMTs (NREMT) introduced a scenario that lasts a minimum of 20 minutes as part of the paramedic practical examination. Paramedic programs should therefore schedule practical lab and exam stations with this in mind.

TEACHING TIP

As a general rule, an instructor should plan 3 hours of preparation time for each hour of instruction.

Suggested Motivational Activity

Learner motivation can vary greatly over the duration of a course. In the beginning, learners are often highly motivated in anticipation of the course. This is especially true for courses leading to a certification level. However, as the course progresses, motivation may wane. Even the most dynamic instructor may find it hard to keep paramedic students motivated after 3 weeks of cardiology. Thus, instructors must continually motivate learners at the beginning and throughout each class session. Lesson motivation serves to increase learner interest in the material of each individual lesson. Most importantly, it establishes the environment, or what is also called the **anticipatory set**, in which learning occurs.

The suggested motivational activity should be designed to appeal to as many styles of learning of the students as possible. It should serve to move the learner emotionally from the external environment to the lesson. It should both pique and focus the learner's attention by stimulating curiosity. Some motivational activities an EMS educator may use include the following:

- Show a picture or video and pause for reflection. The instructor may show a picture or a video clip related to the lesson topic and follow up by asking the learners how this affected them.
- Play a dispatch tape of an actual 9-1-1 call. The instructor may ask the learners whether they feel ready to respond to such a call.
- Role-play a real situation to promote discussion, identify student knowledge, and build the session based on that knowledge.
- Invite a survivor or former patient to address the class, such as a patient with an implanted left ventricular assist device (LVAD). Depending on the topic and the class length, this may not be practical for short lessons.
- Engage the students in an "icebreaker" or anticipatory set activity that relates to the class topic.
- Invite a provider to tell about a significant experience that would be motivational to the learners.
- Administer a pretest (ideally with an audience response or classroom feedback system) to evaluate student knowledge (or to assess whether they have done the required reading).

Regardless of the technique used, instructors must be cautious of two things: patient confidentiality as required by the Health Insurance Portability and Accountability Act (HIPAA) guidelines, and overstimulation of learners to the point that a negative emotional response may be created. An example of the latter would be use of an event that may have emotional and personal ties to the learners.

Body of the Lesson Plan

Once the instructor and learners are prepared and motivated, it is time for the instructor to present the actual material that will allow learners to meet the lesson goal and objectives. To do this, the instructor must have an expert understanding of the lesson objectives and of the depth and breadth of material to be presented. Is material being presented for awareness or for **mastery**? This can be determined by the action verbs used in the course goal and objectives. Each domain of learning has a hierarchy that determines the required level of learning or mastery. The cognitive domain, for example, comprises six levels of mastery: remembering, understanding, applying, analyzing, evaluating, and creating. These six levels can be grouped into the following three levels of understanding:

1. **Simple**: The learner acquires new information or develops a new skill with instructor feedback. It includes objectives that demonstrate remembering and understanding (Levels 1 and 2). This new information may be obtained by the learner on their own by reading the book. The instructor would need to verify students have learned this information without holding up classmates.
2. **Fundamental**: Learners connect the knowledge learned in the basic level with knowledge gained through experience. It includes objectives that demonstrate applying the information (Level 3).
3. **Complex**: Learners move toward learning why events occur as opposed to how to perform a skill. The instructor serves as a facilitator in a coaching or mentoring role. It includes cognitive objectives that require analyzing, evaluating, and creating (Levels 4, 5, and 6).

Often, instructors or institutions assign a level code, similar to these for the cognitive domain, to each objective. This helps the instructor know which level of mastery is required for each objective.

Once the level of instruction is known for each lesson objective, an actual teaching outline, the **declarative material**, is developed. Objectives are arranged and grouped in the order in which they will be taught. This teaching cycle is used to integrate cognitive, psychomotor, and affective objectives. The actual ordering of objectives can be based on a number of different schemes that will determine the order in which declarative material is presented. This will be the actual order of instruction during the class. It is important that the declarative material be presented in a coherent fashion that supports learner understanding and retention. Some examples of schemes include the following:

- Whole-part-whole (practical skill instruction)
- Chronological
- As specified in protocol
- Body-system or organ-system based
- Simple to complex
- Small to large
- Head-to-toe (focused physical exam)
- Dispatch to return-to-service
- Following textbook content

Another simple plan is to "Tell them what you are going to teach them, teach them, and then tell them what you taught them." More specifically, explain the importance of the lesson, deliver the content, allow students to apply or practice the material, gather feedback, provide remediation, and assess performance. An easy way to do this is to open with a quick overview of lesson material and close with the same overview used as a summary.

In creating a lesson plan, the developer chooses a level of specificity for the content portion of the lesson plan. The specificity of the outline, that is, the number of levels used in the outline, varies according to the complexity of the material being presented and the instructor's teaching ability and familiarity with content.

A primary instructor may simply need "B. Start IV" included in the lesson plan, and will be able to teach the entire process. A new instructor, however, will want the lesson broken down to list the various knowledge points and skills necessary to start an IV. The extent of the outline is really a matter of personal preference. However, a lesson plan that is developed for use by various instructors must be adaptable to various levels of instructor expertise; toward that goal, sufficient declarative material must be included in the outline. When one is teaching skills, it is especially important to provide sufficient detail to the learner. Experienced practitioners may be so comfortable doing a procedure that they may not realize the many small steps and nuances that are important to its successful completion; thus, they may not emphasize or share

TEACHING TIP

The instructor should teach Level 1 material before Level 2 information is presented, and Level 2 before Level 3. Students should be evaluated for mastery before they are permitted to move on to the next level.

TEACHING TIP

Instructors can place the pages of their lesson plan in clear sheet protectors. This not only protects the pages, but it allows the instructor to write class-specific notes and comments on the page protectors with a transparency-marking pen. Notes can be wiped clear for use with another class. Additionally, other material such as instructions or protocols can be tucked between the sheets for easy access if needed during class.

these with new learners. It is also good practice to include formulas and drug names in the lesson outline to ensure that they are properly presented to the new learner.

As shown in **FIGURE 10.2**, a good format for a lesson plan is the use of two facing pages with the right page divided into two sections. The left page contains the declarative material in outline form. The first column of the right page includes notes for the instructor. This format allows lesson plans to be easily personalized by different instructors. In the notes space, instructors can include notes and comments that they want to cover in class, additional information that may be needed to answer student questions, drawings to be written on the board, and questions and answers. When teaching formulas or problems, the instructor should include the solving methods and correct answers in this area. This format is especially helpful for new instructors who might become flustered or confused during a lecture. The far-right column is used to list audiovisual aids, handouts, or activities that support the declarative material. Again, it is easy for even the experienced instructor to get off track and forget to use a teaching aid. This format also provides a complete and integrated lesson plan that can be used easily by substitute instructors.

Back End

The remaining parts of the lesson plan constitute the back end, which contains sections that pull the lesson together, check student understanding, and prepare learners for the next lesson.

Summary Session

Regardless of the format used or the complexity of the material presented, the instructor must provide closure to the lesson. Just as the anticipatory set sets the stage for the lesson and the motivational activities focus on relevance and understanding of the material, the summary brings it together for closure. The summary draws from the overview that began the presentation of the declarative material. It is even possible for the motivational activity to be repeated if it is a simple one such as a picture or video clip; this allows students to appreciate the importance of the lesson material and relate it to reality.

Assessment of Learning

To ensure that learning has taken place during a lesson, the instructor must assess learner mastery of the material. Various approaches may be used to conduct such an assessment, and discussion of each is beyond the scope of this chapter. More information on this can be found in Part V, *Student Assessment and Remediation*. However, the instructor should specify in the lesson plan an evaluation method that will be used to determine learner mastery of the material presented. This may be as simple as a few questions asked at the conclusion of the lesson to gauge learner understanding, or it could be student self-assessment undertaken to determine whether a particular objective has been mastered. **Classroom feedback systems** (also called **audience response systems**) or mini whiteboards are a great way to obtain formative feedback throughout the lesson to determine whether students have "got it." Conducting scenarios that relate to the lesson is another way to see if students can integrate content and apply it in context. Alternatively, assessment may take the form of an announcement that a 20-question, multiple choice quiz on the material will be given at the beginning of the next session.

Assignments, Next Lesson, and References

The evaluation section concludes the formal parts of a lesson plan. However, a few additions to the end of the lesson plan that may be helpful to the instructor and to the learners include assignments, the topic for the next session, related readings, and additional references. If the instructor has planned any homework for the learners, it can be assigned or distributed at this time. The next lesson topic serves as a reminder to the learners to prepare for the next session and reinforces any required readings or preparatory assignments. The end of the lesson is also an opportunity for the instructor to announce any schedule changes and to remind students to bring special equipment, such as turnout gear, to the next session. Finally, the instructor can come to class prepared with a list of references, websites, or other sources that may be of interest to learners or that may provide greater detail or explanation of the material already presented. If learners have questions or concerns, they can be referred to this reference list.

Lesson Plan Title	Instructor Notes	References and Aids
Audience: Lesson goal: *After completing this lesson, the student will be able to . . .* Objectives: *Cognitive* *Psychomotor* *Affective* Equipment and supplies: Schedule: Motivational activity/anticipatory set: Guided practice activities:		
Declarative content: Overview Outline Summary		
Student independent/collaborative activity (guided practice): Formative assessments: Assignment: Next session: References: Comment section:		

FIGURE 10.2 Sample lesson plan.

Comment Section

The comment section provides a space for the instructor to reflect on the effectiveness of the lesson plan. This serves as a reminder to change a component of the lesson plan, such as identifying activities that were not effective and need to be changed in future sessions.

Specialized Lesson Plans

The lesson plan presented earlier is a good, universal approach to lesson planning. However, as teaching techniques evolve and change, the instructor may have to adapt or develop lesson plans for specific situations. Two common examples that have become more common in EMS education are online learning and simulation.

Online Learning

The acceptance and recognition of online, asynchronous learning by EMS accreditation and testing agencies have led to increased use of this educational delivery system.

Depending on the nature of instruction, the traditional lesson plan used for in-person instruction may still work online. The front-end components are universal to any instructional activity and thus will not change, with the possible exception of the recommended schedule. Because online learning is most often asynchronous, students can access the lesson at any time. Therefore, the instructor needs to take this into consideration when planning the course. There is also the possibility that not all students enrolled in the course will follow the same schedule, as courses may have open entry points. Examples of this type of course are the National Incident Management System (NIMS) 100, 200, etc. The schedule that an online course follows depends on the length and type of course as well as institutional policy. An online college credit course may be constrained by semester dates and requirements.

Online courses are most often delivered via a **learning management system (LMS)** such as Blackboard. The format and requirements of the LMS may change or limit the methods and strategies used by the instructor to deliver the lesson material. For example, classroom discussion may be replaced by required post to a discussion board, with or without comment by the student on other student and instructor posts. Specialized learning tools such as a Wiki may also be available for online student interaction.

TEACHING TIP

Instructors should be aware that although they will not be spending time in a formal classroom when teaching an online course, they still will need to plan time to evaluate student posts and questions. In the classroom, one student may ask a question that the other students also had in mind. With online learning, every student may post the same or a similar question and expect a response!

The final part of the lesson plan requiring modification to suit online learning is the assessment section. Depending on the features available in the LMS, the instructor may have to modify testing procedures.

Simulation

Simulation is discussed in detail in Chapter 18, *Tools for Simulation*. When creating a plan for a lesson that involves simulation, it is important to include simulation-specific details such as conditions, time frame, participants, equipment, set-up details, grading rubrics, and debriefing topics or questions.

TEACHING TIP

Did you know that word processing programs like Microsoft Word have built-in templates for lesson plans?

Lesson Plan Evaluation

Once the institution or instructor has developed a lesson plan, the development process does not stop there. In addition to initial evaluation of its effectiveness, the

TEACHING TIP

It is handy for an instructor to have a pad of "sticky notes" available while teaching. If the instructor finds a problem with a lesson plan or class, the instructor can jot down a quick note and stick it onto the lesson plan. This technique is also helpful if the instructor needs to find additional material to answer a student's question or for noting areas that need remediation.

CASE in Point

The Last-Minute Lesson Plan

An instructor has just finished teaching a session of EMT to new hires at a commercial ambulance company. As she is walking back to her office, the director of training rushes up to her. She informs her that another instructor who teaches the company's paramedic course is tied up on a long critical care transport and will be at least an hour late for his class that starts in an hour. She asks the instructor to fill in for the absent instructor until he arrives. The instructor hesitates, then says okay.

The instructor asks the director if she has a copy of the class lesson plan. The director says that she does not, but is sure the other instructor has all his lesson plans in his office. The two walk to the instructor's office, and the director lets both of them in. To put it mildly, the other instructor is not organized! Papers, books, teaching materials—everything is strewn about the office. The two cannot even decide where to begin looking for lesson plans. After a quick search, the instructor realizes the situation is hopeless and that time is getting short before class begins. She knows the lesson topic—obstructive pulmonary disease. At least that is the topic listed on the schedule the director had on file. What should she do to prepare for the lesson?

At this point, the fill-in instructor has two major problems. First, she does not know the instructor's plan for that night's class. Are the students expecting a quiz or another activity? She also does not know the level of the students or which topic is scheduled to be covered. Are the students ahead of schedule? Or, are they behind schedule and not ready for this lecture? Her second concern is that her paramedic course lesson plans are at her home because she has only been teaching EMT classes.

To help her plan a class that is on schedule, the instructor can:

- Try to reach the absent instructor.
- Check to see if the training director's office or human resources department keeps copies of attendance rosters (these rosters may list the topics covered in each class session), or the training director may be able to provide a list of students and their contact information; someone can call students to find out what was planned.
- Go to the classroom or another nearby area early to try to intercept a student who is arriving early.
- Begin class by explaining the situation and finding out what was planned; she could work with the students to conduct a meaningful lesson, even if it is a review session of knowledge and skills taught previously.
- Give the students a brief assignment that they can complete on their own or in a small group, and leave the classroom for 15 minutes to prepare a quick teaching outline.

Now that the instructor knows the content scheduled for the class, how can she teach without a lesson plan? She can do the following:

- Ask students if they have an outline for each course lesson. If not, do they have a list of objectives? Any handout materials?
- Use the textbook to create a "down and dirty" lesson plan. Use the chapter heading as the main point, subheadings as secondary points, and so forth. For each heading of the "outline," she can try to think of important facts or ideas to convey. She can jot down these ideas as they come to mind, then skim the text for key points. This approach usually works best if the instructor is familiar with the material and has taught it before. The "lesson plan" will not be extensive or eloquent, but it will provide a rough organizational framework.
- Use the same approach for class objectives. This is more difficult without textual material for elaboration. The same holds true if the instructor has access to a PowerPoint presentation on the lesson topic.
- Use the National Highway Traffic Safety Administration (NHTSA) website (www.ems.gov) to download appropriate parts of the copy of the Paramedic Education Standards. Accompanying materials include instructional guidelines; however, care will need to be taken to identify new and updated information.
- Check the Trading Post on the members-only area of the National Association of EMS Educators (NAEMSE) website to see if a lesson plan or pictures are available.
- Depending on the topic, she can use her EMT lesson plan as a basis for instruction.

The take-home message from this case study is that many options are available by which instructors can quickly produce a basic lesson plan for an instructional crisis. The instructor must be creative and should be sure to be honest with students about "winging it" and needing their cooperation. Who knows? This lesson may turn out to be better than one that was developed with proper preparation time.

CASE in Point

Lesson Plan Disconnect

An instructor has been assigned to teach a paramedic refresher course at the local hospital. The class is made up of experienced paramedics. The instructor is teaching the course because he must obtain instructor certification as a requirement for promotion to supervisor. For maintenance of standardization throughout the institution, he is required to teach from a lesson plan that has been developed and approved by the EMS training officer.

While preparing to teach the unit on cardiac emergencies, he finds that the lesson plan contradicts current ACLS guidelines. He also notes that, although a protocol is in place for handling cardiac patients, the lesson, as written, uses a slightly "modified approach" rather than strictly adhering to the protocol. Because he knows his audience so well, he knows that they will give him a hard time if he tries to teach the material as outlined in the lesson plan. However, he does not want to "make waves" with the training officer because he is coming up for promotional review. What should he do?

This is a situation that involves dynamics beyond the scope of educational instruction. It is also a management issue. For the purposes of this chapter, the alternatives must be examined from an educational delivery perspective. In other words, how should the instructor handle this disconnect in the classroom? Possible approaches include the following:

- Teach the lesson directly as outlined in the lesson plan, and ignore any questions or criticism from the class. Such an approach would ruin credibility and could lead to loss of class control. This outcome would not make the instructor look like a candidate for promotion to supervisor.
- Present the material in the lesson plan and compare it to the institutional policy. Then, ask the class if they have any other approaches to handling such situations. This should lead to discussion of approaches used in the field setting.
- Take a reverse approach to presenting the material. Give the class a scenario in which the responders treat the patient as is really done according to the institutional protocol, in the field setting, then ask them to contrast this with the lesson materials.

An instructor can use these and similar strategies to handle disconnects between the lesson plan and textbooks, protocols, guest lecturers, or other instructors. Regardless of the approach taken, the instructor should never use the podium as a "bully pulpit" to complain or attack others. If an instructor must address a controversy, the instructor should present both sides of the argument impartially so that students can analyze the situation and come to their own conclusions.

lesson plan must be reviewed again periodically for timeliness, correctness, and applicability to the overall local or national curriculum revisions and learner needs.

If an instructor is teaching a new course with newly developed lesson plans, they may be involved more closely in the evaluation process. The initial evaluation process involves a formative evaluation that is ongoing and begins while the lesson plan is being constructed. The instructor should constantly compare the overall goals of instruction, lesson objectives, and content to determine whether performance is in agreement. Tests, audiovisual materials, student materials and activities, and reference materials should be evaluated as well for relevance to the instructional goal.

Even established and published lesson plans should be periodically evaluated throughout their life span. Often, lesson plans are produced to reflect a certain standard or medical protocol that may change over time. The lesson plans that accompany ACLS, for example, must change according to updates in the International Liaison Committee on Resuscitation (ILCOR) *Guidelines for CPR and Emergency Cardiovascular Care* published by the American Heart Association (AHA). A summative evaluation of lesson plans is used to determine the effectiveness of the teaching strategy and to provide information on how future performance of the same strategy and related material can be improved. Again, tests, audiovisual materials, student materials, and reference materials should be evaluated as well.

Lesson Plan Troubleshooting

Regardless of who creates a lesson plan or where it comes from, the potential for problems always exists. Problems usually fall into two broad categories: structural and factual.

Structural problems have to do with the delivery of the lesson material. When structural problems occur, the material to be presented in the lesson plan is correct and up-to-date, but something is wrong with the delivery of the material. Examples include using a lesson plan designed for a 2-hour block of instruction for a 3-hour session, or working alone to teach a skills lesson designed for a four-instructor team. In most cases, the instructor can remedy the problem by keeping the lesson material but rewriting the lesson plan into a more usable format. However, the instructor must be aware of how this lesson fits into the overall scope of the course so as not to disrupt future lessons. Shrinking a 4-hour lesson into a 2-hour session may be possible, but what are the consequences? If enrolled in a certification course, students may be required to have a minimum number of instructional hours in a topic, and this change could affect their eligibility for certification.

Structural problems can often be easily corrected if they are detected in advance of the lesson. However, factual and timeliness issues are more complex. First, the problem has to be discovered. Then, the instructor must investigate to determine the correct information and make changes as needed. This may seem straightforward, but a problem may arise with making changes. If a standardized curriculum is being used, the instructor may not be authorized to make changes. If the program is being taught with other instructors or if the course is being taught in multiple sections, the lesson plan will have to be changed for all instructors. In addition, many programs require that the medical director approve all lesson plans—a requirement that adds another level to the process. To make matters more complex, some medical practices and procedures are not embraced by all medical professionals or groups. For example, the instructor may teach a class on the basics of traditional cardiac arrest management, only to discover that the students have just read in the local newspaper about a study advocating cardiocerebral resuscitation using a pit crew approach. Such research must be verified and studied in greater detail.

Summary

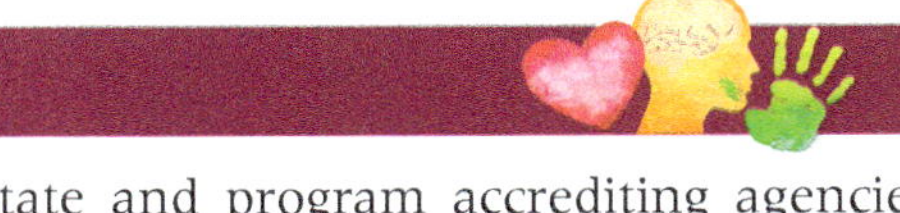

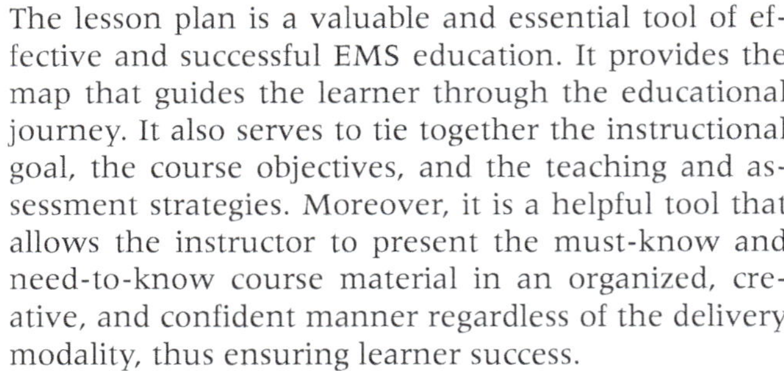

The lesson plan is a valuable and essential tool of effective and successful EMS education. It provides the map that guides the learner through the educational journey. It also serves to tie together the instructional goal, the course objectives, and the teaching and assessment strategies. Moreover, it is a helpful tool that allows the instructor to present the must-know and need-to-know course material in an organized, creative, and confident manner regardless of the delivery modality, thus ensuring learner success.

Lesson planning is essential for many modes of lesson delivery, including face-to-face, online, and laboratory or simulation.

Many state and program accrediting agencies require lesson plans. Before creating a lesson plan, it is important for the educator to conduct a needs assessment to determine the appropriate reading level and related student needs. Every lesson plan should contain certain standard components such as objectives, declarative content, activities, and formative assessments. This can help to ensure that all elements are aligned.

Finally, educators should continually evaluate lesson plans to ensure they remain relevant and effective.

Glossary

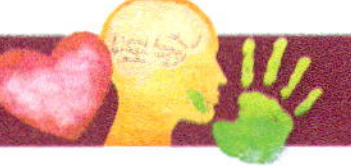

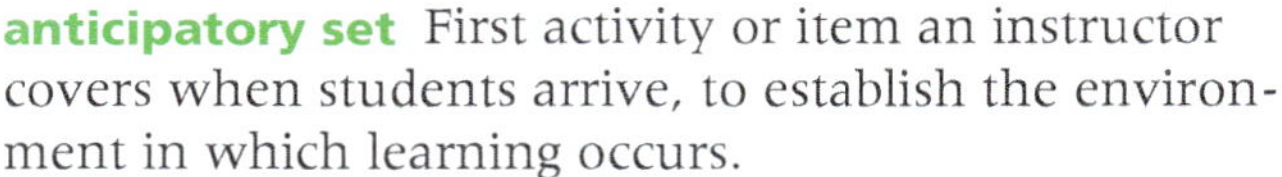

anticipatory set First activity or item an instructor covers when students arrive, to establish the environment in which learning occurs.

audience response systems Systems whereby the instructor receives feedback from the audience or class to specific, posed questions through an electronic device that tallies the responses.

classroom feedback systems Systems whereby the instructor receives feedback from the audience or class to specific, posed questions through an electronic device that tallies the responses.

declarative material Depth and breadth of the content of a lesson; the component of a lesson plan in which objectives and content are arranged and grouped in the order in which they will be taught.

learning management system (LMS) Software package designed to facilitate the delivery and administration of online education.

mastery Achieving goals and objectives established for a specific knowledge area.

Reference

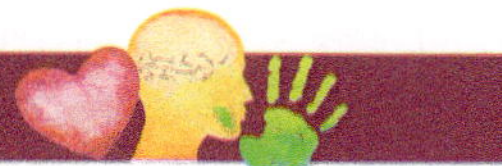

[1] Hodell, Chuck. 2010. *The Basics of ISD Revisited*. Alexandria, VA: ASTD Press.

Additional Resources

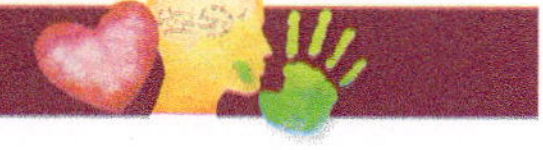

Fautley, Martin, and Jonathan Savage. 2013. *Lesson Planning for Effective Learning*. Maidenhead, UK: McGraw-Hill Education.

Gagné, Robert M. 1974. *Essentials of Learning for Instruction*. Hinsdale, IL: The Dryden Press.

Gagné, Robert M., and Leslie J. Briggs. 1979. *Principles of Instructional Design*, 2nd ed. New York: Holt, Rinehart and Winston.

Gardner, Howard. 2006. *Multiple Intelligences: New Horizons*. New York: Basic Books.

Mager, Robert F. 1975. *Preparing Instructional Objectives*, 2nd ed. Belmont, CA: Fearon Publishers.

Mager, Robert F., and Kenneth M. Beach, Jr. 1967. *Developing Vocational Instruction*. Belmont, CA: Fearon-Pitman Publishers.

Mayer, Richard E. 2011. *Applying the Science of Learning*. Boston: Pearson.

Moore-Cox, Annie. 2017. "Lesson Plans: Road Maps for the Active Learning Classroom." *Journal of Nursing Education* 56, no. 11: 697–700. https://doi.org/10.3928/01484834-20171020-12.

Tyler, Ralph W. 1949. *Basic Principles of Curriculum and Instruction*. Chicago: University of Chicago Press.

Delivering the Message

Most novice and experienced educators would agree that the learning process is a dynamic journey for both the educator and the student. The strategies used to stimulate curiosity and motivate students to learn are as diverse as the student population. A variety of media, as well as independent and group collaborative activities can be implemented to enhance the student-centered learning environment. Whether concepts, skills, or behaviors are the focus of the learning, educators serve as coaches with a single student assessing pulses on a simulation lab manikin, teach proper packaging of a patient with possible spinal injury in the context of a small group, empower students to explore cardiac physiology in a distance learning setting, and model compassionate care for a sick patient experiencing a condition related to substance misuse. Emergency medical services (EMS) educators must tailor their instruction in order to obtain positive outcomes, attain objectives, and ensure lifelong learning for the student.

Sometimes, the most *efficient* method is the least *effective* method of teaching. The evidence-based strategies and techniques described in these chapters will provide the educator with tools that will be useful in everyday practice, whether the instructor's primary role is continuing education, or emergency medical technician (EMT) or paramedic training. The concepts described here are intended to maximize learning and retention. This part of the text introduces teaching strategies for individual students, small and large groups, distance learning, low and high technology simulations, and students in the field experience and clinical settings.

CHAPTER 11

Introduction to Teaching Strategies

OBJECTIVES

At the conclusion of this chapter, the educator will be able to:

Cognitive Domain

1. Explain the difference between teacher-centered and student-centered learning strategies.
2. Describe the role of the educator in a student-centered classroom environment.
3. Describe the role of the student in a student-centered classroom environment.
4. Explain strategies that promote collaboration and teamwork in a student-centered classroom.
5. Describe student-centered classroom strategies that empower and motivate students for self-discovery and lifelong learning.
6. Describe the importance of developing goals and objectives when creating student-centered learning activities.
7. Identify challenges for the educator when implementing student-centered learning strategies in the classroom.
8. Explain effective strategies for the facilitation of small group activities.
9. Compare and contrast various methods to resolve conflict in small group work settings.
10. Identify the levels of conflict resolution that assist with de-escalation of conflict in a group.
11. Describe an example of using the Socratic method of questioning that promotes higher-level thinking.
12. Compare and contrast questioning techniques that build student confidence and foster critical-thinking skills.
13. Describe the five core elements of facilitation that support successful experiential learning.

Psychomotor Domain

There are no psychomotor objectives for this chapter.

Affective Domain

1. Defend the benefits of experiential learning strategies in the classroom.
2. Value alternative methods of presenting information in the classroom environment by implementing student-centered learning strategies in the educator's program.

"Treat people as if they are what they ought to be and you help them become what they are capable of being."

~ Johann Wolfgang von Goethe

CHAPTER GOAL This chapter discusses the evolving teaching strategy of student-centered learning as well as facilitation and questioning techniques to enhance learning.

Teaching strategies vary depending on the setting, the students, and most commonly, the educator. Educators frequently teach the way they were taught, because that is often what they are the most comfortable with. However, that strategy may not be the most effective way for students to learn and to make meaningful changes in knowledge and behavior. Faculty must consciously make instructional method decisions to promote student growth in all domains of learning—cognitive, psychomotor, and affective. There are many techniques that will allow the instructor to become more effective in facilitating learning.

Traditional Education

Traditional education uses as its centerpiece the lecture format, perhaps because it is an efficient way to deliver a large amount of material to any size audience. Because the traditional approach to the classroom of "I teach, you listen" is likely the way many current educators were taught, it is no surprise that it is often the most common technique used by emergency medical services (EMS) educators.

Teacher-Centered Learning

Teacher-centered learning is focused around the teacher and lecture. Although the lecture format itself is not problematic, major reliance on this type of teaching tool can lead to problems because of its teacher-centered approach.

One problem created by the "mostly lecture" approach is that the lecture and the textbook become the major delivery system of information for students. Students are expected to listen, read, and be prepared to take and pass tests. Their success is determined by how well they can memorize the information that is presented. This type of instruction places a high value on memorization, which is usually a low-level learning task. Recall of straight facts is usually at the knowledge level of the cognitive domain, most likely to be forgotten, and least likely capable of being applied to other circumstances in which the student may need to use the information, referred to as transfer of knowledge.

Another problem with "mostly lecture" is that students are less engaged in the educational process and learning is passive. When students need only to sit and listen, and perhaps take notes, they are not fully engaged in the learning process. Again, they are more likely to forget the information and least likely to be able to apply the information when needed, such as in an atypical patient-presentation situation. They may also fail to learn critical-thinking skills.

In classrooms where lecture is the primary delivery model, it becomes difficult to assess the affective component of education. A teacher-centered environment does not provide time or opportunity for the instructor to facilitate development of the whole person. The focus is too often on ensuring that students have the information needed to pass their exams, rather than developing the character and critical-thinking skills needed to apply the information to real-life challenges.

In a classroom focused only on lecture, the lesson plan is typically prepared in advance and facilitated by use of PowerPoint, Prezi, or Keynote. Because these presentations are predetermined, students are not provided the opportunity to be stakeholders in the direction and scope of their education. Instructors act as if they know best, and they dictate the pace and focus of students' education. Instructors who subscribe to this philosophy often believe that students who fall behind must not have the aptitude needed to master the information. However, it is possible that they are bored or have never been engaged in the material by a teacher who has valued the students' life experiences as they may relate to the material at hand.

Trends in Teaching Methods

As the body of evidence grows regarding memory, cognition, and how the brain receives, processes, stores, and retrieves information, all educators from kindergarten teachers to college professors must reevaluate the traditional, teacher-centered approach to education.

Student-Centered Learning

Educators should consider the value of alternate methods of presenting information that put the learner at the center of the educational event. The evidence is becoming increasingly clear—in order to reach higher-level learning goals such as synthesis and evaluation, or what many would call "application, problem solving, and critical thinking," the learner must *do* something with the information. The students must experience the material, relate it to their own life experiences, make judgments about it, and create meaning regarding how the information will be used. It is highly unlikely that those educational events are going to occur during a lecture, because most of what is told to students will be forgotten.

A **student-centered learning** approach uses innovative teaching strategies that create an active and exciting learning environment. This does not mean that traditional approaches such as lecture are abandoned; rather, they are used less frequently to afford time for discussion, group work, case studies, role-play, scenarios, writing assignments, games, and other activities that are known to promote collaboration, communication, and problem solving. A student-centered approach creates a shared experience wherein the student becomes a stakeholder in the educational process and introduces a sense of community to the learning process.

The **flipped classroom** is an example of a student-centered approach in which lectures and activities are posted ahead of time for students to watch and complete before coming to class. This allows students to view lectures and complete some of the assignments on their own time when it is convenient, such as when their children are put to bed in the evening, during their morning commute, or while exercising. Prerecorded lectures and preclass activities also allow learners to review the lecture and speed up or slow down as needed based on their individual needs. The concept of allowing students to engage with the material in different ways and at their own pace is considered *differentiated instruction*. It is an important strategy in K–12 education, and while not often addressed in EMS education, it may facilitate more student success.[1]

One characteristic of the student-centered approach is that the learning process is fluid and should be engaging for both the educator and students. The goal is discovery of information and a shared commitment to excellence. Subjects are explored from a variety of sources inside and outside the classroom.

Students present materials to the class and have some control over the pace of instruction and the amount of material that is shared. If students have a problem understanding a module, more time can be committed to ensure mastery of a particular area. This process minimizes the artificial time constraints that are typically imposed on the learning process.

In the student-centered approach to learning, the experiences of students are respected, and the educator becomes more of a facilitator than the focal point of instruction. Students are viewed as essential to the learning process because they have a wide array of life experiences that they bring to the classroom. The students' own experiences are woven into the instruction so that clarity can be achieved from various points of view. Students are encouraged to relate their life experiences to the material that is presented; this is an example of **anchoring**, or relating new information to ideas with which one is already familiar in regular life. For example, if an educator had a fire fighter in an emergency medical technician (EMT) refresher class, the instructor might relate the concept of septic shock to the student and the class by asking, "What would happen if, after you have primed the line to the fire, I poked holes in the hose with an ice pick?" The student would likely answer that the line will lose pressure. The educator would then ask how the situation could be rectified so that the fire fighters on the nozzle still got enough water pressure. The student would likely answer, "I would have to try to compensate by increasing the pressure." And so, the educator would relate the concept of distributive shock as a loss of vascular tone and pressure from fluid leaking out of the vascular space, causing hypotension and shock. While this could have been a difficult concept to grasp, by using an example that the student and likely many others in the group were familiar with from life experiences, the educator engaged the students. The educator increased the likelihood that the students will be able not only to recall, but to apply the concept, and even begin to problem-solve regarding how the body might compensate during times of distributive shock.

In a student-centered classroom, students are given responsibilities in the classroom, lab, and clinical setting to foster a sense of community, respect, and discipline (**FIGURE 11.1**). The EMS profession requires that students be ready to accept leadership responsibilities. The seeds of leadership can be planted in the classroom by assignment of roles that allow students to practice and improve their leadership skills. The classroom experience can be enhanced by appointment of a class representative or officers, a roll taker, equipment officers, note takers, lab assistants, and team leaders on community service projects. Another

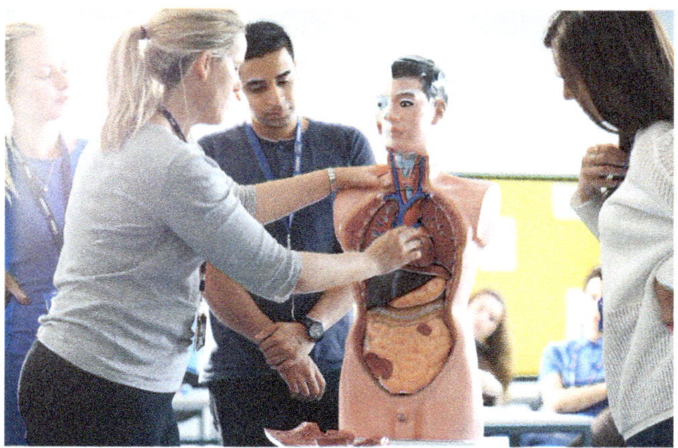

FIGURE 11.1 Student-centered classes bring a sense of personal responsibility to the classroom.

effective technique is to pair advanced students with instructional staff in the lab to help train and educate students who need more help. This cooperative educational technique is a powerful and productive tool for any EMS institution. Although the intended goal is to build leadership skills, the instructor will also note that many positive and powerful attributes in terms of respect, discipline, and a sense of community are realized. In the final analysis, students become a part of the learning process and are better prepared to enter the profession.

In traditional classrooms, a concerted effort is made to develop the whole student through equal emphasis placed on values and character as they relate to academic study. Too many educators believe that the value of an education for students is measured in their success in tackling the cognitive and psychomotor domains. Very little value has been placed on the affective domain, and yet issues around the students' affect, or behavior and attitudes, are the leading cause of complaints, not only from educators and preceptors, but also from employers. While it is true that there is no room for incompetence, the affective domain may be more critical to the quality of patient care and what a student will contribute to the profession than all the knowledge and skills the instructors push students to master. Integrating learning experiences, such as scenarios and simulation throughout the program, provides opportunity for students to demonstrate critical thinking skills and the teamwork required in the profession. Helping students understand their strengths and limitations in relation to their values and character and how that drives their behavior can mean more to a student or an employer than has been previously understood. Values and feelings can impact clinical decision making and judgment about and behavior toward patients more than we realize.[2]

CASE in Point

Classroom Topic: Drug Abuse

Instructor-Centered Method

The instructor tells students to read the substance use disorder chapter in the assigned textbook, and then provides a lecture to support what is in the textbook. Follow-up consists of a written test on the subject.

Student-Centered Method

The instructor gives a scenario and asks the students to decide whether they believe the scenario does or does not represent substance use disorder. Perhaps the scenario is "your babysitter and her boyfriend are caught smoking marijuana in the backyard while the baby takes a nap." If students believe that this is an example of substance misuse, they must physically move to one side of the classroom. If they do not think this is substance misuse, they move to the other side, creating two opposing groups of students. Volunteers are then asked to share their rationale for their opinion. Because the educator is asking the students' opinion, there is no right or wrong answer, and it becomes a safe place to make a decision. However, the physical act of moving to one side of the room forces the student to decide and prohibits indecision, because decision-making capability is an important skill in emergency medicine. Next, the educator gives one or two more examples and asks the students to move to one side of the room or the other, depending on their opinion. Another scenario might be a high school wrestler who uses speed to meet a weight requirement, or a police officer who goes to the local tavern after every shift to have a few beers and wind down.

The instructor then asks students to take out a blank piece of paper and write down in their own words the definition of "substance misuse," as they understand it. Once the students have had 3 or 4 minutes to formulate a response, they are paired with another student in the class to compare answers. Each pair must arrive at an entirely new definition based on input from both students. Once each pair of students has developed a revised definition, the educator requests that each team pair up with another team and repeat the process. The pairing process is repeated until three or four large groups have been formed, each with its own definition arrived at through teamwork and collaboration. At the conclusion of the exercise, each team writes their definition on the board. The educator asks the class to compare and contrast the various definitions until final agreement is reached regarding which definition is most correct given the textbook information and other available resources. A short discussion can then ensue about how their own personal experiences with drugs and alcohol shaped their initial decisions about each scenario, and whether or not it was technically "substance misuse." This exercise allows students to explore their own biases based on positive and negative experiences with drugs and alcohol.

One of the goals of EMS education must be to create lifelong learners and prepare them for a career of self-discovery in a constantly changing and dynamic profession. Because medicine is a science, what providers do for patients and how they practice medicine will constantly change throughout their careers. Students should not view the end of the class as the end of their education. Regular assignments that require students to read about their profession and present topics of interest to their classmates can be crucial to establishing the practice of continuing education and discovery in a complex and changing profession.

The *Case in Point* that follows puts students at the center of the learning process and places the instructor in the role of facilitator. Students remain active throughout the process by formulating responses, defending their position, practicing compromise, and looking at the subject critically. This student-centered, active, multidimensional approach is the very "glue" that will help reinforce the subject matter and make it stick.

Techniques to Enhance Student-Centered Learning

Several techniques and concepts are commonly used to enhance student-centered learning, whether this is done in individual student sessions, small groups, or large groups. These include facilitation techniques, group work, questioning techniques, and **experiential learning**.

Facilitation Techniques

Student-centered instruction places the student at the center of the learning process, and the instructor assumes the role of facilitator. **Facilitation** is an important teaching strategy, and a better understanding of how it is accomplished is important for the educator.

Creation of a relaxed atmosphere that is focused more on the learner constitutes the core of facilitation. In fact, facilitate means "to make easier." Educators can do this by **scaffolding** information for students—this means building upon prior knowledge, relating new ideas to concepts students already know, and helping students make meaningful connections throughout the lesson. (This is discussed further in Chapter 8, *Domains of Learning*.) This strategy allows the educator to create an environment in which student learning is enhanced by interaction and engagement. Coaching, mentoring, feedback, and positive reinforcement represent a variety of techniques that are considered facilitative strategies for learning.

Keys to Facilitation

Facilitation has also been called "the guide on the side" by Allison King, Jon Van Ast, and other adult educational researchers. One of the key elements of facilitation is for the educator to create action in the classroom in which students experience or do something with the information. This is done, in part, by avoiding lectures when possible and engaging learners in activities, such as writing, role-playing, and cooperative group work. Whenever facilitators can design an environment that provokes an emotion, whether the emotion is pride, confidence, happiness, or even stress, this creates additional neural connections throughout the hippocampus via the amygdala, instead of just within the cerebral cortex. This means more opportunities to recall and apply the information when it is needed, during stressful emergency calls.[3]

First, the instructor should consider the layout of the classroom. (See Chapter 7, *The Learning Environment*, for more details.) The arrangement of the classroom sends a signal to students about the class session. The use of groups in facilitation may be made most beneficial when the educator sets up tables and semiprivate work areas, so that greater interaction can take place between students and instructors. The goal of this strategy is to take the emphasis off the educator as the "gatekeeper of information" and to place the burden of interaction with the group. This creates interaction between learners but still allows interaction with the educator, who will manage the learning activities.

The importance of creating the expectation in learners that they are required to participate actively in the learning process cannot be overstated. Students have been conditioned to behave as "tourists" or visitors in the classroom; that is, they have been conditioned to be passive observers, much like people who are on vacation. Tourists follow the tour guide, taking pictures and having minimal interaction with anyone else, then they move on to the next destination. Educators must work to limit tourist behavior in the classroom by actively seeking student participation in the learning process, which may be unfamiliar to many.

In addition, faculty may need to consider the type of class schedule necessary to commit to a student-centered learning environment. For example, an academy-style, 8- to 10-hour class day will not leave much time at home to build a model of the spinal cord and column to share in class, while this task could be easily accomplished by students who meet for 3 hours twice weekly. The full-time class may need to complete the model building in class, using materials provided by the program. The critical elements of the exercise, rather than whether it is done in class or outside of class, are choice of materials to reflect the structures of the spinal cord, engineering and composition to reflect function, and the ability to describe the features of what they have created. Patience, guidance, flexibility, creativity, and positive reinforcement of learners are necessary as they move into this new area. As students succeed, their expectations for learning will change in positive ways.

Promoting active participation of class members is a way educators can increase the success of facilitation in the classroom. One method of increasing participation is to have students assist in some of the day-to-day activities of the course. This may involve something as simple as having them set up the room or bring in equipment. In academic settings, class leaders are often appointed to assist the instructor in maintaining control when breaks begin and end. When not actively involved in a scenario or role-playing exercise, students can act as recorders, time keepers, and note takers. Peer observation allows all learners to gain constructive feedback in a setting where students are actively engaged. Stronger students can serve as mentors or coaches when they study in groups or when they assist others in learning and perfecting skills.

Educators may assign roles, such as leader, scribe, and reporter, to various members in the class. Strategies used to assign roles to learners must be creative so they are as equitable as possible for students. Techniques include alphabetical order, birth date, hiring date (oldest or youngest), color lottery, random numbers, and a sticker on a name tag or chair. Whichever manner is chosen, duties should be rotated equally among the student body so that favoritism and bias are avoided.

Not everyone will agree with or like this new style of learning. Some students will continue to be passive learners despite the instructor's best efforts. The instructor must not be discouraged; it takes effort and persistence to move into the use of facilitation. As the instructor works to include the reluctant learner in the process, eventually the student may choose to willingly participate or may be coerced by fellow classmates to actively participate in the learning process. The student-centered learning approach takes more effort on the part of the student. Educators may find students who simply do not want to exert the effort required to prepare for and participate in class. Grades for affective behavior and participation, as well as clear expectations in the class syllabus, make it clear that such behavior will not be acceptable in the EMS course and will be reflected in grading. It should not be possible to pass the class as a voyeur.

Occasionally other, more traditional faculty will be critical of the facilitation process—facilitated classrooms are livelier, and sometimes louder, appearing as if the instructor has less control of the classroom. EMS educators moving toward facilitation and active learning may find themselves in a position to have to present evidence to colleagues about how retention is more dependent on depth of processing than how many times material is reviewed[4] or other brain-based learning principles in order to defend their more modern, more effective approach to teaching and learning.

Facilitating Discussions

Facilitation requires active learner participation; one of the easiest forms of participatory learning is discussion. This technique is effective for many different types of courses, including continuing education or refresher classes, in which concepts are reviewed and topics involving opinions, experience, and judgment are discussed. Facilitation can also be used to motivate a class start-up or a review. In order to keep all learners actively engaged in the discussion, the instructor could have small groups discuss the same idea. This is effective because all students are actively working toward the solution simultaneously without the anxiety of having to share their response with the large class. It is harder to opt-out of a small group discussion, but if some students become distracted or disengaged, they should be redirected back to the group for participation. It may also be helpful to give each group an opportunity to evaluate each other on their contributions to the group after these exercises, reinforcing the concept of accountability for participation in the group. Rubric-type evaluations can be used at the end to determine the success of the group as a whole and/or individual participation. This may help identify a group problem such as one person dominating the discussion or refusing to share. "Social loafing" can be avoided by encouraging group work but issuing individual grades for each person's contribution.

The educator can keep everyone engaged in the discussion by moving the responses from group to group in an unpredictable pattern. A prop or some other strategy, such as drawing the name of the group out of a hat, will suffice. Facilitating takes more time to accomplish than does simply lecturing to the group. Keep in mind that it is not necessary to comment on each person's contribution; it is more important that students contribute. To check for understanding of the instructor and of the learners, one might paraphrase the responses so that key points can be easily made for the entire group.

The educator should compliment the student on a good comment and redirect an inaccurate or incorrect statement to the group, so students understand, stay on track, and avoid becoming confused. Sometimes many answers are heard but it can be difficult for students to determine which was the "right" answer. If a

TEACHING TIP

One way in which the educator can ensure that students remain focused is to establish a time when the group will come together and report back on its work or progress. With these mini-deadlines in place, students know that they are responsible for giving a progress report and will more readily stay on task. For example, if a set of 10 small cases is provided for students to work through, the educator should not request completion of all 10 at one sitting. Instead, the class should be divided into groups, with three or four cases assigned to each group. Students work on three cases, then the entire class comes together to discuss those cases. The small groups re-form to work on the next three cases. This keeps the class working together, and if one group is not working as it should, the groups can be reconfigured before they reconvene. This can be made to appear as the educator's initial strategy so no one has hurt feelings. This approach also allows the educator to group students who ordinarily would not work together.

right answer is shared according to the objectives or what might be tested, be sure to reinforce it so that every student is clear about that answer.

Similar to diplomats, educators are often required to mediate differences of opinion in the classroom. To perform this delicate balancing act, one must try to keep the discussion going without interjecting oneself as the authority—a move that could damage momentum. Students should be encouraged to back up their statements with facts and evidence, and everyone must be reminded that differing opinions are important to an active and engaged learning community.

Close the session by summarizing what occurred in the discussion and by providing follow-up information for additional studying or reading, so that the group knows where they have been and where they are going in the future.

Facilitation is challenging for educators, and it can be frustrating for students at first. When students encounter difficulty with an assignment, they may be more willing to give up and quit working rather than asking for assistance. The educator must be careful not to do students' work for them. Rather, the educator should be ready to offer assistance to help students locate the necessary resources and should keep learners actively involved in the lesson. In short, a key element of facilitation is to help students become more resourceful and capable of problem solving, with less reliance on an instructor.

TEACHING TIP

One way by which the educator can maintain learner involvement is to invoke the "three before me" technique before intervening. This technique requires that when asking for help, learners must inform the instructor of at least three places where they have looked to find the information. They should be directed to the appropriate resources if they have not located enough information on their own. However tempting, it is not in the learners' best interest for the educator to simply tell them the correct answers, even though this may appear easier.

The goal of the educator is to assist students in becoming critically thinking professionals as they move from lower levels of learning to higher levels of learning. This is nearly impossible to accomplish if learners are not active participants in the learning process. Rarely do they argue with the results of their own learning when they discover the answers themselves. If a topic is learned by this method, students "own it."

Group Work or Collaborative Learning

In real life, EMS problems are often solved by a team approach to a situation. Not every student is comfortable working with others, but teamwork is an important goal of EMS education and included in the evaluation process. Instructors need to create opportunities for students to learn to work effectively in teams. Their teamwork should be evaluated using team leader and team member assessment tools. Some educators identify disadvantages of this method of learning, noting that students typically progress at varying rates and that quiet students may not feel comfortable in a team setting. Additionally, teams may inadvertently increase competition among students, and some students may succumb to conformity just to fit in. Nevertheless, groups frequently devise solutions that are better than the most advanced student could have worked out on their own, and they learn better from each other than from the teacher.[5]

Because time is precious, classroom groups should be identified in a quick and efficient manner. Some situations dictate that groups should stay the same; others do not. EMS personnel will not always work with the same partner or engine company, and variation among members of groups, as well as among skill levels, can enhance the overall performance of individual members and of the team.

Use of randomization techniques such as counting off, drawing numbers, or some other method such as birthday month or zip codes allows learners to maintain some control in the sorting process. If the educator controls selection, it can be done ahead of time based on the instructor's knowledge of the group, keeping in mind student strengths and limitations.

Effective Group Management

For groups to work effectively, written ground rules must be established at the first meeting. Certain mandates should be assigned by the facilitator, including attending class sessions on time; completing all assignments before class and being prepared to discuss them; notifying other group members in advance if class will be missed; willingly sharing information; respecting the values, views, and ideas of others; and abiding by all other rules as agreed on by the group.

One of the most effective strategies for managing a group of learners in a team is to add one additional member whose sole job is to function as a peer facilitator to guide the group and help resolve conflicts. An upperclassman is often an effective facilitator. Members of each group must actively rotate roles within the group so that all students can gain experience in all areas of the activity (**FIGURE 11.2**). The peer leader works to keep the group on track and monitors participation of group members. The recorder, or scribe, records assignments, strategies, unresolved issues, and data, and may convene the group outside of class when necessary. The reporter is responsible for reporting the group's findings to the entire class during discussions and writes a final draft of all assignments. The accuracy coach or timekeeper checks for understanding of the group, locates resources, and manages time.

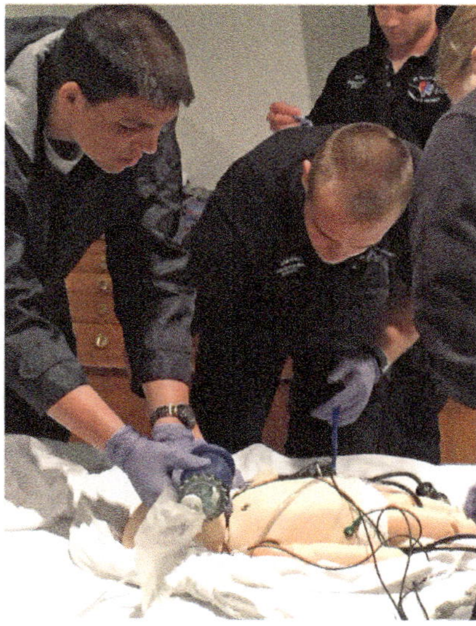

FIGURE 11.2 Creative educators can make meaningful learning easier for students by requiring their active participation.

Courtesy of St. Charles County Ambulance District.

In the beginning of the course, time spent in facilitated learning can be short. Later, it can build to longer segments as students demonstrate their ability to perform appropriately and stay on-task. As a word of caution, do not leave all of the scenario-based, critical-thinking activities for the end of the program, after students have memorized all of the discrete skills. Critical-thinking activities are often most important to conduct throughout the program in the facilitated, supervised environment. The class must be brought together for discussion and clarification of issues at frequent intervals throughout the session. Educators may need to specifically identify which objectives were covered through the group activity or discussion to keep students from feeling like the activity was "a waste of time." In addition, the instructor should plan for individual and group assignments. The opportunity for group members to take the assignment lightly can damage the effectiveness of this strategy. The educator must remain vigilant for behavior that might diminish the group's strength and undermine it. Peer facilitators can be used to assist both the learners and the instructor in maintaining the integrity of this strategy.

Conflict Resolution in Group Work

Not everyone in a family always gets along with one another, and members of the learning community are no different from a family in this regard. In fact, they may actually spend more time with one another than some family members do. Tempers often flare when people spend a great deal of time together in close proximity. The educator can reduce the likelihood that conflicts will escalate at several levels (**FIGURE 11.3**).

The first level focuses on preventing escalation of a conflict. The instructor should monitor the group for early signs of conflict such as raised voices or defensive body language and should intervene immediately to prevent additional problems. Group evaluations can assist the instructor in monitoring individual student behavior that may need correction.

The second level of conflict resolution centers on student empowerment. The educator must listen to students' concerns and encourage them to peacefully resolve any conflicts they may be experiencing. Educators can coach students on strategies for possible resolution of conflicts. If a peer leader is involved, this person should not be undermined in front of the other students or the peer leader will lose authority. The instructor should speak with the peer leader before the leader addresses the other group members to ensure a game plan is in place for resolving the issue.

The next level of conflict requires active resolution of problems that may arise. Each participant must be allowed to present their point while the others actively

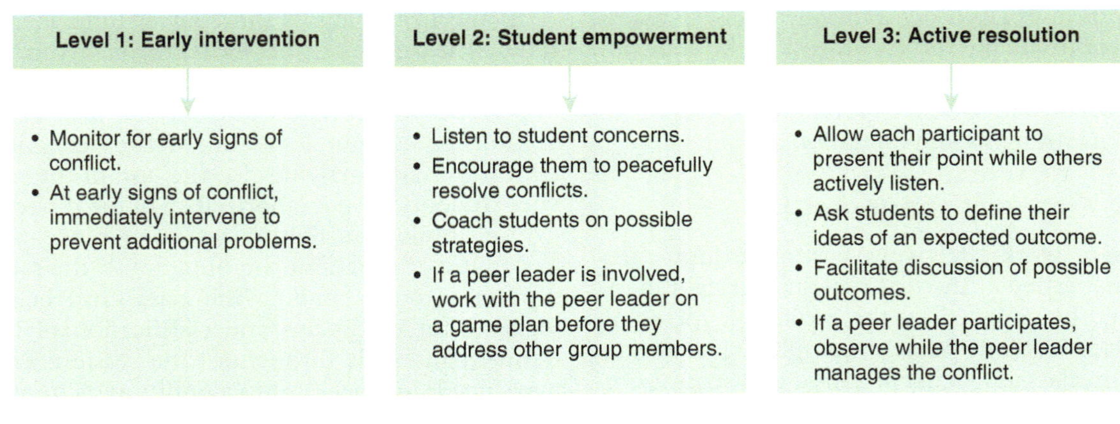

FIGURE 11.3 Levels of conflict resolution.

listen. Students should be asked to define their ideas of an expected outcome, although no guarantees exist that these will be honored. The educator's role is to facilitate the discussion of possible outcomes that may affect those involved in the conflict. If a peer leader participates, the educator may serve as an observer while the peer leader manages the conflict.

Questioning Techniques

Another way by which the educator can move toward a more student-centered classroom is through questioning. Questioning is an inquiry that invites a response. Thought-provoking questions used in the classroom promote active thinking and stimulate higher-level learning and problem-solving skills. This technique increases interaction between the teacher and students and assists with application in the patient care environment.

Socratic Method

The **Socratic method** of questioning is a popular method with law and philosophy professors, but has a place in the EMS classroom, too. The Socratic method of questioning uses the practice of asking, rather than telling, to arouse curiosity in the subject matter so students arrive at their own conclusions rather than being told the "right" answer. The process uses logical, incremental questions designed to challenge assumptions and move students toward greater specificity in their answers as they apply principles on their own. The following is a description of the process: The educator calls on a student who has presumably read the material for this class session. This method has been criticized because it could be embarrassing if a student is not prepared. However, students are allowed an "occasional pass" if they truly do not feel prepared. The instructor asks for the student's *opinion*, which negates the concept that an answer is wholly right or wrong, further making the Socratic method safe to use in the classroom. Next, the student paraphrases the concepts from the reading and the instructor asks if the student agrees or disagrees with the idea. The student is asked to defend the position, backing it up with facts and logic. The educator's role is to continue asking questions, or, some would say "play devil's advocate," until the student is able to conclude confidently that they were justified in the answer based on the facts and logic explored in the questioning.

Building Confidence in Decision Making

Because EMS professionals function in high-stress, time-pressured environments, decision-making ability is imperative to their success. Yet, frequently educators hear from preceptors and field training officers that interns and new employees "just won't make a decision" on scene. New practitioners seem paralyzed by the choices they face and consequences of their decisions. Educators can assist students in learning to trust their decisions by reinforcing the correct choices they make in the classroom. Confidence breeds competence, and competence, or making the correct choices, breeds confidence. Essentially, instructors should make an effort to "catch" students doing things right and reinforce their right decisions with praise and positive feedback. However, just saying "good answer" is not enough. The instructor has to help students see how they arrived at the right answer and that their decision making is solid.

Wait Time

Wait time is an important concept in questioning techniques. It is important that students be given time to think about questions posed to them and to ponder their responses. In practice, however, it is not unusual for an educator to wait only 1 or 2 seconds for students to respond, and when nobody does, the educator gives the answer. When the educator simply gives the answer, students come to see the questions as rhetorical—where the educator was not really expecting a response. In these classrooms, students never bother to think about the question or attempt to formulate a response. Waiting a reasonable amount of time, which has been suggested might be anywhere from 8 to 30 seconds, before calling on a student can increase the number of students who respond and the length of their responses. Before asking a question, the instructor can insist that no one raise their hand to answer. This discourages the situation in which the predictable students raise their hands and others immediately quit seeking the answer. By waiting, students are more likely to consider the question. After waiting, the educator calls on a random student or a volunteer and asks the student to answer (**FIGURE 11.4**). This method allows more students to be involved in the process.[6] The technique is known as **ask, pause, and call**.

CASE in Point

The instructor presents the case of a 54-year-old man with a history of chronic obstructive pulmonary disease (COPD) who is short of breath, speaking in three-word bursts, sitting in tripod position, with circumoral and nailbed cyanosis. The instructor asks the class, "What should we do for him?" A student answers, "Put him on oxygen." The instructor replies, "Yes, that's correct! Why should we put him on oxygen?" Note the strong reinforcement of the correct answer here. If the instructor fails to reinforce that the student has given the right answer, the student is likely to change the answer, seeing it as a challenge to their thinking. Instructors and employers do not want EMTs or paramedics to waffle in their on-scene decision making. Reinforcement that students have the correct answer is essential to building confidence. The student now may answer something low-level, such as "Because he needs oxygen." Encourage the student to elaborate with more questions, such as "How can you tell he needs oxygen?" The student then replies, "Because he looks hypoxic." Instructor says, "Which signs or symptoms demonstrated hypoxia?" And so the exchange goes, reinforcing the right answer and building the student's confidence in their knowledge. Plus, this type of exchange increases the likelihood that the student will answer again in the future.

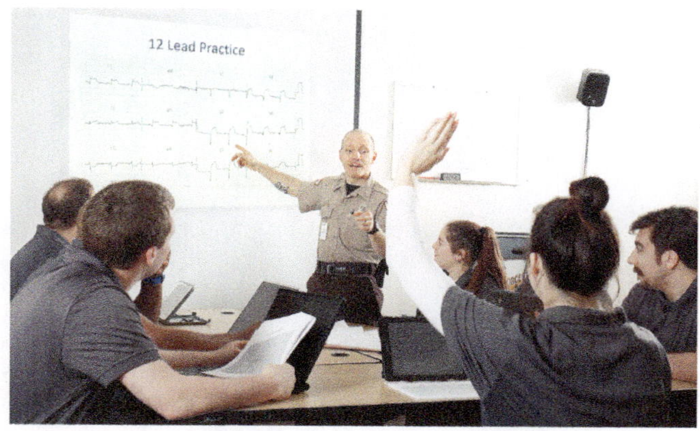

FIGURE 11.4 Effective questioning techniques include the use of thought-provoking questions and the ask, pause, and call technique.

Other Questioning Techniques

Other questioning techniques can be used to engage students. One is the "overhead question," which is given to the whole group and sometimes embedded into the presentation, without calling on someone in particular. After most have written down an answer on paper or a personal dry-erase board (**FIGURE 11.5**), the educator "calls for" an answer. The educator can either ask all students to raise their boards at the same time to see how many had the correct answer, or ask for a volunteer to elaborate on the correct answer. The "relay question" involves calling on different students to add or comment on the previous student's responses until all important information has been obtained. Another technique is the "reverse question," wherein the instructor answers a student's question with another question or asks the class to respond.

Experiential Learning

Another concept important to EMS classroom and clinical educators is the use of experiential learning. Carl Rogers was a pioneering psychotherapist who wrote extensively on the concept of experiential learning.[7] He felt so strongly about the role that experience plays in how individuals learn that he distinguished learning into two distinct types: cognitive (which Rogers described as "meaningless") and experiential (which he deemed as "significant"). He wrote that "all human beings have a natural propensity to learn; the role of the teacher is to facilitate such learning." According to Rogers, learning is facilitated when (1) the student participates completely in the learning process and has control over its nature and direction; (2) it is primarily based on direct confrontation with practical, social, personal, or research problems; and (3) self-evaluation is the principal method of assessing progress or success.

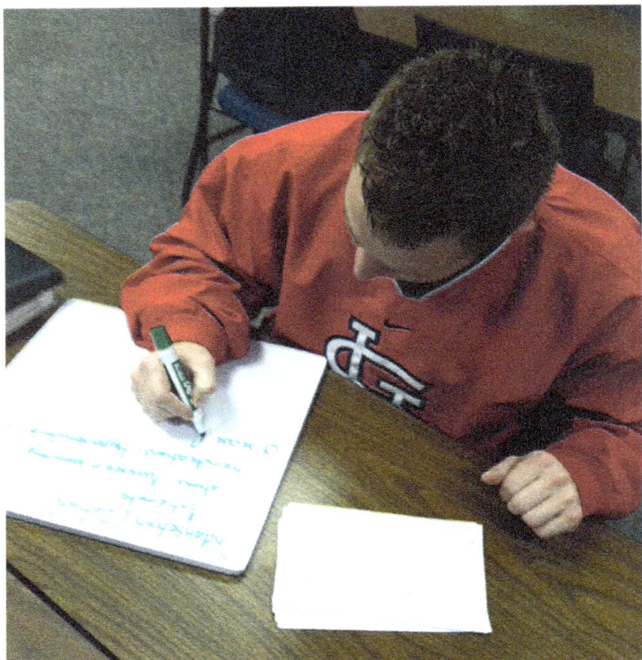

FIGURE 11.5 Having students write their answer on a whiteboard and then share their answers with peers engages students in active learning.

Courtesy of St. Charles County Ambulance District.

Rogers also emphasizes the importance of learning how to learn and being open to change. As medicine relies heavily on continuing education and learning throughout one's career, teaching students how to learn and inspiring curiosity and inquisitiveness ought to be a primary consideration for any health professions educator.

Rogers identified the following five core elements of facilitation that are necessary for successful experiential learning:

1. Setting a positive climate for learning where students understand this to be a safe place to make mistakes. This means not allowing hazing, harassment, or teasing when mistakes are made, and giving regular, timely, honest feedback, including positive feedback for correct decisions and tasks well done.
2. Clarifying the purposes of the learners. These may include why they are taking the class, what they hope to gain, and how they will use this information in their jobs or lives.
3. Organizing and making learning resources available, while teaching students to be resourceful. This might be access to lab equipment, helpful websites to practice ECG interpretation, or referral to a mentor in the field who can help them to navigate the social norms of the profession.
4. Balancing intellectual and emotional components of learning. This can include learning to trust their instincts, to handle the stress of a dangerous emergency situation, or the grief related to a patient who died in their care.
5. Sharing feelings and thoughts with learners but not dominating. This is similar to the concepts of facilitation used in discussion and other classroom activities already explored in this chapter.

In addition to Rogers, the Oregon Technology in Education Council (2007)[8] supports Lave and Wenger (1990)[9] and others such as Clancey (1995)[10] in the proposition that programs that consistently provide situational learning experiences—in which students are active participants in solving problems involving real patient complaints—contribute to progressive learning and achievement of objectives in all domains of learning. Collaboration and engagement in critical thinking to solve a relevant problem enhance student ability to problem-solve in real patient situations.[11] Educators developing these experiential activities need to consider the student's previous and current knowledge, skills, and experience, along with ensuring that the situation in which the student is expected to participate is realistic and provides the opportunity for constructive feedback.

EMS is the ideal discipline by which the benefits of experiential learning can be maximized, because so much of what is done by care providers can be recreated in the classroom through the use of patient care scenarios. In addition, most students will spend valuable time in the clinical and field settings, hoping to apply what they have learned in the classroom. Chapter 19, *Tools for Field and Clinical Learning*, details how instructors can maximize the clinical experience for students. Following are examples of classroom scenarios that can be used to maximize the potential for experiential learning.

For this example, a standard has been taken directly from the 2009 U.S. Department of Transportation National EMS Education Standards for the EMT.

Example 1

It is easy enough for the educator to ask students to read the text on cardiovascular emergencies, then discuss in class the rationale for administering a particular medication for the management of chest pain. However, use of this standard to drive a patient scenario can be much more effective.

"The process whereby knowledge is created through the transformation of experience" is how David Kolb, a leading expert in the study of experiential learning, defines learning. "Knowledge results from the combination of grasping and transforming experience."[12] **Kolb's theory** describes two ways that learners can transform experience into knowledge—reflective observation and active experimentation. Kolb believes that learners transform their previous experience into new knowledge by evaluating and building on this foundation. This reflective practice provides students the opportunity to self-reflect on what they have learned. This strategy is effective throughout the program, and also as their education continues as they care for patients in the work environment. According to Hilliard et al.,[13] student reflection on what they learned is an effective strategy to connect theory and practice for lifelong learning. Many things that are easily done in the EMS classroom can serve as excellent models for these two modes of learning. In the chest pain scenario, students who are actively engaged in a simulated patient encounter learn through active experimentation. The simulated patient is preprogrammed to provide certain responses to help guide students in performing appropriate steps without providing obvious direction. Observers and participants benefit from reflective observation by participating in a follow-up critique of how the patient was treated.

Another example of experiential learning in which the instructor uses active exploration as a means of reinforcing a particular learning objective follows.

Example 2

This objective could easily be approached by lecture and is generally covered quite well in the textbook with the use of illustrations. However, allowing students to experience the practice of assessing pupils and having them see and document their findings will help cement the knowledge through experiential learning.

The examples shown are just a few of the ways in which an educator can use an alternative or student-centered method to meet common objectives. Through the process of trial and error, the educator discovers which methods work best for certain objectives. The challenge for the EMS educator is to identify those objectives with the highest priority and experiment with various methods of delivery. The process of developing a more student-centered approach to the classroom initially requires more work and adds increased risk to what the instructor does; however, the rewards for both students and educator are immeasurable.

Matching Teaching Strategies to Goals and Objectives

Making the conscious decision to become a more student-centered educator is quite different from actually making it happen. It may be comforting for the instructor to know that half the battle has already been decided for EMS educators in that the foundation for

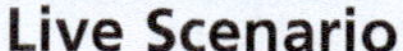

CASE in Point

Live Scenario

Two or three students are selected to play EMTs and are asked to leave the room. Another student is selected to play the role of the patient; this student should be instructed to present with all the classic signs and symptoms of cardiac chest pain, including a recent history of angina. Additional input can be solicited from the class regarding how this patient should present. The patient is provided with a small bottle of medication labeled as nitroglycerin. Small mints or some similar candy is placed in the bottle to represent the medication. The patient is instructed to "pass out" should the EMTs decide to administer the medication before a baseline blood pressure has been established or if the EMT fails to determine how many pills the patient has already taken, or whether or not the patient has taken erectile dysfunction medications such as Cialis or Viagra.

The primary objectives of the scenario are (1) to reinforce the need to establish a minimum blood pressure before medication is administered, and (2) to gather an appropriate history before any medication is given. Several secondary objectives may come up during the post-scenario critique.

The EMTs are brought into the room using a simulated dispatch, such as "Rescue 51: respond code 3 to residence for a man with chest pain." The scenario is allowed to progress until the educator believes it has met the stated objective and concludes with a brief critique. For example, if the students give the nitroglycerin without first assessing a blood pressure, the simulated patient becomes unresponsive and the call can be stopped. The team of responders, beginning first with the team leader, should have an opportunity to critique their own performance and state why they think the patient became unresponsive. Self-assessment is a key element of development in experiential education and should be encouraged; it will be required in the profession of emergency medicine, because most crews do not have an educator or supervisor responding to every call with them, pointing out where there are gaps in their knowledge that require a refresher class. Other members of the team would then be given an opportunity to comment on what went well and what did not relative to the objective of the scenario. Students who are observing are invited to critique the team's performance. The instructor's job is to steer the critique along the path toward the intended objective, encouraging students to think critically and experience the learning, rather than just hearing or reading about it.

CASE in Point

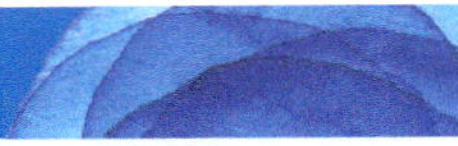

Experimenting with Pupil Reactions

It is difficult for students to actually see pupil changes in a well-lit room. For this reason, it is best for the educator to ask students to pair up and take turns assessing pupil response with a penlight or a similar light source. First, one student should document pupil size and equality on a fellow student. The lights should be turned out for no less than 2 minutes before students are asked to recheck pupil response with the penlight. Both eyes should be checked several times so the pupils can actually be seen to change in response to light. Students should be asked to record their results for each student in the class, then compare their results during a debriefing of the activity. Some students should be positioned in a location where side lighting may affect the readings or the ability to assess pupils. Students should be asked to lie on their backs and look up into the overhead classroom lights. When the educator provides feedback for this activity, the educator should ask students how the position of the patient in the ambulance and light levels will affect their ability to evaluate pupils.

Experiential Tips

Here are just a few examples of experiential techniques that can help reinforce specific learning points:

- Have students feel the pulse of a person with an irregular heart rhythm.
- Use a dual-earpiece teaching stethoscope, or AURiS with Bluetooth technology, to assist students in understanding what sounds they are listening for when taking a blood pressure or auscultating lung sounds.
- To reinforce the importance of the physical exam, have students practice a patient assessment where there are actual simulated injuries to find, such as a bruise on the abdomen, blood on the ground underneath the patient, or subcutaneous emphysema on the chest made out of bubble wrap. (If students do not expose and touch the patient, they will not find all of the hidden injuries.)

the objectives to which they must teach have been defined by such documents as the U.S. Department of Transportation National EMS Education Standards, the National Model EMS Clinical Guidelines,[14] and the scope of practice for each level of care. The challenge for the instructor is to continue to master current teaching methods while developing new and innovative strategies that are best suited for the various standards.

The task of addressing each and every objective included within the standards can be overwhelming. In fact, this is one of the biggest challenges for educators, given the short duration of most emergency medical responder, EMT, advanced EMT, and paramedic programs. The development of objectives from the Education Standard competencies, behaviors, and clinical judgments for the paramedic level could include more than 2,000 objectives that must be addressed at some time during the course of the program. Although it is true that some standards overlap, instructors still must "triage" the components of the standards and select those most worthy of focus during class time. It is impossible to cover every standard in class. Some must be addressed in homework, reading assignments, and activities outside of the classroom.

Educators can maximize their valuable time by ensuring that they understand the instructional level required to attain the chosen objectives. Chapter 8, *Domains of Learning*, describes the revision of Bloom's taxonomy. The taxonomy provides verbs used to describe the behaviors expected at various levels. For example, if an objective begins with "list the signs and symptoms of . . ." then the instructor knows this to be a low-level, or knowledge, or remembering-level objective. Little explanation or classroom activity is likely to be required to achieve competency in this type of objective. A simple reading assignment may accomplish the task. However, if the objective began with "recognize the signs and symptoms of," then this is a higher-level objective and may require photographs, video, or a live-patient demonstration in order to teach the content.

The educator must devise a teaching and evaluation strategy that provides the lower levels of understanding, then allows students to progress toward the upper levels. The old saying, "you must walk before you can run," can be applied here. The wisest EMS educators know that a valuable EMS provider not only understands when to do something, but also knows when not to do something. This level of understanding comes only through a thorough immersion into all aspects associated with the particular concepts. Students must understand all appropriate terminology and be able to see subtle differences between similar terms (factual knowledge). Terminology begins in the lowest levels of understanding within each domain. Terminology concepts are then applied as students begin to understand the subtle differences between words and appreciate their meaning. As students work through problems and scenarios, they use their understanding of the terminology in accurate ways to get their meaning across in words or actions (conceptual knowledge).

For example, many distinct differences can be noted between "ventilation" and "respiration," and students must understand these differences as they evaluate the effectiveness of airway management and adjunct usage (procedural knowledge). However, many educators may have forgotten the differences, or they may not have learned through their educational process how to make the distinction. Students may experience frustration when they encounter an evaluation process that requires that they discriminate among concepts for which they cannot recall differences. If the instructional process does not focus on students learning the difference between these two concepts, but instead focuses only on the development of psychomotor skills, students will be unable to effectively problem-solve an airway management or ventilation issue that differentiates between the two concepts. An example may be a patient with adequate tidal volume and respiratory rate but who remains hypoxic because, despite adequate ventilation, the fluid in his alveoli is preventing proper gas exchange or respiration.

Summary

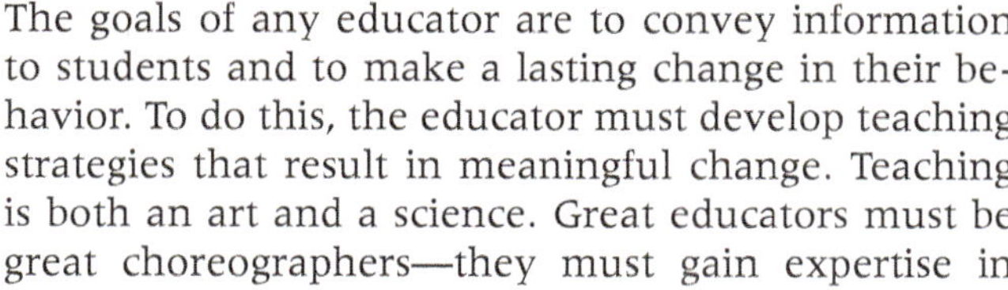

The goals of any educator are to convey information to students and to make a lasting change in their behavior. To do this, the educator must develop teaching strategies that result in meaningful change. Teaching is both an art and a science. Great educators must be great choreographers—they must gain expertise in facilitation techniques that involve groups of students, questioning techniques, and experiential learning (the art). The effective educator also must be adept in using the many teaching strategies that are available and choose which technique will be best for a given situation (the science).

Glossary

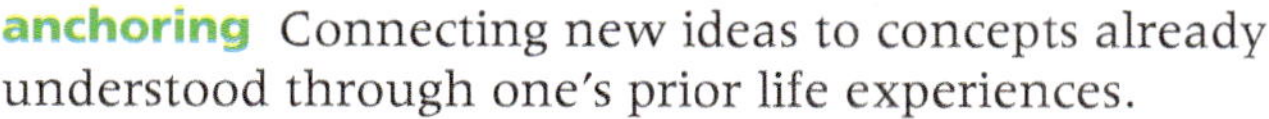

anchoring Connecting new ideas to concepts already understood through one's prior life experiences.

ask, pause, and call Questioning technique wherein the instructor waits for a longer time—up to 30 seconds—before allowing a student to answer a posed question.

experiential learning Learning by doing.

facilitation Teaching strategy in which the instructor creates a relaxed atmosphere that makes it easier for the student to learn.

flipped classroom Student-centered instructional method that uses prerecorded lecture and preclass assignments to maximize class time spent on application and problem-solving activities.

Kolb's theory Theory that describes two ways that learners can transform experience into knowledge: reflective observation and active experimentation.

scaffolding Building upon prior knowledge to aid understanding.

Socratic method Method of questioning that uses the practice of asking, rather than telling, to arouse curiosity in the subject matter so students will arrive at their own conclusions rather than being told the "right" answer.

student-centered learning Instruction that puts the learner at the center of the educational event and incorporates innovative, active teaching strategies such as group work, case studies, role-playing, writing assignments, and so on.

teacher-centered learning Instruction that focuses on the teacher and thus, primarily, the lecture format.

wait time Concept in questioning techniques that gives time to students to think about questions posed to them and to ponder their response.

References

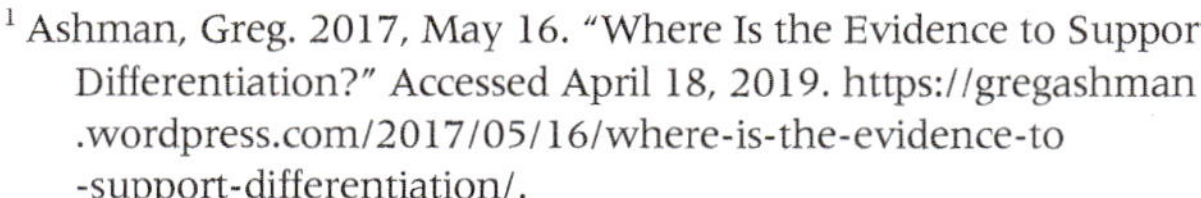

[1] Ashman, Greg. 2017, May 16. "Where Is the Evidence to Support Differentiation?" Accessed April 18, 2019. https://gregashman.wordpress.com/2017/05/16/where-is-the-evidence-to-support-differentiation/.

[2] Croskerry, Pat. 2007. "The Affective Imperative: Coming to Terms with Our Emotions." *Academic Emergency Medicine* 14, no. 2: 184–6. https://doi.org/10.1197/j.aem.2006.08.016.

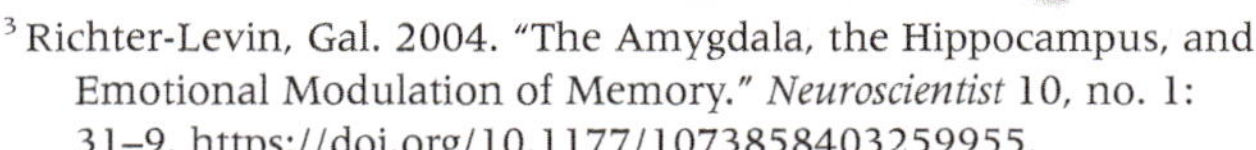

[3] Richter-Levin, Gal. 2004. "The Amygdala, the Hippocampus, and Emotional Modulation of Memory." *Neuroscientist* 10, no. 1: 31–9. https://doi.org/10.1177/1073858403259955.

[4] Craik, Fergus I. M., and Endel Tulving. 1975. "Depth of Processing and the Retention of Words in Episodic Memory." *Journal of Experimental Psychology: General* 103, no. 30: 268–94. http://dx.doi.org/10.1037/0096-3445.104.3.268.

[5] Barkley, Elizabeth F., K. Patricia Cross, and Claire H. Major. 2004. *Collaborative Learning: A Handbook for College Faculty*. San Francisco: Jossey-Bass.

[6] Paulson, Donald R., and Jennifer L. Faust. 1999. "Techniques of Active Learning: Active Learning for the College Classroom." Accessed March 26, 2019. http://www.calstatela.edu/dept/chem/chem2/Active/main.htm.

[7] Rogers, Carl, and H. Jerome Freiberg, 1994. *Freedom to Learn*, 3rd ed. Columbus, OH: Charles E. Merrill.

[8] Oregon Technology in Education Council (OTEC). 2007. "Situated Learning." In *Learning Theories and Transfer of Learning*. Accessed March 26, 2019. http://otec.uoregon.edu/learning_theory.htm#SituatedLearning.

[9] Lave, Jean, and Etienne Wenger. 1990. *Situated Learning: Legitimate Peripheral Participation*. Cambridge, UK: Cambridge University Press.

[10] Clancey, William J. 1995. "A Tutorial on Situated Learning." In *Proceedings of the International Conference on Computers and Education (Taiwan)*, edited by J. Self. Charlottesville, VA: AACE. 49-70. Accessed March 26, 2019. http://methodenpool.uni-koeln.de/situierteslernen/clancey_situated_learning.PDF.

[11] Illinois University, Faculty Development and Instructional Design Center. n.d. "Situated Learning. Northern." Accessed March 26, 2019. https://www.niu.edu/facdev/_pdf/guide/strategies/situated_learning.pdf.

[12] Kolb, David A. 1984. *Experiential Learning: Experience as the Source of Learning and Development*. Upper Saddle River, NJ: Prentice-Hall.

[13] Hilliard, Danya, Kaitlynn James, and Alan M. Batt. 2017, February/March. "An Introduction to Reflective Practice for Paramedics and Student Paramedics." *Canadian Paramedicine*: 17–20.

[14] National Association of State EMS Officials (NASEMSO). 2019, January. "National Model EMS Clinical Guidelines. Version 2.2." Accessed May 6, 2019. https://nasemso.org/wp-content/uploads/National-Model-EMS-Clinical-Guidelines-2017-PDF-Version-2.2.pdf.

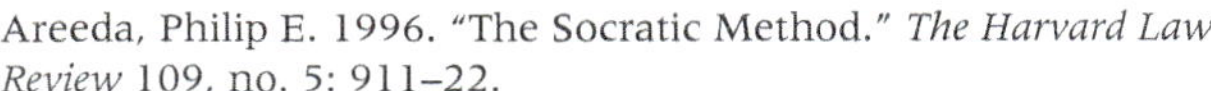
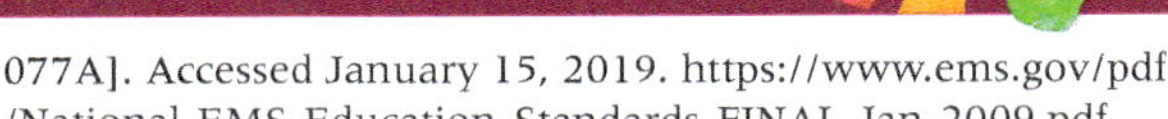

Additional Resources

Areeda, Philip E. 1996. "The Socratic Method." *The Harvard Law Review* 109, no. 5: 911–22.

Brereton, Margot F., Larry Leifer, Greene, J., Lewis, J., and Linde, C. 1993, September. "An Exploration of Engineering Learning." In *Proceedings of the ASME Design Theory and Methodology Conference, Vol. 53*, edited by T. K. Hight and L. A. Stauffer, 195–206. Albuquerque: American Society of Mechanical Engineers.

Combs, Arthur. W. 1976. "Fostering maximum development of the individual." In *Issues in Secondary Education* (NSSE Yearbook), edited by William Van Til and Kenneth J. Rehage, 65–87. Chicago: National Society for the Study of Education.

deWinstanley, Patricia A., and Robert A. Bjork. 2002. "Successful Lecturing: Presenting Information in Ways That Engage Effective Processing." *New Directions for Teaching and Learning* 89: 19–31. https://doi.org/10.1002/tl.44.

Galbraith, Michael W. (Ed.). 1991. *Adult Learning Methods*. Huntington, NY: Robert E. Krieger Publishing.

Johnson, David W., Roger T. Johnson, and Karl A. Smith. 1998. "Maximizing Instruction through Cooperative Learning." *ASEE Prism* 7: 24–9.

King, Alison. 1993. "From Sage on the Stage to Guide on the Side." *College Teaching* 41, no. 1: 30–5. https://doi.org/10.1080/87567555.1993.9926781.

National Highway Traffic Safety Administration. 2009. "National Emergency Medical Services Education Standards." [DOT HS 811 077A]. Accessed January 15, 2019. https://www.ems.gov/pdf/National-EMS-Education-Standards-FINAL-Jan-2009.pdf.

Norman, Geoffrey R., and Henk G. Schmidt. 1992. "The Psychological Basis of Problem-Based Learning: A Review of the Evidence." *Academic Medicine* 67: 557–65.

Nowell, Linda. 1996. "Rethinking the Classroom: A Community of Inquiry." Presented at National Council on Creating the Quality School, Norman, Oklahoma. Fort Worth, TX: Wesleyan University, School of Education. ERIC Document Reproduction Service No. ED350 273.

Reese, Andy C. 1998. "Implications of Results from Cognitive Science Research." *Medical Education Online* 3, no. 1. https://doi.org/10.3402/meo.v3i.4295.

Rideout, Elizabeth. 2001. *Transforming Nursing Education through Problem-Based Learning*. Sudbury, MA: Jones and Bartlett Publishers.

Springer, Leonard, Mary E. Stanne, and Samuel S. Donovan. 1999. "Effects of Small Group Learning on Undergraduates in Science, Mathematics, Engineering, and Technology: A Meta-analysis." *Review of Educational Research* 69, no. 1: 21–51. https://doi.org/10.3102%2F00346543069001021.

Van Ast, John. 1997. "Sage on the Stage or Guide on the Side: An Outcome-Based Approach to the Preparation of Community College Vocational-Technical Faculty for the 1990s and Beyond." *Community College Journal of Research & Practice* 21, no. 5: 459–80.

CHAPTER 12

Teaching in All Domains

OBJECTIVES

At the conclusion of this chapter, the educator will be able to:

Cognitive Domain

1. Compare and contrast the differences in factual, conceptual, procedural, and meta-cognitive types of knowledge.
2. Understand the differences between working memory, long-term memory, and metacognition.
3. Compare and contrast the progressive learning components of the cognitive domain and how they relate to student outcomes.
4. Compare and contrast the progressive learning components of skills development in the psychomotor domain and how they relate to student outcomes.
5. Compare and contrast the progressive learning components of the affective domain and how they relate to student outcomes.
6. Describe the whole-part-whole method of teaching psychomotor skills.
7. Describe strategies to improve acquisition of psychomotor skills during skills lab sessions.
8. Describe how interrater reliability affects the assessment of skills acquisition.

Psychomotor Domain

There are no psychomotor objectives for this chapter.

Affective Domain

1. Value classroom facilitation strategies that promote higher-level thinking skills.
2. Value the inclusion of the affective domain in the assessment of the professional healthcare provider.
3. Defend the value of the team approach in the teaching and assessment in all domains of learning.

“If we don’t model what we teach, then we are teaching something else.”

~ Unknown

CHAPTER GOAL This chapter discusses how to teach critical-thinking skills and how to apply them to the cognitive, psychomotor, and affective domains.

The practice of emergency medical services (EMS) is a complex activity that involves teaching in multiple domains and at multiple levels. EMS educators must prepare future providers to be highly skilled professionals who are able to accurately perform skills and correctly recite treatment protocols, medication dosages, and steps for procedures; the EMS provider also must be a skilled communicator who demonstrates empathy and a deeper appreciation of each patient's social, family, and ethnic background honoring patients' diversity and wishes. This chapter prepares the EMS educator for the challenge of providing a comprehensive EMS education that will produce competent, compassionate care providers.

Types of Knowledge

Anderson and Krathwohl (2001) describe four different types of knowledge: factual, conceptual, procedural, and meta-cognitive.[1] This construct is related to the categories of learning used by EMS educators where factual and conceptual would be categorized as cognitive processes, procedural as psychomotor, and meta-cognitive would be related to the affective domain.

Factual Knowledge

Learning often begins with the accumulation of facts—*factual knowledge*. Objectives for learners at this level include terms such as "define," "recall," "recognize," and "articulate," and cover knowledge of terminology, details, and dates. The ability to identify the structures of the airway before learning intubation is an example of how factual knowledge typically needs to precede conceptual or procedural knowledge.

Conceptual Knowledge

Principles, theories, and models characterize *conceptual knowledge*. Objectives attempting to address conceptual knowledge might include "classify," "assess," "explain," "interpret," and "differentiate." A group of emergency medical technicians (EMTs) attending continuing education should be presented with conceptual knowledge regarding changes in spinal motion restriction procedures based on current literature and the newest joint position paper from the National Association of EMS Physicians (NAEMSP) and the American College of Surgeons Committee on Trauma (ACS COT) before being introduced to a change in spinal motion restriction protocols.

Procedural Knowledge

Techniques, algorithms, and methods are included in *procedural knowledge*. Students being assessed on their procedural knowledge might be asked to "demonstrate," "apply," "execute," or "implement." It is important to note that while almost any learner could be taught the steps of a procedure from bandaging to bag-mask ventilation, learners often need to understand facts and concepts about the procedure they are performing in order to know when to use the skill or which technique to employ.

For example, paramedics need to understand when to use orotracheal intubation versus nasotracheal intubation. It is important to have the conceptual knowledge that nasotracheal intubation is an option for patients nearing respiratory failure but who still have an intact gag reflex. Factual knowledge related to the skill includes that the patient needs to be breathing and that an audible job aid such as the BAAM (Beck Airway Airflow Monitor) is helpful in determining that the patient is breathing. Both factual and conceptual knowledge should be taught before the procedural knowledge and will assist the student in learning, demonstrating, and valuing the skill as a technique for specific patients.

Meta-Cognitive Knowledge

Meta-cognitive knowledge is special because it is how one thinks about their own thinking and learning. Especially important to the affective domain, asking learners to reflect on their own thinking, approach, and progress helps to create lifelong learners who seek mastery orientation of their craft. To gauge students' meta-cognitive knowledge, educators may ask students to plan an approach to studying for the final exam, monitor their progress, then adjust the strategies they are using if success is not inevitable. Suppose a provider has received a notice from the quality improvement department indicating that he failed to treat and transport a patient whom the crew felt was having anxiety but later ended up dying of a heart attack. The quality improvement (QI) manager may ask the crew to use meta-cognitive knowledge to examine their understanding of how an anxiety attack may actually cause a heart attack, reflect on their beliefs about behavioral patients and those with anxiety, and plan a course of remediation for themselves to ensure no such medical error occurs again for this crew.

Application of Anderson and Krathwohl's model of types of knowledge is useful in understanding how to teach thinking and psychomotor skills, as well as teaching and learning in the affective domain.

Teaching Thinking Skills

Widely regarded as the father of modern critical thinking, John Dewey defined **critical thinking** as "the active, persistent, and careful consideration of a belief or supposed form of knowledge in light of the grounds which support it and the further conclusions to which it tends." By using the term "active," Dewey contrasts this method of learning from the more passive method in which the student simply receives information or ideas from someone else. Dewey believed that the attainment of higher-level thinking skills, sometimes called "critical thinking," could be nurtured and developed in students. Approaches to teaching that involve critical thinking require the student to think things through, raise additional questions, and explore solutions for themselves. Dewey believed that educators should pay close attention to each student's life experience and should develop curricula that connect with and extend student experiences to real-world application. Dewey suggested that school should be less about preparation for life and more about life itself.[2]

One way to help students with critical thinking is through the use of flipped classrooms. Use of a flipped classroom model requires students to engage in **active behavior** in their learning process and sets the foundation for critical thinking. In a flipped classroom model, students are assigned reading, slides, or lecture to view; videos to watch; and activities such as building a model of a germ or a section of spinal column ahead of class time. This ensures that the instructor does not spend the precious in-class time they have together lecturing, which is a **passive behavior** experience for the students. Instead, students learn facts and key concepts through exploration of the material, then come to class ready to participate in skills practice, scenarios, discussion, and activities that promote higher-level thinking on Bloom's taxonomy or critical-thinking skills. (See Chapter 15, *Tools for Large Group Learning*, and Chapter 16, *Using Technology to Enhance Classroom Learning*, for further discussion of flipped classrooms.)

It is not enough to simply assume that students will think critically on their own. Although some do, many must be introduced to this skill in the classroom. By keeping alert to available opportunities, educators can begin to develop more meaningful lessons. In the examples given in this chapter and in the following chapters, the common thread is the element of critical thinking. These examples provide a great foundation for new and experienced educators alike.

Teaching thinking strategies requires a careful and deliberate plan of instruction. Educators must determine which thinking skills students have already mastered and which they have yet to learn. Educators must measure thinking skills regularly and should include thinking-skills development exercises and strategies throughout the course. Measuring student achievement is difficult enough when the goal is simply measuring recall of information or psychomotor skills performance, but the process becomes even more complex when one adds to it measuring a student's ability to use information to think critically and to problem-solve. This problem is not unique to EMS education. A study on the evaluation of thousands of test items from K–12 education reveals that nearly three-quarters of these items tested the recall of information (i.e., a low-level cognitive skill), and very few tested the application of **higher-order thinking** skills.[3] Numerous studies in adult and elementary education have had similar findings.

In EMS, instructor-made exams often contain only recall-level items, factual knowledge, or lower-level thinking skills on Bloom's taxonomy (**FIGURE 12.1**). Students may perform well on quizzes and exams in class but then score poorly on the national licensing exam. This is because a national exam used for certification has a robust process for developing higher-level items, which include application of knowledge (conceptual and procedural knowledge) and critical-thinking skills. Instructors must learn about constructing high-quality test items and participate in item-writing activities in order to develop high-quality exams that measure the student's application of facts and ability to transfer that knowledge to new or novel situations that may not have been covered in their textbook or practiced in class. Because learning to write higher-order test items is difficult and time consuming, some programs opt to use a test vendor instead of allowing instructors to write their own exams. Exposure to critical-thinking

Revised Bloom's Taxonomy: Cognitive Domain

Level 1: Remember
Level 2: Understand
Level 3: Apply
Level 4: Analyze
Level 5: Evaluate
Level 6: Create

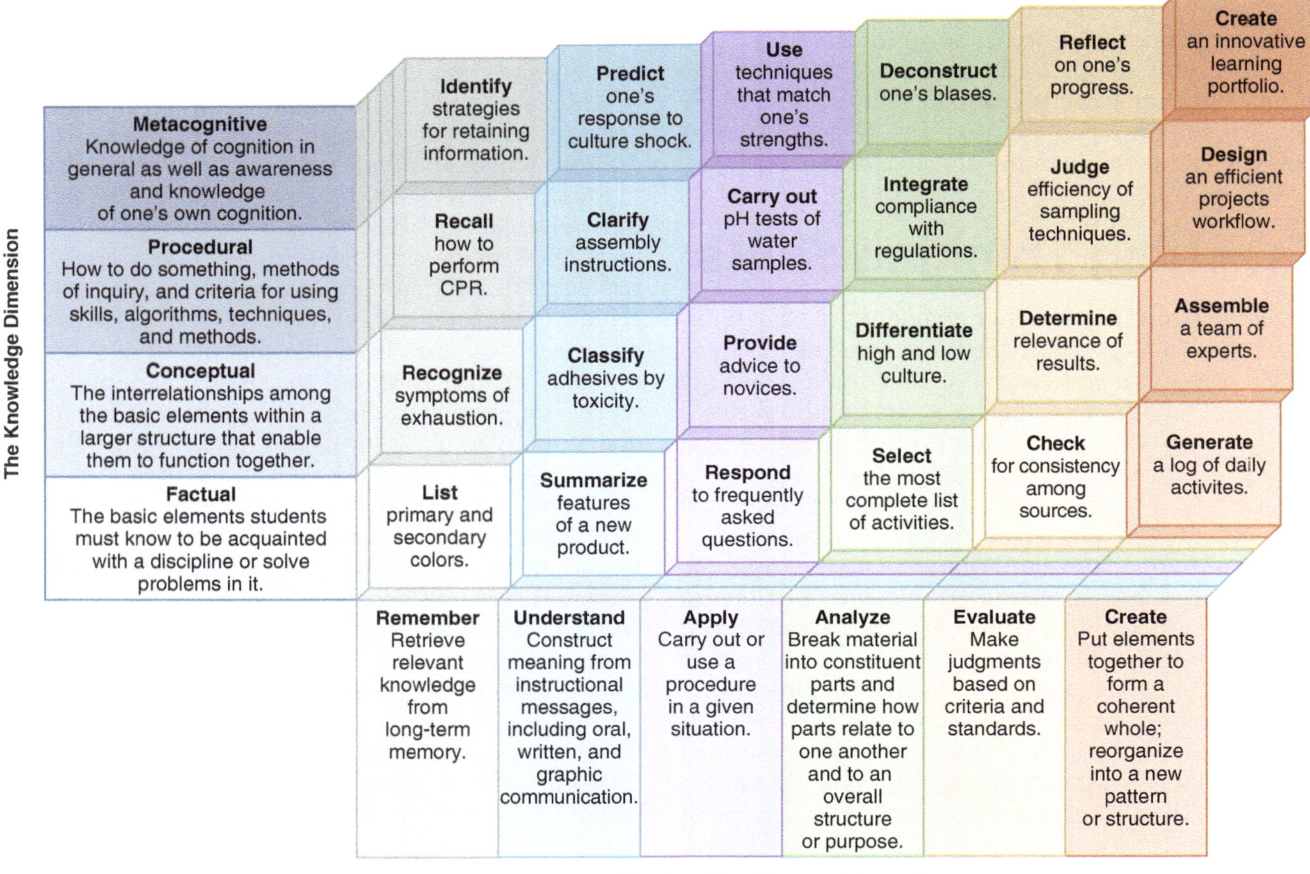

FIGURE 12.1 The colored blocks show an example of a learning objective that aligns with an aspect of the knowledge dimension and the cognitive process dimension.

items throughout the learning process often results in improved performance on standardized or licensing exams.[4]

Three key processes have been identified that enhance an educator's ability to assist students in the development of higher-order thinking skills. Key process 1 involves the implementation by the instructor of various instructional and assessment strategies that teach thinking skills to students, such as preclass work in the flipped classroom model. To do this, educators must have a fundamental understanding of the thinking process and must possess the appropriate tools and techniques to assist students in acquiring the same. Key process 2 requires that students be given ample opportunity to practice these methods. Educators should ensure that they schedule and provide opportunities for students to explore various learning styles and preferences, such as researching and writing a scenario about a diabetic patient that they will present to other students in the class. In key process 3, the educator serves as a role model for critical thinking and problem solving to be emulated by students, by questioning their own thinking, researching emerging trends, or challenging a current policy in their EMS system that is not in line with current evidence-based practice.

Several valid strategies for grouping and classifying thinking skills have been developed. For example, Costa and associates organized thinking skills into the six Rs of thinking: Remembering, Repeating, Reasoning, Reorganizing, Relating, and Reflecting.[5] This

TEACHING TIP

Instructors should provide critical-thinking opportunities that appeal to a variety of student learning styles and preferences.

CASE in Point

After a session in which students learned and demonstrated the ability to ventilate a manikin using a pocket mask, the instructor asked these questions:

- How will you know if your breaths are getting into the patient?
- What does it mean if you do not see good chest rise and fall?

Some students immediately shouted the first answer that came to mind without giving it much thought. For instance, in response to the first question, one student said, "Because I know I gave a good breath." In response to the second question, a second student said, "The patient has something stuck in his throat." These answers may or may not have been correct; however, other conclusions had to be tested before these responses could be evaluated for correctness. To stimulate higher levels of learning, the instructor demonstrated excellent **facilitation** skills by asking follow-up questions, such as, "How can you be sure that the breath you gave is really adequate for the patient?" and "Is a foreign object the only thing that can obstruct an airway?" By offering additional probing questions, the instructor slowed the class down and encouraged students to process information carefully and thoroughly before responding.

model is common to nursing education and is the framework for several of its strategies for the development of critical-thinking skills.

Barry Beyer, working with an inventory of operations common to curriculum developers and educators, classified thinking processes into three distinct groups: thinking strategies, critical-thinking skills, and micro-thinking skills.[6]

Techniques for Teaching Critical-Thinking Skills: The T.H.I.N.K. Model

A common nursing model classifies critical-thinking skills into five modes of thinking: total recall, habits, inquiry, new ideas and creativity, and knowing how you think. It uses the mnemonic **T.H.I.N.K.** and the processes proceed in the order of the spelling of that word.[7] The first two sections of the T.H.I.N.K. model are not actually critical-thinking skills, but rather lay the foundation for critical thinking to come. These first two steps, total recall and habit, establish the reserve from which one will draw.

Total Recall

Total recall is the memorization of facts or remembering where to look for them. As a student practices total recall, it is important to distinguish which information should be recalled instantaneously and which can be looked up. Because patient safety is of the highest priority, it is becoming increasingly more acceptable in health care to use a job aid or reference material to avoid error. Many electronic references are available to providers to search for information such as medication dosages or poison control information at the bedside. Instructors should make clear to students which references may be used in practice and testing and which information is expected to be memorized.

The limits of working memory require strategies to improve processing of information. Working memory is limited in both time and capacity. Most models of working memory suggest that adults can hold three to five pieces of information in their working memory.[8] If the information is not attended to, it will disappear. Rehearsal is one method for keeping information in the working memory, such as reciting the name of a new physician at the hospital over and over. However, recitation is a low-level learning strategy and unless one has time to over-learn that name, the information will be lost. Instead, learners must be taught to utilize meaningful learning strategies such as anchoring, organizing, and elaboration. Instructors can assist learners in developing meaningful learning strategies by scaffolding learning, or building upon already existing knowledge possessed by the students and anchoring to things they already know.[9]

Using patterns, or **mnemonics**, is helpful in improving recall. An example of recall occurs when a person tries to remember the following numbers in order: 5553561809. It looks daunting until they are organized like this: (555) 356-1809. Now, it resembles a phone number and is easier to remember. A common EMS mnemonic is OPQRST (Onset, Provocation or Palliation, Quality, Region and Radiation, Severity, and Time), which is used to obtain the present and past medical histories in patients with pain.

Another example of recall might be asking the learner to look at a list of common words and to try to remember them: apple, car, yellow, pear, bicycle, blue, grapefruit, plane, and green. If the learner sorts the list according to the following patterns, called "grouping or chunking," it is easier to recall:

- Colors: yellow, blue, green
- Fruits: apple, grapefruit, pear
- Transportation: car, plane, bicycle

Another method of recall involves the association of facts with an experience. A person may quickly and easily remember a fact because it is associated with a strong emotion or a funny story. This is called flashbulb memory, as if one's brain took a picture of the time and place this memory occurred.[10] For example, few will ever forget where they were and what they were doing when they learned that commercial aircraft were being flown into buildings in America on September 11, 2001.

Habit

Habit, the second process of critical thinking, is any accepted way that works, saves time, or is necessary for the critical-thinking process to take place. Habits are thinking approaches that become second nature. Within the psychomotor domain, this level of **mastery** is called naturalization. Driving a car to school illustrates this principle for someone who has arrived at class without remembering the journey. Habits in the work environment can make performing a job a lot easier and free the mind to use conscious thought for critical thinking. However, it is important that a person periodically reevaluate performance to ensure that they are not taking inappropriate short cuts, which is considered meta-cognitive knowledge. For example, students should consider whether or not they are actually looking for scene hazards and wearing gloves and goggles or just reciting aloud "scene safety, standard precautions."

Inquiry

Inquiry occurs as the student examines issues in depth and detail and questions what may seem immediately obvious. Although this single process of inquiry is often called critical thinking, the nursing model of thinking requires the action of all five modes of the T.H.I.N.K. model for critical thinking to take place. Inquiry is the primary kind of thinking used to reach conclusions, and conclusions are more accurate if inquiry is used.[11]

Inquiry requires the following six steps:

1. Receive information.
2. Come to a conclusion, but collect additional information to rule in or rule out the immediate conclusion.
3. Compare the new information with what is already known from past experience.
4. Question biases.
5. Consider one or more alternative conclusions.
6. Validate the original or alternative conclusion.

Determining a differential diagnosis is perhaps the most common use of the inquiry step in health care; it is performed daily by practitioners everywhere. Of course, students must have recall of facts related to anatomy, physiology, pathophysiology, signs and symptoms, treatment protocols, and medication dosages as they approach any patient. Next, some of the student's thinking processes will be habit and require little or no conscious thought, such as taking a radial pulse or noting skin signs, freeing the mind for the critical-thinking task ahead. This leads to the steps of inquiry where the provider will first receive information (from a patient, for example). After listening to and confirming the chief complaint and related symptoms the patient is experiencing, the provider will have a short list of possible diagnoses. Using step 2 of inquiry, the provider will then gather additional information, for example from diagnostic tests such as an electrocardiogram (ECG) or lab work, to rule in or rule out the possible diagnosis from their short list. The provider will then compare these findings with what they know from past experience, often needing to consider other possible causes for the patient's complaint. The next step is to consider if any biases are at play. For example, it is known that prehospital providers tend to miss signs of stroke in Asian patients,[12] and signs of myocardial infarction in women.[13]

After gathering and considering all of this information, the provider will determine a diagnosis and establish a treatment plan for the patient.

As one looks ahead to the last two processes in the T.H.I.N.K. system, creativity and **metacognition** are upcoming. Metacognition is the highest of the thinking skills in the T.H.I.N.K. model. "Meta-" means "among" or "in the midst of," and cognition is the process of knowing. A student who attains this level can critically analyze their own thinking process and make adjustments as needed.

In the example of patient diagnosis, creativity could be used if there is not an established treatment protocol for this differential diagnosis or if the patient refused some suggested treatments. Metacognition would perhaps be implemented after the shift when exploring whether or not the treatment for this patient was proper or while exploring how one arrived at the diagnosis in a journaling assignment about the shift required by the professor.

New Ideas and Creativity

New ideas and creativity are the polar opposite of the habit mode of thinking. Creativity allows the thinker to explore different pathways or alternatives for problem solving. A common phrase attached to this process is "to think outside the box." Creative thinking often leads to mistakes or ideas that will not be carried out, but which can provide additional learning opportunities. Creative thinking allows practitioners of health care to individualize care and often to discover new solutions or improved processes. When performed at its highest level, the creative-thinking process allows for individual choices within the framework of medically acceptable behaviors.

Teaching People Skills

It is the affective domain of learning that addresses not what is known about or done for patients, but how the provider goes about it. The affective domain is about how a provider treats patients while treating them. Developing a generation of caring, compassionate providers who are self-motivated to do well and continue learning throughout their careers begins with a classroom environment that respects the learner as an individual who comes with attitudes, beliefs, emotions, and experiences that are of value to the class. Affective skills impact any behavior or decision that one makes, because all behavior includes an emotional component.

Engaging students in active classroom behaviors provides a student-centered learning environment that cultivates critical thinking (**TABLE 12.1**). Educators have long known that the power of emotion can be harnessed to create a memorable learning experience. By tapping into emotion, instructors can build a vibrant classroom that takes students on an exploration of their profession and of themselves. Additionally, it has been shown repeatedly that students learn and remember more and at higher levels of cognition when the lesson was active and involved emotion or the senses. In the end, this student-centered, active-learning atmosphere brings about greater understanding and a more complete student and learning experience. This is why it is critical to begin to change classrooms from passive places of learning to active and engaging ones.

Educators are role models, and they are teaching values whether they realize it or not. Every time an instructor relates a personal experience about how they were empathetic to a troubled patient or family member, communicates verbal and nonverbal reactions to student questions or performance, chooses subjects to be tested, and even emphasizes given topics in a lecture or presentation, the instructor is imposing values. The real issue for the instructor, then, is how to cultivate the ethics and values of the profession while setting aside one's own personal prejudices, beliefs, and emotions. Educators have a much stronger influence on students than they may ever know or appreciate. Students learn from the behaviors that their educators model, including those instructor behaviors that they observe outside the classroom (**FIGURE 12.2**).

Dr. Pat Croskerry, a physician and medical educator who studies and writes about how caregiver attitudes affect judgment and the quality of patient care, says, "Our historical and continuing failure to acknowledge the impact of our feelings on the ways in which we interact with patients ultimately precludes optimal clinical reasoning and decision making."[14] Creating an environment in which students are engaged in activities to explore their emotions and also make critical decisions while under stress and in situations involving strong emotion, such as elder abuse, a workplace shooting event, or a line-of-duty death, is the responsibility of the educator in the development of a more aware, accurate, affective, and ultimately effective medical workforce.

TABLE 12.1 Distinguishing between Passive and Active Behaviors

Passive	Active
Quiet classrooms of note takers	Active classrooms of interactive learners
All work done alone	Work done in cooperative small groups
Rare participation in class	Regular participation to some degree
Classroom-guided materials	Creation of new and challenging assignments
Instructor-controlled lesson	Student- and instructor-controlled lessons
All tasks carried out by the instructor	Classroom responsibilities shared by students

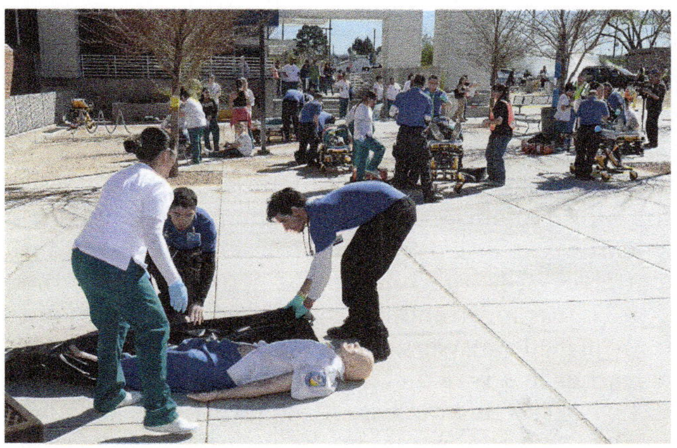

FIGURE 12.2 Educators model values and behaviors by everything they say and do within and outside of the classroom.

To appropriately affect a student's progress within the affective domain, an instructor must be consciously aware of the values, judgments, and beliefs that are inherent in the instructor's teaching but that may not be overtly apparent; then, the instructor must monitor changes in students to detect behaviors that indicate that they are adopting desired values and judgments. For example, in order for patients to feel cared for and respected, it is important to treat patients as human beings, not objectify them as their diseases or symptoms. Educators must be careful not to say things like "we responded on a chest pain last night," but rather to say, "we took care of an elderly patient with chest pain last night." Not only should instructors use the proper form of address and instruction, they must correct students who do not notice themselves treating patients with a lack of respect. This is just one example of how an instructor can model values and affect, but the opportunities to do so are endless—from learning and using patients' and students' names, to covering patients with a sheet or blanket to protect modesty, to wearing a clean uniform or dressing professionally when teaching. Each of these behaviors demonstrates to students the values of the profession of medicine.

TEACHING TIP

Model accountability: Students and other educators cannot break poor habits and lack of accountability unless they replace them with new behaviors such as accepting responsibility and being accountable. Primary instructors should model the desired behaviors they expect of students. This starts by having everyone acknowledge the clear goals and objectives they are striving to meet.

Levels of the Affective Domain

Bloom identified five levels in the affective domain. (See Chapter 8, *Domains of Learning*.) Facilitation is the teaching technique that can be applied at all levels of the affective domain as well as to the cognitive and psychomotor domains. *Facilitation* is the process of assisting learners in discovering information or abilities for themselves. It is a technique distinctly different from lecture or demonstration in that the educator does not simply provide answers, but rather questions or guides the learner in a way that promotes self-discovery.

The next section discusses each level of the affective domain. Typically, students are expected to develop competency in each level throughout their career. The levels of the affective domain include receive, respond, value, organize, and characterize. Development of student affect has become so important to EMS as a profession that affective evaluations are now required elements of the National EMS Education Standards for the paramedic level. Eleven professional behaviors were identified and described as necessary for demonstrating competency in the affective domain (**FIGURE 12.3**). Education programs must operationalize assessment of the affective domain by including the evaluation as a graded element of the curriculum and requiring that competency be met. Many programs require a competent grade on the affective evaluation during each phase of the program before matriculating to the next. For example, a program should not send a student having trouble meeting basic competency in time management to the hospital where their failure to attend might not be noticed by busy hospital staff. Students failing to meet basic competency in any area of the affective evaluation should be counseled and given the opportunity to improve.

Bloom's Taxonomy: Affective Domain

Level 1: Receive
Level 2: Respond
Level 3: Value
Level 4: Organize
Level 5: Characterize

Level 1: Receive

Receiving is where the affective domain begins. It requires no more of the student than that they have awareness of a given piece of information. This is usually cognitive in origin. The student has heard it, seen it, or read it. Receiving is made up of three successive steps. When a student demonstrates any of the actions described by these steps, the student is operating at the receiving level.

These steps include the following:

1. **Awareness**: This step requires only that the student be conscious of the existence of a given piece of information or equipment. For example, the student sees the traction splint in the classroom but does not display any interest in it.
2. **Willingness to receive**: At this step, the student becomes curious enough about the piece of information or object that the student is willing to devote some, but not all, of their attention to it. For example, the student stops to look at the traction splint before sitting down in the classroom, or the student asks questions during the lecture on fracture management.

NATIONAL GUIDELINES FOR EDUCATING EMS INSTRUCTORS
AUGUST 2002

PROFESSIONAL BEHAVIOR EVALUATION

Student's Name: ____________________

Date of evaluation: ____________________

1. INTEGRITY	Competent [ ]	Not yet competent [ ]
Examples of professional behavior include, but are not limited to: Consistent honesty; being able to be trusted with the property of others; can be trusted with confidential information; complete and accurate documentation of patient care and learning activities.		
2. EMPATHY	Competent [ ]	Not yet competent [ ]
Examples of professional behavior include, but are not limited to: Showing compassion for others; responding appropriately to the emotional response of patients and family members; demonstrating respect for others; demonstrating a calm, compassionate, and helpful demeanor toward those in need; being supportive and reassuring to others.		
3. SELF-MOTIVATION	Competent [ ]	Not yet competent [ ]
Examples of professional behavior include, but are not limited to: Taking initiative to complete assignments; taking initiative to improve and/or correct behavior; taking on and following through on tasks without constant supervision; showing enthusiasm for learning and improvement; consistently striving for excellence in all aspects of patient care and professional activities; accepting constructive feedback in a positive manner; taking advantage of learning opportunities.		
4. APPEARANCE AND PERSONAL HYGIENE	Competent [ ]	Not yet competent [ ]
Examples of professional behavior include, but are not limited to: Clothing and uniform is appropriate, neat, clean and well maintained; good personal hygiene and grooming.		
5. SELF-CONFIDENCE	Competent [ ]	Not yet competent [ ]
Examples of professional behavior include, but are not limited to: Demonstrating the ability to trust personal judgment; demonstrating an awareness of strengths and limitations; exercises good personal judgment.		
6. COMMUNICATIONS	Competent [ ]	Not yet competent [ ]
Examples of professional behavior include, but are not limited to: Speaking clearly; writing legibly; listening actively; adjusting communication strategies to various situations.		
7. TIME MANAGEMENT	Competent [ ]	Not yet competent [ ]
Examples of professional behavior include, but are not limited to: Consistent punctuality; completing tasks and assignments on time.		
8. TEAMWORK AND DIPLOMACY	Competent [ ]	Not yet competent [ ]
Examples of professional behavior include, but are not limited to: Placing the success of the team above self-interest; not undermining the team; helping and supporting other team members; showing respect for all team members; remaining flexible and open to change; communicating with others to resolve problems.		

FIGURE 12.3 Eleven professional behaviors necessary for demonstrating competency in the affective domain, according to the 2002 National Guidelines for Educating EMS Instructors.

National Guidelines for Educating Instructors, August 2002, (Excerpt from 1998 EMT-P: NSC), Appendix V: Affective Domain Evaluation Tools, pgs. 3-4

(*continues*)

NATIONAL GUIDELINES FOR EDUCATING EMS INSTRUCTORS
AUGUST 2002

9. RESPECT	Competent [ ]	Not yet competent [ ]
Examples of professional behavior include, but are not limited to: Being polite to others; not using derogatory or demeaning terms; behaving in a manner that brings credit to the profession.		
10. PATIENT ADVOCACY	Competent [ ]	Not yet competent [ ]
Examples of professional behavior include, but are not limited to: Not allowing personal bias to or feelings to interfere with patient care; placing the needs of patients above self-interest; protecting and respecting patient confidentiality and dignity.		
11. CAREFUL DELIVERY OF SERVICE	Competent [ ]	Not yet competent [ ]
Examples of professional behavior include, but are not limited to: Mastering and refreshing skills; performing complete equipment checks; demonstrating careful and safe ambulance operations; following policies, procedures, and protocols; following orders.		

Use the space below to explain any "not yet competent" ratings. When possible, use specific behaviors, and corrective actions.

FIGURE 12.3 *(Continued)*

3. **Controlled or selected attention**: At this point, the student is so interested in the piece of information or object that it momentarily has top priority, despite the fact that other things are of interest at the same time. For example, the student would rather practice with the traction splint than discuss last night's events or is so engrossed in practice that they do not respond to their name when called.

Exactly why the piece of information or object does or does not have top priority is up for interpretation and may be a function of what goes on in the classroom or past experience, such as having been on a call with a patient suffering a femur fracture.

Classroom Implications. An instructor can promote receiving by letting students know what is expected of them. This could be accomplished first by communicating the course objectives. Many times, it is not enough to just hand out the objectives. The instructor may need to explain what they are and how they can be used to the student's benefit.

Making lectures relevant to the student also enhances the receive level. The relevancy of the objectives and of what is being taught may need to be explained. Resources such as equipment, professional magazines and publications, manikins, posters, anatomy charts, and copies of lecture outlines and notes are also invaluable at this level of learning.

Perhaps one of the most important instructor techniques for enhancing the receive level can be accomplished by placing the emphasis on course matter where it belongs, and not where the instructor has a personal preference. Students will emulate what the instructor does without realizing that they are doing it, but they will also disregard what they are supposed to be learning if they perceive no clear reason or rationale for what is being taught. Therefore, when emphasis is placed on a subject, it is helpful for the instructor to explain why the emphasis belongs there. Likewise, instructors must be wary of saying things such as "you don't really need to know that" or "I never do it like that" because in the position of authority and role model that is inherent to the educator, the student may immediately disregard the information and choose not to learn it or have bias against it.

Level 2: Respond

At this level, the student responds to some degree because of an outside influence. This is the point at which an observable change in behavior can first be seen and is often a response to instructor directives, course requirements, or job responsibilities. Responding behaviors are demonstrated when "students act out behaviors consistent with . . . a particular value."[15]

The student has not yet absorbed the value presented but is merely responding to it. Like receiving, responding comprises three steps:

1. **Command response**: This step deals with appropriate responses that the student might not understand or accept the rationale for, and might not perform if certain requirements were not made. For example, the instructor states, "The traction splint must be applied correctly, according to your skills guide, at least once. By the way, you can't leave until you do." The student may call this bribery; the instructor calls this a necessary requirement. Another example of command response would be that the student is required to sign the EMT Oath and Code of Ethics before being allowed to participate in class, regardless of their current value or respect for the content or for following the Code.
2. **Willing response**: This step differs from the first in that the student responds, when asked, without the requirement making it necessary to do so. In other words, the student will respond, when asked, without bribery. The exact motive is not known, but what is important is that the desired response was given. For example, the student actually does sign the EMT Oath and Code of Ethics. The motive for the action comes from outside the person (i.e., the instructor), and the response is made because the student chooses to accept the instructor's request. Note that the reason behind that acceptance is not known, but what is important is that the action was done.
3. **Satisfaction response**: At this step, the voluntary response to sign the Oath or apply the traction splint is accompanied by a feeling of satisfaction or some other type of emotional response. For example, the instructor may want to relate this feeling to the one felt when the application of the traction splint was satisfactorily mastered and a patient demonstrated noticeable pain relief after it was correctly applied, or the student is recognized for ethical behavior. It also could be compared with the student who frequently applies the traction splint because of feeling a sense of satisfaction when performing this skill. This step is directly affected by the response of the instructor, and it has a secondary effect on the student's self-esteem. This effect on self-esteem may be positive or negative depending on performance.

This brings up an important point. The emotional element is present at the respond level in all levels of the affective domain, to different degrees, for the following three reasons: (1) This is the level at which the emotional element most often begins to occur, (2) this is the point where the emotional element becomes part of the motivation (the satisfaction or dissatisfaction gained during the response serves as its own reinforcement; how great a reinforcement it is depends on both internal and external factors), and (3) the emotional element affects the student's overall perception of self.

Respond (Level 2) is directly dependent on successful receive (Level 1). This means that as responding is observed, it may be concluded that Level 1 was attained. The degree to which it was attained may not be readily apparent. The reverse is also true—if responding is not observed in a particular student, the receive level was probably not acquired or was not completed.

Classroom Implications. Because this is the level at which the emotional element most often begins to occur, it has a direct effect on motivation and self-esteem, as stated earlier. Techniques directed toward this level include those that enhance motivation and self-esteem. Perhaps none is as important as ensuring a **safe classroom**. A "safe" classroom refers to an emotionally safe environment where a student will not be ridiculed for asking a question, experimenting with equipment, or failing an evaluation (**FIGURE 12.4**). A great deal of learning can occur from a "failed" attempt. However, adults do not like to fail and often associate a failed attempt with "being a failure" or incompetence.[16]

Another technique for helping students move through the respond level includes leaving equipment out and permitting students to practice in an open-lab environment, instead of having every encounter be instructor-led. The freedom to take equipment apart and put it back together, practice independently and in small groups, and challenge oneself to become faster or more accurate, or perform with more finesse is invaluable at this level.

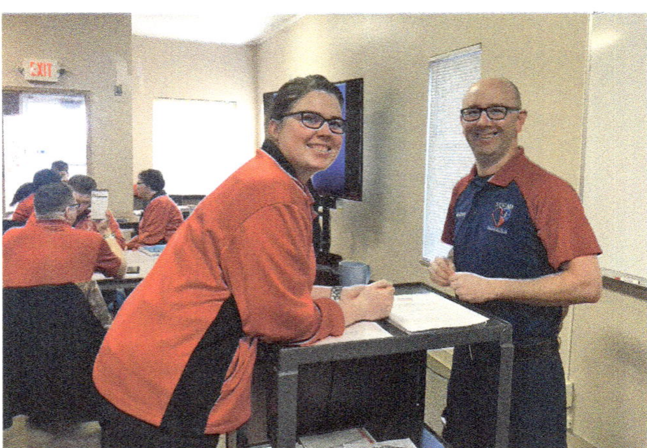

FIGURE 12.4 An emotionally safe classroom, where students are freely allowed to ask questions and reveal their failings, is conducive to a positive educational experience and promotes the respond level of the affective domain.

Courtesy of St. Charles County Ambulance District.

Perhaps no other quality of an EMS instructor at this level is greater than respect for the students themselves. This attitude of respect will guide and support the instructor's choices and, even when unspoken, will be perceived by and communicated to students throughout the course.

Level 3: Value

The third level of the affective domain, value, refers to the point at which the student attaches importance and impact to a subject or phenomenon. In this way, a person's values begin to affect their judgment. These values are internalized slowly, during a process that occurs throughout the student experience, and which includes previous experiences from before the course and interactions with peers, society, and significant others (e.g., instructors, partners, hospital staff, and spouses). The following three steps are involved in incorporation of the value process:

1. **Acceptance (of a particular value)**: This step is similar to the awareness step of receiving, in that the student has become conscious that a particular action, subject, or phenomenon has worth. The instructor can assess whether this step has been reached by observing a student who makes the same or a similar response concerning the value in question when confronted with a number of different stimuli. For example, if the student valued patient advocacy, the instructor would consistently observe the student choosing to do the right thing for the patient whether or not a supervisor was present or the patient was able to state their wishes. Whether anyone would "catch the student doing the right thing" is not the motivator of behavior when the student has reached the valuing level of the affective domain. The motivator is the value itself—in this case, being a patient advocate.
2. **Preference (for a particular value)**: In this step, the student not only has passively accepted the value but chooses to actively pursue it. In other words, when given a choice, the student will choose this value over other values that they may hold. The student typically takes every available opportunity to find out more about this value and those things related to it. Using the patient advocacy example, the student would choose to do the right thing for the patient even if it were inconvenient or uncomfortable

personally, such as transporting the patient to the hospital even if it meant dinner getting cold or missing a potentially more exciting call that was just coming in to dispatch.

3. **Commitment (to a value)**: Here, the student is committed to the belief and may be seen trying to persuade or convince others to accept the value. It is at this point that the student has accepted the value without reservation. In the example of patient advocacy, a student might be observed convincing a fellow classmate to obtain a 12-lead ECG when indicated but not necessarily required, explaining how it may benefit this patient and protect the patient from harm. Or, a student might persist in obtaining an order for pain management when their partner does not want to bother.

Simply put, this level is characterized by two things: a choice and, at its best, consistency between choices.

As with the previous two levels, this level is dependent on the attainment of respond (Level 2) and receive (Level 1). It would be nearly impossible to have a student defend their position for providing pain management to a patient if the student did not first understand the negative effect on the patient both physiologically and psychologically (receiving) and did not possess the skill, ability, and desire to relieve that pain (responding). It is important for educators to be aware that both the student and the instructor can get "stuck" at this level. If an internal valuing process has not developed, students will not progress beyond this level but will appear to do everything that the instructor tells them to do. They will do it the way they are expected to, every time they are observed (i.e., when the instructor is around). What happens when they are not observed or the instructor is not there is another thing.

If the student has adopted the values of a significant other, such as a partner or another instructor or mentor, without examining or testing these values for themself, the values in question tend to be rigid and fixed. This tendency can be observed in the student or in the instructor. In the case of a student, the value may have been developed to gain approval from a rigid instructor, or the student may have lacked the confidence to take a risk. In the case of an instructor, the value may have developed because of lack of recent patient care experience, or the instructor may have perceived a questioning student as a threat. In either case, values tend to be fixed concepts and are rarely examined or tested; as a result, certain values become so rigid that the student or instructor refuses to further their knowledge, even when presented with information that is contradictory. Such individuals tend to feel threatened when their value system is questioned. Student comments that suggest that the student or instructor has gotten stuck include the following:

"That instructor doesn't know what he's talking about!"

"I've worked in the field for 20 years and I'm not going to change now!"

"It doesn't say that in the book!"

Instructor comments or nonverbal clues include:

"Do it this way because I say to do it this way!"

"Who are you to question me?!"

The field of medicine changes rapidly, and keeping up with these changes requires that practitioners go to continuing education events and subscribe to professional journals. Keeping an open mind, experimenting with students, and helping students to develop their reasoning skills all work to keep both the instructor and the student "unstuck." By extending one's own personal experiences to students, the educator can ensure that values are continually being reinforced or modified and kept up-to-date.

Classroom Implications. Elizabeth King maintains "the learning of an attitude occurs when a respected role model makes a verbal communication to the learner regarding desirable choices of action or displays these actions directly."[17] The implications of this statement are clear. Instructors must think about what they, as educators, say and do at all times. Instructors must display an interest in their students and accept, guide, and encourage them while giving them the tools they need to support their own conclusions. If a safe classroom environment has been maintained, students will find the freedom to fail, and in that failing, they will explore the values and choices the instructor has shown them in the classroom. Students need the chance to analyze and synthesize for themselves, so they can claim values as their own. Students can be helped in this process by an instructor who supplies them with a good background in general knowledge, and then forces them to explore new concepts and ideas, to analyze what they are learning, and to synthesize new ideas and concepts on "their own." An instructor may teach the definition of substance use disorder and associated signs and symptoms. But in order for all students to make decisions about their values associated with this population of patients, instructors will need to allow students to explore this topic further. For example, the instructor may ask students to create their own definition of a patient with substance use disorder or give scenarios where the student must judge the description of behavior in the scenario against the definitions created, possibly forcing students to explore (with instructor

CASE in Point

It was that unpopular time of year when the "last-minute crowd" registers for the required refresher courses. The EMS educator always dreaded these refreshers because they are heavily populated with the most experienced and hardened EMTs and paramedics—those who have waited until the last possible minute to register for their continuing education and refresher courses. To make matters worse, these experienced field providers view instructors as "ivory tower" has-beens who do not do the job anymore and do not even remember what it was like being in the field. To cap it off, the director made improvement of evaluations of the refresher courses one of the EMS educator's performance goals for the year. She was losing sleep over what to do, so she decided to stay up and read the EMS educator's textbook, where she found a few ideas that she thought might help her manage the situation.

As a first step, she set aside 5 days over 2 weeks to get out into the field and ride along with the crews. Second, she made a conscious decision to show respect for the EMS providers and their issues. She took the huge step of seeing situations from their perspective. After all, they are doing the job competently on a full-time basis all year and then they have to go into a classroom and practical labs to listen to a rehash of material that they believe they already know. Then they have to pretend to run codes and perform routine skills on plastic manikins. How boring it must be, she realized. This led her to a breakthrough concept. She decided to go out on a limb and redesign the presentation format. She kept the same course objectives, the same content, and the same presentation and reference resources, but she changed the way everything would be presented.

On the first day of class, she mingled with the participants over coffee, chatting about the calls that she had been on over the previous 2 weeks. Next, she handed out the course materials and went over the objectives and schedule. Then she made an announcement: "I'm not going to do any lecturing for this refresher. Because this is a refresher course, you are all very familiar with the content and how to do all the procedures. I'm going to ask you to 'discuss' the topics based on your experiences on calls. The only requirement will be that we all need to discuss every required topic in full. The way we do this will be up to you."

Everyone looked around uncomfortably. Most thought that it was going to be a complete disaster. To everyone's surprise, however, the group became animated, and a lively discussion began. Some participants tried to hijack the course and turn it into a social jam session, and others tried to become invisible, but most got on track and drove it in the right direction.

The result was a successful course that covered all course objectives and had a 100% pass rate on the final performance testing. The instructor, of course, was a nervous wreck after it was over, but the excellent course evaluations made it all worthwhile.

In this case, the EMS instructor took some real risks and allowed herself to be vulnerable. First, she spent rare and precious time in the field with crews, which helped to dispel the ivory tower stigma. Second, she decided that she would respect the responders and trust them. When she communicated this sincerely, they picked up on it and respected her and the process in return. Finally, she gave up the "security blanket" of presenting topics through traditional lectures in favor of letting participants form discussion groups and present their knowledge to each other. She realized that this approach might not work for every group or in every system, but she also suspected that opportunities for nontraditional approaches that incorporated trust and empowerment could probably be found in nearly every course, once she decided to look for them.

facilitation) the emotional issues around identification and care of these patients. All of this forms the basis for the next level.

It has been said that good judgment comes from experience, and experience comes from bad judgment. If this is true, wouldn't it be best to start the student's experience from bad judgment in the classroom so they will have good judgment in the field? One way to start this process is to present challenging, realistic simulations in the classroom, where it is safe for students to fail. After all, the patients are actors or plastic manikins, and their emergencies are not real. For simulations to be effective in helping students move through the valuing level of the affective domain, the same choices that they will face in the field must be made available in the classroom. Careful planning and coordination are necessary if students are to make the most of simulations in the classroom that will have real-world applicability in the field, clinic, or hospital.

Students who are stuck at this level are often found in continuing education classes. They are the ones who already have a strong value and belief system that they have formed over years of experience and other training. To get through to these students and really offer them a worthwhile educational experience, the educator must appreciate their educational experiences from the students' perspective. First, such students not only have ideas and concepts that are already deeply rooted and that work for them, they also frequently are fearful, and fear of failure is very strong for adults.[18] Their fear does not need to be realistic or rational from the perspective of the educator to be very real to the adult student learner. This fear need involve only a perceived threat. The most likely threat is that to the student's esteem and self-perception of competence, as failure is associated with incompetence. Therefore, the ideal strategy for the educator is to calm the fears of these students by making the classroom and laboratory a safe place to make and learn from their mistakes. This means that not only will instructors respect students, they will also insist that students respect each other. No horseplay, teasing, or ridicule should be tolerated if a student's performance is sub-par.

To achieve a change at this level when students are stuck, the educator can go back to the receive level and use techniques that have already been suggested, such as making the information or change relevant by conveying to students why the training is necessary. The educator can then move to the respond level by showing examples and asking for student responses to specific situations, then creating activities that require a response. The educator can then move to the value level, where learners will have a chance to tear the subject matter apart and put it together again (analysis and synthesis of the value in question). These activities generally are best accomplished through the use of challenging and realistic scenarios, case studies, or problem-based learning activities.

Level 4: Organize

During the formation of values and attitudes, students begin to recognize several values that apply to the same situation. Students begin to categorize these by how much worth the new value has in relationship to the other things they value that apply to this situation. By doing this, students establish an order of values that they can defend and justify. The more concretely the student can justify and defend their choices and actions, the more confident they will become. When this is done, the student is operating at Level 4, organize.

Classroom Implications. Information that instructors provide should allow students to begin to reason out the "whys." Instructors should start the reasoning in the classroom by monitoring and correcting student actions when necessary. For example, the instructor may ask students to compare patient situations, given two patients, both of whom are complaining of abdominal pain. One patient is a 25-year-old female, and the other is a 65-year-old female. Students can then be asked to discuss the keys of assessment (physical examination and history), explore the differential diagnosis, and compare treatment options. Then, the instructor can make the patient a 45-year-old with a history of alcohol use disorder and ask students to explain how this changes their answers and treatment choices.

Use of scenarios to force students to examine two values facilitates organization of knowledge, behaviors, and attitudes according to sound medical reasoning. Consider this example: A patient falls and twists her neck. Upon assessment, she is not breathing adequately. Clearing her airway does not improve her ventilations. The student is faced with performing spinal motion restriction with the patient in the position found, or gently moving her head and neck into alignment. What should the student choose and why? The instructor should have students justify their answers. The instructor should have discussions involving two choices, exceptions to the rule, and immediate life threats. These approaches help students to organize their decision-making process.

Use of scenarios is especially helpful at this level. Discussions of why certain signs and symptoms appear, what (if appropriate) expected signs/symptoms are not apparent and why that may be, and which treatment should be selected and why, all contribute to helping students justify their actions with the use of sound medical reasoning.

Level 5: Characterize

At this level, the value system is so ingrained in student behavior patterns that it becomes part of their lifestyle, and student values become integrated into a total philosophy of care. Experience is required to attain this level. Therefore, this level is not usually observed in the classroom unless continuing education is being taught to a group of seasoned providers.

The two steps that constitute this level help describe a person who has attained it:

1. **Consistency**: This means that when the student is confronted with a number of situations that involve a reaction based on the same value system or characteristics, the student's reactions are automatic and predictable. The key here is consistency. When confronted by a situation that demands a choice between values, the student is consistent in their choice and is able to consistently defend that choice with sound medical knowledge and judgment based on balancing of values, book learning, skills, and

experience. The instructor is able to predict how the student will act in a given situation. For example, a student who believes in treating all patients with dignity will consistently complete a full assessment and care plan for the intoxicated homeless patient regardless of how many times that same patient has called EMS. The instructor, or later, coworkers and supervisors, will be able to accurately predict that this provider will not take shortcuts or dismiss the patient simply because they have cared for the patient many times before.

2. **Characterization**: At this point the student is so closely associated with the value or characteristic in question that people use the characteristic to describe that student, like ALS Amy who tends to err on the side of caution and ride in with advanced life support measure in place on nearly every patient, or Safety Sam who always wears gloves and eye protection no matter how clean the patient appears. The student has integrated attitudes, values, and ideals into a total philosophy. Typically, this level is associated with a high level of student pride in accomplishment, as well as a high degree of satisfaction in work performed.

It is important for the instructor to recognize that student experiences may greatly contribute to their attaining this level in one area but not in all. For instance, students may attain the characterize level with behavioral patients, but they may attain only the first steps of the value level with pediatric patients. This may be because of the population groups they serve, or it may be a result of where their interest lies. The student interest and comfort levels dictate choices, such as a provider preferring to care for behavioral patients and preferring to have their partner care for pediatric patients.

Life events and peers, especially partners, receiving hospital staff, and administrators, may directly affect attainment of this level. A provider may demonstrate characteristics of this level but then vacillate between levels, depending on what is going on in their life. For instance, a provider may be on his way to acquiring the characterize level when the provider is suddenly faced with the death of a coworker, a divorce, administrative decisions that negatively affect their ability to deliver patient care, or a receiving hospital staff whose attitudes are demeaning. If enough stress is introduced that basic value systems are called into question, an individual may revert back to the receive or respond level. Personal stressors may become powerful inhibitors to acquiring or maintaining this level.

Classroom Implications. The most important action instructors can take is to model this level. Participating in continuing education as students, belonging to professional organizations, reading professional journals and discussing articles with students, extending their knowledge base to other disciplines, ensuring that classroom topics are relevant and applicable to the field, and being sensitive to what happens to students when they leave the classroom, all help to contribute to the acquisition of this level by instructors—not only for themselves, but also for students.

TEACHING TIP

Scenarios should provide the student with a problem to solve that can be achieved with choices in strategies.

Teaching Psychomotor Skills

The learning, mastery, and performance of skills are, and will remain, an important part of the medical field—from the medical assistant who takes vital signs to the surgeon performing a delicate operation. Therefore, it is imperative that medical educators be proficient in the teaching and evaluation of skills performance.

Psychomotor skills development is crucial to good patient care. All of the effort put forth at the scene of an EMS incident is dependent on the provider's ability to select the right skill, at the right time, and to carry it out in the right manner. In addition, many of the skills routinely performed at an EMS call are critical to patient survival and leave little or no margin for error. As an example, correct placement of an intraosseous infusion is vital to securing and maintaining a route for fluids and medications in an infant. However, this procedure allows no margin for error. The device must be placed in the correct location or the patient will not get needed medications. Thus, teaching paramedics to place intraosseous infusions must be done correctly, efficiently, and in a manner that ensures learner success. This can be accomplished only when the instructor has a solid understanding of psychomotor skills training, mastery, and performance.

Understanding the Psychomotor Domain

The psychomotor domain comprises the skill, action, muscle movement, and manual manipulation related to performing a physical action. Similar to all domains, the physical activities addressed in the psychomotor domain also have affective and cognitive dimensions. A learner who is being taught to start an intravenous line (IV) not only needs to learn the physical movements and manipulations needed to insert an IV catheter, but must also appreciate the discomfort the procedure causes, an element of the affective domain, as well as the why and when associated with starting an IV, which is the "psycho," or cognitive, part of the psychomotor domain. In addition, the context or environment in which the skill will be performed is important. Many medical procedures are carried out in a field environment that is very different from that of a hospital or classroom. As one of the basic parts of a behavioral objective, a condition is specified under which the desired behavior is to occur. (See Chapter 9, *Goals and Objectives*, for further discussion.) When psychomotor skills are taught, it is imperative that the instructor stress, and if possible simulate, the various conditions in the classroom in order to prepare the student to perform those skills in real-world settings such as with the patient seated in a lab chair, lying in a hospital bed, or ambulatory at the scene of a motor vehicle crash. It would be unfair for a learner to master a technique while not wearing personal protective equipment (PPE), and then suddenly find that they are unable to perform, or feel awkward performing, the same skill in a field setting wearing PPE. And, as with all learning experiences, modeling plays an important part. It is imperative, therefore, that the instructor and all other instructional personnel carry out skills and procedures in a manner consistent with that expected of the learner. In this example, the instructors should therefore wear gloves and goggles while demonstrating the skill.

When teaching psychomotor skills, the instructor must consider learner "prerequisites" needed if the student is to learn the cognitive material. The ability of the learner to actually perform a skill is dependent on a number of parameters. The instructor should consider the following:

- **Physical strength of the learner**. Can the learner, for instance, lift a stretcher containing a 150-pound patient? Can the student carry equipment and equipment containers up a flight of stairs?
- **Physical endurance**. Can the learner perform cardiopulmonary resuscitation (CPR) at the proper rate and depth for several minutes at a time?
- **Coordination**. Does the learner possess significant coordination and fine motor control, or is the student "all thumbs"?
- **Sensory acuity**. Can the learner see fine detail? Exhibit sufficient depth perception? Does the student wear bifocal glasses that make intubation difficult? Can the student hear well enough to note different heart tones or breath sounds?
- **Composure**. How does the learner perform under stress? Does the student develop tremors that interfere with delicate procedures? Does the learner become impatient, and thus tend to perform skills hastily or without proper attention to detail? Conversely, if the skill produces discomfort for the patient, does the student freeze and fail to complete the skill?[19]

The instructor is cautioned that when these parameters are assessed, measures appropriate to the actual job description of the provider should be followed, as should the requirements of the Americans with Disabilities Act. (For more information on the Americans with Disabilities Act, see Chapter 25, *Legal Issues for EMS Educators*.)

Levels of Psychomotor Skills Development

It would be convenient if learners could see a skill demonstrated once and then be able to exactly reproduce the skill immediately and permanently. However, this is not the case. Learning a skill and assimilating it into a rote response involves a number of developmental steps. As with the other domains of learning, a taxonomy of psychomotor skills development has been devised. For the purposes of this textbook, Bloom's taxonomy of psychomotor skills development is used.

Bloom's Taxonomy: Psychomotor Domain

Level 1: Imitation
Level 2: Manipulation
Level 3: Precision
Level 4: Articulation
Level 5: Naturalization

Imitation

The most basic psychomotor skill is repeating or modeling a skill that is demonstrated to the learner by an expert. In this "see one, do one" approach, the instructor demonstrates the skill, then asks learners to repeat it. Usually, the instructor talks or guides the learner through the steps of the skill. This method works best for skills that are simple and can be understood easily through observation. For more complex skills, the instructor begins the learning process at the imitation stage by breaking down the complex skill into simpler, more easily learned skills that can be modeled by the beginner. Because learners are receptive to modeling the behavior of the instructor or another expert, it is important that the instructor avoid modeling incorrectly. This can be difficult because the instructor has progressed to the naturalization level and may not be cognizant of how they are performing the skill. However, should a skill be modeled incorrectly, it will take many more practice attempts to "untrain" the incorrect behavior than it would have taken to teach the behavior to mastery level in the first place.

Manipulation

The second phase of skills mastery is manipulation. During this stage, learners move away from simple modeling to performing the skill according to guidelines, such as skills sheets. They "manipulate" the various parts of the skill in such a way as to develop their own basis or foundation for doing the skill. Because learners are still exploring the skill, mistakes are common and are to be expected. Mistakes help learners to better understand the skill through the corrective actions needed. It is important for the instructor to closely monitor learners as they practice skills to ensure that no incorrect actions or bad habits are learned as part of the skill. Because each learner is different, some variation in performance may occur, but by and large, the learner must perform the skill as modeled by the instructor or according to the skills sheet or established standard. It is also important at this stage for the instructor to explain to learners why a particular action or technique is used. This is especially important if skills taught later in the program will require this action. For example, proper placement of limb leads in obtaining an ECG may not be critical for a 4-lead ECG, but it becomes more important when a 12-lead ECG is obtained.

This is also the period during which the learner begins independent practice of the skill. It is important that skills sheets or procedures be explained clearly and in sufficient detail. Practice sessions should be observed closely, and any incorrect behaviors should be immediately identified and corrected. Because the learner is discovering the new skill, peer practice with a lab partner may provide a supportive environment and can allow learners to explore the new skill together.

Precision

At the precision stage, the learner can perform the basic skill without coaching or the skills sheet and with few, if any, mistakes. However, the learner still has not developed the expertise to perform the skill in various contexts. For example, the learner may be able to splint a fractured arm on a simulated patient who is sitting up without angulation. However, any variation of the patient position or severity of injury, such as the patient lying down, will reduce the learner's precision. Precision is often the level students are at when they are tested on a psychomotor skill. They can perform the skill correctly without the skills sheet, but only in a controlled environment without distraction or variation.

Specific feedback and **deliberate practice** will help develop precision. Specific feedback is given so learners can deliberately practice that component of the skill performance without an instructor or evaluator having to be present.[20] One must be thoughtful in order to give feedback specific enough to allow deliberate practice. For example, if a student were not successful at intubation, to say that they "are holding the laryngoscope at the wrong angle" would be accurate feedback. However, it is not enough information to allow the student to correct their behavior without further intervention by the instructor. In this situation, specific feedback might sound something like, "hold the laryngoscope and aim for where the ceiling meets the wall in your line of sight; that will always give you the correct angle to view the structures of the airway."

Articulation

Articulation blends psychomotor skills development with the cognitive and affective dimensions of a skill or procedure. The learner understands why the skill is done in a particular way and knows when the skill is indicated. The learner can now evaluate the context in which the skill is performed and can adjust performance to the situation. In the earlier example, the learner would now be able to splint an arm, regardless of patient position or other conditions. The learner is now performing the skill without mistakes and without the assistance of aids such as skills sheets or instructor prompting. This is the level of psychomotor skills performance that is expected of an entry-level provider. However, students are often never tested at this level. Given constraints on classroom and lab time, students may not get past the precision level in class. Often, clinical time, internship, or even on-the-job-training is required to reach the articulation level. Instructors should be aware that potential employers may be expecting a higher level of performance than can be delivered by a new graduate of their medical educational program.

In an attempt to assist with this expectation mismatch, the National Registry of EMTs has implemented integrated out-of-hospital scenario-based testing of paramedic candidates. Because this is how students will be tested for licensure, many programs have begun practicing more challenging scenarios to develop the integration of cognitive, psychomotor, and affective skills of students in order to assist them in passing the exam. As a result, employers of these new graduates have been reporting that they feel the recent graduates are more field-ready than in the past when testing was primarily focused on discrete skills.

Naturalization

At this stage, the learner can perform the skill flawlessly and without much conscious effort. In a scenario, simulation, or actual patient care situation, the learner will be able to perform the skill while continuing to monitor the context and environment. The learner will be able to multitask effectively (**FIGURE 12.5**). The learner has achieved what is known as "muscle memory"; that is, the skill has become rote and can be initiated and performed with minimal sensory awareness. A common example of this level of mastery is the provider who is seen performing a manual skill, such as a pulse or neuro-check, while obtaining an oral history from the patient. This level is rarely seen in the classroom learner or entry-level provider. It develops later as the provider gains experience on the job.

Psychomotor Skills Instruction

Effective teaching of psychomotor skills involves more than just demonstrating a skill and having learners practice. As with any instructional activity, preparation and teaching technique are important aspects of the overall experience. This is especially true in the psychomotor domain because of the complexity of many EMS skills.

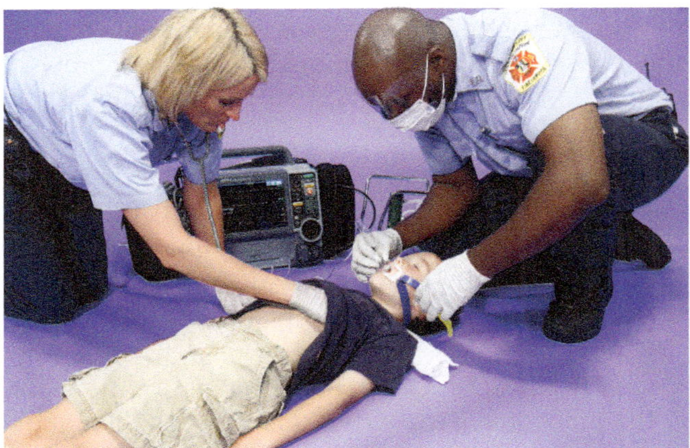

FIGURE 12.5 Naturalization of a psychomotor skill is achieved when the student is able to multitask effectively.

Because EMS skills almost always involve equipment and, to be effectively demonstrated, usually require special teaching aids or manikins, preparation is important. To begin, the instructor must review the lesson goal, objectives, and lesson plan to ensure that they are familiar with the lesson. Necessary equipment, supplies, and teaching aids should be identified and secured. The instructor is cautioned not to assume that equipment and materials will be available in the classroom. This is especially true in multiuse facilities, where different instructors and different classes may meet in the same facility. If the instructor arranges for an in-service unit to provide lesson props, a backup plan should be in place in the event the unit suddenly becomes unavailable. The same applies to lessons planned for outdoors that may be canceled or modified because of weather.

When setting up the classroom or drill ground, the instructor should consider the following:

- **Safety**. The instructor should consider safety, not only in terms of practice by the learners, but as it relates to any inherent danger associated with demonstrating the skill. For example, caution is needed when demonstrating automobile extrication skills. Vehicles and equipment can shift or parts may fly off during certain activities. The instructor should clearly define and mark safe zones. Other safety considerations include sharps, medical waste, restraining of simulated patients on hard surfaces, and lifting and moving exercises.
- **Visibility**. For the learner to model and imitate a skill, the learner must be able to see all aspects of the process. Therefore, it is important that the instructor provide visibility. This may involve moving learners, breaking into small groups, using video demonstrations, or using special, large-scale models or cameras and video projectors.
- **Rehearsal**. Regardless of how many times an instructor has performed a skill or how well an instructor can do it, it is always prudent to practice the skill before class. This is especially true when using special models or equipment that differs from routinely used equipment. Nothing kills an instructor's credibility more readily than an inability to use the equipment that the instructor is using to teach. If something is to go wrong, it will surely happen during the class session.
- **Classroom preparation**. The instructor should arrange the classroom to ensure visibility and to accommodate the equipment and instructional props.

The instructor should check in advance for electrical or oxygen connections, venting, and so forth.

- **Practice space**. If learners are to practice a particular skill, the instructor must ensure that sufficient space and appropriate equipment are provided at each skills practice area. If learners will rearrange a classroom before they begin practice, the instructor must ensure that the furniture can actually be moved and that doing so will not be disruptive to the learning process.
- **Group size**. Most physical or psychomotor educational programs recommend no more than a 10:1 student to instructor ratio to ensure students are properly supervised, can see all demonstrations, and will receive adequate practice time and feedback from the instructor. However, many programs find that 6:1 is a more realistic ratio, and that regardless of group size, students will rarely get enough practice to reach precision, articulation, or naturalization levels during class time. A skills disclaimer or statement in the course policy manual alerting students to the fact that they will need to practice outside of scheduled classroom and laboratory hours will help set this expectation.

Whole-Part-Whole Instruction

The standard technique used for teaching EMS skills is the **whole-part-whole method**. To use this technique, the student is exposed to the skill three times:

1. **Whole**. The instructor demonstrates the entire skill from beginning to end, either live or via prerecorded video, while briefly naming each action or step. If possible, the skill should be performed under the conditions specified in the psychomotor behavioral objective, such as "The paramedic student will successfully demonstrate initiating an IV line on a patient in the emergency department with no critical errors." Because it is so important that the initial imprint is a perfect demonstration, many instructors choose to use a video of the skill for the first "whole" demonstration. Because video can be edited, the instructor can ensure that the demonstration is a match for the established technique or standard.
2. **Part**. The instructor demonstrates the skill again, step-by-step, explaining each part in detail. It is important that the instructor select proper size "bites" of the skill. If the information is too specific, the learner can be overloaded with detail; too broad, and the learner may not be able to make the connection from step to step. The instructor should be cognizant of the limits of working memory and choose bites of the skill with no more than 3 to 5 steps.
3. **Whole**. The instructor demonstrates the entire skill from beginning to end, without interruption, and usually without commentary.

This technique provides repeated, accurate examples of how the skill is done. If a learner was not completely focused on the skill demonstration the first time, two other opportunities for observation are provided. This approach also provides a rationale for how the skill has been performed. During the part presentation, the instructor can integrate affective and cognitive objectives and encourage student interaction and questions. Finally, it has been proven that the technique works well for both analytic and global learners. Analytic learners appreciate the step-by-step instruction, and global learners get the chance to see the skill performed in context.

Progression through the Psychomotor Domain Levels of Skills Acquisition

As has been discussed, the learner moves through a progression of increasing proficiency, eventually reaching the mastery level. When teaching psychomotor skills, the instructor must provide an environment that fosters this development.

The instructor should first work with learners to move from novice to expert, that is, being able to perform the skill at the precision level. When moving learners in this direction, the instructor should keep the following in mind:

- Learners should be allowed to progress at their own pace. If learners are moved too quickly, they may not understand what they are doing and will not acquire good thinking skills.
- Although the demonstration may provide information on the performance of the entire skill from start to finish, learners should be allowed to learn the individual parts of the skill before pulling it all together and demonstrating the whole skill. For example, learners may need to learn how to hold or operate a piece of equipment before they can be taught the sequence of applying or using the device.

- Learners should be at the precision level of individual skills before being placed in the context of a scenario or simulation.
- Instructors should implement skills in context or use mini-scenarios as students demonstrate proficiency in the discrete skill steps but before moving to complex simulations. Mini-scenarios involve a small amount of decision making and incorporate the skill. For example, the mini-scenario might be that the student arrives to find a bleeding patient already loaded into a basic life support (BLS) ambulance but in need of an IV. The student must decide needle size, type and quantity of fluid, and location to start the IV but does not have to complete an assessment beginning with the primary and moving all the way through loading the patient into the ambulance.
- Learners should be allowed ample time to practice a skill before they are tested. Some programs allow students to declare to the instructor when they feel ready to test skills.
- The need for constant direct supervision should diminish as practice time increases and skill level improves. Research shows that peer evaluation is accurate and effective at improving practice and performance.[21]

Taking these factors into consideration, the instructor should plan skills learning to follow a sequence similar to the following:

1. The instructor provides demonstration of the skill to learners three times using the whole-part-whole method, either live or via video.
2. Learners attempt the skill under direct supervision of the instructor, who can correct sequencing or technique mistakes before or as they happen.
3. Learners practice with a lab partner using a skills check sheet.
4. Learners practice the steps of the skill until they can verbalize the sequence without error.
5. Learners perform the skill, stating each step as they perform it.
6. Learners perform the skill while answering questions about their performance.
7. Learners perform the skill in context of a scenario or an actual patient situation (FIGURE 12.6).

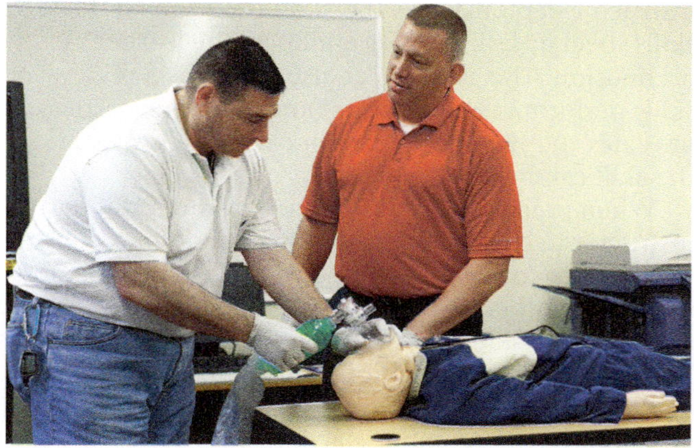

FIGURE 12.6 Learners should move through a progression of increasing proficiency and achieve mastery before using skills on real patients.

Honest feedback about the learner's performance should be provided regularly. The instructor should not hesitate to correct improper performance, but whenever possible the instructor should also include positive feedback, to ensure that the learner continues the correct behaviors while modifying the actions that were not quite right. This is especially critical during the early stages of skills development. If incorrect behaviors are not effectively corrected, mastery or muscle memory of the wrong technique will occur, and correcting this later on will be more difficult. The instructor may allow advanced learners to identify and correct their own errors under limited supervision. To reinforce correct behaviors, the instructor could end practice sessions with a demonstration of correct performance.

As a learner becomes proficient at a skill, it is important for the instructor to appreciate the level of performance required of the learner at this stage in their education and career. Too often, instructors and practical test evaluators expect a learner to perform a skill at a level beyond that attainable by an entry-level provider. Some instructors and evaluators expect performance that matches their own level of mastery. This is not only an unrealistic expectation, it is also unfair to the learner. It is important for instructors and evaluators to accept that many skills may be performed in a number of different but medically acceptable ways. Just because a learner performs a skill in a way that differs from the instructor's performance does not mean that the learner's performance is wrong, unless it is medically incorrect or may harm the patient.

Skills Sheets

When new skills are taught, it is important for the learner to know clearly what is involved in the skill, in terms of both actions and sequence. Although the instructor demonstrates the skill, the use of a detailed skills sheet or task analysis enhances the learner's comprehension. The skills sheet also serves as a review for skills performance. For visual and concrete learners, it provides the needed framework on which mastery of the skill can be built.

When preparing a skills sheet, it is important for the instructor to clearly list the various steps of the skill at a level consistent with that used in the teaching demonstration. In other words, if six steps are demonstrated in completing a skill, the skills sheet should list six steps. The skills sheet should not be used to break the skill down to a level that is more finite than the one taught, or conversely, to compress actions into fewer steps. It is also important for the instructor to design the skills sheet with emphasis on areas that are critical to proper skills performance and subsequent skills evaluation. If process is important, it should be included. Likewise, if sequence is important, sequencing should be delineated on the skills sheet, and it should be clearly communicated to the learner that it is important.

A common practice is for instructors to provide students with the practical evaluation skills sheets of the National Registry of Emergency Medical Technicians (NREMT) for use during practice. While it is appropriate for students to have and use the National Registry skills sheets, it should be remembered that these were intended as evaluation tools, not teaching tools, and they lack sufficient step-by-step detail for the student new to the skill to understand how and why each step is executed. A skills video, skills manual, or skills textbook may be necessary in addition to the skills sheets.

Improving Psychomotor Skills Development during a Skills Session

Skills sessions provide valuable time for the learner to practice and master skills. However, for full support of skills mastery, it is important that the skills session be used to maximum advantage. To accomplish this, the instructor should keep the following in mind:

- Have all necessary equipment set up before the session begins. However, if the set-up is complicated or the class is large, the instructor may have the learners retrieve equipment from a storage area and set up the practice stations. In a similar manner, learners can be asked to put away the equipment.
- Use realistic and current equipment that is in proper working order. Do not expect learners to master a skill if they do not have the right equipment to use.
- Use standardized teaching tools such as skills videos and skills sheets.
- Allow ample practice time in class, at breaks, and during other times. However, ensure that all practice sessions are conducted safely and with proper supervision as needed.
- Always model correct psychomotor skills behavior.
- Keep learners active and involved. This can be difficult, especially as learners become more proficient; they may not wish to engage in repeated practice of a skill. Consider adding context to practice, such as placing the manikin on the floor, or in a chair, or under a table to simulate different positions in which patients may be found.
- Insist that learners respect equipment and skills as part of the affective evaluation.
- Ensure competence in individual skills before using scenarios. Scenarios should be designed to tie together basic skills, once they have been mastered.
- Consider videotaping a skill and allow students to review their performance.
- Add realism. It is important for the instructor to place skills in the context of on-the-job situations. When using scenarios, do the following:
  - Limit the objective of the scenario to three learning points.
  - As learners become more sophisticated with the use of critical-thinking skills, add dimensions to the scenario.
  - Make the scenario realistic, especially in terms of the performance objective and the safety requirements, such as wearing PPE.
  - Insist that students perform every step; do not allow only verbalization.
  - Consider the use of moulage, props, background noises, and so forth.

TEACHING TIP

When practicing skills, students perform all aspects of the skill; the instructor should not allow students to only verbalize some parts of the skill. For example, if the student is practicing intubation, it is not enough to say, "I would apply capnography." The student must have a device or prop to apply so their motor memory develops. If the student does not perform the steps of the skills in practice, they are less likely to do so in real life.

Managing the Skills Session

Skills practice time is an essential component for skills mastery to occur, especially in certification courses like

EMT. It is imperative that the instructor plan practice time to provide maximum opportunity for the learner to master skills. This is best achieved when some degree of structure is provided during the session. Simply providing a room full of equipment and instructing students to practice skills will usually result in chaos and little active practice. This is especially true when learners are reviewing skills that they believe they have already mastered. Instructors teaching refresher or renewal courses are often faced with the challenge of motivating learners to perform skills they believe they already know. To ensure maximum use of practice time, the instructor should plan activities to keep the whole class engaged for the entire length of the practice session. This is especially important if only one or two instructors are managing a large class.[22]

After appropriate introductory material and with adequate resources such as skills checklists, some student groups can be independently assigned for peer evaluation. A few issues about the use of assistant instructors must be mentioned. Assistants can be a great help to an instructor, and they may provide direct assistance and feedback to learners. However, it is important that the lead instructor and assistant instructors teach the same skill in the same manner. Instructor development meetings where the teaching tools, skills sheets, equipment, and evaluation tools can be reviewed together can go a long way in helping assistant instructors remain consistent with program goals. **Interrater reliability (IRR)** exercises should be conducted for all evaluators. IRR is the process of calibrating instructors to the evaluation tool so that each instructor is grading exactly the same way. Often, a video of a medical skill is played, then the student in the video is rated by all instructors present. Scores for the student are shared; often they are wildly different. A lead instructor or program director then reviews the skill, the standard, and the evaluation tool with the instructors. The group then watches the same video again, grading according to the instruction they just received. Usually, the scores among all instructors are now much closer together. If necessary, the process can be repeated several times until all evaluators understand which behaviors should and should not be counted as correct.

Maximizing Skills Session Time

To ensure that practice time is used as efficiently as possible, instructors should plan activities to fill the entire instruction time. Instructors should consider assigning roles to learners during skills practice. In this way, learners will have the chance to practice different skills and rotate through different roles during the skills practice. This approach works well to occupy learners who otherwise would be waiting to practice a skill or to move on to the next skill. Detailed skills sheets allow students to self- and peer-evaluate during the skills sessions.

Learners can be assigned to the following roles, depending on the size of the practice group:

- **Evaluator**. The evaluator uses a skills sheet or records steps as they are performed. This allows learners to appreciate the challenge of evaluating a skill and reinforces learning through observation of the skill that is being performed.
- **Facilitator**. The facilitator uses a script and provides information as it is requested—for instance, vital signs appropriate for the scenario when they are taken.
- **Team leader**. The team leader is the primary patient care provider and leader of the team performing the skills.
- **Team members**. The team members assist the team leader and perform care as directed by the team leader; depending on practice parameters, they may be silent or may be able to suggest and interact with the team leader. More than one team member or partner may be needed for safety, such as during spinal motion restriction or patient restraint. Team members are expected to perform delegated tasks competently and in a manner consistent with the principles of **crew resource management** (**FIGURE 12.7**), utilizing appreciative inquiry to alert the leader if they observe a dangerous mistake or omission.[23]
- **Patient**. The patient faithfully portrays signs and symptoms according to the scenario and may be moulaged for realism. This role also familiarizes the learner with the experiences of the patient and promotes empathy.
- **Bystander**. Additional practice team members can assume the role of bystanders and can act as distracters or helpers. It is important for the instructor to monitor learners in this role to ensure that they do not get too carried away with their role-playing, thereby disrupting the actual practice of the skill in a realistic setting.
- Additional roles, if groups are large, might include first responders, members of the fire department or law enforcement, or a hospital charge nurse to whom the report will be given. Scribes who are recording the performance of discrete skills within the scenario such as bag-mask ventilation or IV initiation are needed to ensure skills performed during scenarios are added to the student's psychomotor portfolio.

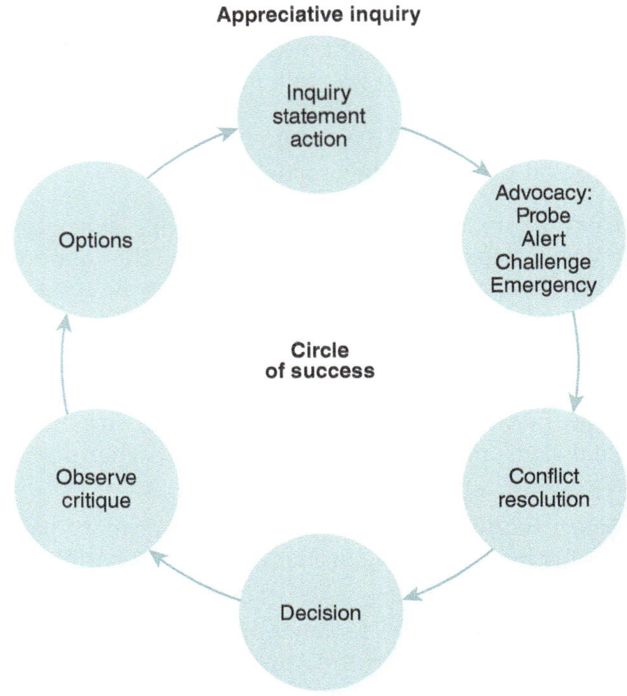

FIGURE 12.7 The principles of crew resource management.

When designing a practice session, the instructor should either assign students to write scenarios or distribute a written scenario to practice groups. The scenario should be realistic for the learner's level of expertise and local operational capability. It should also match the performance objective that is being reviewed. Sources of scenarios include actual calls, medical scenario books, EMS textbooks, instructor resources, and professional organization websites.

To begin the practice session, the instructor should have the facilitator read the dispatch information. Whenever possible, learners should be allowed to complete the scenario without interruption. At this point, the learner should have mastered individual skills, so stopping for correction should not be necessary. Once the scenario has been completed, the group as a whole should evaluate skills performance, beginning with the team leader. By allowing the team leader to identify their own mistakes, the instructor is able to determine the degree of self-awareness possessed by the team leader. Additionally, the instructor can compare the learner's self-assessment to the instructor's own assessment of the same, helping to calibrate the learner to the standard of professional performance.

The various role players should next be called on to critique the performance. Remember that learners are often their own greatest critics. They should be encouraged to look for the positive aspects of their performance. Otherwise, they may focus on what they perceive as poor performance. The team members, patient, and bystanders should all take turns providing feedback. Finally, the evaluator should comment on timing, sequencing, prioritization, and skills performance.

Regardless of how an evaluator is issuing the critique, it should be a positive learning experience—not a learner bashing. To provide a positive experience, a positive-negative-positive format is often used; however this method has come under scrutiny in recent years. It has been suggested that the positive-negative-positive approach, or "feedback sandwich" as it has been called, is manipulative and minimizes the value of anything positive said because the listener already knows something negative is coming and will focus only on the negative.[24] To make sure this does not happen, the positive feedback should be specific and personal, focused on a single behavior in a single discussion. The instructor should next move to constructive feedback and areas for improvement, citing specific actions or decisions of concern. Comments must be consistent with what learners have been taught, and they must follow the skills sheet. The instructor should end the review with a positive comment such as: "I was especially impressed by how you applied the traction splint, given the location of the fracture."

Once the scenario has been critiqued, learners should change roles. Sufficient scenarios and time should be provided for all learners to have at least one chance to play each role. However, time constraints may not permit this, so it may be helpful for students to develop a rotation in their group where the roles are rotated not just during one skills lab, but each time the students are practicing skills. Additionally, instructors may want to script the scenarios to ensure that by the end of the course each group has participated in a sufficient variety of patient care situations.

Tracking of skills and scenarios is a requirement for paramedic program accreditation. Programs will, in concert with their medical directors and community stakeholders, set minimum requirements for patient complaints and presentations, as well as individual skills performed. Skills and assessments are to be completed in a variety of settings, from the lab and scenarios to real patients during clinical and field internship experiences. These experiences should be recorded in each student's psychomotor portfolio and represent the student's developing competency over time and in a variety of settings. Each performance should be a measured encounter, graded either by a peer, instructor, or preceptor.

CASE in Point

The EMS instructor was conducting the cardiac arrest skills session for six EMT students. He began by asking, "Who wants to be the team leader first?" A lively, bright, and aggressive student jumped up to the head of the manikin and said, "I'll do it." The information provider presented the case of a witnessed arrest with bystander CPR and no on-scene automated external defibrillator (AED) present when the crew arrives.

"The first thing I'm going to do is standard precautions and scene safety, and I'll determine whether I need any help. Are there any other patients? Any hazards, like downed electrical lines? He didn't get electrocuted, did he?" He immediately gave out team assignments to check for unresponsiveness and signs of breathing, assess for the presence of a pulse, start CPR beginning with chest compressions, and apply the AED. After the AED indicated a need for shock, everyone stood clear while it delivered a shock. Chest compressions were restarted and the other team member alternated with bag-mask ventilation until the next shock was indicated. The instructor then conducted a brief critique of the session, allowing the patient care provider to go first, then allowing others in the group to provide input.

Addressing the team leader, he said, "Your initial steps and team management were well organized and effective. Well done." To the team member who managed the airway, he said, "Your assessment and ventilations were fine, but you didn't use an oropharyngeal airway. I was wondering why not?" After the team member shrugged and looked around for support, the instructor said, "I understand you may have overlooked it, but realize that the oropharyngeal airway is the most neglected adjunct in the basic life support tool kit. Everybody should keep it in mind. Can you think of why?" The discussion went on with the instructor providing constructive nonjudgmental feedback in a positive learning environment.

This was a typical cardiovascular skills assessment session in which realistic manikins, an AED, and airway and ventilation devices were provided. The instructor's feedback to participants was nonjudgmental, honest, and helpful. The organized setup, combined with a qualified and prepared instructor, provided the next best learning environment after actual clinical settings.

Summary

Comprehensive EMS education involves teaching in every domain and at all levels. Educators must be conscious of the three domains of learning and must apply appropriate teaching methods for the purpose of developing competent, compassionate care providers. In addition to giving attention to each domain, the educator must be aware of the multiple levels of learning that students go through in becoming fully competent. Each level requires that the instructor (1) be aware of the signs of progress and (2) know the teaching methods that help move students toward higher levels of learning and critical thinking.

Critical thinking skills can be encouraged through models that encourage active behavior, such as use of a flipped classroom, use of the T.H.I.N.K model, and inclusion of thinking-skills development exercises implemented throughout the course. It is important for educators to gain a sense of which thinking skills students have mastered and which ones they have not, then craft strategies to build such skills. In terms of assessment, quizzes and exams should include a range of items that test both lower- and higher-level knowledge and skills, in order to position the student for success on national licensing exams.

Teaching people skills is also critical to developing a generation of caring, compassionate providers. Instructors must be aware of the values, judgments, and beliefs that are inherent in their teaching. Educators must have a solid understanding of the eleven professional behaviors that reflect competency in the affective domain, and must model these behaviors.

In addition to affective skills, psychomotor skills are crucial to good patient care. Learning a skill and assimilating it into a rote response involve a number of developmental steps. Instructors should develop skill instruction such that sessions move students through the levels of skill acquisition, from novice to expert, in progressive steps, providing feedback on a regular basis. It is important to invest in preparation to ensure equipment, materials, and logistics are addressed in advance. To prepare students for licensure, once students have reached the articulation level, it may be useful to practice challenging scenarios to develop integration of cognitive, psychomotor, and affective skills.

Glossary

active behavior Student is actively thinking or doing something to learn.

command response Requirement of the student.

crew resource management Team management strategy to ensure safety in environments that have a high acuity for human error.

critical thinking Higher-level cognitive skills or problem-solving skills.

deliberate practice Practice of specific components of psychomotor skills based on specific feedback.

facilitation Assisting a learner in discovering information or their own abilities.

higher-order thinking Relating to Bloom's higher cognitive levels, including analysis, synthesis, evaluation, critical thinking, and problem solving.

interrater reliability (IRR) Consistency among evaluators or evaluation methods.

mastery Possession of a skill.

metacognition Thinking about thinking; literally, "in the midst of knowing"; an awareness and control of one's thinking.

mnemonics Patterns that are used to assist in recall and that are made from the first letter of each word in a phrase; for example, OPQRST to obtain present and past medical histories in patients with pain.

passive behavior Student is not engaged or active but only receives information or ideas.

safe classroom Environment in which the student feels little risk of emotional harm while actively participating in learning activities.

satisfaction response Voluntary response that brings on a sense of self-esteem.

specific feedback Feedback or critique of a skill with enough direction and detail to allow the learner to practice and correct performance without the instructor having to be present.

T.H.I.N.K. A model or system; a mnemonic used for a model to teach critical-thinking skills that stands for "T," total recall; "H," habits; "I," inquiry; "N," new ideas and creativity; and "K," knowing how you think.

whole-part-whole method Teaching technique that first provides the big picture, then breaks it into separate parts and steps, then completes the technique with another overview of the big picture.

willing response Students respond of their own accord.

References

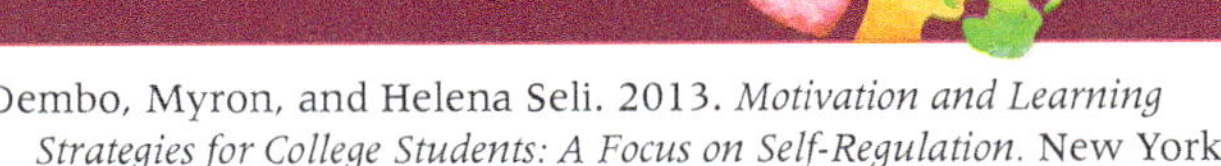

[1] Anderson, Lorin W., and David R. Krathwohl (Eds.). 2001. *A Taxonomy for Learning, Teaching, and Assessing: A Revision of Bloom's Taxonomy of Educational Objectives*. New York: Pearson.

[2] Dewey, John. 1963. *Experience and Education*. New York: Collier.

[3] Stiggins, Richard J., Evelyn Rubel, and Edys S. Quellmakz. 1986. *Measuring Thinking Skills in the Classroom*. Washington, DC: National Education Association.

[4] Lawler, Ron, Elias Frick, Ben Getsug, Brian Hendrickson, Sara Houston, Evelyn Hunter, Andy Lovell., et al. 2015. "Early Exposure to Valid Test Items Improves EMT Student Performance on Summative Exams." *Prehospital Emergency Care* (PEC) abstract. Accessed February 19, 2019. http://www.fisdap.net/research/projects/early_exposure.

[5] Costa, Arthur L., Robert Hanson, Harvey F. Silver, and Richard W. Strong. 1985. "Building a Repertoire of Strategies." In *Developing Minds: A Resource Book for Teaching Thinking*, edited by Arthur L. Costa, 141–3. Alexandria, VA: Association for Supervision and Curriculum Development.

[6] Beyer, Barry K. 1987. *Practical Strategies for the Teaching of Thinking*. Boston: Allyn and Bacon.

[7] Rubenfeld, M. Gale, and Barbara K. Scheffer. 1995. *Critical Thinking in Nursing: An Interactive Approach*. Philadelphia: J. B. Lippincott.

[8] Cowan, Nelson. 2010. "The Magical Mystery Four: How Is Working Memory Capacity Limited, and Why?" *Current Directions in Psychological Science* 19, no. 1: 51–7. https://doi.org/10.1177/0963721409359277

[9] Dembo, Myron, and Helena Seli. 2013. *Motivation and Learning Strategies for College Students: A Focus on Self-Regulation*. New York: Routledge.

[10] Brown, Roger, and James Kulik. 1977. "Flashbulb Memories." *Cognition* 5, no. 1: 73–99. https://doi.org/10.1016/0010-0277(77)90018-X.

[11] Beyer, Barry K. 1988. *Developing a Thinking Skills Program*. Boston: Allyn and Bacon.

[12] Govindarajan, Prasanthi, Benjamin T. Friedman, James Q. Delgadillo, David Ghilarducci, Lawrence J. Cook, Barbara Grimes, Charles McCulloch, and S. Claiborne Johnston. 2015. "Race and Sex Disparities in Prehospital Recognition of Acute Stroke." *Academic Emergency Medicine* 22, no. 3: 264–72. https://doi.org/10.1111/acem.12595.

[13] Kudenchuk, Peter J., Charles Maynard, Jenny S. Martin, Mark Wirkus, and W. Douglas Weaver. 1996. "Comparison of Presentation, Treatment, and Outcome of Acute Myocardial Infarction in Men versus Women (The Myocardial Infarction Triage and Intervention Registry)." *The American Journal of Cardiology* 78, no. 1: 9–14. https://doi.org/10.1016/S0002-9149(96)00218-4.

[14] Croskerry, Pat. 2007. "The Affective Imperative: Coming to Terms with Our Emotions." *Society for Academic Emergency Medicine* 14, no. 2: 184–6.

[15] Lorber, Michael A., and Walter D Pierce. 1983. *Objectives, Methods, and Evaluation for Secondary Teaching*, 2nd ed. Englewood Cliffs, NJ: Prentice Hall.

[16] Norman, Geoffrey R. 2000. "The Adult Learner: A Mythical Species." *Academic Medicine* 75, no. 3: 217–8. https://doi.org/10.1097/00001888-199908000-00011.

[17] King, Elizabeth C. 1984. *Affective Education in Nursing: A Guide to Teaching and Assessment*. Rockville, MD: Aspen System.

[18] Wlodkowski, Raymond J. 1999. *Enhancing Adult Motivation to Learn*. San Francisco: Jossey-Bass.

[19] Sage, George H. 1984. *Motor Learning and Control: A Neuropsychological Approach*. Dubuque, IA: W.C. Brown.

[20] Ericsson, K. Anders. 2004. "Deliberate Practice and the Acquisition and Maintenance of Expert Performance in Medicine and Related Domains." *Academic Medicine* 79, no. 10: S70–81. https://dx.doi.org/10.1097/00001888-200410001-00022.

[21] Field, Max, Joanne M. Burke, David McAllister, and David M Lloyd, 2007. "Peer-Assisted Learning: A Novel Approach to Clinical Skills Learning for Medical Students." *Medical Education* 41, no. 4: 411–8. https://doi.org/10.1111/j.1365-2929.2007.02713.x.

[22] Zipp, Genevieve P., and A. M. Gentile. 2010. "Practice Schedule and the Learning of Motor Skills." *Journal of College Teaching and Learning* 7, no. 2: 35–42. https://doi.org/10.19030/tlc.v7i2.87.

[23] LeSage, Paul, Jeff T. Dyar, and Bruce Evans. 2011. *Crew Resource Management: Principles and Practice*. Sudbury, MA: Jones and Bartlett Publishers.

[24] Johnson, Spencer, and Constance Johnson. 1986. *The One Minute Teacher: How to Teach Others to Teach Themselves*. New York: William Morrow.

Additional Resources

Amato, Teresa. 2007. "Respecting the Power of Denial." *Academic Emergency Medicine* 2: 184. https://doi.org/10.1197/j.aem.2006.05.027.

Ambrose, Susan A., Michael W. Bridges, Michele DiPietro, Marsha C. Lovett, and Marie K. Norman. 2010. *How Learning Works: Seven Research-Based Principles for Smart Teaching*. San Francisco: Jossey-Bass.

Croskerry, Pat. 2002. "Achieving Quality in Clinical Decision Making: Cognitive Strategies and Detection of Bias." *Academic Emergency Medicine* 9: 1184–204. https://doi.org/10.1197/aemj.9.11.1184.

Croskerry, Pat. 2005. "Diagnostic Failure: A Cognitive and Affective Approach." In *Advances in Patient Safety: From Research to Implementation*. AHRQ publication No. 050021, Vol. 2, 241–54. Rockville, MD: Agency for Health Care, Research and Quality.

Croskerry, Pat. 2005. "The Theory and Practice of Clinical Decision Making." *Canadian Journal of Anaesthesiology* 52: R1–8. https://doi.org/10.1007/BF03023077.

Damasio, Antonio R. 1994. *Descartes' Error: Emotion, Reason and the Human Brain*. New York: Grosset/Putnam.

Docheff, Dennis M. 1990. "The Feedback Sandwich." *Journal of Physical Education, Recreation and Dance* 61: 17–8. https://doi.org/10.1080/07303084.1990.10604618.

Kassirer, Jerome P., and Richard I. Kopelman. 2002. *Learning Clinical Reasoning*. Baltimore: Williams and Wilkins.

Krathwohl, David R., Bertram B. Massie, and Benjamin S. Bloom. 1964. *Taxonomy of Educational Objectives Handbook. II: Affective Domain*. New York: David McKay.

McCombs, Barbara L., and Sharon McNeely (Eds.). 1996. *Psychology in the Classroom: A Series on Applied Educational Psychology. Teaching for Thinking*. Hyattsville, MD: American Psychological Association.

Musinski, Barbara. 1999. "The Educator as Facilitator: A New Kind of Leadership." *Nursing Forum* 34, no. 1: 23–9. https://doi.org/10.1111/j.1744-6198.1999.tb00232.x.

Regehr, Glenn. 2004. "Self-Reflection on the Quality of Decisions in Health Care." *Medical Education* 38: 1025–7. https://doi.org/10.1111/j.1365-2929.2004.01979.x.

Sternberg, Robert J. 1985. *Beyond IQ: A Triarchic Theory of Human Intelligence*. New York: Cambridge University Press.

Wlodkowski, Raymond J. 2008. *Enhancing Adult Motivation to Learn: A Comprehensive Guide for Teaching All Adults*, 3rd ed. San Francisco: Jossey-Bass.

CHAPTER 13

Tools for Individual Learning

OBJECTIVES

At the conclusion of this chapter, the educator will be able to:

Cognitive Domain

1. Describe the role of self-regulated learning in student success.
2. Apply learning theory to assist students in becoming self-regulated learners.
3. Discuss how utilizing reflective practice in the classroom builds student confidence and lifelong learning.
4. Use an evidence-based approach when advising students toward improving performance through individualized strategies.

Psychomotor Domain

There are no psychomotor objectives for this chapter.

Affective Domain

1. Demonstrate awareness of the need to develop self-regulated learners.
2. Create a learning environment that fosters self-regulated learners.

> **"You cannot teach a man anything; you can only help him find it within himself."**
>
> ~ Galileo Galilei

CHAPTER GOAL The goal of this chapter is to introduce methods for promoting self-regulated learning in emergency medical services (EMS) education.

Although adult students have likely made the choice to acquire new knowledge and independently seek out ways to improve, research has shown that even in higher education, students are not always aware of their strengths and weaknesses and often select strategies that are less likely to support their learning and improvement.[1] Recent education research demonstrates that **self-regulated learners**, those who are aware of their motivation and learning skills, and who employ techniques toward self-improvement, are more likely to succeed than those who do not.[2–4] Self-regulation can be a challenge, because students are exposed to a wide variety of Internet, social media, and multimedia resources that are available within a few finger taps on a smartphone, tablet, or keyboard. The benefit of accessible information is that students can investigate topics of interest independent of textbooks and additional instructional materials provided in the traditional classroom setting or through an online learning management system. The disadvantage of the vast amount of accessible information is that the student can easily become lost or distracted from the primary objectives of a lesson and waste time discovering information that is not relevant or is contradictory to EMS best practice. An instructor becomes the guide through the vast maze of information that a student might access in the course of their EMS training, whether it is initial or continuing education, in a classroom, lab, or patient care environment.

This chapter is organized into sections starting with a description of self-regulation and reflective practice, and their applications to individual student performance. The remainder of the chapter provides examples of tools for individualized learning using a variety of specific learning modalities, including distance education applications. Examples of tools for individualized learning include reading assignments, case reviews, practice tests, and targeted clinical shifts. Whether the instructional delivery is face-to-face, online interactive, or through other media such as podcasts, smartphone applications, or virtual reality programs, the principles of self-regulation and the strategies to engage students are the same. Retrieval and application of content is key to retention. Also included are examples of techniques used inside and outside the classroom that encourage self-regulation and promote long-term learning. Common issues and pitfalls are addressed in each section where relevant.

Self-Regulated Learning

Most educators can recall a student whose performance did not seem to match the time and effort spent studying. This student is the one who had stacks of flashcards bound by a thick rubber band, well-worn textbooks with highlighted text, and notebooks filled cover to cover with written notes (and coffee stains). Yet this same student performed poorly on tests. How does this happen? Highlighted text and note taking might be evidence of reading, studying, and rereading, but are not necessarily indicative of student engagement and learning.[5–7]

Decades of research from education and psychology have demonstrated that learning and retention are enhanced through frequent, spaced retrieval practice (practice testing) and metacognitive (self-reflection) strategies throughout various stages of learning, and that these practices are superior to restudying and rereading course content.[8–10] Several intercepting theories on student self-regulation and engagement have also been applied to medical education environments.[11,12] Improvements in student outcomes are most notable when students apply strategies designed to enhance engagement and self-regulation. Phases of individual student self-regulation include specific goal setting, task monitoring, and efforts to control and regulate learning. Metacognition is the awareness and monitoring of one's own learning, thinking, attitude, and performance. Metacognitive exercises such as reflective journals and self-assessments are embedded within each of the phases of self-regulated learning as the student reflects on personal objectives (planning), during active task performance (monitoring), and as an after-action learning activity.[11]

The role of the instructor is to teach the student how to self-regulate using strategies that encourage advanced goal setting, self- and peer monitoring, and reflection on performance and improvement.[13] An instructor may even begin a course or program with an introductory assignment that describes the current research on how adults learn, prompting the students to become aware of their prior knowledge and study habits, and to develop an individual plan that will encourage engagement and self-regulation. Some instructors use a screening questionnaire, such as the Motivated

Strategies for Learning Questionnaire (MSLQ), to assess the learning strategies and academic motivation of individual students.[13] Others have taken this a step further and demonstrated improvement in student learning outcomes by using strategies that improve student self-regulation.[14]

Critical Thinking and Reflective Practice in Adult Education

Rote memorization of facts and performing calculations were the most common educational modalities and the guiding principles for all education for centuries. In recent decades, however, the emphasis has shifted from fact-based learning to critical thinking and reflection.[15] These two principles expand and elevate the levels of education and the capacity of the practitioner to advance toward self-actualization and independent evaluation of evidence and self-determination of practices, as a professional.[16,17]

Critical thinking involves challenging ideas by actively considering all points of view and counterarguments, and weighing the strengths and weaknesses of each idea on the merits of logic, evidence, and sound reasoning.[16,17] The major emphasis on EMS education and practice in prior decades had been on learning to perform cognitive and psychomotor skills and execute algorithms.[18] Today, evidence-based practice and the evaluation of sources for clinical validity and detection of biases are standard inclusions in course curricula.

Reflective practice involves viewing situations and practices through varied lenses, other than from the perspective of just one's own point of view. For instance, rather than taking care of a patient and performing interventions based on treatment protocols and strict narrow policies and system guidelines, the provider also considers each patient's wishes and concerns, along with the patient's past medical history and prognosis. The responder also considers the wishes of the family, the receiving physicians and nurses, the payer agencies, and the public perspectives on the actions of the crew. Furthermore, the reflective EMS responder also has to keep in mind quality assurance reviewers, lawyers and courts, and future and past providers and managers. The EMS responder must consider the past, because traditions and standards of practice weigh heavily on judging performance. The EMS responder must consider the future managers, because setting precedents can have a policy, economic, and quality of care impact for months and years to follow. In other words, EMS practitioners are not just performing a skill on a single patient at any one time; they are practicing in a complex milieu of clinicians, administrators, educators, researchers, economists, politicians, media specialists, and community advocates. The reflective provider is always cognizant of the greater, complex ecosystem. Likewise, the EMS educator is also cognizant that in teaching an EMS student, the educator is reflecting on the views and needs of the educational institution, future employers, the recruitment of future students, the program alumni, future patients, state officials, accreditation agencies, and the media. It is the ability to see situations through various frames of reference and through the eyes of others in differing roles that is the hallmark of the professional reflective practitioner and educator.

Reflective education is often facilitated through having students journal (i.e., record their reflections daily, especially during clinical and internship rotations), group discussions (where challenging situations have occurred, often where no right pathway was evident), and deliberative exercises (such as practicing how to manage a model patient who is near death or a model family member who has been abusive, etc.).

Professional and educational reflection is constructive, in that it examines events and internal reactions deliberatively and with a goal of gaining an understanding of how and why events occurred, as well as possible strategies for avoiding or handling future occurrences. It is productive, in that rather than endeavoring to explain away unfortunate events, or conversely, celebrating fortuitous events, it examines underlying elements, including causes and responses. Ultimately, the reflective professional considers how the event will be viewed in the future and whether the course of action will have a lasting positive or negative impact.

The following sections discuss common tools that students use for individual study and learning that can improve self-regulation and reflective practice.

Reading Assignments

One of the most common sources of educational material is text (print or digital). Most EMS instructors assign reading to supplement content presented during the class or to prepare students prior to participating in classroom activities. Research suggests that students who value and complete reading assignments have better exam scores, increased class participation, and increased understanding.[6] Despite these benefits, in many classrooms a substantial number of students fail to complete the required reading. Some researchers determined that less than 30% of the college students they studied completed the assigned reading.[7,19]

Students may not complete course readings for the following reasons:

1. Unpreparedness
2. Lack of motivation
3. Time constraints
4. Underestimation of reading importance[6]

There are several possible approaches to increase student reading. To start, the instructor must read and engage with the text that the student is expected to read. In doing so, the instructor will attach value to the reading assignments and allow for rich classroom discussion and interaction. An instructor who is familiar with content of the text can better prepare and anticipate student questions, particularly around controversies and conflict within and among various sources of reading material.

In some cases, students read the material but fail to comprehend or retain the content. This student may be underestimating the time and effort required for deep reading. In many instances, these students do not have effective habits for engaging in reading before they enter the EMS classroom. Research has demonstrated that students who read a section of text and then explain the content either verbally or in writing will retain the learned content more successfully than those who read and highlight or take written notes as they read.[20] This is not to say that note taking and highlighting are not effective practices. In fact, these commonly used techniques can make relevant text and passages stand out so when the student needs a later reference, that information is easier to find and retrieve. However, there are strategies to get the most out of highlighting text.

A common study habit among students is to highlight text as they are reading. If all students do is highlight as they read, then very little is gained in actual learning and retention. Some researchers suggest that highlighting can give an "illusion of knowing" to the student who focuses on the words rather than the meaning.[21] Others state that highlighting benefits learning because the simple act of highlighting can help process the text at a deeper level than if the student simply read the text without highlighting. Benefits are gained from retrieving information, and the ease of finding that information is realized by highlighting. Notice that it is the *retrieval* of content and meaning that improves learning!

No matter the source of text content (textbook, journal articles, program handbooks, online blogs), an instructor can make the most of reading assignments by holding students accountable and by rewarding compliance.[22] It should be mentioned here that the same principles will hold true for flipped classrooms, when the learner draws content from other sources of media such as audio or video clips. (A flipped classroom is one in which the presentation of material is "flipped"—the lesson content [readings, lectures, video clips] are given as homework preparation, and time in class is reserved for active learning activities such as skills labs, case studies, and simulations.)

> **TEACHING TIP**
>
> Here are some tips to give to students who use highlighting as a study habit during reading:[20]
>
> 1. First read or skim the text without highlighting. Then go back and decide on the key concepts, using the highlighter to organize and emphasize content on the second pass.
> 2. Make flashcards or questions out of the highlighted text and use them to self-test later.
> 3. Be selective about what you highlight.
> 4. Do not use highlighting as your only study habit.

Here are two strategies that instructors can use to engage students in content:

1. Self-reflective writing before, during, and after reading (or after reviewing audio or video content in the flipped classroom environment).
2. Assignment to the student to write test questions based on the content that can then be used in class to test other students. To accomplish this most effectively, the students should first be taught how to write effective test questions.

McGuire demonstrated the effectiveness of The Study Cycle in his college classroom by having the students first preview the reading before class; attend class and review their notes within 24 hours, asking why, how, and what-if questions during the review; and then assess their own learning on a regular basis through teaching of content to other students.[23] This method is consistent with other research on the effectiveness of **SQ3R** (survey, question, read, recall, review) to enhance student learning and retention. Students survey (skim) the text and answer either instructor or student-developed questions or prompts related to the assigned reading. This process encourages deep reading with a focus on answering these questions. Later, through teaching other students, the student recalls or retrieves information and reviews it at spaced intervals. This retrieval practice is also known as the **testing effect**[24] and is a practice well supported in the educational literature. Practice tests are examined in a later section of this chapter (see *Practice Tests*). The testing effect is demonstrated in self-reflective reading

CASE in Point

Self-Reflection Activity

An instructor wanted to use a self-reflection activity to promote his students' awareness of their mastery level in a particular subject area through a series of self-reflections. The instructor was using a flipped classroom approach, so he first assigned the students to read, highlight, and take notes on key points from a segment of video viewed before coming to class. (The instructor had used this technique with audio and text assignments in the past, with success.) The instructor then had the students free-write personal reactions to the material, key points, most confusing points, and questions remaining. He also instructed students to document their confidence level with mastering the content. Finally, he added motivational factors for the student to reflect upon, such as barriers to completing the content review, prior knowledge and experiences, and feelings or attitudes about the content.

This free-write self-reflection activity allowed the students to observe and monitor themselves as they learned and were tested on content. After it was completed, the instructor collected and reviewed these reflections to shape his teaching and adjust strategies to fill gaps in student learning.

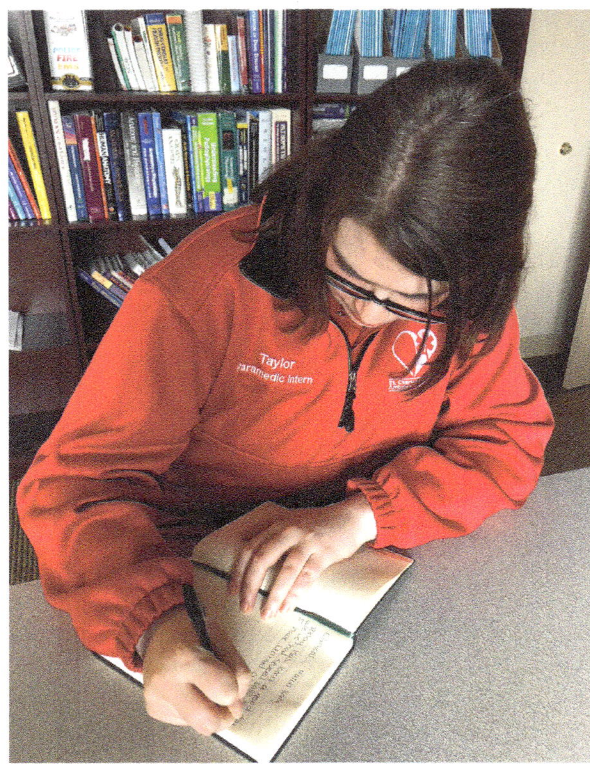

FIGURE 13.1 Journaling allows students the opportunity to reflect on their experiences and explore their feelings.

Courtesy of St. Charles County Ambulance District.

assignments as the student first reads and recalls, then forgets, and then retrieves and applies content.

Self-reflective assignments should not only ask about content knowledge, but also about motivational factors and confidence levels of the student in mastering the content (see Case in Point: Self-Reflection Activity) (**FIGURE 13.1**).

These strategies, when used appropriately, can increase the students' ability to attach meaning and to incorporate the new material within their **schema of knowledge** related to that topic.[22] The next section looks at specific sources of text and some of the built-in strategies students can use to improve engagement and learning.

Textbooks

Although the usefulness of textbooks in education is often debated in the literature, a textbook can be an important tool for individual learning if it is used appropriately.[25] Before the educator can begin to maximize the potential of a textbook, however, an understanding of the book and its elements should be reached. Educators should view a textbook as a tool for organizing key content. They must always ensure that the content is consistent with the national education standards. Textbooks are not commonly used as the sole source of information, especially considering the digital world of information accessible to students outside of the traditional educational setting. But, the textbook can provide a foundation of content from which an educator can expand and enhance the student learning experience, and it can be used as a tool for answering questions and providing feedback.[22] The educator should assign the textbook a role in the overall learning experience, using it as a baseline for knowledge and a reference for questions or clarifications.

Many textbooks have specific elements designed to scaffold student learning and retention. Organizational elements like tables of contents, glossaries, and appendices allow for ease in navigating through the content. Elements such as learning objectives, case scenarios, review questions, and enrichment information all offer opportunities to enhance individual learning. The instructor can enhance student self-regulation by deliberately utilizing these built-in tools as outside-of-class assignments and prompts for student reflection.

Learning Objectives

A reliable EMS textbook has learning objectives that directly reference and map to the national EMS education standards. This structures the content and identifies intended graduate outcomes for EMS educational programs. These standards determine the minimum educational content and the desired cognitive, psychomotor, and affective student outcomes at the four levels of EMS provider education (emergency medical responder, emergency medical technician, advanced emergency medical technician, and paramedic). Although it is not always the case, a reliable EMS textbook maps the content objectives directly to the national education standards, including the breadth and depth of individual subjects.[26]

One way to engage the student is to direct the student to read the objectives before reading the content and to write questions and reflections in anticipation of learning the content. While reading, the student can then refer back to the objectives to ensure that they are identifying the most important information. Reflective writing prompts can ask the student to pinpoint content that is unclear or conflicting with their current knowledge of local protocols. This way, the student comes to class with specific goals for learning. Through interactive class discussion, the instructor can identify areas of student need and provide additional assignments in a variety of formats (for example, podcasts, articles, and protocols) that can clarify and expand on the subject matter.

When using objectives for individual learning, the instructor should direct students to review them again before taking a cognitive or skills exam. Students can use the objectives to develop their own test questions, which can then be reviewed by the instructor and used to test other students. At the conclusion of a lesson (or course), the instructor can use the objectives to develop a student survey as students reflect on whether the lesson content allowed them to meet the objectives stated in the textbook.

Case Scenarios

Written case scenarios are another common element of many textbooks. For example, some textbooks begin each chapter with a scenario to provide meaningful context for the student. The case study also serves as a motivational tool to help the learner attach value to the topic of a chapter or section of a textbook. Scenarios can be excellent tools for students as they learn to think critically and improve their problem-solving skills. One caveat is that the elements of a written textbook scenario should map directly to the objectives of the lesson. Student-developed scenarios used in simulation exercises may be helpful as formative tools to assist the student in the application of content learned in the course of their EMS education. This is a subject of a later section in this chapter (see *Case Reviews*).

> **CASE in Point**
>
> **Prompting with Review Questions**
>
> An instructor selected three review questions to begin a lesson to encourage students to discuss or find the answers. She selected questions pertaining to the next class lesson. Even though students have not yet covered the related material, this encourages them to complete the assigned reading. Having found that a higher percentage of students were prepared for class as a result of her using this technique, the instructor made a practice of beginning her lessons with some of these questions, so students would be more likely to read the questions ahead of time and formulate a response.

Review Questions

Textbooks often contain review questions at the end of the chapter, interspersed throughout main sections of a chapter, or at the end of the textbook. In addition to student-developed questions, the student can use these review questions to guide their learning, and the instructor can periodically use these as prompts in the context of the classroom lecture to promote interactive discussion and better engagement with the material.

As mentioned earlier, students can develop exam or review questions to share with other students. A student-developed test question bank can be used to initiate and promote discussion. Instructor-vetted student questions can then be put onto index cards or into classroom presentations and used as review prior to formative or even summative exams.

Before the time of clicker questions and personal response systems in the classroom, Mazur measured great gains in student learning through the use of mini-lectures (15 to 25 minutes) interrupted by slides containing multiple choice questions.[27] Students would individually answer and gauge confidence level and then engage in discussion with neighboring students on the content of the question and correct answer. Classroom clicker technology and smartphone applications now allow personal interactivity from student to projected question in the presentation, but the benefits are the same. Remember that these tools can not only test content knowledge but also improve metacognitive skills and self-awareness. Together this can align student confidence level with actual performance on a test.

Textbook Companions

Textbooks can have many ancillary tools or companions that undergird the main content contained within the textbook. Audiobooks, student workbooks, websites, and learning management systems are some examples of textbook companions.

At one time, audiobooks were only considered for students who had difficulty with reading written text. More recent research shows the all students benefit from using a variety of learning modalities (audio, video, text) on the same content.[28] Publishers may also include access to these audiobooks on a companion website linked to the purchase of the textbook package. Ancillary products such as pocket guides and exam review manuals have been replaced with the online versions found on the companion website. Some publishers continue to offer printed workbooks that accompany the textbook when there is a market need. These workbooks also offer a way for the student to retrieve information (self-test) and deepen learning.

Many publishers have created online tools that are ideally suited for individual learning and exploration. These tools typically are contained on a website that has been developed and is owned by the publisher for a specific book, hence the name "companion website" (**FIGURE 13.2**). These sites generally contain information such as learning objectives and various activities that reinforce content from the text. Instructor tools are also available, including instructor manuals, lesson plans, and test banks.

A textbook may also link to an online learning management system (LMS) which differs from a companion website in that the LMS is designed to increase student engagement with the content. An LMS may be sponsored through the educational institution or already designed by a textbook publisher. The LMS contains interactive materials such as images, video clips, links to podcasts, quizzes, discussion boards, and practice exams. Such materials provide multiple presentations of the same content, a practice that has been shown to improve student learning and retention.[28] Instructors who run their own LMS through their educational institution might do so using technology-enhanced, hybrid, or fully online coursework. (See Chapter 17, *Tools for Distance Learning*.) However, none of these materials will be effective tools for individual learning unless the student engages with the content, no matter which format; therefore, it is imperative that the instructor assign, hold accountable, and reward students for engaging and completing assignments in an LMS.

Most LMSs allow the instructor to measure the level of student engagement through online course activity reports. Some even have early warning detectors that flag the instructor to check in with a student who is falling behind. The instructor can then prompt students who have not been completing online reading, assignments, or content review or who are falling behind on the coursework. This simple act of prompting can redirect the student to the content and improve student engagement and outcomes.

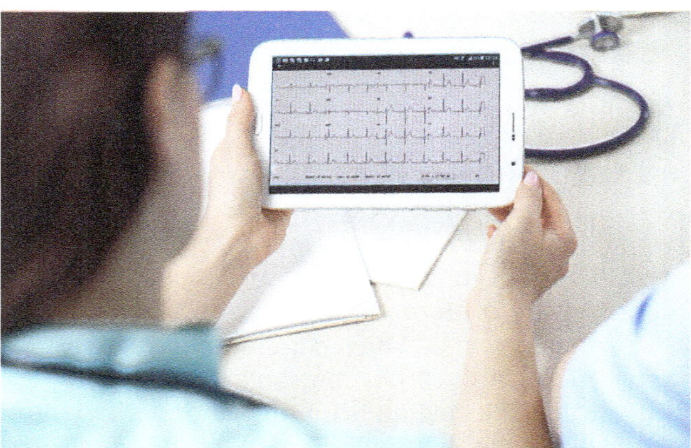

FIGURE 13.2 Studying on a companion website may suit the needs of younger students because of the advantages of audio and visual content.

TEACHING TIP

Not all students have smartphones or access to computers; therefore, an overreliance on digital media presents important student equity and access issues. Instructors need to work with the educational institution to ensure that all students have access to these learning materials through computer labs, libraries, educational discounts, and financial aid resources. Instructors can also build in the time for students to complete digital assignments during class sessions and reassess the need for backup written assignments if needed.

Journal Articles

Most textbooks provide an overview of content within a specific area. While this is important for student understanding and organization of content, the textbook may lag behind current research or lack sufficient detail in an emerging field. Assigning reading from professional journals can ensure that students are aware of recent updates and current controversies in prehospital care.

When assigning reading from journals, instructors must distinguish between review articles from trade journals and peer-reviewed journals, and between opinion pieces and original research. Assigning reading from a trade journal has its advantages, because the material is written in a popular style that appeals to front-line EMS personnel. These journals often contain reviews of recent research and continuing education articles written by those with expertise in specific aspects of prehospital care.

Assigning reading of an original research article from a peer-reviewed journal can pose a challenge for students who are not accustomed to reading this type of literature. It can benefit the instructor to first gauge students' confidence and comfort levels with reading original research. Ways to increase engagement with original research might include assigning an article that has an accompanying review article from a trade journal that summarizes key points in plain language, or one that has an accompanying podcast that dissects and examines the key elements of the research itself as well as the implications for practice. Other ways to improve research literacy among EMS students can include free online self-paced courses on research basics, engaging students in a guided research project, and using library resources for workshops on conducting journal searches and on how to evaluate a research article from the medical literature. Instructors and students can review research in a journal club activity using a recent or controversial research study, and they can even participate as a class in a live journal club webinar or podcast. This not only deepens engagement with content; it also introduces the principles of EMS research.

TEACHING TIP

Assign a project where students must examine the case for and against an issue related to prehospital emergency care. This requires them to find relevant articles to support and refute their position. Topics could include emergency care issues such as prehospital advanced airway management, spinal motion restriction, or the use of lights and sirens during emergency response. Other topics could include the role of EMS in public health issues, prevention of work-related burnout, and diversity of the EMS workforce. Students may also review educational research related to performance and outcomes of EMS students using different educational interventions.

Program Handbooks

Instructors may not commonly think of the program handbook as a tool for individual student learning; however, it can be consistently called upon to support student learning, much like a syllabus supports an individual course. Program handbooks not only contain policies, but also a list of resources available at the educational institution that support student learning and achievement. Also, overall program goals and graduation or completion requirements are outlined in the program handbook. Typically, the program handbook is reviewed during the first week of class, marking the start of a contract between educational institution and student. During the course of an educational program, students can lose track of overall goals and program requirements as they delve into the workload. Continuously redirecting the student to the program goals, competencies, and graduation requirements can ensure that a student stays on the path to successful completion.

Online Blogs and Social Media Links

In addition to textbooks and ancillary text materials, students commonly follow links posted on social media and read online blogs on subject matter from class. Free Open Access Meducation (FOAM) is increasingly being used as a platform for individual learning and collaboration and has gained an international audience of EMS students and professionals.[29] This is an exciting opportunity for students to engage in clinical, educational, and technical content in a global arena, and instructors should become involved in the conversations or at least the oversight to ensure that content is supported by referenced primary source material. Instructors may also need to help students prioritize content knowledge for the purpose of program success and delineate that which is primary educational content aligned with the education standard and objectives, and that which is more appropriate for a continuing education audience.

Case Reviews

Most allied health profession standards are expressed in terms of what the provider will do or be able to perform once on the job. The standards or objectives are expressed using verbs. These determine the level of performance and, therefore, the breadth and depth of teaching and learning. As noted in the revised Bloom's taxonomy, verbs like "recall," "list," or "name," reflect a basic level of learning, whereas verbs such as "distinguish" or "create" express critical thinking and higher complexity of cognitive competency.[30] The cognitive, psychomotor, and affective domains can be developed and assessed in the context of a more complex learning environment such as a case review, scenario, simulation, or clinical environment.

When designing a case review or scenario-based activity, the instructor should avoid cognitive overload, a situation in which the educator gives too much information or too many tasks for the student's capabilities. This can happen when placing a student into a complex simulation too soon, before the student has the baseline competencies to handle many tasks (for example, taking a history and delegating to team members) or many sources of information (for example, bystander historians and medication lists). Instead, the instructor may first begin with classroom case review projects designed to test knowledge at these higher-level thought processes. For example, students may be given a scenario, corresponding dispatch data, and specific information about a patient's complaint. Instead of providing all information on a case in a single data set, students can work through each step of the assessment and treatment as they learn to prioritize, ask relevant history questions, obtain objective data from a physical exam, and determine most appropriate prehospital actions. This is also an opportunity for students to develop a view of the care they provide as a critical phase on the continuum of medical treatment for a type of patient. It is also a chance for students to understand the value of an accurate verbal and written report made to the hospital staff who will base their treatment decisions on the prehospital report.

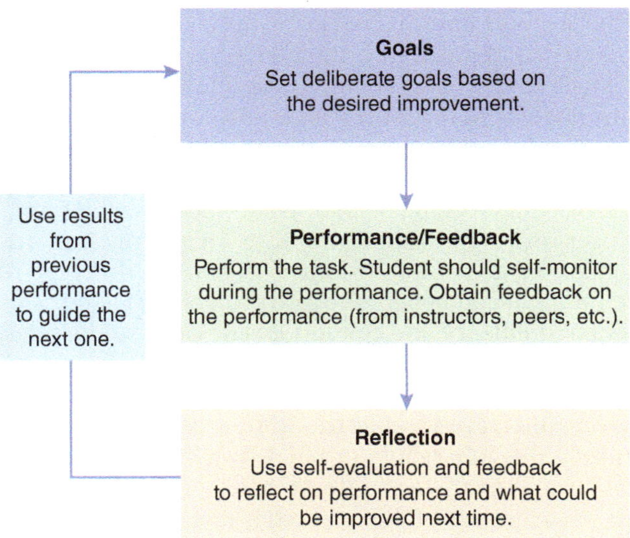

FIGURE 13.3 Example of self-regulation pattern.

Kirk, Karin. n.d. "What Is Self-Regulated Learning?" Accessed February 22, 2019. https://serc.carleton.edu/sage2yc/self_regulated/what.html.

CASE in Point

Student-Developed Scenarios

An instructor was seeking an effective way to engage students in specific content. After talking with colleagues, he decided to have the students write and develop targeted scenarios that he could then evaluate for accuracy and use as a pilot test for other students who would act as responders. During the scenario, the instructor considered his role to be to ensure integrity of the scenario and to monitor the safety of students involved. In fact, in order to ensure student safety, he assigned a student to the role of safety officer once he realized the scenario's complexity required it.

During the activity, the instructor divided the students into teams and had the teams rotate through roles in each scenario. One team served as the responder group; another group served as the actors and scenario builders. Finally, he collected a group of students to act as peer evaluators to assess specific skills, leadership, and communication. The students were engaged through the design, participation, response, and evaluation of the scenario. The scenarios were timed and videotaped for later review by faculty, the medical director, and the student responders. As the final step, the instructor held postscenario reflections following video review to allow the students to examine, critique, and improve their performance.

Case studies can be mapped or linked to specific objectives to ensure that they are met upon completion of the project. In addition, the case can be an opportunity to enhance student self-regulation using the following steps. First, have students gauge their confidence related to the patient's differential diagnosis and their proposed treatment plan. Second, students can discuss alternative possibilities with classmates monitoring performance and developing a rationale for the treatment. Third, have students review the outcome of the patient, reflecting on what they learned and how that will impact their next approach to a patient case review. This pattern of planning, performance, monitoring, reflecting, and feedback is a self-regulation pattern that can then be carried from classroom to simulation and into the clinical setting during initial and continuing education (**FIGURE 13.3**).

Practice Tests

The most common reason instructors test students is to assess competency; however, research also supports the use of testing as a pedagogical strategy to enhance student learning. In fact, the testing effect has been demonstrated repeatedly at a variety of levels and settings, such as cognitive psychology labs, classrooms, simulation, and practical settings. In health professions education programs, frequent testing (also known as retrieval practice) has proven superior to studying or rereading content. The testing effect is stronger with frequent, repeated tests that are spaced over time, and when accompanied by feedback, so students learn from their mistakes.[10]

Many resources are available for practice tests both online and in print with a growing number of digital options that can be accessed easily from a smartphone or tablet. One of the most important aspects of practice testing is self-regulation before, during, and after answering a practice test item and while reviewing the response and performance on the item. Practice testing is important for students to compare their level of confidence in mastering the material with actual performance in specific areas. Instructors can use tools of self-regulation to assist students to become aware of areas for improvement.

SRL to Diagnose Problems with Testing

Why do some students perform poorly on tests? Methods for remediation of students who perform poorly on written tests are not well supported by evidence. Andrews, Kelly, and DeZee developed a tool using self-regulated learning (SRL) theory to diagnose issues of task, metacognition, causal attribution, and adaptation in a medical education program.[14] Such a tool might help reveal which aspect of student learning (content knowledge, application, problem-solving, confidence) requires attention.

Targeted Clinical Experiences

A **targeted clinical experience** is a focused (hospital or field) assignment through which a specific aspect of learning is enhanced or remediated. Such experiences require personalized, measurable learning objectives for the rotation, tasks, or activities to complete, and tools for measuring outcomes. Consider the following examples: a student with either an interest in, or who lacks experience with, patients suffering from behavioral disorders may be placed in the in-patient psychiatry area to observe how patient behavior changes after an acute episode. Students who struggle with electrocardiogram (ECG) interpretation may benefit from clinical experience in a cardiac unit, where they can observe many ECGs over time and interact with subject matter experts. A student who is interested in rural EMS may be interested in spending focused time with a rural EMS unit. The primary goal of targeted rotations, however, is to enhance and measure learning and achievement of specific outcomes. These rotations can be valuable for a student who needs specific attention as identified during the capstone field internship by directly honing in on the area of weakness (for example, intravenous [IV] access failures) and designing an intervention toward improvement (for example, a shift with an IV team). The outcome measures should be specific and measurable (for example, 16 successful IVs out of the last 20 attempts) and should also include student self-reflections on their learning and confidence in the task before and after the experience.

CASE in Point

Individual Tools for Learning during the Capstone Field Internship

A field preceptor has identified that her student has difficulty making rapid decisions about the patient priorities and has been inconsistent when assessing patients. She comes to you for help and advice. One of the program faculty suggests that the student be assigned to the intake/triage area of a busy hospital alongside a trained nurse preceptor where the student can develop a systematic assessment process and learn to prioritize rapidly. Three shifts and 40 patients later, the student shows marked improvement in field performance, and student self-reflections show increasing confidence with patient assessments.

Techniques for Students to Make the Most of Learning

1. Study information in "chunks" that contain no more than seven key concepts.
2. When reading, summarize each paragraph in one sentence using your own words.
3. Organize key concepts into sequences, pictures, models, or algorithms as you study them.
4. When reading new material, consciously relate it to something you already know.
5. Motivation to succeed and the students' belief that they can succeed are essential elements to success in learning. Focus on your end goal so you will put in the work needed to learn the material. Break content into small pieces so it is manageable to learn.
6. Think about how you learn most effectively, and try to use those strategies. When given an assignment, consider what will be involved and what parts of it you might find difficult. Then identify the steps needed to complete it successfully.
7. Meaningful learning does not occur if you play a passive role. To really learn something, you must actively participate in the learning process.
8. Your instructor guides the instruction, but you must work to understand new knowledge and to see how it fits in with what you already know.
9. Apply what you are learning to a situation you might see on the ambulance and predict how the scenario would progress. Ask yourself, what would this patient look like? What would her vital signs be? How might her condition change as time passes if no interventions are performed? How would I manage the situation?
10. When learning a new concept or fact, strive to know the "why" associated with it. For example, a patient with a heart rate of 30 beats per minute is likely to have signs of shock. Ask yourself why that is.
11. Practice the new concepts and skills you have learned often and in as many different situations as possible.
12. Monitor your progress. If you are struggling with specific knowledge or skills, change your learning strategy to be more successful using input from class peers or instructors.
13. Learning new complex material takes time and repetition—plan for both.

Summary

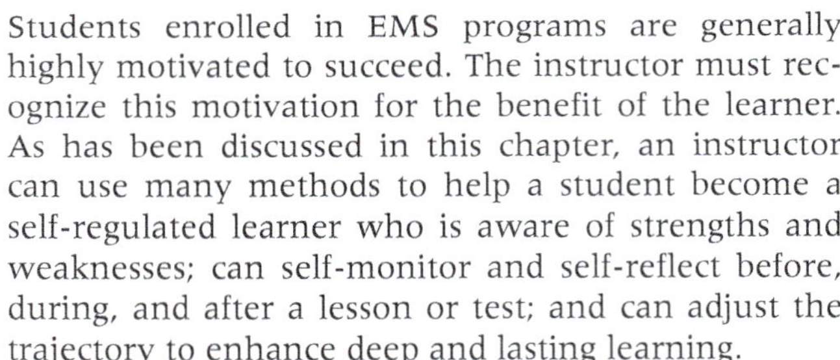

Students enrolled in EMS programs are generally highly motivated to succeed. The instructor must recognize this motivation for the benefit of the learner. As has been discussed in this chapter, an instructor can use many methods to help a student become a self-regulated learner who is aware of strengths and weaknesses; can self-monitor and self-reflect before, during, and after a lesson or test; and can adjust the trajectory to enhance deep and lasting learning.

The educator should become familiar with the many tools available for individual learning and institutional learning resources that can assist struggling students. Instructors must remember that not all learning occurs within the classroom, and the modern student has access to a wide variety of digital resources and a constant flow of social media communication. EMS students often are eager to extend their learning beyond the classroom and to develop critical thinking skills that will remain useful throughout their career. Instructors can guide the student through honest self-assessment, continuous monitoring, and the development of individual strategies to promote lifelong learning.

Glossary

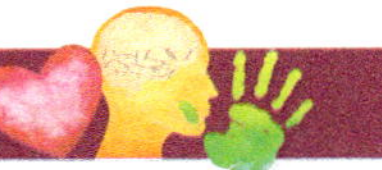

reflective practice Act of viewing situations and practices through varied lenses, other than from only one's own point of view; in EMS education, involves using a wider mental lens when teaching, considering the views and needs of the institution, future employers, future patients, and other stakeholders.

schema of knowledge Patterns of thought and behavior related to categories of information and relationships between and among them.

self-regulated learners Learners who are aware of their own motivation and learning skills, and who employ techniques toward self-improvement.

SQ3R Method for enhancing student learning that involves survey, question, read, recall, and review.

targeted clinical experience Focused (hospital or field) assignment through which a specific aspect of learning is enhanced or remediated.

testing effect Practice in which students read or recall content; are then tested on it so they can retrieve and apply it; and finally, feedback is provided so they can learn from their mistakes.

References

[1] Pintrich, Paul R., and Akane Zusho. 2007. "Student Motivation and Self-Regulated Learning in the College Classroom." In *The Scholarship of Teaching and Learning in Higher Education: An Evidence-Based Perspective,* edited by Paymond P. Perry and John C. Smart, 731–810. Dordrecht, The Netherlands: Springer.

[2] Artino, Anthony R., Ryan Brydges, and Larry D. Guppen. 2015. "Self-Regulated Learning in Healthcare Profession Education: Theoretical Perspectives and Research Methods." In *Researching Medical Education,* edited by Jennifer Cleland and Steven J. Durning, 155–66. Hoboken, NJ: John Wiley and Sons.

[3] Zimmerman, Barry J. 2010. "Self-Regulated Learning and Academic Achievement: An Overview." *Educational Psychologist* 25, no. 1: 3–17. https://doi.org/10.1207/s15326985ep2501_2.

[4] Zimmerman, Barry J., and Dale H. Shunk. 2011. "Self-Regulated Learning and Performance: An Introduction and an Overview." In *Handbook of Self-Regulation of Learning and Performance,* edited by Barry J. Zimmerman and Dale H. Shunk, 1–12. New York: Routledge.

[5] Sappington, John, Kimberly Kinsey, and Kirk Munsayac. 2002. "Two Studies of Reading Compliance among College Students." *Teaching of Psychology* 29, no. 4: 272–4. https://doi.org/10.1207/S15328023TOP2904_02.

[6] Bean, John C. 2011. *Engaging Ideas: The Professor's Guide to Integrating Writing, Critical Thinking, and Active Learning in the Classroom.* Hoboken, NJ: John Wiley & Sons.

[7] Kerr, Mary M., and Kristen M. Frese. 2017. "Reading to Learn or Learning to Read? Engaging College Students in Course Readings." *College Teaching* 65, no. 1: 28–31. https://doi.org/10.1080/87567555.2016.1222577.

[8] Svinicki, Marilla D. 2004. *Learning and Motivation in the Postsecondary Classroom.* San Francisco: Anker Publishing.

[9] Cromley, Jennifer. 2005. "Metacognition, Cognitive Strategy Instruction and Reading in Adult Literacy." *Review of Adult Learning and Literacy* 5: 187–220.

[10] Ariel, Robert, and Jeffrey D. Karpicke. 2018. "Improving Self-Regulated Learning with a Retrieval Practice Intervention." *Journal of Experimental Psychology: Applied* 24, no. 1: 43–56. http://dx.doi.org/10.1037/xap0000133.

[11] Zimmerman, Barry J. 2015. "Self-Regulated Learning: Theories, Measures, and Outcomes." In *International Encyclopedia of the Social and Behavioral Sciences,* 2nd ed., edited by James D. Wright, 541–6. Amsterdam: Elsevier.

[12] Leggett, Heather, John Sandars, and Trudie Roberts. 2017. "Twelve Tips on How to Provide Self-Regulated Learning (SRL) Enhanced Feedback on Clinical Performance." *Medical Teacher* 11: 1–5. https://doi.org/10.1080/0142159X.2017.1407868.

[13] Duncan, Teresa, Paul Pintrich, David Smith, and Wilbert J. McKeachie. 2015. "Motivated Strategies for Learning Questionnaire (MSLQ) Manual." *ResearchGate.* Accessed February 5, 2019. https://www.researchgate.net/publication/280741846.

[14] Andrews, Mary A., William F. Kelly, and Kent J. DeZee. 2018. "Why Does This Learner Perform Poorly on Tests? Using Self-Regulated Learning Theory to Diagnose the Problem and Implement Solutions." *Academic Medicine* 93, no. 4: 612–5. https://doi.org/10.1097/ACM.0000000000001422.

[15] Slavich, George M., and Philip G. Zimbardo. 2012. "Transformational Teaching: Theoretical Underpinnings, Basic Principles, and Core Methods." *Educational Psychology Review* 24, no. 4: 569–608. https://doi.org/10.1007/s10648-012-9199-6.

[16] Perry, William G. 1970. *Forms of Intellectual and Ethical Development in the College Years: A Scheme.* New York: Holt, Rinehart & Winston.

[17] Kitchener, Karen S., and Patricia M. King. 1981. "Reflective Judgment Concepts of Justification and Their Relationship to Age and Education." *Journal of Applied Developmental Psychology* 2: 89–116. https://doi.org/10.1016/0193-3973(81)90032-0.

[18] Glavin, Chris. 2014. "Reforms in the 1980s." *K12Academics.* Accessed July 3, 2018. https://www.k12academics.com/education-reform/reforms-1980s.

[19] Bembenutty, Héfer, and Marie C. White. 2013. "Academic Performance and Satisfaction with Homework Completion among College Students." *Learning and Individual Differences* 24: 83–8. https://doi.org/10.1016/j.lindif.2012.10.013.

[20] Yue, Carole L., Benjamin C. Storm, Nate Kornell, and Elizaebeth L. Bjork. 2015. "Highlighting and Its Relation to Distributed Study and Students' Metacognitive Beliefs." *Educational Psychology Review* 27, no. 1: 763–7. https://doi.org/10.1007/s10648-014-9277-z.

[21] Bjork, Robert A. 1999. "Assessing Our Own Competence: Heuristics and Illusions." In *Attention and Performance XVII. Cognitive Regulation of Performance: Interaction of Theory and Application,* edited by Daniel Gopher and Asher Koriat, 435–59. Cambridge, MA: MIT Press.

[22] Nilson, Linda B. 2013. *Creating Self-Regulated Learners: Strategies to Strengthen Students' Self-Awareness and Learning Skills.* Sterling, VA: Stylus Publishing.

[23] McGuire, Saundra. 2008. "Using Metacognition to Effect an Extreme Academic Makeover in Students." In *National Association of Geoscience Teachers (NAGT) Workshops.* Northfield, MN: Carleton College.

[24] Roediger, Henry L., and Andrew C. Butler. 2010. "The Critical Role of Retrieval Practice in Long-Term Retention." *Trends in Cognitive Sciences* 15, no. 1: 20–7. https://doi.org/10.1016/j.tics.2010.09.003.

[25] Knight, Bruce A., and Mike Horsley. 2013. "The Ecology of Change and Continuity in the Use of Textbooks in Higher Education." *Text,* 23. Accessed February 5, 2019. http://www.textjournal.com.au/speciss/issue23/content.htm.

[26] National Highway Traffic Safety Administration. 2009. "National Emergency Medical Services Education Standards." [DOT HS 811 077A]. Accessed January 15, 2019. https://www.ems.gov/pdf/National-EMS-Education-Standards-FINAL-Jan-2009.pdf.

[27] Mazur, Eric. 1997. *Peer Instruction: A User's Manual.* Upper Saddle River, NJ: Prentice Hall.

[28] Rose, David H., Wendy S. Harbour, Catherine S. Johnston, Samantha Daley, and Linda Abarbanell. 2008. "Universal Design for Learning in Postsecondary Education: Reflections on Principles and Their Applications." In *Universal Design in Higher Education: From Principles to Practice*, edited by Sheryl E. Burgstahler and Rebecca C. Cory, 45–59. Cambridge, MA: Harvard Education Press.

[29] Mason, Paige, and Alan M. Batt. 2018. "#FOAMems: Engaging Paramedics with Free, Online Open-Access Education." *Journal of Education and Health Promotion* 7: 32. Accessed April 5, 2019. http://www.jehp.net/text.asp?2018/7/1/32/226486.

[30] Anderson, Lorin W., and David R. Krathwohl (Eds.). 2001. *A Taxonomy for Learning, Teaching, and Assessing: A Revision of Bloom's Taxonomy of Educational Objectives*. New York: Pearson.

Additional Resources

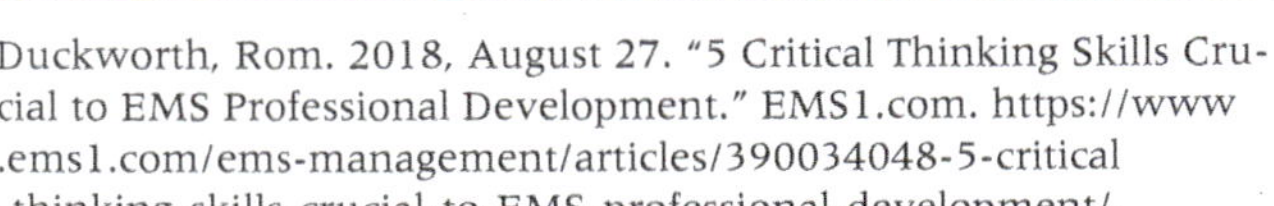

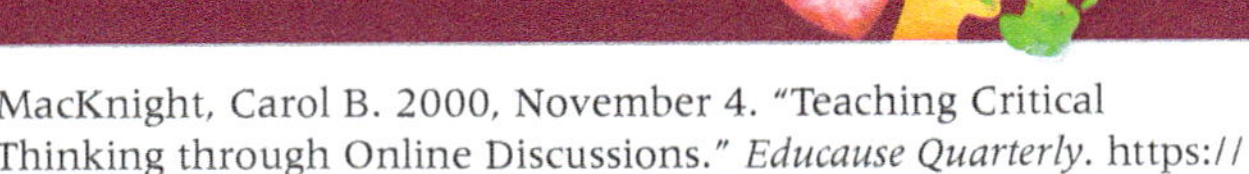

Duckworth, Rom. 2018, August 27. "5 Critical Thinking Skills Crucial to EMS Professional Development." EMS1.com. https://www.ems1.com/ems-management/articles/390034048-5-critical-thinking-skills-crucial-to-EMS-professional-development/.

FISDAP. 2019. "Research 101." http://www.fisdap.net/support/other/research_101.

Global Health Training Centre. 2019. "Short Courses." https://globalhealthtrainingcentre.tghn.org/elearning/short-courses/.

MacKnight, Carol B. 2000, November 4. "Teaching Critical Thinking through Online Discussions." *Educause Quarterly*. https://er.educause.edu/~/media/files/article-downloads/eqm0048.pdf.

University of Kent. 2012. "Learning: Reflective Learning." https://www.kent.ac.uk/learning/PDP-and-employability/pdp/reflective.html.

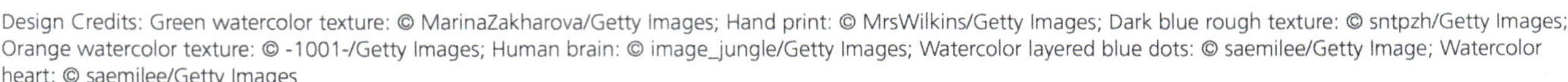

CHAPTER 14

Tools for Small Group Learning

OBJECTIVES

At the conclusion of this chapter, the educator will be able to:

Cognitive Domain

1. Describe key elements of learning in a small group.
2. Describe the benefits and disadvantages of small group learning.
3. List the steps to assign groups for formal and informal activities and short- versus long-term assignments.
4. Distinguish characteristics of cooperative versus collaborative group activities.
5. Outline key elements of small group learning techniques, including problem-based learning, tutorials and seminars, case discussions, role-plays, peer-review activities, and simulations.

Psychomotor Domain

There are no psychomotor objectives for this chapter.

Affective Domain

1. Perceive the need to actively incorporate elements of physical and psychological safety within the lab setting.

"It is the long history of humankind (and animal kind, too) that those who learned to collaborate and improvise most effectively have prevailed."

~ Charles Darwin

CHAPTER GOAL This chapter explores the concepts of facilitation in small groups and provides examples of different strategies that educators can use when teaching small groups.

According to the United Nations Educational, Scientific and Cultural Organization (UNESCO), educators in all fields must teach students to be global learners. This encompasses four principles: learning to know (cognitive knowledge), learning to do (skills-based), learning to be (ethic, values, self-awareness), and learning to live together.[1] Learning to live together is at the heart of team-based learning. Small group learning with effective facilitation will help learners to build these essential prehospital skills.

Small group learning is a team-based approach to learning that allows students to work together to achieve shared learning objectives. A small group format encourages learners to express their understanding of a topic and compare their ideas with others, thereby deepening their knowledge of the subject. The basic tenet of small group teaching focuses on teamwork and cooperation; educators and students work together to solve problems and develop critical and higher-order thinking skills. Educators should facilitate learning within small groups and provide the opportunity for students to monitor their progress and become more self-directed.[2]

A group can consist of two or more students working together.[3] However, the size of the small group is relative to the educational environment. If an educator is used to teaching groups of 100 to 200 or more students, a small group may consist of 40 to 50 students. Alternatively, if a large group consists of 35 to 40 students, the small group may comprise fewer than 10 students. For the purposes of this discussion, a small group is defined as consisting of 2 to 10 students; however, 4 to 5 students is ideal.[4]

The Cornell University Center for Teaching Innovation states that small group learning activities are most often based on four principles:[4]

1. The learner or student is the primary focus of instruction.
2. Interaction and doing are of primary importance.
3. Working in groups is an important mode of learning.
4. Structured approaches to developing solutions to real-world problems should be incorporated into learning.

Small group learning has many characteristics that set it apart from other models of teaching and learning in both approach and delivery method. This chapter details the different types of small group learning models and suggests strategies to employ them in the classroom.

Advantages of Small Group Learning

Active engagement in the learning process for all learners is the main advantage of using the small group format within a course. Lectures often cannot hold the attention of a large group due to the passive learning model this format is based on.

Student engagement in learning is one of the essential elements to reduce attrition in higher education.[5,6] An active classroom teaching environment that integrates cooperative and collaborative learning has been found to improve retention.[7,8] In fact, group work is seen as so valuable that learning with peers (collaborative learning; discussions with diverse others) is one of the four themes measured annually on the National Survey of Student Engagement (NSSE). The NSSE states that "collaborating with peers in solving problems or mastering difficult material deepens understanding and prepares students to deal with the messy, unscripted problems they encounter during and after college."[9]

Small group learning allows learners to bring their own experiences to the learning process and increases active learning. Group learning has been found to outperform individual learning with regard to transfer of higher-level cognitive knowledge.[10] Additionally, it encourages creativity, stimulates discussion, and has been shown to improve confidence and performance.[11] Furthermore, small groups encourage and assist students to develop transferable skills such as teamwork, communication, collaboration, and leadership. This is particularly true in healthcare education, where small groups are used in continuing education environments such as journal clubs and case reviews.[12]

Working in small groups allows students to learn from others—from the examples they offer and their insights, opinions, and mistakes. The educator facilitates the learning objectives. For example, one student may learn a task more quickly than others and then may offer to demonstrate to others how the skill was mastered. Although some schools of thought claim that small group learning requires more instructor time and preparation, others claim that it actually decreases lecture load and overall workload.[3,11,13]

The primary purpose of teaching and learning in small groups is to develop student knowledge, skills, and attitudes so that they can meet desired educational outcomes. This is done in association with the learning outcomes that are described in the curriculum. Because of the intensive nature of the instruction provided with a ratio of one instructor to a small number of students, small groups afford the student the opportunity to learn the finer details of the profession.[14]

Disadvantages of Small Group Learning

It is estimated that it takes approximately 500 to 600 hours of faculty time to provide for 130 hours of lecture. That number remains consistent whether the class size is 10 or 500.[15]

However, while a single instructor can lecture to a large group, small group learning in any form requires a much lower instructor-to-student ratio. The challenges are not limited to the facilitation of these small group activities. Effective delivery of small group learning requires a significant commitment of many hours outside of the classroom designing activities, creating "simulations," or developing problems for the students to solve.

Management of group dynamics can become an issue, and workloads within groups may not be equally distributed. (See Chapter 11, *Introduction to Teaching Strategies*.) The small group learning format requires that more time be spent on a lesson, and educators may not be able to cover all subject matter if using a traditional curriculum. Facilitation may be complex because of the diverse range of learning preferences as well as variation in abilities, personalities, age, and cultural backgrounds, and because students may be unmotivated or passive learners.[14]

Creating Successful Small Groups[3,13]

- Design challenging exercises to be done in a limited time frame.
- Ensure that work assignments are clearly defined.
- Assess both individual and group work.
- Use both peer evaluation and self-assessment.
- Monitor and facilitate small group work (remain visible).
- Ensure that the learning environment is suitable to the task.

Most of the cited disadvantages, however, can be overcome with effective planning and time management. The *Creating Successful Small Groups* box lists some techniques for successful small group learning.

Small Group Dynamics

As individuals, human beings are each different; they have different needs, wants, perspectives, beliefs, and values. Similarly, students differ from each other. Within small group teaching and learning environments, the effective educator will notice the way in which the group interacts. Some students might not readily verbalize their ideas in class and might appear withdrawn and passive. Alternatively, other students might dominate discussions about their experiences and opinions. This may result in negative arguments, group dissension, and personality difficulties that can cause ineffective group productivity.

At times, the instructor will need to employ skillful group-management actions to arbitrate the potential challenges they might experience in association with dysfunctional collaborative learning groups. Some students might complain that others in their assigned group have not contributed equally to the learning exercise. Other students might express their dissatisfaction when their grade is less than what they anticipated due to another student's weaker submission. Therefore, it is essential that clear guidelines be given to students both to ensure that each student knows what is expected and to define the criteria for grading. When assigning a group project, the instructor should consider structuring the scoring rubric in a way that elicits peer feedback about the contribution of each group member. This can minimize the tendency of some group members to "hitchhike" on the work of others. Structuring the grading so the group grade is the goal, with the possibility that those who do not contribute earn less, may incentivize participation.

To encourage a productive, collaborative learning environment, the successful educator will do the following:

- Ask each student a given number of questions.
- Ask open-ended questions as a strategy to engage quieter students.
- Seek clarification or ask probing questions so that students can expand their thoughts.
- Moderate the amount of time and frequency that eager students proffer their discussion, that is, "shared air time."
- Promote students to work toward a common goal—the success of their learning.

CASE in Point

The instructor poses the scenario to which students are to respond.

"Matthew is wheezing really badly—he's an asthmatic and is having trouble breathing!"

As a group, students research information that explains the following content:

- Anatomy and physiology of the respiratory system
- Causes of asthma—what triggers an asthma attack, how asthma develops
- Home management to maintain healthy lifestyle—"reliever and preventer" inhalers
- Pharmacology to relieve the impact of asthma—how these medications work on the body
- Medical intervention in asthma crisis/respiratory arrest—oxygenation, invasive or noninvasive ventilation, medication administration
- Hospital treatment of acute asthma
- Patient education to manage asthma

Types of Groups

Small groups can be formal or informal. Formal groups typically have a planned purpose, require a formal selection process, and assign roles to each group member (FIGURE 14.1). A formal small group, for example, may be used for problem-based learning, case discussions, or simulations. Informal groups can work over a much shorter duration without assigned roles

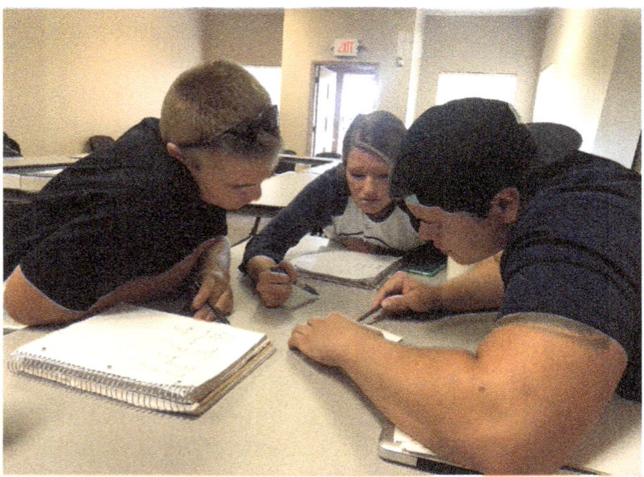

FIGURE 14.1 Small groups can be formal, with a planned purpose and roles, as in problem-based learning.

Courtesy of St. Charles County Ambulance District.

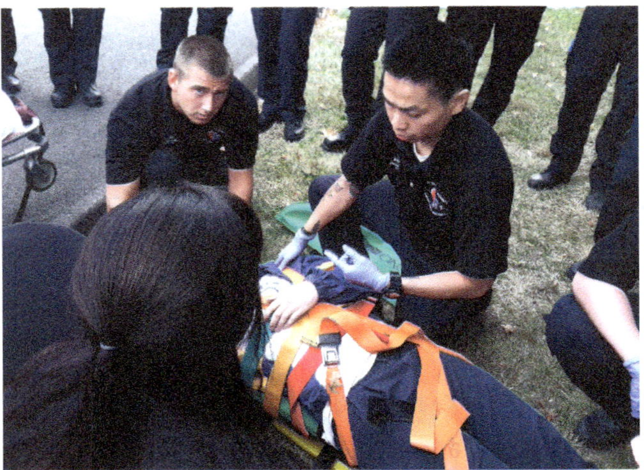

FIGURE 14.2 Groups can be informal, as in a skills practice laboratory. Both formal and informal groups can promote effective learning.

Courtesy of St. Charles County Ambulance District.

(FIGURE 14.2). For example, breaking up a large class by having learners turn to their neighbors to discuss a concept or problem is one example of an informal small group approach.[13] Having students move between different lab stations to learn isolated skills is another example.

Many educators deliver lectures to larger groups, then subdivide students into smaller tutorial groups to create a manageable environment, particularly when the goal is psychomotor development within practical skills laboratories. Ideally, these smaller groups comprise a mix of different types of students (e.g., age, cultural background, personality) and skill levels; the diversity of students adds a dimension of richness to the group.

Small Group Learning Models

There are several structures for small groups. Each of these can be used in either formal or informal learning experiences. A key element for learning success is that group members collaborate with one another and build on each other's strengths to achieve success. Students working in groups may struggle initially with group diversity and may be unwilling to accept differing opinions. Therefore, it is important to encourage students to embrace the many diverse opinions of the group and challenge them to try to include some aspect of each group member's input. Remind students that the world is made up of widely varying points of view, so in order to relate to everyone, each point of view must be respected and considered.

Terms related to group learning, such as *cooperative learning* and *collaborative learning*, are often used synonymously although there are small differences. The cooperative group tends to be more structured and under greater faculty direction.[10]

Cooperative

Cooperative learning is characterized by positive interdependence, where students perceive that better performance by individuals produces better performance by the entire group.[16] Each student makes an individual contribution that contributes to a shared goal. By employing cooperative techniques, students learn real-world communication skills as well as the learning objectives presented. Specific types of activities are discussed later in this chapter; one example of a cooperative learning activity is "Think-Pair-Share." This technique promotes collaboration and cooperation among students. The instructor can pose different questions to different groups, or one main question to all. Each student is required to think about the potential solution, then after a period of time, students convene to work out the best solution to the problem. Students then present their findings to the entire class. Cooperative learning is similar to collaborative learning in that it promotes communication and critical thinking among colleagues.

CASE in Point

A 28-year-old female patient with severe abdominal pain calls 9-1-1. The patient says she might be pregnant. To provide appropriate patient care, students must learn about abdominal pain associated with ectopic pregnancy. If five students constitute the group, a specific learning task should be allocated to each student, such as the following:

- Normal anatomy and physiology of the female reproductive system
- Pathophysiology of ectopic pregnancy
- Clinical presentation of ectopic pregnancy
- Clinical problems and complications that may be anticipated
- Patient care required before time of arrival at the hospital

In turn, each student presents his or her findings to the whole group. If additional students are available, the educator has the option to subdivide tasks (e.g., one student is allocated the anatomy of the reproductive system, and another is asked to find out about the physiology). Alternatively, two students could be allocated to work on a task together.

Features of Cooperative Learning[17]

- **Intentional group formation**. Group members are selected, according to predetermined criteria. For example, recent high-school graduates mix with older students.
- **Continuity of group interaction**. Members have regular group meetings to deal with the assignment, and, in turn, a social network develops. For example, the group may elect to meet in the cafeteria, where, over coffee, they can divide out the work.
- **Interdependence among group members**. Groups work toward a common goal; each member is assigned a specific role associated with the learning process.
- **Individual accountability**. Students are graded individually to reduce "social loafing." Each student makes an independent contribution to the learning; therefore, each assignment is graded on an individual basis.
- **Instructor as facilitator**. The instructor circulates in the group to clarify the task and to offer encouragement.

Collaborative

Employers expect graduates hired from emergency medical services (EMS) programs to be flexible, to be team players, and to have good interpersonal skills. **Collaborative learning** experiences encourage students to think for themselves, compare their thinking with others, and engage in higher-order thinking processes.

Collaborative learning involves the following:

- Discussion
- Negotiation
- Problem solving
- Clarification
- Interpretation

Collaborative learning, in contrast to cooperative learning, focuses on learners working together on a task, problem, or project and being jointly responsible for successful learning outcomes.[18] It encourages active student participation in the learning process by requiring that individual students do an assigned task and think about the approach they must take. Each student must participate in discussion and justify his or her position. Collaborative learning is one way that students can learn from each other—it is a powerful learning tool. Collaborative learning contains an element of subliminal peer pressure that develops between students when one student is seen to be more knowledgeable than the others. Each member of the group researches a section of the task to find information that assists other members of the group.

Team-Based Learning

Team-based learning is a longer-term assignment where a group of students is assigned to a permanent team. Instructors should choose team members thoughtfully, ensuring that a diversity of skills, academic backgrounds, and relevant personal characteristics are selected. Periodic group homework or in-class activities can be assigned to the team. These teams, or squads, as they are sometimes called, can be assigned to classroom tasks that build job-related attributes such as reliability and thorough completion of tasks. The aims of the team are to enhance academic, professional, and interpersonal skills.[16]

Team-Based Learning[19]

Team-based learning is another method of group learning. In this process, the instructor divides the class into permanent teams. Team readiness for activities is ensured using the following:

1. Preassigned reading
2. Individual multiple choice assessment
3. Multiple choice assessment repeated with group
   - Assessment self-graded by group using a progressive disclosure method until all correct answers are known
4. Teams may appeal answers with instructor
5. Mini-lecture by instructor based on material with which students are struggling

Each team is assigned an in-class activity (4 Ss) as follows:

1. *Significant* problem to solve collaboratively
2. *Same* problem is assigned to each group
3. *Specific* choice (answer) is developed by each group
4. *Simultaneous* report-out is conducted, in which:
   a. Each group defends its choice using evidence.
   b. Each group describes how they came to their conclusion.

Summative peer evaluation is conducted several times throughout the semester.

Problem-Based Learning

Problem-based learning (PBL) is an instructional method by which the instructor creates a complex, well-structured real-life problem that a group of students works together to solve. Although the term *problem-based learning* is used loosely as an educational tool for any real-life patient problem or situation, the true form of PBL is well defined and structured. The problem presented is realistic and serves as the catalyst for learning. Students first work to uncover the facts and basic science behind the problem. In subsequent steps, students create possible explanations (hypotheses) about the problem and propose ways to solve some of the issues presented.[20,21]

PBL is not a new concept in education. Socrates and Plato pushed their students to think and search for answers and debate their hypotheses in an educational environment. In 1968, PBL was more formally established by Barrows and colleagues at McMaster University in Ontario, Canada, as a way of helping students apply basic scientific methods to clinical problems.[21,22]

The educator in PBL serves as a coach (also referred to as a "facilitator," "guide," or "tutor") and helps balance and guide the direction of student inquiry. As a facilitator, the educator sets the tone for a positive and respectful exchange and for critical discussion of ideas. Feedback is essential to this facilitation.[22,23]

The belief behind this method is that by discovering the issues and processes that characterize a problem, students acquire basic knowledge and immediately apply that knowledge to solve the problem. Successful PBL teams demonstrate effective self-directed learning, reflection, and teamwork.

Research evidence has been steadily mounting to show that PBL improves clinical reasoning skills and helps students better organize and apply clinical knowledge. This type of group learning fosters cooperative working and improves assessment skills.[24–27] Some studies have shown that PBL reduces the stress of intense medical education.[24]

Advantages of PBL include the development of interpersonal skills, research approaches, communication techniques, prioritization of time and resources, teamwork, and, potentially, learner confidence. Additionally, students are motivated by working on a relevant real-life problem, and they are given the opportunity to be self-directed to some extent. Some disadvantages of PBL include the difficulty of stepping back from a traditional information-delivery model, the time and resources needed for set-up, and the ongoing need for facilitation.[25] Also, scheduled time for independent research and study is essential and may not be available because of the requirements of the curriculum.

Sample Class Sessions with Problem-Based Learning Technique

Class 1

Morning: Group meeting to (a) review case, (b) review terminology, (c) identify critical data, (d) discuss possible explanations, (e) discuss group action plan, and (f) identify learning issues for group and individual students
Afternoon: Lecture or lab to support problem

Class 2

Morning: Independent research to support problem: reading on core issues, writing down individual issues
Afternoon: Lecture or lab to support problem

Class 3

Clinical experience to support problem

Class 4

Morning: Independent research to support problem
Afternoon: Lecture or lab to support problem

Class 5

Morning: Group meeting to discuss how new learning applies to the analysis and resolution of the case

Parameters for Problem-Based Learning

Although PBL units can be presented in various formats, the following principles remain consistent:

- In a PBL unit, the ill-structured problem, as described below, is presented first and serves as the organizing center and context for learning.
- The problem on which learning centers should:
  - Be ill structured
  - Be presented as a "messy" situation
  - Often change with the addition of new information
  - Not be solved easily or formulaically
  - Not always have a "right" answer
- In PBL classrooms, students assume the role of problem solver; teachers assume the roles of tutor and coach.
- In the teaching and learning process, information is shared, but knowledge is a personal construction of the learner. Thinking is fully articulated and is held to strict benchmarks.
- Assessment is an authentic companion to the problem and the process.
- The PBL unit is not necessarily interdisciplinary in nature but is always integrative.

Preparing for Small Group Teaching

Within any classroom, the role of the educator is to engage students in learning. Because of the intimacy of small groups, the educator may take on various roles as needed, such as instructional guide, content expert, examiner, facilitator, teacher, learner, and advocate. Each role is determined by the dynamics of the group and the topic that is being presented. On one hand, a firm or semiauthoritative approach may be needed when student requirements for successful completion of the course are outlined; on the other hand, a relaxed, friendly, and casual approach may be used to create a comfortable learning environment when that is the goal.

Assigning students to specific groups is more effective when dealt with ahead of time. If this is not possible, it should be quickly attended to at the commencement of class so as not to waste time.

The instructor can use several methods to assemble groups. Randomization techniques such as counting off or drawing numbers allow learners to maintain minimal control in the random-sorting process. The educator can control the selection before class time based on knowledge of the group, keeping in mind individual strengths and limitations. The educator might assign groups according to students' age, sex, relative ability, or study major. Student control of selection allows individual or collective formation of groups based on the wishes of group members. However, student self-selection is generally not recommended, as students might not consider the demands of the study task when choosing fellow group members. This option may prove to be less effective because the student strengths might not match the task at hand.[28]

TEACHING TIP

Remember that EMS personnel will not always work with the same partner or crew. Variation in the memberships of groups, as well as in their skill levels, can enhance the overall performance of individual members and of the team.

CASE in Point

Example of a Problem for PBL

Scene

EMS is dispatched on a Saturday evening to an affluent shopping mall for a "girl who is acting strangely and talking out of her head." The dispatcher says that mall security initiated the call, and that the patient is somewhat verbally aggressive. When the crew arrives, they meet a provocatively dressed young woman who is smoking a cigarette and says she is 20 years old and was just pushed by a man she met inside the bar. She says she is "fine" and would be "better if the ?@** police would stay out of her life and leave her alone." Mall security indicates they smell alcohol on the patient's breath. The police officer on the scene states that this could be her cologne and that she appears to be constantly staring at the floor.

Assessment

The patient admits to occasional drug use but says she has not taken anything recently. EMS notes that she has an abrasion on her knee and a medic alert bracelet on her wrist, indicating allergy to haloperidol and benzodiazepines. The police have searched the patient for weapons and have given EMS empty bottles of rifampin, metformin hydrochloride, and valproic acid. The patient is refusing to be treated and states that she is being "set up" for another hospital bill because the "police said the detox unit is full." She just wants to go home. Her blood pressure is 160/90, pulse is 124, respirations are 20 per minute, and SpO_2 is 80% on room air.

In their own defense, the police privately admit that the county detoxification unit is full, but they are willing to arrest her for disorderly conduct if the EMS crew medically clears the patient.

Questions for the First Group Meeting

1. What key elements are included and/or missing in the patient assessment?
2. What physiological mechanisms might be responsible for the symptoms present?
3. What field impressions should the EMS crew consider?
4. What legal principles are at play? What psychosocial issues are implicated between each of the agencies responding to the call (mall security, police, and EMS)? How would each of those be managed?
5. What is the patient's possible medical history based on the assessment findings?

Complications to Be Discovered after the First Discussion Is Completed

Case continuation: As the crew questions the patient, she has a tonic seizure (arms only); afterwards, she is unresponsive to any stimuli.

- How should EMS manage this patient?
- Should the patient awaken and become violent, what type of physical and alternative restraint systems might be used?

Planning Classroom and Lab Sessions

With any teaching assignment, the instructor must first consider what students need to achieve so that learning objectives can be identified. These learning objectives should be clearly defined and attainable within the scope of the session activities. Each step of the learning process must include clear tasks so that students can build on existing knowledge and relate new information to previous learning. Each step must be delivered at a level that students understand, and students must comprehend relationships at each point. Therefore, special attention must be paid to the materials being used for each teaching session, and when used, scenarios and assessment instruments must fall in line with the session's objectives.

Chapter 10, *Lesson Plans*, provides details on how the instructor should develop lesson plans for a standard class session. Methods of delivering instruction to small groups are consistent with the basic techniques used for a group of any size. The instructional session should begin with an introduction that sets the scene and provides a focus for the learning that is to come. The introduction should include a statement that illustrates the significance of what is to be learned and explains why it is important for students to develop knowledge and skills associated with the learning objectives of the session.

The body of the instruction is set out in a logical and sequential manner. The instructor is challenged to design the instruction in such a way that new knowledge is constructed by building on existing knowledge. Various activities that involve students are incorporated into the lesson. Examples of such activities include student identification of cases for discussion, simulations, and role-playing.

The conclusion of the lesson brings together its significant features. The conclusion provides an opportunity for the instructor to restate the main components. This statement reminds students of the important items they need to study to consolidate their learning. At the end of the session, it is a good idea for the instructor to describe the students' original knowledge base and point out the new knowledge that they have acquired since the lesson began.

Additional Small Group Applications[13]

- Begin class discussion with small groups to motivate learners and set the stage for learning.
- Break up a lecture with small groups to deepen and assess understanding.
- End class discussion with small groups to summarize the learning tasks of the day.
- Use small class format for exam review.
- Work in small groups for exam debriefing.
- Use small group activities as an adjunct to audiovisual presentations.

Etiquette and *Practice Like We Play* Mentality

Special emphasis should be made for participants to "practice like they will play." In other words, participants should perform all activities in the classroom and the lab with the help of simulation in as close to the manner they would use in a real situation. Doing this avoids the possibility of preprograming bad behaviors or actions that can affect patient care.

Of the considerations that should be made, safety and professionalism should take top priority. Participants may need to be reminded of the importance of professional behavior during group activities in order to eliminate any potential unprofessional programing that could show up during real situations.

Culture of Safety

EMS educators play essential roles in recognizing safety knowledge gaps and infusing safety culture within all learning activities.[29] Every classroom and lab activity should foster a culture of safety by clearly outlining the real or potential hazards. It should be clear that every participant is responsible for the safety of the patient as well as the entire group. This means that every student not only has the ability to stop any activity when a crew or patient safety concern arises, but is expected to stop an activity any time crew or patient safety is called into question. Additionally, participants are encouraged to confirm their findings and actions with each other (regardless of training level) in order to reduce the possibility of medical errors. The culture of safety practice needs to be heavily integrated into every aspect of EMS education so it will become completely engrained into each participant.[30]

In the lab or classroom setting, faculty have the added responsibility to ensure the psychological and physical safety of students, patient models, and others involved in the learning activity. The instructor must intervene immediately to stop the activity and take corrective measures. If it is not possible to reasonably ensure safety, the activity should be abandoned to avoid potential for injury and a claim of negligence directed toward the instructor.[31]

Common Small Group Strategies

Diverse types of learning activities can be used with small groups. Included here is a discussion of tutorials and seminars, case discussions, role-plays, peer-review activities, and simulations. As mentioned earlier, the formats of cooperative, collaborative, team-based, and problem-based learning can be applied when performing various small group strategies.

In general, it is best to move from simple to complex group activities to allow students to build team learning skills. Many small group exercises can be employed in the online learning environment as well as within the traditional classroom setting. **TABLE 14.1** illustrates examples of simple small group activities.

Tutorials and Seminars

Lectures presented to large groups of students are usually planned to work hand in hand with tutorials and

TABLE 14.1 Examples of Simple Small Group Activities

Method	Activity
Aaronson's Jigsaw Method[32]	Each person in a group is assigned a subtopic to investigate; they investigate then meet with the "expert" members of other groups assigned the same subtopic to compare notes and refine their knowledge before returning to the group, where the information is combined to form the whole conclusion.
Catch-Up[33]	Lecture is stopped at a predetermined point. Students turn to one or more group members to review the content, identify areas of confusion, and develop questions if needed.
Group Investigation Method[34]	A topic is assigned and the group decides how to study it. The work is divided among the group members and then assembled and presented to the class.
Numbered Heads Together[35]	Students are assigned to a group and given a question to answer. Together the group determines the answer to the question. One member of the group presents their findings to the class.
Scripted Cooperation[36]	Students in each group are assigned a topic and one member summarizes material while the other member(s) notes any errors or missing information. Then they change roles.
Think-Pair-Share[37,38]	The instructor poses a question. First, students consider the question by themselves and make notes related to their thoughts. Then the students assemble in their group to compare answers, considering where their responses agree or differ, until they reach consensus on an answer that is then shared with the entire class.

seminars. The lecture provides the formal academic point of view, whereas the purpose of tutorials and seminars is to transfer theory into applications for clinical practice. It is common for tutorials and seminars to be included within the format of a class.

The **tutorial** is achieved primarily through discussion. The educator usually leads the tutorial, and students are expected to provide input. The tutorial provides a wealth of opportunities through which students can learn. It is in this class that the relevance and meaning of what students are doing become apparent.

TEACHING TIP

The main task that the educator faces is getting the discussion going; this can be a challenge for the new instructor. As with most other teaching methods, getting students involved creates a functional learning environment. One of the most disappointing situations that the instructor can experience is a silent group. If no one offers to start a discussion, the instructor must take the lead. The instructor should ask students for their opinions and have students share experiences with the group. Students do not always recognize what they do not know. The tutorial provides a means by which students can identify shortcomings, so they can review and work on those areas. For this purpose, the wise instructor pays attention to the tutorial preparation.

Effective tutorials require clear guidelines that enable students to achieve expected learning outcomes, along with expectations that everyone will participate in the learning process and that decisions will be made by group consensus. In smaller class settings, tutorial activities may be integrated between or within the lectures.

In situations in which questions and statements for discussion are drawn from the lecture content, the educator should have an outline prepared in advance. This outline is the roadmap that guides the learning process. Development of questions for the tutorial requires thorough attention to the preceding lecture content. If another faculty member has delivered the lecture, it is useful for the instructor to liaise with this person to ensure that the outcome is in accordance with overall curriculum requirements.

A **seminar** is typically led by students while the instructor facilitates the learning theme. Seminars, like tutorials, are usually associated with a parallel lecture; a seminar provides a forum in which students can raise learning issues by working through allocated tasks. During seminars, students and educators discuss a topic that is part of the course content in an environment that does not demand the rigor of academia.

At the commencement of the course, seminar tasks are usually allocated to students who are required to prepare a theme for discussion. For example, if the focus of the lecture is myocardial infarction (MI), the seminar could address topics such as physical exercise and nutrition for a healthy heart, or associated physiology of time-related activity of cardiac markers after an MI. Or, if the focus of the lecture is heat-related illness, the seminar could address topics such as the effects of high humidity in hot environments or the long-term physiological effects of prolonged heat exposure.

Handouts distributed at seminars and tutorials provide insights into the content discussed. Handouts help the student recall the topic as discussed in class; a reference list of available texts and resources for independent study can be provided as part of the handout. Students are encouraged in this way to read more about the topic than is provided in the handout.

Case Discussion

The relevance of bringing together theory and practice has impact when each student is asked to describe a particular case that they have experienced as part of field internship. The case can be dissected into specific sections for analysis.

A diabetic crisis is used to illustrate how each section can be analyzed. For example:

- **The situation in which the patient was found**. What clues provide information that could assist EMS personnel to determine the cause of the incident?
- **The clinical features of the patient**. What were the clinical features, and how do they relate to the underlying pathophysiology?
- **Associated medical conditions of the patient**. Some medical conditions such as diabetes may be accompanied by retinopathy, a vision problem. How and why does this develop?
- **Prehospital care**. What care was provided? Why was this done? What could or should have been included when this care was provided?
- **Patient education**. What does the patient need to learn to manage his or her diabetes at home?

Because each student has a personal interest in the case, the student group and the instructor provide detailed discussion that creates a great learning opportunity. Additionally, case studies can provide a great opportunity for the program medical director to become involved in the learning process.

Role-Play

Role-playing is a group-oriented process that involves at least two participants in a classroom dramatization. Role-plays can involve as many as 7 to 10 characters but are usually limited in duration and scope. This type of classroom drama can be used to investigate and bring alive almost any topic. The technique is meant to create a situation in which each participant adopts a realistic character, or type of patient, and interacts with others in the role-play according to how the character would act in real life.

Adequate preparation and facilitation skills are essential for the successful use of a role-play. In general, the extent to which the acting performance is realistic determines the degree of learning that will occur. Instructors should set the stage so that students take the exercise seriously. Giggling, joking, and outbursts of laughter are often related to discomfort on the part of the role-players, or students. These outbursts tend to diffuse needed tension and can break the concentration of players, minimizing the importance of the event. It is important for the instructor to remind students that they may face this very situation in an actual patient care environment. Debriefing and discussion are key elements in reinforcing important learning points and integrating the performance into the lesson plan. Acknowledgment of the stress involved in the performance and appropriate use of humor can be encouraged once the goals of the role-play have been achieved.

Care should be taken to respectfully diffuse the anxiety of participants so that a safe learning environment is created. Students may try to psychoanalyze the players based on their roles; it is important for everyone to be reminded that these are only dramatizations and improvisations—not necessarily the real feelings or actions of the participants. Inviting guests such as past patients, acting students, local crisis team workers, Community Emergency Response Team (CERT) members, or EMS program graduates to play a role can often lead to a higher level of intensity and learning. Videotaping can enhance this activity, allowing for retrospective group or individual performance review and evaluation.

Role-plays differ from scenarios in that very little medical equipment is used. (Scenarios are covered in Chapter 18, *Tools for Simulation*.) Role-plays focus on human interaction, case presentation, symptomatology, interview approaches, deescalation, and communication skills. Crisis intervention, therapeutic communication, and courtroom-testifying skills are particularly well suited to this type of group process.

Essential Elements of Role-Playing[39]

- **Briefing students**. Explain the subject, goals, and key elements of the situation. If particular physical behaviors are needed, such as facial expressions or body position, the instructor should coach the role-players on a realistic way to reenact actual patient presentations.
- **Conducting the drama**. Act, or set the stage and environment so others can act.
- **Debriefing**. Identify key concepts that have been learned, and facilitate a constructive conversation about the performance of the players.

Some types of role-playing include the following:

- **Student–student scripted role-play**. A group of 2 to 10 students dramatizes a patient encounter, taking on the roles that would be involved—from patient(s), family members, and bystanders, to first responders and EMS crew members.
- **Student-directed improvisational role-play**. A group of students creates a situation to which another student (or team of students) must respond. Students prepare the dramatization in advance, researching the signs, symptoms, and possible actions or reactions that might occur during such an event. Students who prepare the role-play might anticipate what occurs when a patient is treated inappropriately or is not treated at all.

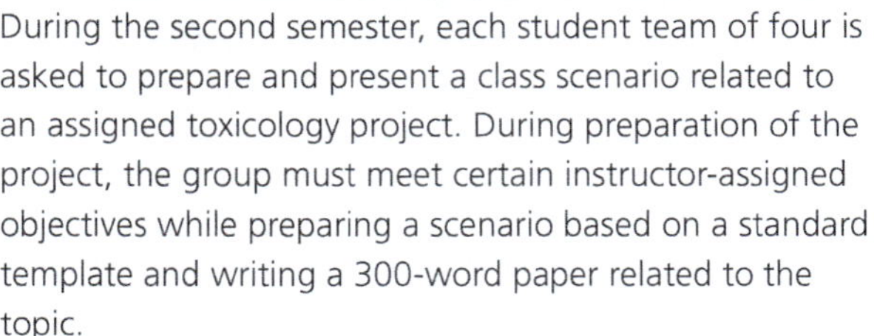

During the second semester, each student team of four is asked to prepare and present a class scenario related to an assigned toxicology project. During preparation of the project, the group must meet certain instructor-assigned objectives while preparing a scenario based on a standard template and writing a 300-word paper related to the topic.

The group must present the scenario (which must be approved by the faculty member 48 hours in advance) and supply all actors and props. Students are given a grading rubric that details expectations for the scenario and the paper. In addition, each team member must complete a separate team participation evaluation for each of their teammates (including themselves).

Team 4 is assigned organophosphate poisoning. They craft a scenario that undergoes minor revisions based on faculty feedback. Team members participate fully in developing the scenario. Amina writes the paper, gathers props, and helps the team set up. Jeremy helps gather references and writes up the scenario. In addition to gathering research on the topic, Mateo dresses up in a pest-control uniform he borrowed from his uncle and plays the role of the patient while another team plays the role of responder. Mateo's teammate Jasmine serves as the scenario facilitator, giving any additional prompting or feedback needed to the responding crew. All team members reviewed both the paper and the scenario before submission. Their group scored 94% on the project, and based on the peer evaluations, it was determined that each group member participated fully and was also awarded the full score.

- **Instructor–student role-play**. The instructor pretends to be a patient and interacts with two or more students as they try to interview and take care of the instructor.
- **Guest role-play**. A person unknown to the class is invited to dramatize a case. Students are placed in the role of EMS responders who try to provide care to the guest.

Peer-Review Activities

A **peer-review activity** allows students to assume the role of evaluator and view the activity from a different perspective. For instance, reviewing a fellow student's patient care documentation or his or her draft version of a research paper can prove to be mutually beneficial. Peer-review activities have been found to increase the knowledge of the topic in both the peer reviewer and the classmate whose work is being reviewed.[40] This benefit is especially true of peer-reviewed lab skills. During these activities, participants evaluate other classmates of like knowledge and skill level using standardized assessment instruments.[41] Ideally these activities should reflect how an instructor assessment of the same activity would be performed.[42]

An instructor should supervise peer-review activities to reduce the risk of participant bias and to ensure that the environment is reflective of an instructor-led review activity. If left on their own, participants have a tendency to either be overly lax or overly strict toward each other.

In order to give participants an opportunity to practice the activity in an assessment environment without the risk of receiving a poor grade, peer-review activities should precede similar instructor-reviewed activities. These activities allow participants to hone and refine their skills while still receiving valuable feedback on their performance. However, students should be held accountable to both their performances and their assessments of other participant performances. Students who make perfect scores on their peer reviews should be expected to perform equally as well when being assessed by an instructor. When there is a disconnect between peer and instructor reviews, the participant and their peer evaluator should be held accountable.

Peer performance feedback can be helpful and important; however, peer comments need to be monitored to ensure that they reflect the activity requirements and are given in a constructive manner. This is an area where students who have filled the role of evaluator can sometimes feel overly empowered and add personal thoughts or opinions rather than relying on objective and relevant information. The overarching goal of peer-review activities is to foster a culture of learning that includes continuous patient safety and best practices.[41]

Simulation

Simulation exercises provide an excellent opportunity for students to incorporate cognitive, psychomotor, and affective skills while working in groups (**FIGURE 14.3**). The purpose of simulation is to create problem-solving situations like the ones that students can expect to manage during their careers. It is useful to base the problem around student's current learning and clinical experiences to ensure that the scenario is within reach of each student's level of training and degree of expected competence.

Similar to role-plays, simulations require a patient actor or high-fidelity manikin, a responding crew, bystanders, and a facilitator. Using **moulage** to simulate illness or injury can enhance the realism of this experience. Simulations can be used to open a class by stimulating discussion, or to close a class by evaluating student understanding of the covered material. Simulations can be done as remediation during clinical or field rotations when similar cases have been seen. Finally, they can be done during lab time as a "put it all together" activity for students. Simulation is discussed more fully in Chapter 18, *Tools for Simulation*.

Simulation exercises offer many benefits. Each scenario can be stopped at any time to draw attention to certain aspects to which the participant must give due attention. Because the demands associated with real-life events are not a part of the exercise, each part of the scenario can be discussed at the point of activity, and each can be supportively debriefed at the conclusion.

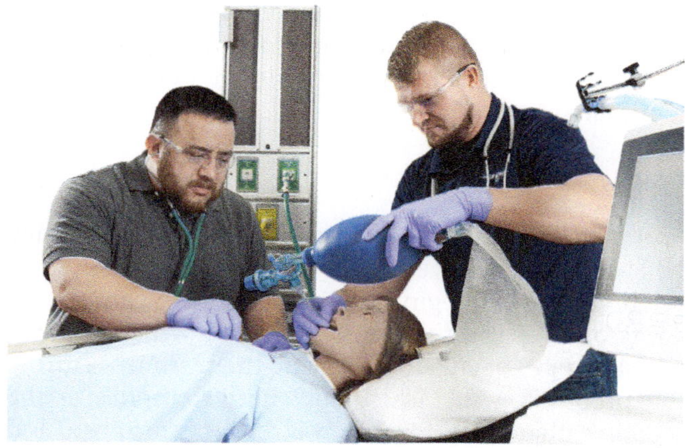

FIGURE 14.3 Simulation exercises are typically popular with students because they give students the chance to practice what they have learned and to self-assess.

Courtesy of CAE Healthcare.

CASE in Point

Vehicle extrication is one example of a simulation exercise. Although it might be difficult to acquire or use actual car wrecks, the simulation is effective when an actual vehicle is used. With relevant training equipment, each student takes the role of the victim to be extricated from the vehicle. If different types of vehicles are available, it is beneficial to repeat the exercise in different vehicles to enhance student awareness of the problems to be encountered in various real-life situations.

Different scenarios can be created to dramatize problems of advanced complexity that must be solved—extrication of the patient who has spinal injuries, or a potential leg fracture, or a major hemorrhage and crushed chest. Each scenario will require actions and practices that demonstrate standard competencies of prehospital care.

TEACHING TIP

To make simulations more realistic, move students to a different location such as outdoors, in the hall, or in the bathroom. Use moulage, background noise, and props such as medical supplies, medication vials and bottles, or other products; have simulated patients follow a scripted storyline.

Teaching Psychomotor Skills

Teaching psychomotor skills provides an excellent opportunity for the instructor to teach in small groups. Psychomotor skill development is crucial to good patient care. All the effort put forth at the scene of an EMS incident depends on the provider's ability to select the right skill at the right time and to carry it out in the right manner. Many of the skills routinely performed at an EMS incident are critical to patient survival and leave little or no margin for error. Details of teaching psychomotor skills can be found in Chapter 12, *Teaching in All Domains*.

Skill Sequencing

Special consideration should be made for the sequence in which participants are introduced to new skills. New skills should be introduced in a logical sequence that matches the sequence and progression of cognitive learning materials in order to foster a deeper understanding of how and why a skill should best be utilized for the benefit of a patient. Proper skill sequencing also aids in retention of new skills and materials.

Prebriefing

Prebriefing is used to prepare students for what they will be doing in a given small group or lab session. Prebriefing helps to begin building trust with the participants by preparing them mentally for what they will be asked or expected to do during the session.[43] During the prebriefing the instructor should emphasize the session's objectives, explain the session's purpose, and outline the rules that participants are expected to follow.[43] Prebriefing is an essential part of the learning process because it reduces participant confusion and frustration by explaining in detail what is expected before the session begins. The prebriefing is also a good time to review and reinforce relevant information and materials that have been taught up to the present point in the course.

Demonstration

Prior to allowing students to practice psychomotor skills independently in the lab, it is essential that they know what proper performance of the skill looks like. This can be accomplished by having the instructor demonstrate the skill, by having the students watch a video of the skills being taught, or by a combination of the two. While instructor-led demonstrations have a proven track record, video-based skill demonstrations have been shown to enhance learning, improve skill understanding, and assist with revision and retention.[44] Generally, it is recommended that instructors use skill demonstration videos in order to reduce the possibility of errors during the learning phase that can be difficult to correct.

Documentation

Documentation of every skill or scenario performed in the lab should be maintained as a part of the participant's permanent course record. These records include both peer and instructor assessments.

Skill Assessment

Skill assessment requires the use of valid assessment instruments. These instruments should be detailed enough to document vital aspects of the performance and have a format that is logical and easy to understand. This minimizes the risk that the evaluator will be distracted by the instrument and lose focus on the participant's performance.

Determining Student Competency

Participant skill competency should ideally be determined through the use of success ratios. Rather than measuring competency by the number of times a skill is performed successfully, a success ratio measures a student's cumulative performance throughout the course.[45] So, instead of deeming a student competent after the student successfully performs 5 or 6 attempts at a given skill, a success ratio requires that the student maintain a level of success. Ratios are generally set at 8 of the last 10 or 5 of the last 7, meaning the student must successfully perform the skill 8 of the last 10 times or 5 of the last 7 times that they attempt the skill. If a student fails to meet the success ratio, the student should complete more lab practice until skill mastery is demonstrated. Once the success ratio is met, the student is considered competent in that particular skill within the context of where the assessment was performed.

Debriefing

Debriefing is a way for students to critically reflect on the experience in a constructive manner to solidify lessons learned from the experience so they can be applied to real patient care events.[46,47] According to Fanning and Gaba proper debriefing is "the cornerstone of the experiential learning experience."[43] During the debriefing process, participants discuss what took place during the event (good and bad) in a nonthreatening, nonjudgmental way. Debriefing is intended to assist the students to reflect on their actions and how those actions positively or negatively impacted the event. During debriefing sessions, one person's input is not more or less valuable than another's. It is important for the process to remain educational and nonthreatening.

Throughout the debriefing, the instructor acts as a facilitator, gently guiding the direction of the discussion while acting as a resource for the students.[43] However, if the students are disengaged with the debriefing process, the facilitator may need to become more involved by directing the actions of the group and asking specific questions or providing a detailed review of the session.

Not every laboratory session requires or would benefit from the debriefing process. In general, individual or team skills that are relatively straightforward (i.e., intubation, applying a splint, etc.) do not benefit from the debriefing process. However, sessions utilizing team training, multidisciplinary training, or crew resource management skills typically benefit from a debriefing session.[43]

Debriefing should be a planned event and scheduled as a part of the overall session. The length of the debriefing session depends on the complexity of the event. Generally speaking, debriefings should occur directly following the event so that student actions are still fresh; however, if video and paper documentation is used, debriefings may prove beneficial days or even weeks after the event. Delayed debriefings are useful for reviewing documentation practices or to prepare students for how documentation is used in the legal process, should they be called upon as a legal witness during their career.

Lab Session Planning and Preparation

Lab sessions should be planned weeks in advance so that proper preparations can be made prior to the lab session. The first step is to determine what skills need to be taught and in what sequence in order to meet the objectives of the topics that are being covered. Next, an inventory list of supplies, props, and equipment should be developed that includes enough items to teach all participants in a timely manner. Maintain a manikin-specific inventory of consumables (skins, veins, batteries, lubricants, etc.). A list of objectives should be available for each lab as well as directions for the lab instructor regarding the specific expectations for the session. Any relevant skill assessment sheets (paper or electronic) must be provided as well as supportive explanatory material for the instructor to refer to if needed.

If utilizing a nonstandard lab location such as a hallway, office, dining area, or exterior location, be sure to reserve the location in advance. Location background should also be considered, because background that appears out of place can be unrealistic and distracting to the students. Consider the use of partitions or premade scene backdrops to aid with realism where needed.

Ideally, these steps should be completed far enough in advance so that any needed items can be ordered or secured prior to the scheduled lab day.

Summary

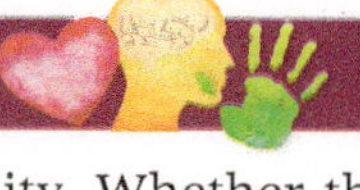

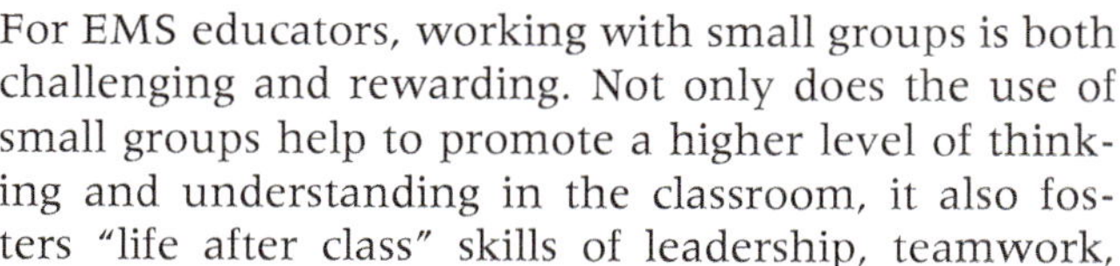

For EMS educators, working with small groups is both challenging and rewarding. Not only does the use of small groups help to promote a higher level of thinking and understanding in the classroom, it also fosters "life after class" skills of leadership, teamwork, communication, and accountability. Whether the entire curriculum is designed around small groups, or they are simply used to break up lectures or to teach psychomotor skills, small group instruction can be an extremely effective educational strategy.

Glossary

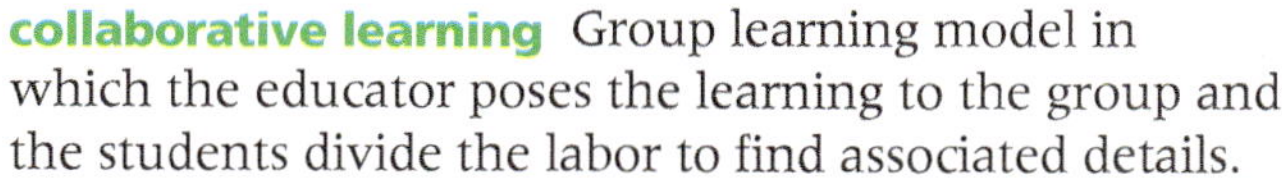

collaborative learning Group learning model in which the educator poses the learning to the group and the students divide the labor to find associated details.

cooperative learning Group learning model in which the educator poses the learning to the group and the students work together and are jointly responsible for learning outcomes.

debriefing Session that occurs at the end of a small group activity, in which students reflect on and discuss what was learned.

moulage Application of makeup and props to simulate injuries or signs of illnesses.

peer-review activity Type of small group activity in which a student reviews work by another student and provides feedback.

prebriefing Information provided by an instructor, for example, verbally at the beginning of a skills session or simulation, which prepares students by explaining what to expect in the session.

problem-based learning (PBL) Instructional method by which the instructor creates a complex, well-structured problem that a group of students tries to solve.

role-playing Group process that involves students in a dramatization.

seminar Recurring small group discussion session comprised of an educator and students.

team-based learning Learning model in which a longer-term assignment is given to a group of students assigned to a permanent team.

tutorial Discussion-based session led by the educator, which occurs in small group format, in which decisions are made by group consensus, and in which students are expected to provide input.

References

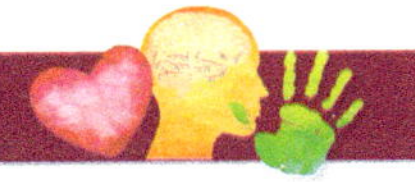

[1] UNESCO (Ed.). 1996. *Learning: The Treasure Within: Report to UNESCO of the International Commission on Education for the Twenty-First Century*. Paris, France: UNESCO Publishing.

[2] Jaques, David. 2000. *Learning in Groups: A Handbook for Improving Group Learning*, 3rd ed. London, UK: Kogan Page.

[3] Healey, Mick, Hugh Matthews, Ian Livingstone, and Ian Foster. 1996. "Learning in Small Groups in University Geography Courses: Designing a Core Module around Group Projects." *Journal of Geography in Higher Education* 20: 167–81. https://doi.org/10.1080/03098269608709364.

[4] Cornell University Center for Teaching Innovation. n.d. "Group Work: How to Create & Manage Groups." Accessed November 24, 2018. https://teaching.cornell.edu/resource/group-work-how-create-manage-groups.

[5] Tinto, Vincent. 1993. *Leaving College: Rethinking the Causes and Cures of Student Attrition*, 2nd ed. Chicago: University of Chicago Press.

[6] Tinto, Vincent. 1975. "Dropout from Higher Education: A Theoretical Synthesis of Recent Research." *Review of Educational Research* 45, no. 1: 89–125. https://doi.org/10.3102/00346543045001089.

[7] Braxton, John M., Amy S. Hirschy, and Shederick A McClendon. 2004. "Understanding and Reducing College Departure." *ASHE-ERIC Higher Education Report* 30, no. 3: xi–99.

[8] Pascarella, Ernest T., and Patrick T. Terenzini. 2005. "Educational Attainment and Persistence." In *How College Affects Students, Volume 2*, 373–444. San Francisco: Jossey-Bass.

[9] Center for Postsecondary Research and Indiana University School of Education. 2018. "NSSE: National Survey of Student Engagement." Accessed November 24, 2018. http://nsse.indiana.edu/html/engagement_indicators.cfm.

[10] Pai, Hui-Hua, David A. Sears, and Yukiko Maeda. 2015. "Effects of Small-Group Learning on Transfer: A Meta-Analysis." *Educational Psychology Review* 27, no. 1: 79–102. https://doi.org/10.1007/s10648-014-9260-8.

[11] Sobral, Dejano T. 1998. "Productive Small Groups in Medical Studies: Training for Cooperative Learning." *Medical Teacher* 20: 118–21. https://doi.org/10.1080/01421599881219.

[12] Jaques, David. 2003. "Teaching Small Groups." *British Medical Journal* 326: 492–4. https://doi.org/10.1136/bmj.326.7387.492.

[13] Cooper, James L., and Pamela Robinson. 2000. "Getting Started: Informal Small-Group Strategies in Large Classes." *New Directions for Teaching and Learning* 81: 17–24.

[14] Cooper, Lesley, Mike Lawson, and Janice Orrell. 1997. *Raising Issues about Teaching: Views of Academic Staff at Flinders University.* Adelaide, Australia: Flinders Press.

[15] Donner, Robert S., and Harmon Bickley. 1993. "Problem-Based Learning in American Medical Education." *Bulletin of the Medical Library Association* 81, no. 3: 294–8.

[16] Johnson, David W., Roger T. Johnson, & Karl A. Smith. 2014. "Cooperative Learning: Improving University Instruction by Basing Practice on Validated Theory." *Journal on Excellence in University Teaching* 25, no. 3&4: 1–26.

[17] Maughan, Caroline, and Julian Webb. 2001. "Small Group Learning and Assessment: UKCLE Seminar, 'From Little Acorns . . .'" Accessed January 18, 2018. http://ials.sas.ac.uk/ukcle/78.158.56.101/archive/law/resources/teaching-and-learning-practices/grouplearning/index.html.

[18] Mayer, Richard E. 2011. *Applying the Science of Learning*. Boston: Pearson.

[19] Sibley, Jim, and Sophie Spirdonoff. 2014. "Introduction to Team-Based Learning." The University of British Colombia Faculty of Applied Science. Centre for Instructional Support. Accessed February 5, 2019. https://cdn.ymaws.com/teambasedlearning.site-ym.com/resource/resmgr/Docs/TBL-handout_February_2014_le.pdf.

[20] Center for Problem-Based Learning, Illinois Mathematics and Science Academy. Accessed February 5, 2019. https://www.imsa.edu/problem-based-learning/.

[21] Wang, HsingChi, Amy Cox, Patricia Thompson, and Charles Shuler. 1998. "Essential Components of Problem-Based Learning for the K-12 Inquiry Science Instruction." School of Dentistry University of Southern California. Accessed February 6, 2019. https://www.academia.edu/1535735/Essential_Components_of_Problem-Based_Learning_for_the_K-12_Inquiry_Science_Instruction.

[22] Barrows, Howard S. 1996. "Problem-Based Learning in Medicine and Beyond: A Brief Overview." In *Bringing Problem-Based Learning to Higher Education: Theory and Practice, Volume 68*, edited by LuAnn Wilkerson and Wim H. Gijselaers, 3–12. San Francisco: Jossey-Bass.

[23] Wilkerson, Luann. 2004, September. "An Introduction to Problem-Based Learning." *2004 National Association of EMS Education Symposium*. Los Angeles: NAEMSE.

[24] Kaufman, David M., David Mensink, and Victor Day. 1998. "Stressors in Medical School: Relation to Curriculum Format and Year of Study." *Teaching & Learning in Medicine* 10: 138–44. https://doi.org/10.1207/S15328015TLM1003_3.

[25] Whitfield, Carol F., Elizabeth A. Mauge, Jeffrey Zwicker, and Erik B. Lehman. 2002. "Differences between Students in Problem-Based and Lecture-Based Curricula Measured by Clerkship Performance Ratings at the Beginning of the Third Year." *Teaching & Learning in Medicine* 14: 211–7. https://doi.org/10.1207/S15328015TLM1404_2.

[26] Walters, Janice A., Lila G. Croen, Zoe Brown Weissman, and Michael J. Reichgott. 1999. "A Small Group, Problem-Based Learning Approach to Preparing Students to Retake Step 1 of the United States Medical Licensing Examination." *Teaching & Learning in Medicine* 11: 85–8. https://doi.org/10.1207/S15328015TL110205.

[27] Kilroy, D. 2004, July. "Problem-Based Learning." *Emergency Medicine Journal* 4: 411–3. http://dx.doi.org/10.1136/emj.2003.012435.

[28] Cross, K. Patricia, and Mimi Harris Steadman. 1996. *Classroom Research: Implementing the Scholarship of Teaching*. San Francisco: Jossey-Bass.

[29] Friese, Greg (Ed.). 2018. "Examine Your EMS Agency's Safety Culture to Improve Patient Outcomes." Center for Patient Safety and Medtronic. Accessed February 8, 2019. https://www.ems1.com/ems-products/Ambulance-Safety/articles/392773048-Your-guide-to-improving-your-EMS-agencys-safety-culture-eBook/.

[30] EMS.gov. 2013, October 3. "Strategy for a National EMS Culture of Safety." Accessed February 6, 2019. https://www.ems.gov/pdf/Strategy-for-a-National-EMS-Culture-of-Safety-10-03-13.pdf.

[31] Goudreau, Kelly, and Eileen Chasens. 2002. "Negligence in Nursing Education." *Nurse Educator* 27, no. 1: 42–6.

[32] Aronson, Elliot. 2002. "The Jigsaw Classroom." In *Improving Academic Achievement: Impact of Psychological Factors on Education*, edited by Joshua Aronson, 215–9. San Diego: Academic Press.

[33] Cornell Center for Teaching Innovation. n.d. "Examples of Collaborative Learning or Group Work Activities." Accessed January 18, 2019. https://teaching.cornell.edu/resource/examples-collaborative-learning-or-group-work-activities.

[34] Sharan, Yael, and Shlomo Sharan. 1992. *Expanding Cooperative Learning through Group Investigation*. New York: Teachers College Press.

[35] Kagan, Spencer. 1989. "The Structural Approach to Cooperative Learning." *Educational Leadership* 47, no. 4: 12–5.

[36] O'Donnell, Angela M., Donald F. Dansereau, Richard H. Hall, and Thomas R. Rocklin. 1987. "Cognitive, Social/Affective, and Metacognitive Outcomes of Scripted Cooperative Learning." *Journal of Educational Psychology* 79, no. 4: 431–7. http://dx.doi.org/10.1037/0022-0663.79.4.431.

[37] Lyman, Frank. 1981. "The Responsive Classroom Discussion: The Inclusion of All Students." In *Mainstreaming Digest*, edited by Audrey Springs Anderson, 109–13. College Park, MD: University of Maryland Press.

[38] Johnson, David W., Roger T. Johnson, and Karl A. Smith. 1991. *Active Learning: Cooperation in the College Classroom*. Edina, MN: Interaction Book Company.

[39] Orlich, Donald C., Robert J. Harder, Richard C. Callahan, and Harry W. Gibson. 2001. *Teaching Strategies: A Guide to Better Instruction*, 6th ed., 296–7. Boston: Houghton Mifflin.

[40] Cho, Young Hoan, and Kwangsu Cho. 2011. "Peer Reviewers Learn from Giving Comments." *Instructional Science* 38, no. 5: 629–43. https://doi.org/10.1007/s11251-010-9146-1.

[41] Haag-Heitman, Barb, and Vicki George. 2017, September 13. "Nursing Peer Review: Principles and Practice." *American Nurse Today*. Accessed February 5, 2019. https://www.mghpcs.org/eed_portal/Documents/ProfDev/Nursing-Peer-Review-Article.pdf.

[42] International Literacy Association (readwritethink.org). 2019. "Strategy Guide: Peer Review." Accessed January 18, 2019. www.readwritethink.org/professional-development/strategy-guides/peer-review-30145.html.

[43] Fanning, Ruth M., and David M. Gaba. 2007, Summer. "The Role of Briefing in Simulation-Based Learning." *Society for Simulation in Healthcare* 2, no. 2: 115–25. Accessed January 18, 2019. http://multibriefs.com/briefs/aspeorg/Debriefing2.pdf.

[44] Lynch, Kathy, Nigel Barr, and Florin Oprescu. 2012. "Learning Paramedic Science Skills from a First Person Point of View." *Electronic Journal of e-Learning* 10, no. 4: 396–406. Accessed January 18, 2019. https://files.eric.ed.gov/fulltext/EJ986672.pdf.

[45] Nielsen, Jakob. 2001, February 18. "Success Rate: The Simplest Usability Metric." Nielsen Norman Group. Accessed January 18, 2019. https://www.nngroup.com/articles/success-rate-the-simplest-usability-metric/.

[46] Dreifuerst, Kristina Thomas, Sara L. Horton-Deutsch, and Henry Henao. 2014. "Meaningful Debriefing and Other Approaches." In *Clinical Simulations in Nursing Education: Advanced Concepts, Trends, and Opportunities*, edited by P. R. Jeffries, 44–57. Philadelphia: Wolters Kluwer, Lippincott, Williams & Wilkins.

[47] Decker, Sharon, Mary Fey, Stephanie Sideras, Sandra Caballero, Leland Rockstraw, Teri Boese, Ashley E. Franklin, et al. 2013. "Standards of Best Practice: Simulation Standard VI: The Debriefing Process." *Clinical Simulation in Nursing* 9, no. 6: S26–9. https://doi.org/10.1016/j.ecns.2013.04.008.

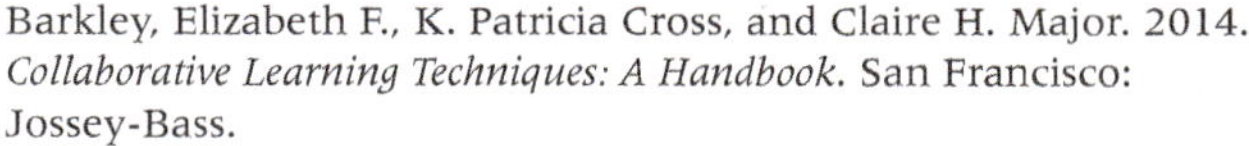

Additional Resources

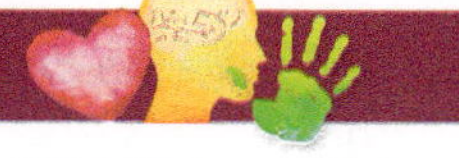

Barkley, Elizabeth F., K. Patricia Cross, and Claire H. Major. 2014. *Collaborative Learning Techniques: A Handbook*. San Francisco: Jossey-Bass.

Dolmans, Diana H. J. M., Sofie M. M. Loyens, Helene Marcq, and David Gijbels. 2016. "Deep and Surface Learning in Problem-Based Learning: A Review of the Literature." *Advances in Health Sciences Education: Theory and Practice* 21, no. 5: 1087–112. https://doi.org/10.1007/s10459-015-9645-6.

Roschelle, Jeremy, and Stephanie Teasley. 1995. "The Construction of Shared Knowledge in Collaborative Problem Solving." In *Computer-Supported Collaborative Learning*, edited by Claire E. O'Malley, 69–97. Heidelberg, Germany: Springer-Verlag.

CHAPTER 15

Tools for Large Group Learning

OBJECTIVES

At the conclusion of this chapter, the educator will be able to:

Cognitive Domain

1. Describe the advantages and disadvantages of teaching large groups.
2. Describe the advantages and disadvantages of lecture as a teaching strategy.
3. Outline the process for developing an effective lecture.
4. List strategies for effective presentation to a large group.
5. Describe the use of effective questioning to promote learning.
6. List benefits of audience feedback systems.
7. Outline small group strategies to use within large group settings.
8. Describe the concept of the flipped classroom.

Psychomotor Domain

1. Given a topic, conduct a large-group learning session incorporating the strategies described within this chapter.

Affective Domain

1. Value the need to receive feedback during large group teaching.
2. Appreciate the need to incorporate active learning strategies within the lecture.
3. Modify teaching strategies in large group settings based on student feedback and learning outcomes.

"Those who know, do. Those that understand, teach."

~ Aristotle

CHAPTER GOAL This chapter offers teaching strategies for instructors to use when they face the challenge of teaching large numbers of students.

Teaching large groups can be challenging for the educator. What is meant by a **large group** in the context of teaching? A review of the literature shows that there is no consensus as to this definition. Much of the constraint inherent with instructing large groups depends on the content that is being taught. For example, delivering a pathophysiology lecture is generally easy to accomplish with any number of students either in person or online. Teaching students to perform a patient assessment is much more difficult if instruction of this psychomotor skill depends on only one educator. For the purposes of this text, a large group is defined as a greater number than can be easily handled for small group activities.

The default mode for most large classes is the lecture. This limits the amount of active learning that the student is able to take part in and impairs the instructor's ability to ensure student understanding after the lecture. Other techniques should be incorporated into the large group setting to address the limitations inherent with using lectures only. For example, thanks to technology, even the shyest student can actively participate in large classes. Although a large class can be a challenge to teach, skilled educators can be successful by identifying and applying effective teaching strategies. With careful planning as well as with a little creativity, teaching large groups can also be fun.

Lecture

The process of using the **lecture** to teach has been around since the dawn of time. During the Middle Ages, instructors viewed their students as having empty brains waiting to be filled with knowledge and experience.[1] At that point, student education involved attempting to memorize every word spoken by the instructor. Although beneficial for the lower levels of learning that leaned on rote memorization, this strategy did not foster higher levels of critical thinking.

Lecture continues to be the most common mode of information delivery in healthcare classrooms today. This is despite abundant research indicating that lecture is the least effective method of learning.[2] If, as the research shows, lecture is such an ineffective manner of teaching, why does it continue to be relied upon so heavily in the classroom? There may be several reasons. First, when compared to the amount of work required to prepare and execute a student-centered approach to teaching, a lecture is almost always easier to prepare.[3] As instructors progress in their teaching career, it becomes much easier to stand in front of a class and verbally regurgitate to the students. With this type of content delivery, less preparation is needed. A second reason for the over-reliance on lecture could be that this is how many educators were taught; the emergency medical services (EMS) educator may not be aware of better alternatives available for teaching.

Lecture is described as a method of teacher-centered learning.[4] It is only one style of presentation. EMS educators must understand that the use of lecture is like the use of any medication. There are indications for it and, when used properly, it can be an outstanding teaching tool. Used improperly, however, little or no learning may take place. It is possible to make lectures more interactive even with large groups. Later, this chapter presents an array of options that will help facilitate active student involvement during the lecture. Regardless of the method of presentation used, it is imperative that the student—not the presenter—be the center of the teaching and learning process.

CASE in Point

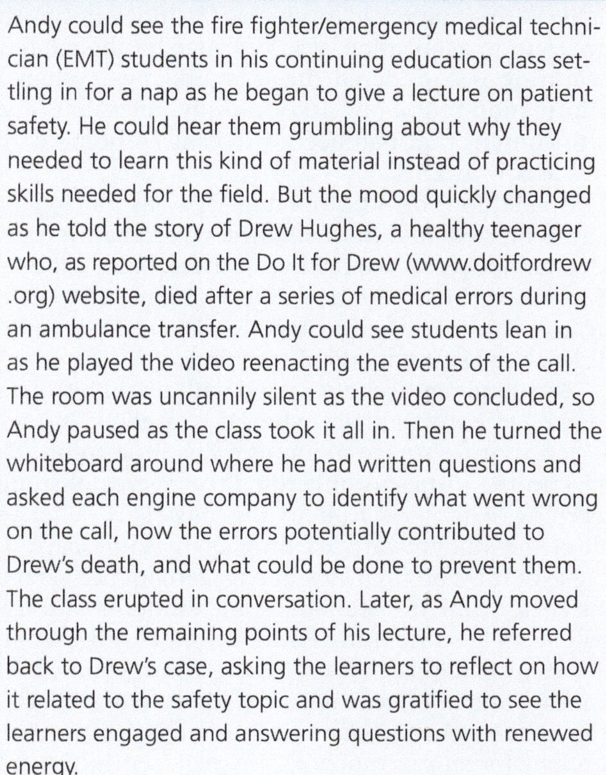
Andy could see the fire fighter/emergency medical technician (EMT) students in his continuing education class settling in for a nap as he began to give a lecture on patient safety. He could hear them grumbling about why they needed to learn this kind of material instead of practicing skills needed for the field. But the mood quickly changed as he told the story of Drew Hughes, a healthy teenager who, as reported on the Do It for Drew (www.doitfordrew.org) website, died after a series of medical errors during an ambulance transfer. Andy could see students lean in as he played the video reenacting the events of the call. The room was uncannily silent as the video concluded, so Andy paused as the class took it all in. Then he turned the whiteboard around where he had written questions and asked each engine company to identify what went wrong on the call, how the errors potentially contributed to Drew's death, and what could be done to prevent them. The class erupted in conversation. Later, as Andy moved through the remaining points of his lecture, he referred back to Drew's case, asking the learners to reflect on how it related to the safety topic and was gratified to see the learners engaged and answering questions with renewed energy.

Advantages and Disadvantages of Lecture in Large Groups

The most notable advantage of lecture is that the cost to deliver the content per student drops dramatically. Colleges and universities often have general education classes, such as English or general science, with 200 or more students in large lecture halls. In these types of courses, the use of lecture is efficient and, from a cost perspective, economical.

Lecture is effective in the dispersal of large amounts of information to students and may be useful when teaching large groups of people in a short period of time. The effective and judicious use of lecture can often emphasize the value of the topic via the degree of enthusiasm presented by the educator during the presentation.

Other advantages of the use of lecture include the following:

- They allow the instructor maximum control of the learning experience.
- They present little risk for students who may be shy or worry about being embarrassed by not knowing the answer in a more student-centered approach.
- Lectures are appreciated by those who learn primarily via the auditory approach.

There are some major detriments inherent with the use of lecture. Although lecture allows an instructor to deliver information to students, this does not always translate to acquisition of knowledge by the students. Lecturing is considered the least effective system for information retention.[5] In one study, retention of lecture content that had been provided 24 hours earlier was as low as 25%.[6]

In addition, healthcare education has a heavy emphasis on psychomotor activities. Overreliance on lecture hampers the acquisition of these skills, especially if it is the primary method of teaching used by the educator. Another disadvantage is that students tend to dislike the lecture mode of teaching.[7]

The disadvantages associated with use of lecture are magnified exponentially when it is used exclusively.[8] When lecture is used alone, there is little to no feedback to the instructor regarding the degree of student learning. This may lead to the mistaken belief that all of the students are learning at the same pace. Because of this potential lack of engagement between the instructor and the student, some students' attention will begin to wander in as little as 8 to 10 minutes after the lecture begins.[9] When lecture is not coupled with another mode of teaching, especially when teaching complex or abstract material, this may result in the student forgetting much of the acquired information within 24 hours after the class ends[10] (**FIGURE 15.1**).

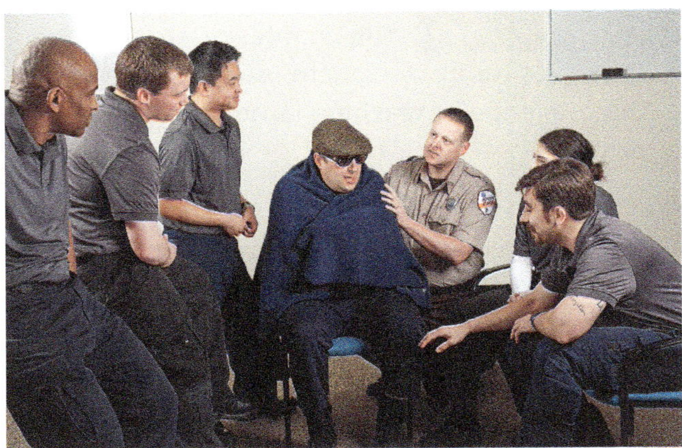

FIGURE 15.1 Techniques can be used to enhance lecture format and contribute to student learning.

Using lecture places an emphasis on learning by listening, not by doing. This is disadvantageous to students with other learning preferences. Lecture alone without visual aids may work well with auditory learners, but can lose the attention of visual and kinesthetic learners. When possible, lecture should be presented with some type of visual accompaniment.

Finally, lecture is not the best method of introducing a multifaceted academic argument regarding a topic. Therefore, the educator should only use lecture to cover one topic, and sparingly at that.

According to Brookfield, students have identified features that improve lecture delivery, which include the following:[11]

- Educators should use a variety of teaching strategies and communication processes.
- Educators should be organized so learners can follow the train of thought.
- Educators should model behaviors they expect students to demonstrate.

Lecture 101

Regardless of how an educator intends to deliver the content, all of the methodology should invite students to begin a mindful journey toward the solution of a problem or issue. The role of the educator is much more involved than simply "covering the material" or going over what will be on the test. Instead, the prime directive should be to instill in the students a deeper curiosity about the subject. In doing so, the goal will be to motivate the student to explore the topic in greater depth outside of the lecture time.

When lecturing, the aim is to deliver information in a conversational, relaxed format. The instructor must be comfortable with the content of the lecture. Students typically do not appreciate being read to; nor do they learn well with this approach.[12] This practice often causes students to mentally "check out" during the lecture.

Instead, when instructors allow themselves to think out loud, it suggests that it is acceptable for students to do the same when struggling with the topic or when they have questions. By modeling this behavior, the instructor makes the environment safer for students who do not grasp the topic easily or on the first pass. The educator should not only allow for questions from the students, but should encourage it by setting the standard for this early in the delivery. More on the Socratic method of lecture will be presented later in this chapter.

Preparing for the Lecture

The fact that an instructor is a subject matter expert in a healthcare topic does not mean that the instructor is ready to present a lecture on that topic. In 1950, it was estimated that medical knowledge doubled every 50 years. By 2020, that time frame will drop to 73 days.[13] The ever-expanding, continually evolving field of medicine necessitates some extra preparation on the part of the instructor. Preparing for a lecture by reviewing material and seeking newer evidence is essential so the educator can present with more self-confidence while enhancing the efficacy of the lesson.

Several hours of preparation time are needed for each hour of lecture.[14] To prepare, an instructor should develop an introduction to the topic that will quickly grab students' attention and entice them to listen to what the instructor is about to say. The use of stories is helpful in taking the lecture information from theoretical to practical. The introduction should outline to the audience what the instructor is going to teach during the lecture. The introduction is important in framing student expectations. The educator can then meet those expectations through the use of a well-developed lesson plan, so that the critical information is delivered. (See Chapter 10, *Lesson Plans*.)

Fine Tuning the Focus of the Lecture

The main points in the lecture should be limited to a maximum of one for each 10 minutes of content. The instructor should plan on 5 minutes for the introduction as well as another 5 minutes for the conclusion. In a 50-minute lecture this leaves approximately 40 minutes to build the presentation and present the evidence to support the conclusions made during the lecture.

The objectives should be highlighted when the relevant content is covered. Doing so will provide one more point of emphasis to the student and will help ensure that all key points are addressed. Objectives can be referenced again as content is summarized at the end of the lecture. An educator should not attempt to deliver all of the needed information during the lecture time. The purpose of the lecture is to redirect students to study outside of class with the provided resources. Doing so enables the student to better encode the information for later recall.

In preparing a lecture, an educator should identify which concepts are most important and which concepts can be relegated to a lesser role. The instructor should develop a study guide that identifies the gaps in the lecture and directs students to areas of the textbook that cover critical concepts. Some lecture time may be used to emphasize the importance of proper use of the textbook and other supplemental reading or resources assigned.

In slide presentations, the amount of text included on each slide should be minimized.[15] Slide presentations are most effective when they include photos or other illustrations to augment the presentation.

Making the Presentation

It is not necessary for the instructor to be a charismatic presenter in order to get information across to an audience in a systematic, concise manner. However, there are some simple public speaking rules that promote success. The instructor should make regular eye contact with members of the audience. This should be done slowly rather than by a rapid scan. Eye contact is most effective when sustained for about 5 seconds; research shows that this amount of time is the most comfortable for the audience member.[16] The instructor should face the audience when presenting, in order to facilitate eye contact. Instructors should spend only a small portion of time writing on the board or looking at the slides. New instructors may consider recording the lecture during a practice session. When replaying it, the use of "filler" words such as "uh" or "em" will become evident. An effective method for minimizing the use of filler words when presenting is to take a breath when sensing the need to use such words.[17]

Including the Audience While Speaking

When lecturing, the use of the **Socratic method** of teaching signals that the students are expected to be an active part of the lecture presentation.[18] Named after the Greek philosopher Socrates, this method of teaching is based on the premise of asking and answering questions with the primary purpose of stimulating critical thinking. It is from this process that other information is discovered by both the educator and the student.

Two important caveats must be provided if the educator intends to use this method of instruction. First, when implementing the Socratic method, the instructor must be prepared for the discomfort of silence. If students have previously been taught in a strictly one-way method of lecture, they must be able to learn the new ground rules that require them to participate by answering questions or coming up with questions of their own. The inevitable silence must become more uncomfortable for students than for the educator. According to Weetman, "Pause procedure provides a vessel for an instructor to incorporate various active learning strategies during their lecture in order to improve teaching and learning process."[19] Second, even after students have become familiar and comfortable with this style of teaching, the educator must allow enough time for them to process the questions, retrieve the information from their short-term and long-term memory, and formulate their responses. The instructor must not let the discomfort of silence derail an effective method of teaching.

Obtaining Student Feedback

Feedback from students can be either verbal or nonverbal in nature. For nonverbal cues, the instructor should watch the behavior and, especially, the facial expressions and body language of the students. Are they actively engaged in understanding the content and responding with nods of the head, note taking, and active involvement of asking and responding to questions? In other words, are they "tracking" along with the instructor? Later, this chapter examines some applications that help educators obtain real-time feedback from students during the lecture presentation.

Handling Questions

Taking questions from the audience is highly recommended.[20] Student questions provide valuable information about whether the information from the lecture was understood. Therefore, questions from the audience should rarely be discouraged. There are multiple methods of handling questions. Early in the presentation, the instructor should set the ground rules about whether questions may be submitted during the lecture or if it is preferred that they be held until the end (**FIGURE 15.2**). Each approach has positive and negative aspects. Allowing students to ask questions during the lecture often adds to the quality of the information and minimizes the chance that the student may forget the question while waiting for the lecture to be completed. When taking student questions during the

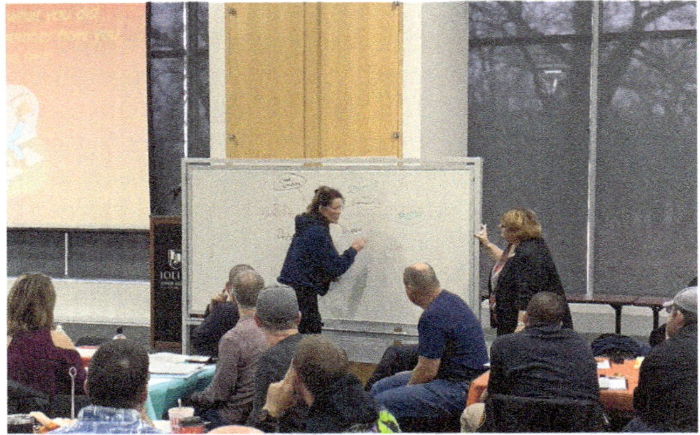

FIGURE 15.2 Effective questioning techniques can be used in a large group. However, the instructor must be prepared to manage the discussion.

lecture, it is important to manage the amount of time allocated. Student questions should not be allowed so much time that they cause the instructor to run out of time, leave out important points, or rush through the presentation to complete it. To avoid these situations, some instructors prefer to wait until the end of the lecture to address questions.

A number of applications can be used as a middle ground to minimize negative outcomes. For some instructors, using the "parking lot" method of addressing questions is helpful. This method can turn a one-sided lecture into an interactive feature. During the presentation, have students write their questions regarding the presentation on a sticky note. At an appropriate time, near the end of the lecture, allow them to bring the questions forward and place them within an assigned location on the wall or board. Some instructors will even have a graphic of an actual parking lot for this. During the lecture preparation, be sure to allow adequate time to address the more commonly asked questions. If a common thread appears regarding particular topics, use that to either help direct the preparation of the next lecture, or provide a short audio or video recording for the students, addressing the issue. Educators without much experience may wish to avoid questions for fear that they might not be able to

TEACHING TIP

Some instructors prefer to take questions electronically. Platforms for backchannel communication such as Mentimeter, GoSoapBox, or BackChannel Chat can be used to facilitate this. When using this strategy, it is helpful to have a moderator to monitor the content.

TEACHING TIP

Students have grown up with television, the Internet, and social media, and therefore, with interruptions. The lecturer should include summaries and illustrative points during the presentation in order to allow students to process information in chunks.

answer them. This should not be a deterrent from using this valuable tool! When posed with difficult questions, the instructor can say, "That's a great question, and I don't readily have an answer for it. However, if you send me your email address, I'll be happy to research it for you and share what I find." Such honesty in handling difficult questions enhances the instructor's approachability as well as their validity as an expert. It also gives students permission to not have all of the answers themselves.

When choosing to accept questions during the lecture, the instructor should stop when facial expressions or body language indicates that the audience is confused. Educators should not simply say, "Are there any questions?" Instead, the educator should make a generalized statement noting the confused looks and should express a genuine desire to clear up any confusion. Instructors should avoid calling out an individual to ask if they are confused, unless they have a good working relationship with that student. Doing so risks embarrassing the student and can lead to the audience turning against the instructor. When lecturing in a large class, instructors should ensure that questions are repeated so all students have an opportunity to hear what was asked prior to the question being answered.

Dressing for Success

Most educators can point to several important influences in their lives that helped them determine that teaching was their calling. Therefore, educators should never underestimate the influence their words and tone (either positive or negative) will have on students. An instructor's attire has an influence on students as well. Research supports this conclusion in a 2015 study completed by Choi and Mattila, who researched how customers would respond depending on how restaurant waitstaff were dressed. They found that customers had a much more favorable impression of their waitstaff when they were dressed formally compared to when they were dressed for comfort.[21]

It is not difficult to apply this concept to educators and their students. First impressions may not be the most accurate, but they are generally formed within a few minutes. These impressions often last long into the relationship.[22] By spending a few moments to ensure one's own professional appearance, an instructor will convey the initial impression of a subject matter expert. This leads to self-confidence, which enhances all presentations.[23]

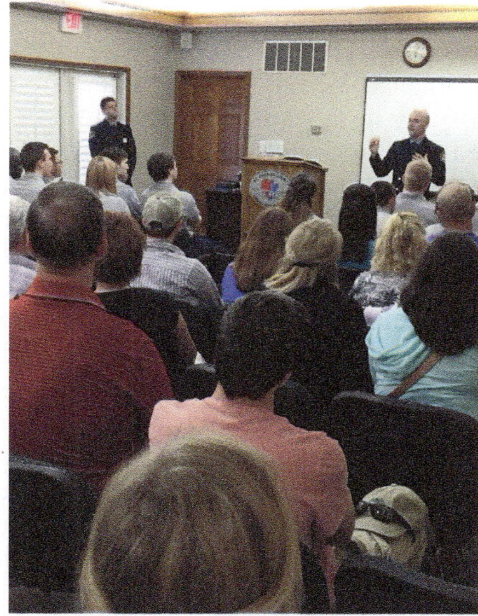

FIGURE 15.3 The educator's attire should present a professional image to the audience.

Courtesy of St. Charles County Ambulance District.

If possible, determine the typical manner of dress of your audience prior to your arrival. One school of thought is that the educator should be dressed a little more formally than the audience (**FIGURE 15.3**). Regardless, the instructor's attire should be both comfortable and functional. The conservative approach to clothing is generally a safe approach.

Parts of the Lecture

Instructors are expected to be proficient in the grasp and understanding of their topic. Most of what an instructor is asked to present will be simple and easy for the instructor to understand. The presenter may or may not have any input into what the lecture topic will be, but that does not prevent the instructor from determining the "angle of attack" to take during its preparation. Rather than trying to tell every detail about the subject in the allotted time, the instructor should narrow down the scope of the topic. Instead of trying to have students "drink from a fire hydrant," the educator must distill the presentation down to the three or four main concepts. The following steps can help accomplish this.

In the very early stages of lecture preparation, the first question to answer should be, "What are the most important thing(s) that the students need to learn and apply from this presentation?" By not answering this basic question early in preparation, an instructor increases the risk that the lecture will be unfocused and will take longer than the allotted time. The more specific the answer to this question, the more likely it is to attain the defining goals.

An instructor should not be afraid of structure, for it is an instructor's friend! Knowing the order of presentation of each of the subtopics reduces the possibility for any confusion during the delivery of the lecture. The instructor must ensure that the progression of the lecture makes sense. If it does not, the students will likely find it confusing as well! During this phase of development, instructors should know that no one structure fits all. The structure selected should match the desired goals of the lecture. For example, the use of a modest list of points presented in a linear progression may be satisfactory for a simple anatomy or physiology lecture. When teaching higher order, critical thinking topics, using a *chained* structure may be preferable. In this format, students are challenged with an argument toward the correct information by using multiple proofs of support. **Chaining** in education is the process of breaking down the objectives and linking them together in a progression of learning.[24] Rather than having one large task to complete, the educator should proceed objective by objective. On successful completion of all objectives, what might have been viewed as an insurmountable activity has actually been made easier. An example of this might include teaching anatomy and physiology early in the class; later on, the presentation transitions to pathophysiology. If the student fails to grasp the basics in the first part of the presentation, they are likely to struggle when they begin to make a care plan for a pathological condition. In reality, instructors often use more than one of these structures for the same lecture.

Once the lecture structure is determined, it is helpful to provide students with a roadmap of where the lecture will be taking them. Much like taking a trip, it is almost always more enjoyable if the traveler knows where they are and what the next stop will be. In terms of a lecture, the map may be as simple as a list of objectives or may be an entire set of slides presented during the lecture. The use of repetition to emphasize important aspects or objectives is helpful for students to identify topics that they will need to highlight for further study. Keep in mind that it is the lecturer's responsibility to lead students to where they need to be while, at the same time, making sure that no one is left behind.

Some instructors present their class from an outline; others prefer to use something more akin to a script. Regardless of the method chosen, it is imperative to include the right amount of information to fit into the time allotted. As a general rule, instructors have a tendency to select too much information to present in the time given. As a result, when they try to present all of the information, they rush through the latter part of the lecture or even skip portions. When an instructor rushes through content, it signals to the student that the content is not that important. Skipping material may confuse students, especially when points in the lecture build upon each other. It is much easier to narrow a lecture before class than when standing in front of a group of eager undergraduates waiting to learn!

Much can be learned from the training that professional speakers and actors undergo. For example, think about the pace of speech. Talking at the same speed without variance is just as bad as speaking in a monotone voice. One of the greatest dangers, especially for new instructors who may be nervous, is the tendency to speak too quickly. When an instructor talks slowly, the audience has more time to grasp the information, and the instructor sounds confident and in control. A good approach is to speak slowly enough so that, if giving someone a phone number, they would be able to write it down without asking the speaker to slow down.[25]

The instructor should arrive before the students. This allows time to set up materials and avoids cutting into valuable teaching time. If using computer and projection equipment for the first time, arriving early allows the instructor time to become familiar with the devices and to seek assistance if there is a problem.

The advent of cloud storage services makes it seem that the days of the USB drive are gone. However, instructors should not get rid of them yet. Problems with Internet connectivity can render access to the presentation impossible. Backup plans for this type of problem include bringing a paper copy of the presentation, in addition to a digital drive with a copy of the presentation. A presentation should never have to be canceled due to a lack of properly functioning equipment.

TEACHING TIP

One method of gauging the number of slides needed for the time allotted is to use the 10/20/30 rule. This calls for the instructor to use 10 slides for every 20 minutes of lecture, using a 30-point font.[15]

TEACHING TIP

Instructors should get to know their audience. When presenting at a conference, prior to the presentation instructors should mingle with members who have come to participate in the session. This allows the instructor to begin building rapport and will introduce some familiar faces to focus on while speaking.

Introduction: Tell Them What They Are Going to Be Told

Educators must make opening statements unique and memorable. A lecture that begins with a memorable opening statement sends the message, "This is important! Pay attention!" As a result, learners will be more likely to give their full attention and retain more of the content presented. How the first 5 minutes of lecture is handled will often have a direct effect on how the students engage for the remainder of the presentation time. The introduction should engage, stimulate, and challenge students. The instructor should also set the expectations for the students. Sharing little-known facts that pertain to the subject can ignite curiosity right at the beginning. The instructor's passion, or lack thereof, for the subject being presented will be contagious.

The Body of the Lecture: Tell Them

As the body of the lecture begins, the instructor should refrain from the temptation to fill the allotted time with the sound of their own voice. Limit the number of objectives to be covered to five or less. Whether or not to share the slides with the audience prior to the presentation is up to the instructor. Many instructors are concerned that doing so decreases the student's engagement with the lecture and encourages passive learning. However, research completed by Worthington and Levasseur found that the practice of instructor-provided slides had no impact on class attendance or overall course involvement.[26]

The new instructor should not worry about being a charismatic presenter; however, there are some basic speech and presentation skills that need to be mastered. First, an instructor should *never* read the presentation verbatim. Often, this action solicits anger from those in the class, and they will quickly disengage from the lecture. This is not to say that the instructor cannot refer to notes on a regular basis; however, the presenter must be seen as the subject matter expert. Preparation should minimize the need for this.

Scanning the room just above the heads of the students suggests that the presenter is nervous. From the point of view of the students, the natural inference may be that the instructor is not well prepared. Looking another person in the eye sends a message of confidence in both oneself and the material. As noted, the amount of time for such eye contact should be between 3 and 5 seconds. Anything longer can tend to make the student begin to feel uncomfortable.[27]

The Conclusion: Tell Them What You Told Them

An instructor can finish the lecture in a meaningful way by highlighting key take-home points discussed during the lecture. This is most effective when active formats that involve the learners are used. This can be done using Socratic questioning techniques, learner feedback tools, or other strategies, or by presenting a case study or exercise that incorporates key elements of the lecture. This reflection on learning is essential to promote retention of information.

After the Lecture: Self-Review and Adjustments

At the conclusion of the session, the instructor should complete a self-review of the presentation for positives and negatives as to how it was received and whether the methods chosen deepened the students' understanding of the topic. One of the most useful methods, but perhaps most painful, is for the instructor to view a video recording of the presentation. Doing so will allow an instructor to see exactly what the students experience. Educators should use this information to improve future presentations. Educators should be open to making whatever changes are needed, even if it means overhauling the presentation. The time and effort spent on this is an investment that will save significant time and effort in the future.

Involving the Audience during the Presentation

As stated earlier, lecture is the most passive form of teaching among all of the options. However, regardless of its size, instructors can engage an audience through the use of small group activities or technology. The next section will review a few strategies available at the time of printing of this book. Most of these come with a free version that limits the number of students that can be engaged, the number of questions shared, or the number of features, such as reports, offered.

Audience Feedback Systems

The use of **audience feedback systems** (clickers) in the classroom has been a longstanding practice by educators (**FIGURE 15.4**). A benefit of some audience feedback systems is that there is nothing for the student, instructor, or educational facility to purchase, unless they desire more options. This feature alone makes these devices very valuable in the classroom. While these systems can be used for assessment, they can also be used to promote educator/student interaction, as discussed here. The value of these tools is instructor-dependent. Instructors should not let the technology become the center of the presentation, only a means of enhancement.

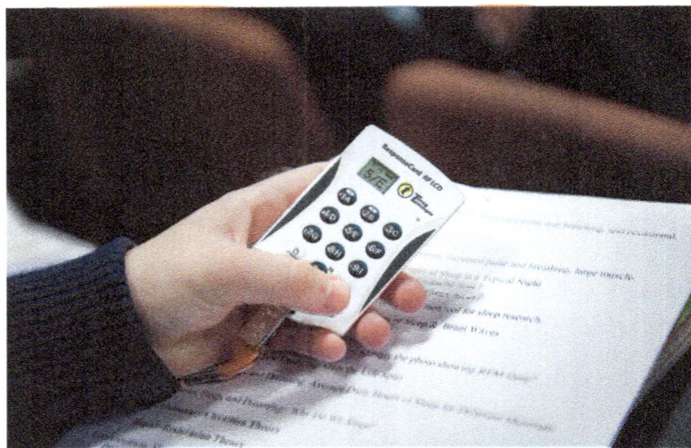

FIGURE 15.4 Audience feedback systems can be used to promote interaction between the students and instructor.

Courtesy of Turning Technologies.

Poll Everywhere

Poll Everywhere, found at www.polleverywhere.com, is an online service that is functional with any operating system and is relatively simple to implement. During the development of a lecture, the instructor can embed a question that is shared with the class during the lecture presentation. Poll Everywhere allows students to anonymously respond to multiple forms of questions, including open text, multiple choice, and rank order. Responses can either be publicly shared in real time (not recommended for open text) or hidden from the students. The use of open text is particularly valuable, as it allows students to ask questions of the presenter in real time. This is more effective when another person acts as a facilitator and screens the questions for appropriateness. The latter method (in which responses are hidden from the students) is a better approach for a more accurate assessment of student comprehension, as peer pressure can sway a student to select the most popular answer instead of the one the student believes is correct. With Poll Everywhere, the instructor can download a plug-in for Microsoft PowerPoint and develop questions within the presentation software without having to switch from the slide to the website. Upon completion of the lecture, the instructor has access to multiple levels of reporting. This application is best suited for implementation in formative quizzes that will give feedback to the instructor on how well the class is understanding the content.

Socrative

Taking its cue from the Socratic method of teaching, the application Socrative is a bit more robust than Poll Everywhere. As it is cloud-based, it can be used across all platforms of computer technology. The basic features of Socrative are free, but educators can upgrade to gain more robust reporting features.

The types of formative assessments cover the entire gamut of multiple choice, true/false, or open-ended responses. The speed of the presentation can be controlled by either the educator or the student. Educator-paced activities, such as those that may be used to encourage discussion among the participants, are especially valuable to help offset some of the negative characteristics of lecture. Through the use of Socratic questioning, both the student and the instructor are able to gauge the amount of retention on the part of the class. This will be helpful when developing and delivering examinations.

A particularly appealing feature of Socrative is that it uses a game called "Space Race" to allow teams of students to compete against each other. The objective in this game is to determine who is able to launch rockets into space fastest by answering the highest number of multiple choice or true/false questions correctly. After the participants complete the game, the educator can log in and view, as well as download, a report that shows areas of strength and weakness among the students. This is especially valuable as it quantifies the areas that the educator will need to review.

TEACHING TIP

A low-tech audience response system can be constructed by having the local hardware store cut 12- × 12-inch squares from 8- × 4-ft white tileboard sheets. Each student is given a whiteboard, a paper towel, and a dry-erase marker. After asking a question, the instructor has the entire class hold up their whiteboards at the same time. This involves the class in the lecture and provides insight regarding whether the class is mastering key concepts. It also permits students the chance to show creativity, as some answers can be drawn, rather than written.

Additional Interactive Strategies

Think-pair-share (TPS) is a student-centered, collaborative learning strategy in which students pair together to answer a question about the lecture content. This approach works well when using medical case studies as a major part of the lecture process. As noted by the title, the student will first think, on an individual basis, about the problem or question. In doing so, students depend on their level of recall to begin to formulate a potential solution. If TPS is used on a regular basis, students may be led to maintain a greater degree of attention during the presentation.[28] According to Cobb, students reported a higher level of self-esteem by being listened to by a fellow classmate.[29] Another potential benefit is that that it can help the student build communication skills as they share the potential solution(s) that they have developed individually.

To use TPS, the instructor decides what questions will be used. Educators must ensure that these questions are based on key concepts in the text as well as in the lecture. The instructor then describes the process of TPS to the students, keeping in mind that this learning concept may be foreign to them and they may, initially, resist it or simply respond with silence. Don't give up! Instructors should show the students what they are supposed to accomplish with TPS by modeling it first. As students think about the question, it may be helpful for the instructor to require them to put their thoughts on paper. After a preset period of time, the instructor should pair up students so they may share their thoughts about the solution with their partner. Ultimately, the instructor should expand this pairing into a whole class discussion. Having a partner to help with the sharing may take some of the fear out of students presenting to the entire class.

CASE in Point

Brioni, who was instructing paramedics for her third year, understood that shock was confusing to students. She began the class with an online quiz related to their assigned reading on the topic. To break the material into measurable "chunks," she delivered a brief 20-minute lecture to review the concepts in the reading materials, making sure to emphasize the points that students struggled with on the quiz. After the brief lecture, Brioni asked five high-level multiple choice questions using an audience feedback system to check in and ensure that most of the class had mastered the points she reviewed. Their responses made it evident that the concept of obstructive shock was still not clear, so she asked the class to take 5 minutes to do a TPS related to the causes of this type of shock. Within moments the room was buzzing with discussion. Brioni was pleased to see that scores were high on this topic on their next quiz.

Buzz Groups

A **buzz group** consists of three to six people who are assigned a specific question or problem to be researched and answered in a short period of time. Buzz groups are effective in the development of possible solutions to problems. It is best for the instructor to assign members of the group based on their grasp of the content. In doing so, the instructor will minimize the potential for one person to monopolize the discussion. The instructor should have each group appoint a recorder who will report out the group's findings to the larger class. The instructor should watch the dynamics of the groups while circulating through the classroom. A benefit of a buzz group is that some students may feel more comfortable openly sharing their thoughts and ideas in a small group, but may be hesitant when placed in the larger context.[30]

Doceri

Doceri is a presentation app that allows the educator to record both screen and voice as well as have access to an interactive online whiteboard. Doceri interacts with the desktop, and the instructor can control all desktop functions from their tablet devices. Using a stylus, instructors can highlight important content, create new slides, draw on the screen, and broadcast to the entire class. The entire presentation can be recorded for sharing with the students or to implement in the flipped classroom. Doceri can be found at https://doceri.com/. Doceri can make a slide presentation to a large group more interactive. Other presentation technology is discussed in Chapter 16, *Using Technology to Enhance Classroom Learning.*

Flipping the Classroom

It is difficult to determine the actual originator(s) of the flipped classroom concept. Most point to Jonathan Bergmann and Aaron Sams as the earliest, most visible proponents of this approach to teaching.[31] Bergmann and Sams were high school science teachers in rural Colorado who, when frustrated with the number of student absences due to sports, band, and other activities during regular class hours, developed a new approach to lecture delivery. They discovered that they were able to record a PowerPoint presentation and embed audio and notes. At that time, they began sharing the videos with students via a DVD. Their original name for this project was "pre-broadcasting." The plan was for their students to watch the video outside of class and be ready to work on their homework assignments during the scheduled time in school. This allowed Bergman and Sams to provide more concentrated, one-on-one instruction to each student.

Flipping the classroom is not without its detractors; however, research studies have shown that the results are positive.[32] Bergmann and Sams state that "when teachers aren't standing in front of the classroom talking at students, they can circulate and talk with students."[33] The two primary questions that must be answered are, does the flipped classroom make an academic difference, and what is the degree of acceptance by students in the change from a traditional classroom lecture to one that is flipped?

A group of educators at the University of North Carolina looked at these questions. These professors flipped a first-year pharmaceutical course for students who were majoring in pharmacy. They provided all lectures ahead of time, streamed video, and used in-class time for active learning activities. They found that 82% of their students watched the videos prior to attending class, with 79.3% watching them more than once. As for student attitudes toward this flipped method, "93.1% agreed or strongly agreed that teaching and learning methods in the flipped classroom promoted understanding and application of key concepts."[34]

Summary

Lectures remain the primary tool of teaching in academic institutions. The instructor must keep in mind, however, that the presentation must be about student learning. The prime directive should be to encourage the process of thinking critically and learning actively. Lecture can be an effective method for delivering a large amount of content. However, the astute educator will remember that delivery does not always equate to understanding on the part of the student. Using the lecture as a method of teaching should always be a work in progress. Educators must dedicate themselves to continual self-improvement, adjusting presentations as needed to ensure they are effective in deepening student understanding. Instructors should always seek better methods to make presentations interactive. By taking these steps, teaching large groups can become engaging and can result in more meaningful learning.

Glossary

audience feedback systems Technological systems that allow a presenter and an audience to interact, for example, by providing feedback or answering questions via an electronic device or clicker.

buzz group Group typically consisting of three to six people who are assigned a specific question or problem to be researched and answered in a short period of time, for example, within a lecture.

chaining In the context of education, the process of breaking down the objectives and linking them together in a progression of learning.

large group For the purposes of this text, defined as a greater number of students or audience than can be easily handled for small group activities.

lecture Teaching session in which the instructor is the principal teacher.

Socratic method Method of teaching based on the premise of asking and answering questions with the primary purpose of stimulating critical thinking; from this process, both the educator and students discover other information.

think-pair-share (TPS) Collaborative, student-centered learning strategy in which students pair together to answer a question about lecture content.

References

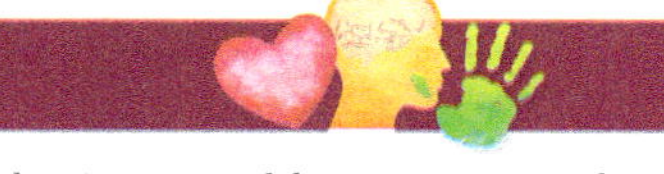

[1] Butterfield, Herbert. 2018. *Origins of History*. Abingdon, UK: Taylor & Francis.

[2] Ahmadi, Seyed-Foad, Hamid R. Baradaran, and Emad Ahmadi. 2014. "Effectiveness of Teaching Evidence-Based Medicine to Undergraduate Medical Students: A BEME Systematic Review." *Medical Teacher* 37, no. 1: 21–30. https://doi.org/10.3109/0142159X.2014.971724.

[3] Henderson, Michael, Neil Selwyn, and Rachel Aston. 2015. "What Works and Why? Student Perceptions of 'Useful' Digital Technology in University Teaching and Learning." *Studies in Higher Education* 42, no. 8: 1567–79. https://doi.org/10.1080/03075079.2015.1007946.

[4] Dole, Sharon, Lisa Bloom, and Kristy Kowalske. 2015. "Transforming Pedagogy: Changing Perspectives from Teacher-Centered to Learner-Centered." *Interdisciplinary Journal of Problem-Based Learning* 10, no. 1. https://doi.org/10.7771/1541-5015.1538.

[5] Merritt, Chris, Brendan W. Munzer, Margaret Wolff, and Sally A. Santen. 2017. "Not Another Bedside Lecture: Active Learning Techniques for Clinical Instruction." *AEM Education and Training* 2, no. 1: 48–50. https://doi.org/10.1002/aet2.10069.

[6] Emke, Amanda R., Andrew C. Butler, and Douglas P. Larsen. 2016. "Effects of Team-Based Learning on Short-Term and Long-Term Retention of Factual Knowledge." *Medical Teacher* 38, no. 3: 306–11. https://doi.org/10.3109/0142159X.2015.1034663.

[7] Mohan, Lalit, Smita Shenoy, B. R. Eesha, Anoopkishore, K. L. Bairy, and Navin Patil. 2014. "Students' Attitude toward Didactic Lecture Versus Problem-Based Learning in Pharmacology: A Questionnaire Based Study." *International Journal of Basic & Clinical Pharmacology* 3, no. 4: 619. https://doi.org/10.5455/2319-2003.ijbcp20140810.

[8] Petrović, Juraj, and Predrag Pale. 2014. "Students Perception of Live Lectures Inherent Disadvantages." *Teaching in Higher Education* 20, no. 2: 143–57. https://doi.org/10.1080/13562517.2014.962505.

[9] Ward, Adrian F., and Daniel M. Wegner. 2013. "Mind-Blanking: When the Mind Goes Away." *Frontiers in Psychology* 4: 650. https://doi.org/10.3389/fpsyg.2013.00650.

[10] Sousa, David A. 2017. *How the Brain Learns*, 5th ed. Thousand Oaks, CA: Corwin, Sage Publishing Company.

[11] Brookfield, Stephen D. 2015. *The Skillful Teacher: On Technique, Trust, and Responsiveness in the Classroom*. San Francisco: Jossey-Bass.

[12] Entwistle, Noel James, and Paul Ramsden. 2015. *Understanding Student Learning*. London: Routledge.

[13] Poorman, Elizabeth. 2017. "Staying Current in Medicine: Advice for New Doctors." *NEJM Knowledge*. Accessed November 22, 2018. https://knowledgeplus.nejm.org/blog/staying-current-in-medicine-advice-for-new-doctors/.

[14] Mohammadjani, Farzad, and Forouzan Tonkaboni. 2015. "A Comparison Between the Effect of Cooperative Learning Teaching Method and Lecture Teaching Method on Students' Learning and Satisfaction Level." *International Education Studies* 8, no. 9: 107. http://dx.doi.org/10.5539/ies.v8n9p107.

[15] Bradbury, Neil A. 2016. "Attention Span during Lectures: 8 Seconds, 10 Minutes, or More?" *Advances in Physiology Education* 40, no. 4: 509–13. https://doi.org/10.1152/advan.00109.2016.

[16] Parada, Francisco J., and Alejandra Rossi. 2017. "Commentary: Brain-to-Brain Synchrony Tracks Real-World Dynamic Group Interactions in the Classroom and Cognitive Neuroscience: Synchronizing Brains in the Classroom." *Frontiers in Human Neuroscience* 11: 554. https://doi.org/10.3389/fnhum.2017.00554.

[17] Laserna, Charlyn M., Yi-Tai Seih, and James W. Pennebaker. 2014. "Um . . . Who Like Says You Know: Filler Word Use as a Function of Age, Gender, and Personality." *Journal of Language and Social Psychology* 33, no. 3: 328–38. https://doi.org/10.1177/0261927X14526993.

[18] Dillon, James J. 2016. "Socrates Structures the Course." In *Teaching Psychology and the Socratic Method*. New York: Palgrave Macmillan; 27–33.

[19] Weetman, Pauline. "Accounting Standards: A Pause for Reflection." *Accounting and Business Research* 7, no. 27: 168–76. https://doi.org/10.1080/00014788.1977.9728700.

[20] Bakker, Arnold B., Ana Isabel Sanz Vergel, and Jeroen Kuntze. 2014. "Student Engagement and Performance: A Weekly Diary Study on the Role of Openness." *Motivation and Emotion* 39, no. 1: 49–62. https://doi.org/10.1007/s11031-014-9422-5.

[21] Choi, Choongbeom, and Anna S. Mattila. 2015. "The Effects of Other Customers' Dress Style on Customers' Approach Behaviors." *Cornell Hospitality Quarterly* 57, no. 2: 211–18. https://doi.org/10.1177/1938965515619228.

[22] Holtz, Brian C. 2014. "From First Impression to Fairness Perception: Investigating the Impact of Initial Trustworthiness Beliefs." *Personnel Psychology* 68, no. 3: 499–546. https://doi.org/10.1111/peps.12092.

[23] Chollet, Mathieu, Torsten Wörtwein, Louis-Philippe Morency, Ari Shapiro, and Stefan Scherer. 2014. "Exploring Feedback Strategies to Improve Public Speaking." *Proceedings of the 2015 ACM International Joint Conference on Pervasive and Ubiquitous Computing*.

[24] Snodgrass, Melinda R., Hedda Meadan, Michaelene M. Ostrosky, and W. Catherine Cheung. 2017. "One Step at a Time: Using Task Analyses to Teach Skills." *Early Childhood Education Journal* 45, no. 6: 855–62. https://doi.org/10.1007/s10643-017-0838-x.

[25] Sprenger, Marilee. 2018. *How to Teach so Students Remember*. Alexandria, VA: Association for Supervision and Curriculum Development.

[26] Worthington, Debra L., and David G. Levasseur. 2015. "To Provide or Not to Provide Course PowerPoint Slides? The Impact of Instructor-Provided Slides upon Student Attendance and Performance." *Computers & Education* 85: 14–22. https://doi.org/10.1016/j.compedu.2015.02.002.

[27] Pejsa, Tomislav, Sean Andrist, Michael Gleicher, and Bilge Mutlu. 2015. "Gaze and Attention Management for Embodied Conversational Agents." *ACM Transactions on Interactive Intelligent Systems* 5, no. 1: 1–34. http://dx.doi.org/10.1145/2724731.

[28] Maisyura, C. M. Zubainur, and T. F. Abidin. 2018. "The Quality of Mathematics Learning Material Using a Modification of Think Pair Share (TPS) Model." *Journal of Physics: Conference Series* 1088: 012097. http://dx.doi.org/10.1088/1742-6596/1088/1/012097.

[29] Cobb, Paul, Terry Wood, Erna Yackel, John Nicholls, Grayson Wheatley, Beatriz Trigatti, and Marcella Perlwitz. 1991. "Assessment of a Problem-Centered Second-Grade Mathematics Project." *Journal for Research in Mathematics Education* 22, no. 1: 3–29. https://doi.org/10.2307/749551.

[30] Roland, Damian, and Thomas Balslev. 2015. "Use of Patient Video Cases in Medical Education." *Archives of Disease in Childhood—Education & Practice Edition* 100, no. 4: 210–14. http://dx.doi.org/10.1136/archdischild-2014-308030.

[31] Bergmann, Jonathan, and Aaron Sams. 2015. *Flipped Learning: Gateway to Student Engagement*. Moorabbin, Australia: Hawker Brownlow Education.

[32] Christopher, Sarah V. E. 2018. "Students' Perceptions of a Flipped Classroom Approach to Paramedic Theory." *British Paramedic Journal* 2, no. 4: 1–9. https://doi.org/10.29045/14784726.2018.03.2.4.1.

[33] Bergmann, Jonathan, and Aaron Sams. 2012. *Flip Your Classroom: Reach Every Student in Every Class Every Day*. Washington, DC: ISTE, and Alexandria, VA: ASCD.

[34] McLaughlin, Jacqueline E., Mary T. Roth, Dylan M. Glatt, Nastaran Gharkholonarehe, Christopher A. Davidson, LaToya M. Griffin, Denise A. Esserman, and Russell J. Mumper. 2014. "The Flipped Classroom: A Course Redesign to Foster Learning and Engagement in a Health Professions School." *Academic Medicine* 89, no. 2: 236–43. http://dx.doi.org/10.1097/ACM.0000000000000086.

Additional Resources

Brown, George, and Michael Manogue. 2001. "AMEE Medical Education Guide No. 22: Refreshing Lecturing: A Guide for Lecturers." *Medical Teacher* 23, no. 3: 231–44. https://doi.org/10.1080/01421590120043000.

Courneya, Carol A. 2017. "Heartfelt Images: Learning Cardiac Science Artistically." *Medical Humanities* 44, no. 1: 20–7. http://dx.doi.org/10.1136/medhum-2016-011140.

CHAPTER 16

Using Technology to Enhance Classroom Learning

OBJECTIVES

At the conclusion of this chapter, the educator will be able to:

Cognitive Domain

1. Understand the historical foundations of technology in education.
2. Categorize the use of educational technologies using the SAMR model.
3. Evaluate a technology to determine if it is suitable to use in the emergency medical services (EMS) classroom, using a rubric.
4. Distinguish advantages and disadvantages of selected presentation software tools.
5. Recognize how apps and other technology can be used to enhance case-based learning.
6. Outline the advantages of digital assignments.
7. Describe strategies and tools to promote learning in Web-enhanced classrooms.
8. Discuss the role of social media in education.

Psychomotor Domain

There are no psychomotor objectives for this chapter.

Affective Domain

1. Recognize the need to be selective in the use of technology as a tool to enhance a solid educational plan.
2. Display a commitment to using technology in educationally sound ways.

"Sometimes you have to travel a long way to find what is near."

~ Paulo Coelho

CHAPTER GOAL The chapter quote from Paulo Coelho is often true of finding the right educational technology tools. The goal of this chapter is to make your educational technology journey shorter than it might otherwise be.

A review of the history of educational technology (edtech) is important for context and to address the perceptions of edtech enthusiasts, technophobes, and edtech cynics. For as long as there have been advances in technology, there have been both enthusiasts predicting its transformative powers and cynics predicting its ability to undermine learning or subvert teaching. Socrates, who lived between 470 and 399 BCE, was one of the best known Greek philosophers and made significant contributions to the field of epistemology. Yet were it not for the writings of Plato and other students of Socrates, which were, at the time, considered a technology, we would not know of his teachings. He felt that writing would melt the brains of Athenian youths by undermining their willingness to memorize.[1]

Fast forward to the 20th century with the invention of the television, which promised to bring experts into the classroom and threatened the existence of books. Some felt it might even pose an existential threat to the teaching profession. In the early 20th century, Thomas Edison famously predicted: "Books will soon be obsolete in the public schools. Scholars will be instructed through the eye [television]."[2] These threats never came to pass, and television, like most technologies, has come to supplement rather than replace learning in the classroom. While television might not be thought of as a tool for supplementing EMS education, video from a variety of sources can be used in the classroom. For example, reality TV shows like *Nightwatch* or *Recruits: Paramedics* (Australia) can be viewed over the Internet and shared with students for case-based discussions.

More recently, extreme predictions were made about the concept of **massive open online courses (MOOCs)** such as those offered by *Coursera* and *Udacity*. MOOCs are courses available online over the Internet, frequently offered for free, from a variety of reputable universities, to a large number of people. With the sudden popularity of MOOCs, some predicted that brick and mortar schools would be replaced, or that, at the very least, MOOCs would be a viable alternative to colleges and universities for low-income students.[5,6] The reality is that MOOCs will likely continue to play a role, but they are unlikely to pose a threat to EMS or traditional higher education. On the other hand, MOOCs could become an invaluable edtech tool for continuing education in EMS.

This chapter will discuss how technology can be supportive, transformative, disruptive, or simply novel with no added benefit to the learner. Other chapters address the pedagogical principles that should be first and foremost in the educator's mind before selecting an edtech

Disruptive Technologies in the Classroom

Technology has a long history in the classroom. In *The Visual History of Classroom Technology*, Jeff Dunn lists some of the most "disruptive" technologies, such as: the magic lantern in 1870 that projected images that were printed on glass frames, the chalkboard in 1890, the pencil in 1900, the film projector in 1925, the television in 1927, the overhead projector 1930, the ballpoint pen in 1940, the hand-held calculator in 1970, the interactive whiteboard in 1999, and the iPad in 2010.[3] The phrase "disruptive technologies in the classroom" has come to refer to any technology that disrupts current practices (**FIGURE 16.1**).[4]

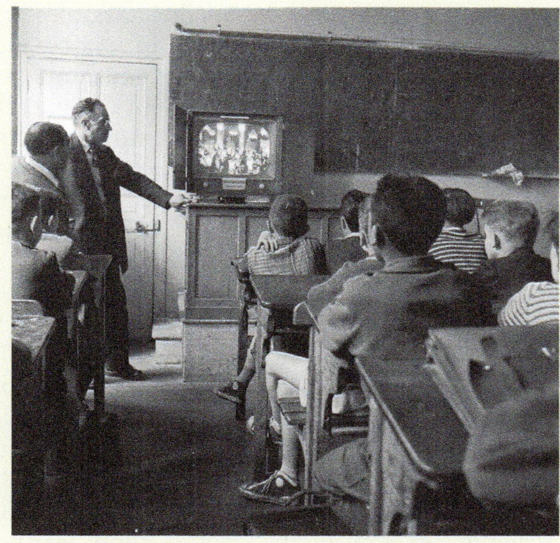

FIGURE 16.1 The television was once a disruptive technology in the classroom.

tool. To master a new edtech tool and to fairly evaluate its effectiveness, educators should be prepared to commit to using it with one or more courses.

TEACHING TIP

If you feel timid about trying a new educational technology, try keeping your experimentation to one tool per course. To help you get started, YouTube and instructional blogs contain endless resources.

Technology-Enhanced Classroom

It is a common perception among educators that personal electronic devices are a source of student distraction and disengagement.[7] Many educators are ambivalent about how to manage student use of technology in the classroom. The results of studies on the use of laptops or tablets in the classroom have been mixed.[8–10] Indeed, mobile devices can be a distraction. William and Pence suggest that one way to manage the misuse of smartphones, laptops, and tablets in the classroom is to have a portion of the class designated as "technology on" and a portion designated as "technology off."[11] But is it fair to restrict or prohibit the use of technology, given the many benefits of having continuous access to mobile technology for activities such as electronic note taking, annotation of digital slide handouts, and literature searches? Despite the potential challenges of keeping students on-task, the tools available through digital devices allow learning to be immediate, flexible, robust, and personalized.[12] The role of the instructor is to keep students engaged, either despite the potential distractions or by leveraging the technology (**FIGURE 16.2**).

CASE in Point

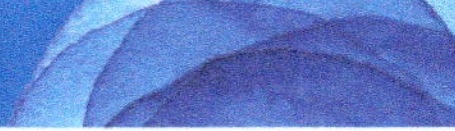

An instructor notices that some students are taking notes on their smartphones in class. The instructor decides to try integrating mobile devices into the classroom learning. The instructor observed that student engagement in the discussion increased with active participation. The instructor successfully used mobile devices to engage students, and devices empower student learning, without allowing the technology to create chaos in the classroom.

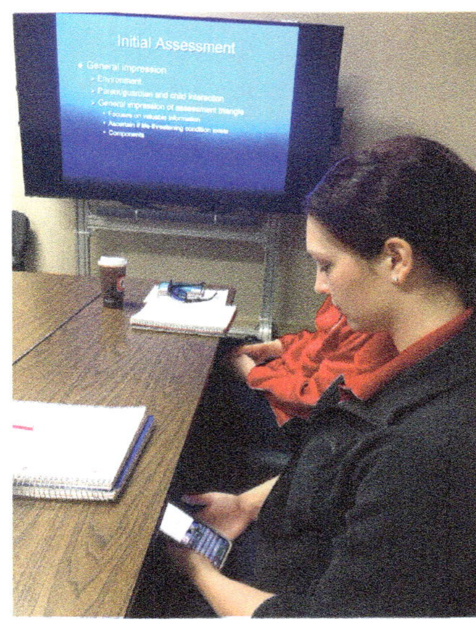

FIGURE 16.2 Personal electronic devices in class can be a source of distraction.

Courtesy of St. Charles County Ambulance District.

Which Technologies "Work"?

With the ubiquity of smartphones, tablets, and **apps**, educators who wish to leverage these learning technology tools in the classroom need a framework to help them determine whether an app or a piece of hardware is simply novel or whether it enhances the learning experience. Dr. Ruben Puentedura created a taxonomy for categorizing technologies. This taxonomy is called the **SAMR model** (**TABLE 16.1**). The acronym SAMR stands for:

Substitution

Augmentation

Modification

Redefinition

While the SAMR model has been criticized for a lack of supporting peer-reviewed research,[13] it is nonetheless worth considering at face value. It is simply a taxonomy that prompts educators to think about educational technology through a pedagogical lens.

The following is a brief description of each of the SAMR levels: At the **substitution** level, the technology replicates a task that was previously done without a computer or a learning technology; there is no functional change. An example is moving from a typewriter to a word processor to type documents. At the **augmentation** level, the technology offers a more effective tool to perform common tasks. For example, a prescription drug reference app might be considered

TABLE 16.1 The SAMR Model

SAMR Level	Description
Substitution	Technology replicates a task that was previously done without a computer or a learning technology; no functional change.
Augmentation	Technology offers a more effective tool to perform common tasks.
Modification	Technology allows tasks to be done in a completely new way.
Redefinition	Technology allows new tasks to be performed, which were not possible before.

Modified from Puentedura, Ruben R. n.d. "SAMR and the EdTech Quintet: A Hands-On Introduction." Accessed January 24, 2019. http://hippasus.com/rrpweblog/archives/2018/11/SAMRAndTheEdTechQuintet_AHands-On Introduction.pdf.

FIGURE 16.3 A QR code. This particular QR code goes to the NAEMSE website (https://naemse.org/).

Courtesy of Rob Theriault.

an augmentation compared to a paper-based reference book, because the app will be updated frequently, will always be current unlike its analog counterpart, and the search functions make it arguably faster than the paper-based alternative. At the **modification** level, technology allows tasks to be done in a completely new way. A quick response (QR) code is an example (**FIGURE 16.3**). A QR code might be used to take a student from a document to a website, a video, a quiz or some other relevant content that might otherwise occupy too much space on a single worksheet. Another example of modification might be the ability to highlight and annotate in digital documents such as e-books or PDF files, and be able to edit and search for annotations and highlights. Yet another example of modification would be the ability for students to interact and collaborate with shared documents such as in a wiki page or using Google docs. Finally, at the **redefinition** level, students can perform new tasks that were not possible before. For example, students might create multimedia-enriched and interactive documents using iBooks Author, or may collaborate on the creation of a Web-based mind map when face-to-face collaboration is not possible. Learning through interactive virtual reality is considered an example of redefinition because of its immersiveness and the sense of presence a student experiences when wearing a head-mounted display and entering a 360-degree video environment.

The University of Waterloo created a rubric for evaluating eLearning tools. This rubric is broken down into the components shown in **TABLE 16.2**.

New learning technologies are coming to the market faster than their true value and impact can be assessed. For this reason, it is important for educators to put pedagogy first and determine what, if any, technology facilitates the achievement of the learning outcomes in either a more efficient or effective way.

The next sections discuss different technologies individually, with a focus on the benefits, and include tips and suggestions to keep the edtech experience positive.

Presentation Technology

Before discussing presentation technology, a brief discussion of the art of presentation is in order. The lecture has received significant criticism over the years as research has shown that students learn more efficiently and effectively when they spend less time listening and more time discussing, thinking, and doing.[14,15] Nonetheless, the lecture can and should be an effective part of the student learning experience, provided it is not the only means by which the students learn in the classroom.

A lecture does not require a set of slides. In fact, one small study found that students performed better on testing when they took longhand notes and the lecturer did not use slides.[16] However, slides and videos, when designed well and used wisely, can be engaging and can provide imagery that can otherwise only be seen in the field during real patient encounters. When creating slides, it is important to understand that slides should be designed to support and complement what is being said, explained, or discussed. They should never be used as a teleprompter for the lecturer.

Deeper learning is observed when relevant graphics are used or words are presented alone in a slide presentation.[17] Some people refer to this as the

TEACHING TIP

When it comes to designing slides, images enhance and words distract.

TABLE 16.2 Rubric for Evaluating New Technology for Use in the Classroom

Category	Subcategory	Works Well	Minor Concerns	Serious Concerns
Functionality	Scale			
	Ease of use			
	Tech support/help availability			
	Hypermediality (links to audio, video, or hyperlinks to websites, surveys, or documents)			
Accessibility	Accessibility standards			
	User-focused participation			
	Required equipment			
Technical	Integration/embedding within a learning management system (LMS)			
	Operating systems			
	Web browser			
	Additional technical requirements			
Mobile design	Access			
	Functionality			
	Offline access			
Usage and account set-up	Sign up/sign in			
	Cost of use			
	Archiving, saving, and exporting data			
	Data privacy and ownership			
Social presence	Collaboration			
	User accountability			
	Diffusion (level of familiarity among audience who will use the new technology)			
Teaching presence	Facilitation			
	Customization			
	Learning analytics			
Cognitive presence	Enhancement of cognitive task(s)			
	Higher-order thinking			
	Feedback on learning			

Modified from Anstey, Lauren, and Gavan Watson. 2016. "Rubric for eLearning Tool Evaluation." Accessed January 11, 2019. http://elearningtoolkit.uwo.ca/eLearning-Toolkit-Rubric.pdf.

TEACHING TIP

Knowledge and passion for a subject can communicate more effectively than a colorful, jazzed-up slide presentation.

"Goldilocks Rule," which is to present the "just right" amount of data so that slides enhance a presentation and do not become a distraction. In *Presentation Zen: Simple Ideas on Presentation Design and Delivery* by Garr Reynolds and *Slide:ology The Art and Science of Creating Great Presentations* by Nancy Duarte, the authors remind us that when there is a lot of text on the screen while an instructor is talking, students preferentially read the text and do not listen to what the instructor is saying. This finding is based on cognitive load theory, which indicates that a human cannot effectively perform these tasks at the same time. Therefore, each complete presentation should contain relevant images and as few words as possible (fewer than six objects per slide). Bullet points should be used sparingly, and they should be animated to appear on the screen one at a time, then fade so that the student focuses on the current bullet point and not the previous one. Based on the same principles, presentations should be kept short and address only one message per slide and only one theme per presentation (e.g., it is better to create and deliver a short presentation on croup than a presentation that covers multiple causes of airway compromise such as croup, epiglottitis, airway burns, and foreign body airway obstruction). Short presentations allow students to better assimilate the information. This is called "chunking" and is described in *Make It Stick: The Science of Successful Learning* by Peter C. Brown (see Additional Resources).

Most educational publishers offer presentation slides as part of their online resource library. Slides can be purchased from a publisher or vendor, or downloaded from a website (such as the NAEMSE Trading Post, available to NAEMSE members at www.NAEMSE.org), or educators may develop their own slides. Each option has advantages and disadvantages. When presentation slides are purchased from a vendor, they are usually generic and cover only the basic points of a lesson.

Making Slides Available

Should you make slides available to the students? In short, the jury is out. Researchers have found that attendance is higher when slides are available before the lecture and that students participate more in class, but overall exam performance is no different.[18,19] When planning to use slides, as most instructors do, the time it takes for students to write down salient points when slides (or notes) are not made available in advance can slow the pace of the class.

Presentation Software

Microsoft PowerPoint has been the go-to software for most presenters for over two decades. It has served and continues to serve educators well, especially those who have learned to keep their slides simple and short, use contrasting colors, and minimize animations and transitions. Other applications such as MS Office Sway, Apple's Keynote, emaze, Haiku Deck, Prezi, SlideDog, Visme, Videoscribe, and Google Slides, to name a few, offer different features. Some applications such as Prezi, Visme, and Videoscribe offer enhanced video animations, which can be engaging if used tastefully and sparingly. Educators are encouraged to explore and try different options to see what works well in the classroom.

Most slide programs permit numerous features, such as the ability to zoom in on a specific section and the ability to draw on the slides. These features help to focus the student's attention on key points, but are often underutilized. They are described in the software's help sections and tutorials, and they can be used to help illustrate dynamic processes such as drawing a dotted line below the oxyhemoglobin dissociation curve to demonstrate how it shifts according to the patient's condition.

TEACHING TIP

Try using one new slide feature per week, such as drawing on slides or using the zoom function.

Other Presentation Tools

Presenting is not restricted to slide decks. Numerous laptop, tablet, and smartphone options are available to make presentations more engaging than was previously possible. For example, 3-D anatomy apps allow the instructor to explore organs with the students from multiple angles and to zoom in and out to highlight key structures (**FIGURE 16.4**). Many of these apps are low cost or free, allowing the instructor to present while the students follow along with their own apps.

TEACHING TIP

You can connect your tablet or smartphone to a data projector to display anatomy and other medical apps to your students. This sometimes requires an adaptor.

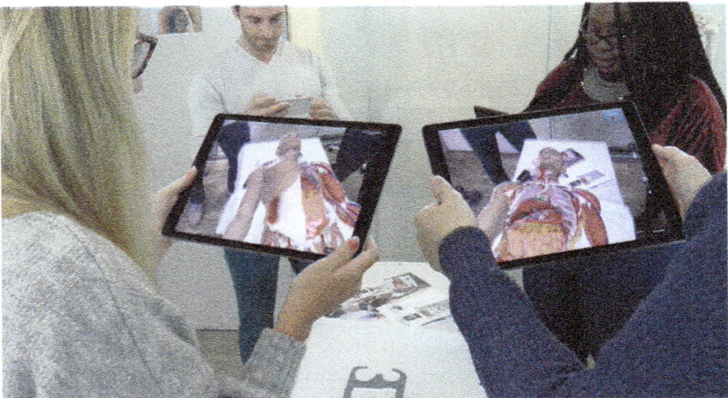

FIGURE 16.4 A 3-D anatomy app allows instructors and students to study anatomy from multiple angles.

Courtesy of 3D4 Medical.

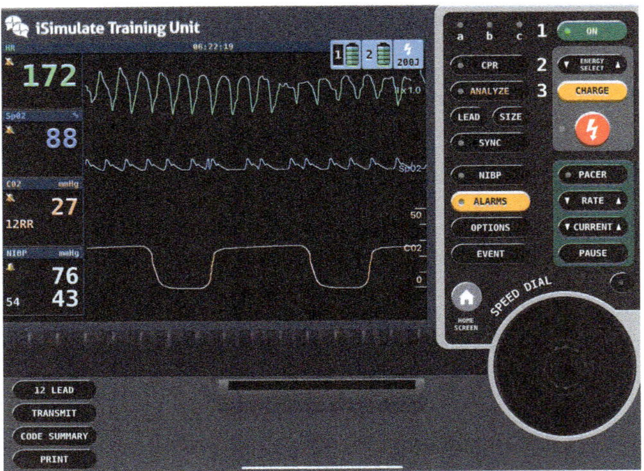

FIGURE 16.5 A monitoring app such as the iSimulate screen shown here gives various readings and can be used to enhance case-based discussions in the classroom.

Courtesy of iSimulate.

Another example of alternative presentation apps are electrocardiogram (ECG) monitoring apps. Presenting ECGs on a slide deck is a good starting point, but there are a number of ECG apps that allow the instructor to show both static and dynamic ECGs and even show full-scale cardiac monitors. Monitor apps such as iSimulate's REALITi (**FIGURE 16.5**) and DART Sim provide a dynamic ECG, heart rate, respiratory rate, blood pressure, oxygen saturation and waveform, and end-tidal carbon dioxide. These apps are great for case-based discussions where the student can see all of the essential vital signs on the screen and the instructor can change the vital signs as the cases progress through treatments and responses to treatments.

Other apps that can be used in the classroom for both presentation and interaction include resuscitation simulation apps such as ACLS Simulator by Anesoft Corporation, Full Code by Minerva Medical Simulation, and Resuscitation! by EM Gladiators. Several triage apps are available to help students master the basics of sorting patients before participating in a mock disaster.

Manipulatives

Manipulatives, such as bag-mask devices, oropharyngeal airways, syringes, and other medical devices, while not digital technologies, are important **analog technologies** for the EMS educator. They enable students to see and touch the tools that they will be putting into practice in their lab, clinical, and field training. This makes in-class education more experiential.

Podcasting an Instructor Presentation

In the classroom, students write down what they hear and what they perceive. What they perceive is not always an accurate reflection of what the educator said. A **podcast** provides a way to stop, rewind, and review the original information, which reinforces learning. Podcasts provide immense value to students, especially when made available through platforms called really simple syndication (RSS) sites that allow students to subscribe to and download their instructor's podcasts to their device automatically and for free. Examples of such sites include iTunes, GooglePlay, Stitcher, or Spotify, to name a few.

With a podcast, students receive the presentation information verbatim. They can relisten to the classroom content anywhere and at any time. Students believe that podcasts are a more effective way to review information than using textbooks, and they are able to write and rewrite notes and learn more efficiently.[20] Several studies have shown that students who listen to podcasts perform better than students who do not.[21–23]

It has been argued that listening to podcasts is not an ideal learning method because most people are not auditory learners. While it is true that many people prefer to learn visually and through tactile experiences, it is also important to bear in mind that the concept that every individual has a specific, innate learning style has largely been debunked.[24] Instead, every person learns by various means.

Podcasts have the added advantage that they can be listened to at any time, often while doing other activities such as driving, working out, or simply sitting and taking notes (**FIGURE 16.6**).

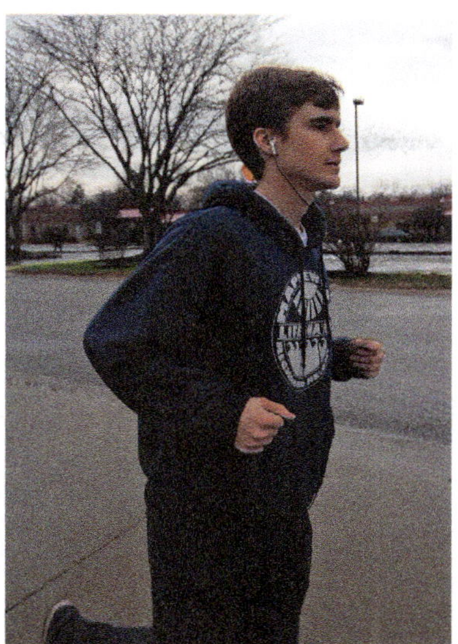

FIGURE 16.6 A student can listen to a podcast anywhere and at any time, as long as they have technological access.

Courtesy of St. Charles County Ambulance District.

Podcasting need not be restricted to recording lectures. If case-based learning or group work activity is being used, an educator might consider recording the resulting discussions after the group activities are done. This captures the salient points that come out of the students' work.

Inevitably, when recording lessons in the classroom, the voices of some students will be captured in the recordings. At most institutions and training agencies, this requires obtaining a signed student consent form.

Digital Apps for Capturing Student Work

Flip charts, when used effectively, are a great tool for getting students out of their seats and working collaboratively to brainstorm, problem-solve, and exercise their higher-order thinking skills. Although the flip chart is an analog tool, technology may be used as an adjunct to the work students do. For example, instead of transcribing the students' flip chart work onto a computer, the instructor (and the students) can take photos of the work for later viewing or to display using a data projector. The app TextGrabber can be used to convert the handwritten work into digital text, or instead of flip charts, the instructor can have the students use sticky notes and capture them digitally with an app like Post-It Plus for display.

How to Podcast

Step 1: Create the recording. Identify the recording device. Any smartphone or small hand-held recorder can be used. A Bluetooth earpiece with microphone can also be used, which gives the instructor the freedom to wander around the classroom and results in student voices being only faintly audible. The instructor must remember to repeat each student's question before answering it, so that the podcast listener knows what question is being answered.

Step 2: Transfer and manage audio files. If you are unable to transfer recordings directly from your phone to a podcast-hosting platform, you may wish to transfer the audio files to a laptop or desktop to more easily manage the files. Some instructors like to be able to edit their recordings with an editing program such as GarageBand (iOS) or Audacity. Editing is especially helpful to remove periods of silence, for example, while the instructor or students are writing on the board. However, editing requires additional time. The instructor can also use the pause function while recording to eliminate long silences and for parts of discussions that should not be recorded.

Step 3: Host, store, and link audio files. Audio files must be stored once they are recorded. The platforms mentioned previously are publishing sites from which students can download the podcasts. Not all publishing sites also allow upload of audio files. For hosting files, an instructor may need a separate site to upload and obtain a link that can be embedded in the publishing site. Examples of hosting sites include the free sites Internet Archive, Anchor, or other sites that may have limited free hosting such as Podomatic, Podbean, Libsyn, or SoundCloud. A search for a podcast hosting site is worthwhile to see what additional features are offered.

Step 4: Post the podcast and alert the students. Take the link you created at the podcast hosting site and embed it in the podcast publishing site such as iTunes, GooglePlay, Stitcher, or Spotify. Finally, provide your students with the name and a link to your publishing site and the name of your podcasts.

Student Response Systems

Repeated retrieval practice is an effective way to help students transfer information from short-term to long-term memory and is far more effective than rereading the information.[25–30] This type of practice can be done by simply adding questions at the end of each lesson (e.g., on slides) and having the students write down the answer after reflecting on what they have learned. Alternatively, there are a number of **student response system** apps that can be used both to quiz the students throughout a lesson and for students to write a short answer or fill out a multiple choice form to reflect on what they have learned. To be effective, questions used for these purposes must be representative of what students will see on summative tests. This requires considerably more work for the instructor, but the return on investment in time will be reflected in the students' improved performance. In addition, research has shown that use of student response systems is effective only if used consistently.[31] This makes intuitive sense but should not discourage educators from using technology for formative assessments. Student response systems, when used consistently, also increase student participation and engagement.[32]

Student response systems vary in functions and features. Some require hardware in the form of individual "clickers," as well as software. For adult learners, clicker systems are unnecessary for the most part, as the majority of adult students possess smartphones or tablets with which they can access app-based response systems. A search for the best (and free or least expensive) response systems will yield the information needed for an instructor to get started. Some of the better known systems include NearPod, Socrative, Kahoot, Google Forms, and PearDeck, to name a few.

Case-Based Learning Using Technology

Thanks to mobile learning, gone are the days of uniform pockets laden with reference books. Everything from calculators, to drug references, to e-textbooks can now be accessed through a smartphone and are available wherever and whenever the student or the practicing EMS provider needs them (**FIGURE 16.7**). Use of reference apps is a growing trend in medicine to guide physicians, nurses, paramedics, and allied health professionals in their everyday work.[33,34] Using digital references and checklists has "the same potential to save lives and prevent morbidity that it did in aviation over 70 years ago by ensuring that simple standards are applied for every patient, every time."[35]

Apps can make the work of healthcare providers easier. They are the digital counterpart to the past analog world. Whereas students once relied on printed textbooks that they carried to class and to the field setting, many of these large and easily damaged reference tools have been replaced with digital apps in a single, lightweight digital device. In health care, the knowledge required to be a competent provider is broad and continuously changing and advancing. Unlike books,

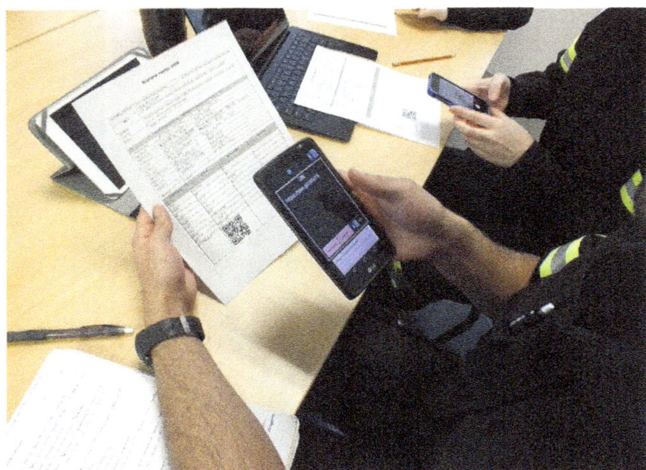

FIGURE 16.7 Apps make current reference information easily accessible to healthcare professionals.

Courtesy of Rob Theriault.

apps are updated frequently and provide students and practitioners with current information.

The use of apps in the learning environment, especially in case-based learning and clinical patient encounters, enables students to explore, inquire, and acquire knowledge in a constructivist way. Case-based learning is a means of giving students a situated learning experience in the classroom. Students score significantly higher through case-based learning.[36] With case-based learning, students collaborate and discuss real medical cases, and in doing so, develop their problem-solving and critical thinking skills. In the past, students sat together at desks with stacks of reference books and documents spread before them. These included textbooks (e.g., pathophysiology, physical assessment, medical math), several different drug references, books on differential diagnosis, and a variety of other medical books. Today their desks are, or should be, free of clutter.

For a case-based learning handout, to conserve space and keep the case to one double-sided page, you can use QR codes that direct students to images (e.g., wounds, car crashes, ECGs), videos, quizzes, or other information relevant to the case. Al-Shatti and Alhammad (2014) described the use of two-dimensional barcodes (QR codes) for a similar purpose and found that 59% of students felt that interacting with QR codes made the material more accessible; 77% indicated that being able to link to a video made it easier to visualize problems in class.[37]

TEACHING TIP

There are many free apps that create QR codes. A YouTube search will provide videos demonstrating how to create QR codes.

Reality Television

One of the shortcomings of case-based learning, even with the use of apps, is that it is difficult for students who are new to EMS to visualize cases described in the classroom. This is changing with reality TV shows about EMS. If the instructor is able to navigate the copyright obstacles (see Chapter 25, *Legal Issues for EMS Educators*), students can see and discuss the general principles of assessment and care based on real calls. Alternatively, because many reality TV episodes are available on YouTube or the TV Network website, the instructor can assign a particular episode along with a series of reflective questions that can later be discussed in the classroom. Television shows such as *Recruits: Paramedics* from Australia, the U.S. series *Nightwatch* and *Boston EMS*, or the Canadian series *Paramedics: Emergency Response* are examples the instructor can consider showing, with copyright permission. An instructor can play select sections, then ask students to reflect and discuss what they have seen and how it fits or does not fit into their understanding of how patients should be assessed and treated. In the classroom setting, this might be the closest thing to experiential learning.

Types of apps that can be useful in case-based learning include the following:

- Drug references
- Calculators
- Differential diagnosis guide
- Pediatric guide
- Triage guide
- Emergency response guide
- HazMat guide
- PDF reader
- e-textbooks

To help discern what apps are best for the students, the instructor can consult a rating system for medical apps called the mobile app rating scale (MARS), which is available through an Internet search. This rating scale is a complex system that requires expert peer reviewers.[38] EMS faculty may wish to collaborate to explore this rating scale.

Note Taking

Most students still prefer writing notes by hand, and some research has shown that students who take notes by hand perform better on conceptual questions than their laptop keyboarding counterparts.[39] The theory is

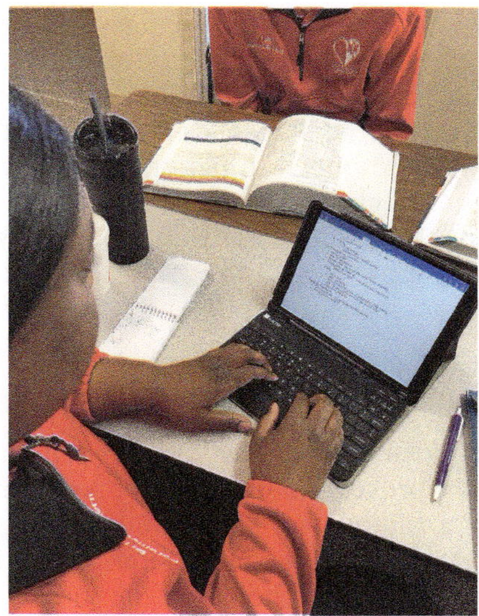

FIGURE 16.8 Writing notes on a digital device allows students the benefits of taking notes by hand, the convenience of decreased clutter, and the accessibility of the online format.

Courtesy of St. Charles County Ambulance District.

that because keyboarding is faster than writing, students who keyboard tend to type notes verbatim, whereas students who write are more selective about what they write and therefore pay greater attention to what is heard. In this study, the students were tested on their knowledge immediately after they took notes. It is not known how students using these two notetaking approaches fared a few days or a week after the note taking when both groups would have had a chance to study the material. Further research is needed to determine whether keyboarding the class content verbatim results in equally accurate information and better test results after both groups have more time to review their notes.

Digital note taking does not require keyboarding. Numerous apps enable handwritten notes (**FIGURE 16.8**); many apps will convert handwriting to block lettering if desired. One of the advantages of having everything written on a device, be it a laptop, tablet, or smartphone, is that it can be accessed and repurposed at any time. There is no paper cost, no clutter, and no backpacks bulging with binders and notepads. Students can keep all of their scholarly works on the device or in the cloud (e.g., Google Docs) so that they can access their work at any time, from anywhere, and from any device.

Digital Assignments

In the 21st century, there are few reasons to use paper in education other than that it remains a preference for most people. To reduce costs and the carbon footprint, some or all assignments can be offered digitally. For example, essays can be submitted electronically. Some schools use tools such as Turnitin that allow students to submit their paper, and it is compared to millions of papers and journal articles around the world for similarities. This reduces plagiarism and improves student originality in writing. Papers can be graded digitally as well using the "review" functions in MS Word, Apple's Pages, Google Docs, and Adobe PDFs and then returned to the student via e-mail. Some word processing programs even allow the addition of audio notes to a document to avoid having to type feedback.

Green and Efficient

Instructors and students can reduce waste, clutter, and cost, and achieve greater efficiencies by using the following:

- Digital handouts
- Digital assignments
- Software that analyzes essays for plagiarism
- Digital means of grading and returning essays to students
- e-textbooks
- Online exams
- Online courses (reduced travel)

Video and Audio Assignments

Audio and video assignments can be used in a number of ways to improve student performance. For example, one of the challenges in any EMS program is to help students learn the art of the handoff report. For an assignment, students can be given the task of recording handoff reports based on patient simulations in the lab setting or patient encounters in their hospital or field placement. The instructor can provide them with an outline of the information and sequence of information expected in a medical report and create a rubric to show how the reports will be evaluated. Unlike in the lab or in clinical placements, where students are expected to give reports spontaneously and with little preparation, audio reports give them time to think about, prepare, and rehearse reports before they are submitted. Spacing the time between submitted audio reports allows the instructor to provide feedback for each report so that the students can make improvements in this important skill.

Another example of an audio or video assignment that can be given in class or as homework is to have the students practice assessing the OPQRST of pain, or practice taking a patient's history while recording the exercise with either audio or video. Students can pair up, with one playing the patient and the other playing the care provider. The instructor can provide the student playing the patient with a sheet containing the responses; the provider's goal would be to ask all of the appropriate questions. The recordings could either be reviewed in class, making this a formative assessment, or be submitted as a summative assessment assignment. Another audio/video assignment is to place students in groups to record journal club discussions of relevant and timely research papers, then play them for the class for further discussion and debate.

There are many other ways audio and video assignments can enhance the learning experience for students. Brainstorming with other instructors or students can provide additional audio/video assignment ideas.

Digital Office Hours

Students feel more invested in a course when there is a personal connection between them and their instructor. However, it is sometimes difficult to make a personal connection with all students when there is limited time available for office hours. To try to correct this situation, some instructors hold virtual office hours using an online communication platform such as Skype or Google Hangout. Some potential benefits to this method include (1) a higher percentage of students may contact the instructor with questions, as it gives them the freedom to make contact with the instructor from anywhere, and (2) students sometimes study together; when they come across something on which they cannot all agree, one of them may contact the instructor via their computer or smartphone. This usually leads to a virtual office tutorial with the whole group, and additional questions arise from this engagement. Students love the quick access, but like any form of communication with students, hours of availability should be made clear in a syllabus.

Web-Enhanced Classroom

Learning Management Systems

A **learning management system (LMS)** is a software application for all activities related to a course, including posting of all course-related learning materials, assignments, quizzes, performance and progress tracking, threaded discussions, student grades, communication tools such as announcements, email, and more. An LMS can be used to enhance the classroom delivery in a face-to-face class or to deliver online courses (discussed in Chapter 17, *Tools for Distance Learning*). The advantage to delivering materials via an LMS rather than via email is that once all of the course materials are loaded into the LMS, they are stored there for the duration of the course or program.

This allows instructors and students to access all of the materials from one location. As a quality assurance measure, the instructor can track which students have viewed which documents and track assignment progress and completion. If students lose documents, they are always accessible on the LMS. This can save the instructor (and students) a great deal of time. Other advantages for students include the ability to collaborate on assignments online, communicate with their instructor, and access the LMS from anywhere and on any device. Its cloud-based nature makes an LMS an ideal mobile learning platform.

Most colleges and universities have an LMS; however, smaller training agencies may not be able to afford an expensive platform. The good news is that there are alternatives, some of which are free and some that are more affordable. Google Classroom is a free LMS that became available to educators outside of the K–12 system in 2017. CourseSites by Blackboard is a free LMS that allows an instructor to create up to five courses and restrict enrollment to their own students or to open courses to anyone. With the unlimited access feature, instructors can create a MOOC. Moodle is another free open source LMS, but may require internal technical support. Sakai is a free open source LMS specifically intended for educational institutions. Other examples of free open source, low-cost LMSs include WizIQ, Latitude Learning, Dokeos, Schoology, ELMSLN (built on Wordpress), MyiCourse, Open edX, Claroline, and Totara. Additionally, some educational publishers provide LMS platforms to accompany their textbooks. See Chapter 17, *Tools for Distance Learning*, for additional information about LMSs.

Webinar Platforms

The primary benefits of having access to a **webinar** or synchronous online learning platform is to be able to invite subject matter experts from a distance into your class or to host online tutorials to supplement the in-class learning. See Chapter 17, *Tools for Distance Learning*, for more on synchronized online learning platforms.

Use of Podcasts to Supplement Instructor Lectures

As mentioned earlier, educators can create podcasts of their classroom lectures for students to use as a study tool. Podcasts from other sources across the Internet can also be used to supplement student learning. Podcasts give students access to some of the most knowledgeable physicians, paramedics, and allied health experts on the planet. In the past, this type of access was possible only for those who were able to attend conferences where the best speakers were invited to present.

Podcasts have become increasingly popular in higher education.[40,41] Whether they are instructor-recorded podcasts or one of the thousands of podcasts available online, they give students verbatim information for note taking and allow time to pause, reflect, and mentally process the words and meanings.

Screencasting

A **screencast** is a digital audio-video recording of whatever is on the computer screen, be it a narrated slide presentation or a simple explanation of an image or graph. The screencast allows the instructor to capture lectures or explain difficult concepts. Like a podcast, one of the appealing features of the screencast is that the student can stop, rewind, and replay as needed. There are several free or low-cost screencasting tools available, such as Screencast-O-Matic, Jing, Snagit, and Screencastify. A quick search will reveal numerous screencasting apps for multiple operating systems.

The ideal length of a video or screencast tutorial is debatable. Plaisant and Shneiderman (2005) say that the ideal video length is between 15 and 60 seconds.[42] However, most other studies suggest that 3 to 10 minutes is the ideal length.[43,44]

While a screencast may be more engaging than text-based homework, it is still a passive form of media. To make it truly engaging, questions can be embedded into the screencast using Camtasia or Adobe Captivate, or by uploading the screencast to YouTube and then using programs such as PlayPosit or Edpuzzle. Alternatively, the screencast can be embedded into a quiz using Google Forms. While it is not clear at this time if interactive video improves learning outcomes, it certainly improves the interaction between the student and the screencast, and increases the time spent with the learning materials.[45]

Sal Khan of Khan Academy acknowledges that screencasts alone are not an effective tool through which students can learn.[46] Kahn suggests that "where the meat is" (i.e., the engagement and experiential learning) is in the exercises and feedback that complement the videos. Students prefer interactive screencast/video homework over text-based homework.[47]

Flipped Classroom

Some instructors use screencasts to "flip" the classroom by recording core content such as anatomy, physiology, pathophysiology, pharmacology, or patient care theory to be viewed online. Students are expected to access these screencasts prior to class, then engage in case-based learning in the classroom. Whatever an educator's reason for flipping the classroom, it takes some time to plan and execute. In a traditional math class, for example, the instructor discusses math concepts and the students practice equations at home. The concept of the **flipped classroom** was born out of the idea that the instructor could enable the students to view the lectures at home and then have them spend their time in the classroom solving problems. This enables the instructor to spend more one-on-one time with the students and support students as they apply the information.

The concept of the flipped classroom makes more sense for some subjects than for others. For example, math, chemistry, and physics are well suited to the flipped approach, because the hands-on component is critically important, and time in class can be better spent "doing" instead of discussing. The same might be said in EMS education in areas such as patient care theory where a review of patient conditions, assessment criteria, and interventions might be well-suited for screencasting while case-based discussions could occur in the classroom. This might also be an ideal approach for continuing education, where EMS providers can review core material through screencasts and discuss cases in the classroom.

Open Educational Resources

Do educators in higher education have an obligation to offer an equivalent electronic textbook (e-textbook) to students who prefer digital materials or wish to save money? Consider that the consumer—the student—does not choose the textbook; it is chosen for them by the professor. Some describe this as a "broken market" because the professor chooses the book but does not pay for it. This allows the publisher to set prices for a captive audience.[48] In addition, consider that when a book is published, some of its information may be out of date by the time of printing. Students recognize this by finding more current sources of information online through scholarly journals and social media. For these reasons, an educator may want to consider offering alternatives to printed textbooks.

Publishers typically offer textbooks in various forms, including printed hard-copy textbooks and digital e-books, giving instructors and students a choice. With the rising cost of school and the rising cost of textbooks, many students choose to buy used books, share a single text, rent or buy an e-textbook, or attempt to get by without a textbook. In fact, according to the U.S. Public Interest Research Group, 65% of college students chose not to buy a textbook because of the high cost.[49] Giving students an e-textbook alternative, particularly if it is free, or even handouts or links to relevant information can help minimize student costs.

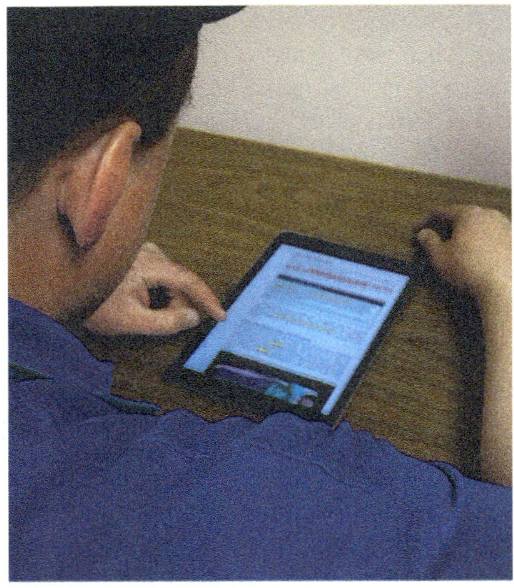

FIGURE 16.9 E-textbooks offer interactive features such as the ability to highlight, take notes, and bookmark, and may also include links to videos, animations, or other multimedia content.

Courtesy of St. Charles County Ambulance District.

The value of e-textbooks is their digital interactivity. Most e-texbooks permit the student to highlight, annotate, and bookmark, and they may also contain hyperlinks to key terms and associated information such as drug profiles (**FIGURE 16.9**). To attract more students to the e-textbook market, some publishers add more interactive multimedia, and this will be critically important for publishers to develop, whether they are open source like OpenStax or from the traditional publishing industry.

Text to Voice

When it comes to studying, students do not always have time to read large amounts of text for a given subject. One of the advantages of some e-readers and apps is that they can convert **text to voice**. Apps such as Voice Dream and NaturalReader Pro can read PDF files aloud while the student does other activities such as driving or exercising. Although the voices sound somewhat robotic, these apps allow students to take in information when reading is not possible or if listening is their preferred method of learning.

Cloud Computing

Cloud computing is the practice of using remote servers to host and manage computer files, instead of storing files on one device. The advantage of using cloud computing is that these files can be accessed via the Internet, from any device. Most cloud services allow synchronization of local files with cloud-stored files, so they can be used even when there is no Internet access.

Most Americans own two computer devices, and 36% own three or more, according to the Pew Research Center.[50] When students do school-related work on more than one device, they quickly discover the inconvenience of having to move files from one device to another. The advantage to using cloud-based platforms such as Google Drive, Dropbox, or OneNote is that homework, notes, and assignments can be accessed in one place from any device.

Another advantage of cloud-based computing is that the user can elect to keep documents, spreadsheets, slides, and other forms private, or can choose to share files or collaborate in the files with classmates. A student can also share a link to an assignment with an instructor to grade in the cloud.

Mobile Learning

Unlike any other period in time, the digital age permits instant, mobile access to information ranging from news to scholarly papers. With smartphones and tablets, students are not restricted to studying in their room, a commons area, or the library. They can read, listen, view, research, and write anywhere and at any time. This is the benefit of mobile learning: It gives the student unrestricted access to learning from the world's entire knowledge base wherever they might be. Students can experience differentiated learning through multiple online sources—from e-textbooks, to blogs, to videos, to podcasts—from the best schools and the best educators in the world. Students create their own learning networks using social media. They connect with experts in their field of interest from around the globe. While this is exciting, it also poses a dilemma. Students need help finding information that is most suitable and appropriate to their learning needs. This is where digital literacy plays a critical role.

Digital Literacy

It is vitally important that students develop the skills necessary to find relevant and credible information on the Web. The reality, however, is that this is not given much thought by most organizations and institutions. But who should be responsible for teaching students digital literacy? The instructor? The library? The educational institution or agency? Furthermore, students need the skills to be able to critically analyze information. In an age of evidence-based medicine, educators must help students develop their digital literacy skills, not just for their current studies, but for lifelong learning.

It is the educator's responsibility to help their students learn where to search for and find primary and high-quality secondary research sources through search engines such as PubMed and Cochrane, and to respect copyright laws. It is also the educator's responsibility to help students become skeptics in an information-rich world.

Digital-Only Materials

Is it possible for a student or educator to use only digital materials? Yes. Digital-only is definitely not for everyone, but for those who are willing to try, it is possible. Alternative digital books can be suggested for students who prefer digital content. Some students prefer reading digitally and learning from blogs, educational videos, and podcasts. Students can also use text-to-voice apps for reading articles or books when traveling or exercising. Note taking and assignments can be completed digitally and if the educator is willing to accept digital assignments, these can be submitted digitally as well. When possible, let the student decide what medium they prefer. Digital-only is cheaper, lighter (e.g., tablet vs. books), and better for the planet.

The Role of Social Media in Education

Social media is a relatively recent phenomenon. It has its origins in the social media site Six Degrees that was created in 1997.[51] This ushered in the era of Web 2.0, where the Internet was no longer a static display of text, images, and video, but became a place where people could interact with the Web and with each other. For educators, students, and lifelong learners, this meant that their sphere of influence expanded on a global scale.

As far as information goes, social media provides the access and ability to connect with billions of people around the world and millions of experts in any field of interest. The question is, with billions of blogs, podcasts, Twitter accounts, YouTube channels, Facebook groups, and more, how does one discern between truth, belief, opinion, consensus, best practices, evidence-based assertions, and bunk? Whereas some information sources in social media are opinion-based, many sources, such as medical blogs, contain hyperlinks to evidence. Students should be encouraged to follow the cited evidence to judge its authenticity and credibility.

Peer Learning Networks

In an age of mobile learning and with experts across the Internet, students learn from their instructors and from social media sources. Differentiated learning is beneficial, and students should be encouraged to build **peer learning networks** using podcasts, blogs, video channels, apps, and social media. Chances are, students are part of such a network before coming to class for the first time. The instructor's role should be to help steer students toward credible learning and to help them to discern between what is and what is not credible.

As educators, social media should also be a source of knowledge and medical news for lifelong learning. According to one study: "Over 90% of all [college] faculty are using social media in courses they're teaching or for their professional careers outside the classroom."[52]

The following is a guide for assessing sites and their content for credibility:

- **Cross-check the facts**: When learning something new from a site, students and educators should cross-check it with other sites to see if there is agreement. Students can also do a PubMed or Cochrane database search to see if research evidence exists to confirm their findings.
- **Peer reviewed**: Is the site peer reviewed? Life in the Fast Last, for example, is a blog by Dr. Mike Cadogan, an emergency room physician from Australia who, with a couple of other colleagues, coined the term *free open access meducation*, also known as #FOAM or #FOAMed. His site has multiple physician authors and is peer reviewed by other physicians and physician-researchers.
- **Currency**: Does the information seem new or dated? Are pages and information updated as new information becomes available? In medicine, research changes practice frequently, and content on blogs and other social media sites should be updated accordingly.
- **References**: Does the site or author provide references to their sources? These sources should be primary research evidence or secondary evidence of the highest quality, such as critical reviews or meta-analysis.
- **Disclosures**: Do the sites have sponsors? Are the authors paid? Any conflicts of interest should be disclosed up-front. Otherwise, the credibility of the content is questionable.
- **Balance**: Does the site present conflicting research or concede in some circumstances that more research is needed on a given subject?

Emerging Technologies

Humans are on the precipice of a technological evolution like never before. Everything is changing at an exponential pace that is only at the "knee" of the exponential curve. All of the advances of the 18th to 20th centuries combined will pale in comparison to what will emerge in the first half of the 21st century. To put it simply, in the words of Marc Prensky, "everything is changing much faster than in the past."[53]

What kind of changes can educators expect in the future of learning in higher education? For one, it will become increasingly mobile, automated, and unbundled, from "fixed timing and courses of study to more competency-based approaches."[54] Textbooks and lectures are becoming less relevant as students have multiple sources of learning at their fingertips and can choose to learn from the best professors in the world instead of ones who work nearby. This will continue into the future. As an example of what is to come, at Georgia Institute of Technology **artificial intelligence (AI)** is currently taking on the role of the teaching assistant, performing tasks such as grading papers, answering student questions in a forum, reminding students of important dates over email, and providing instructional correspondence—sometimes without the students knowing that they are being helped by technology with AI capabilities. Because of its human-like conversational style that blends into online discussion threads, students are not only unaware they are communicating with an AI, some students even exhibit a bond with their AI tutor through conversation that extends beyond the tutoring.[54–56]

Artificial Intelligence and Adaptive Learning

AI will be the next disruptive technology that will forever change the way humans learn. AI is already a part of most digital devices, from the autocorrect function on phones to digital assistants such as Cortana, Siri, and Alexa. There is software that evaluates university papers, and AI that is writing sports columns. As AI improves, it will be truly pervasive, becoming a component of every digital medium. Currently there are intelligent tutoring systems that provide immediate and customized instruction and feedback to learners, usually without intervention from a human instructor. These AI systems use interactive tutorials combined with sophisticated algorithms to identify student strengths and weaknesses, target the weak areas, and generate remedial learning. Examples of AI are found in programs from Khan Academy; examples of AI with adaptive learning are found in programs from Knewton. In both cases, the student takes a lesson and attempts to solve some problems. If the student is unsuccessful, new lessons are offered that are different from the first (differentiated learning), and the student is able to try new problems. The differentiated and adaptive learning ability of AI-enabled software enables student-centered and individualized learning.

AI is typically designed for a specific task or tasks, in contrast to **artificial general intelligence (AGI)** which can perform any task. AGI is machine intelligence that is able to perform the same intellectual work as humans, as opposed to machine ability to only perform certain cognitive tasks. In the book *Life 3.0: Humanity in the Age of Artificial Intelligence*, Max Tegmark predicts that AGI will not happen in the foreseeable future. However, when AGI does happen, it will likely outperform humans. In other words, these will be thinking machines with an intelligence comparable to the human mind. Why might this be valuable in education? The student-centered approach of AGI will outperform what any human instructor can do.[57] Will this mean the end of teaching and educators? That's unlikely. While AI or AGI may be become great tutors on many levels, educators will be needed to teach critical thinking, creativity, and emotional intelligence. In a TED talk in 2010, Conrad Wolfram argued that it is pointless to teach calculus or complicated mathematics when a smartphone can do the work, adding that educators should instead focus on helping students to be creative with math and solve real-world problems.[58] Perhaps this is the lesson educators must learn to keep pace with technology.

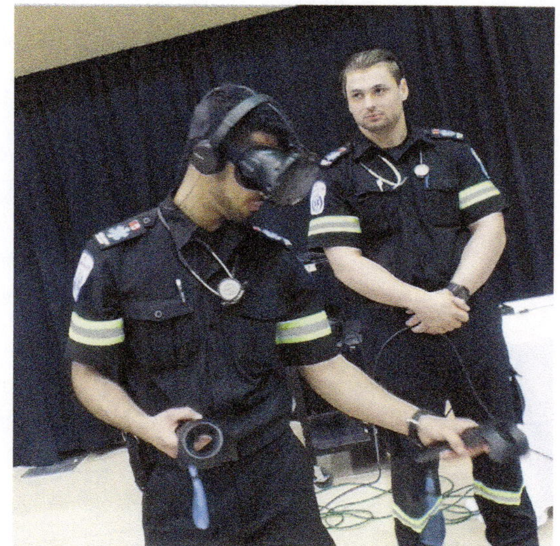

FIGURE 16.10 Virtual reality applications in education include stress inoculation, teaching to the affective domain, and exposure to more types of patients and conditions than can be achieved in real-life training.

Courtesy of Rob Theriault.

Virtual, Augmented, Mixed, and Extended Reality

What if classroom learning could be immersive? More situated? More experiential? Virtual, augmented, mixed, and extended reality are poised to profoundly transform education.[59] These immersive and heuristic approaches to learning will be a disruptive pedagogy.

Virtual reality (VR) is a 360-degree, immersive, computer-generated environment in which participants can interact with objects and the environment (**FIGURE 16.10**). To truly understand how VR places a person in a different world, one needs to experience it firsthand with a head-mounted display. As an example, students can learn human anatomy through adventures inside the human body. Immersive virtual patient simulations, unlike animated simulations on a computer screen, give the student a sense of "presence," or actually being with a real patient who is seriously ill or injured. That sense of presence gives the learner a feeling of urgency that cannot be replicated on a computer screen or even in the lab setting. Short of seeing patients in the hospital or the field, what VR offers is a multitude of patients, conditions, and environments. VR enables students to learn how to assess, think critically, and manage patients in a safe environment while still providing a sense of suspended disbelief. Because of the sense of presence that one experiences in VR, this learning environment can be used for stress inoculation. In this method the student is immersed in simulations with escalating levels of stress. VR also offers the ability to teach in the affective domain. This is arguably the most challenging and elusive of the domains. VR can place the learner in the shoes of someone else so that they can experience what it is like to be, for example, an elderly patient or a schizophrenic, or what life is like for someone living in a refugee camp. VR is a new frontier in health education, and it will be transformative because, unlike current modalities, it will be possible to alter the way students feel and to help them to develop empathy or to shape what they value in a measurable way.[60,61]

Augmented reality (AR) is a technology usually associated with the use of AR glasses, which superimpose 3-D digital images/holograms on a user's view of the real world, and/or add other elements such as sound, weather, etc. Another term, **mixed reality (MR)**, refers to AR technology with interactive physical elements (**FIGURE 16.11**). A static manikin, for example, could appear as a living, breathing, distressed patient. The fact that the student can also touch or perform procedures on the manikin makes this an MR experience. MR provides the advantage of making a simulation seem more realistic, and because the learner sees images superimposed on real objects (e.g., manikin), they are able to perform tactile skills

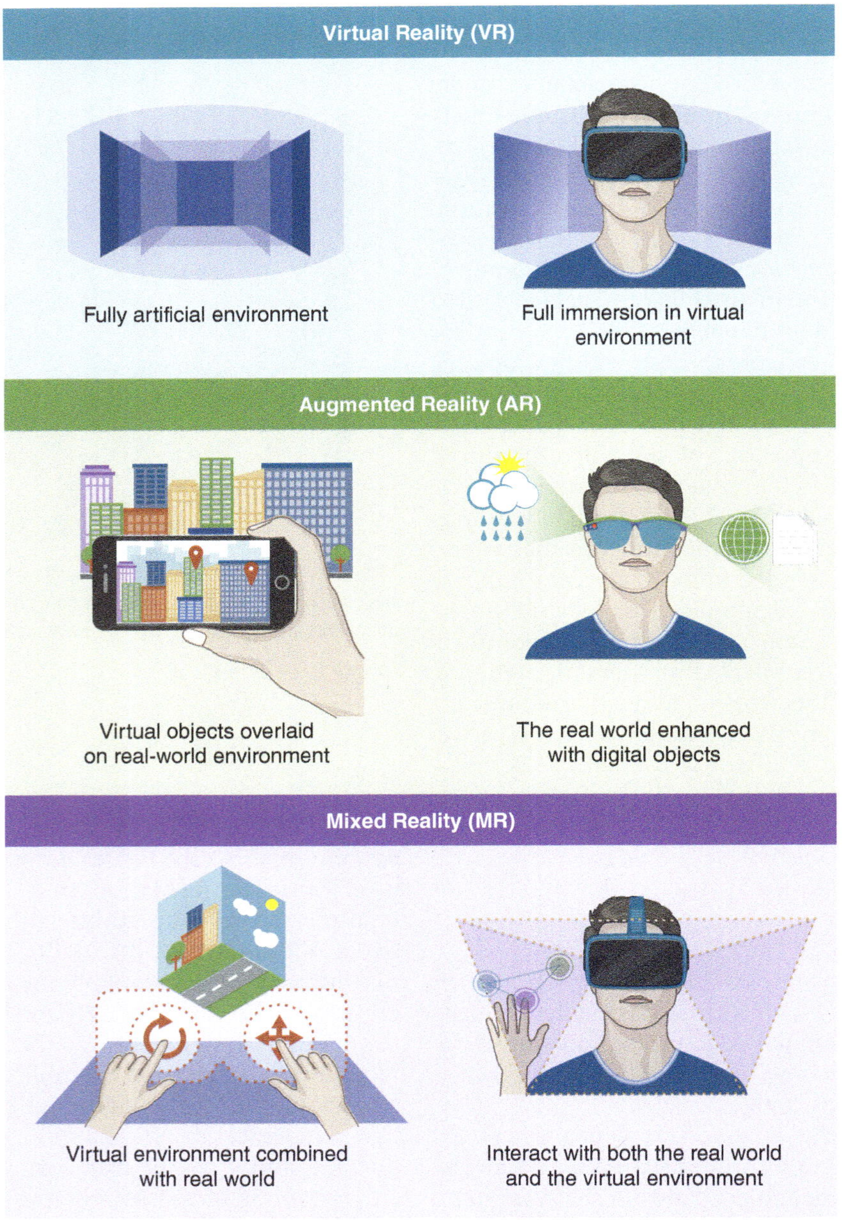

FIGURE 16.11 Comparison of virtual reality, augmented reality, and mixed reality.

such as intravenous cannulation. The disadvantage is that with AR and a static manikin, the perception of patient movement is incongruent with the tactile assessment of the manikin. Nonetheless, this may provide advantages over animated patients encountered in the VR environment that lack a true tactile element to enable the practice of psychomotor skills. Another advantage of AR or MR is that students can interact with each other and can touch and manipulate objects in the AR world for truly interactive learning and feedback.

To address some of the confusion with VR, AR, and MR, leaders in the field have come up with the term **extended reality (XR)**. XR is an umbrella term intended to capture the blending of real- and virtual-world elements. Because these are still nascent technologies, there will be continued advances, and the terminology may evolve with time.

Summary

The potential for educational technology to transform how students learn is both exciting and undeniable. However, all educational technology-related matters come down to four basic questions:

1. What are the learning objectives?
2. What is the best pedagogical approach to help students achieve those objectives?
3. Is there a technology that will help students meet those objectives in a more efficient or effective way?
4. Is there qualitative and, ideally, quantitative evidence that the technology is effective in helping students achieve their objectives and improve learning outcomes?

If a technology does not add anything to the learning experience, either in efficiency or improved outcomes, then it is probably not worth pursuing.

Technology is advancing rapidly. Choosing an edtech tool requires careful consideration and a willingness to use it for a long enough period to achieve mastery and survey students for their feedback. Because many educational technologies are at the nascent stage, educators should be willing to explore the potential of new technologies to enhance learning, be willing to gain experience with technologies, and finally, play an active role in the development of edtech tools.

Glossary

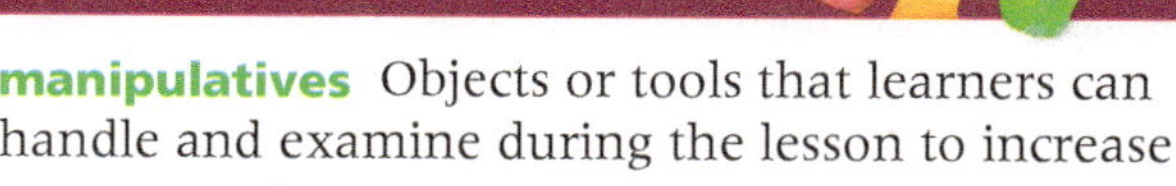

analog technologies Tools such as whiteboards, flip charts, and manipulatives that are used for teaching and learning.

apps Software programs that are typically downloaded by a user to a mobile device.

artificial general intelligence (AGI) Machine intelligence that is able to perform the same intellectual work as humans, as opposed to machine ability to perform only certain cognitive tasks.

artificial intelligence (AI) Machine intelligence that is able to perform a specific cognitive task or tasks.

augmentation SAMR level at which a technology offers a more effective tool to perform a common task.

augmented reality (AR) Technology in which special eyeglasses usually need to be worn, which superimpose 3-D digital images or holograms on a user's view of the real world.

cloud computing The practice of using remote servers to host and manage computer files.

extended reality (XR) An umbrella term that refers to the elements of virtual reality, augmented reality, and mixed reality.

flipped classroom Educational model in which an instructor assigns lectures to students as prework, then uses class time to apply the information.

hypermediality Links to audio, video, graphics, or hyperlinks to other Web pages.

learning management system (LMS) Software application for all activities related to a course.

manipulatives Objects or tools that learners can handle and examine during the lesson to increase engagement.

massive open online courses (MOOCs) Courses of study made available over the Internet at minimal to no cost to a very large number of people.

mixed reality (MR) Technology in which special eyeglasses usually need to be worn, which superimpose 3-D digital images or holograms on a user's view of the real world and in which digital elements are able to react to real-life elements.

modification SAMR level at which a technology allows tasks to be done in a completely new way.

peer learning networks Groups of social media participants that engage in online learning together, usually without the presence of an instructor.

podcast Recording of an audio presentation that is made available online and that can be downloaded.

redefinition SAMR level at which a technology enables a new task to be performed, which was not possible before.

SAMR model Taxonomy for categorizing technologies.

screencast Recording of a computer presentation that is made available online and that can be downloaded.

student response system Type of technology in which students answer questions or provide feedback via a technological device, such as a clicker.

substitution SAMR level at which a technology replicates a task that was previously done without a computer or a learning technology; there is no functional change.

text to voice Technology that converts written prose to audio.

virtual reality (VR) Immersive 360-degree, computer-generated environment in which participants interact with objects and the environment through use of a head-mounted display.

webinar Live presentation given online, in which an audience can listen and participate through a technological device with Internet access.

References

[1] Andrew-Gee, Eric. 2018, January 6. "Your Smartphone Is Making You Stupid, Antisocial and Unhealthy. So Why Can't You Put It Down?" *The Globe and Mail*. Accessed February 6, 2019. https://www.theglobeandmail.com/technology/your-smartphone-is-making-you-stupid/article37511900/.

[2] Hoffelder, Nate. 2014. "Books Will Soon be Obsolete in the Public Schools." *The Digital Reader*. Accessed February 6, 2019. http://the-digital-reader.com/2012/05/08/books-will-soon-be-obsolete-in-the-public-schools/.

[3] Educational Technology and Mobile Learning. 2014, March 19. "A Wonderful Visual Timeline of the History of Classroom Technology." Accessed January 24, 2019. https://www.educatorstechnology.com/2014/03/a-wonderful-visual-timeline-of-history.html.

[4] Flavin, Michael. 2012. "Disruptive Technologies in Higher Education." *Research in Learning Technology* 20. https://doi.org/10.3402/rlt.v20i0.19184.

[5] De Langen, Frank, and Herman van den Bosch. 2013. "Massive Open Online Courses: Disruptive Innovations or Disturbing Inventions?" *Open Learning* 28, no. 3: 216–26. https://doi.org/10.1080/02680513.2013.870882.

[6] Pence, Harry E. 2012. "When Will College Truly Leave the Building: If MOOCs Are the Answer, What Is the Question?" *Journal of Educational Technology Systems* 41, no. 1: 25–33. https://doi.org/10.2190/ET.41.1.c.

[7] Hassoun, Dan. 2014. "'All Over the Place': A Case Study of Classroom Multitasking and Attentional Performance." *New Media & Society*. https://doi.org/10.1177/1461444814531756.

[8] Wurst, Christine, Claudia Smarkola, and Mary Anne Gaffney. 2008. "Ubiquitous Laptop Usage in Higher Education: Effects on Student Achievement, Student Satisfaction, and Constructivist Measures in Honors and Traditional Classrooms." *Computers & Education* 51, no. 4: 1766–83. https://doi.org/10.1016/j.compedu.2008.05.006.

[9] Grace-Martin, Michael, and Geri Gay. 2001. "Web Browsing, Mobile Computing and Academic Performance." *Educational Technology & Society* 4, no. 3: 95–107.

[10] Fried, Carrie B. 2008. "In-Class Laptop Use and Its Effects on Student Learning." *Computers & Education* 50, no. 3: 906–14. https://doi.org/10.1016/j.compedu.2006.09.006.

[11] Williams, Antony J., and Harry E. Pence. 2011. "Smart Phones: A Powerful Tool in the Chemistry Classroom." *Journal of Chemical Education* 88, no. 6: 683–6. http://dx.doi.org/10.1021/ed200029p.

[12] Romrell, Danae, Lisa C. Kidder, and Emma Wood. 2014. "The SAMR Model as a Framework for Evaluating mLearning." *Online Learning* 18, no. 2. Accessed February 6, 2019. https://eric.ed.gov/?id=EJ1036281.

[13] Linderoth, Jonas. 2013. "Open letter to Dr. Ruben Puentedura." Accessed February 6, 2019. http://spelvetenskap.blogspot.com/2013/10/open-letter-to-dr-ruben-puentedura.html.

[14] McGregor, Debbie, and Andrew Tolmie. 2009. "Group Work in Science Classrooms." *Education in Science* 234: 30–1.

[15] Tsay, Mina, and Miranda Brady. 2012. "A Case Study of Cooperative Learning and Communication Pedagogy: Does Working in Teams Make a Difference?" *Journal of the Scholarship of Teaching and Learning* 10, no. 2: 78–89.

[16] Kiliçkaya, Ferit. 2016. "Information Comprehension from Longhand Notes and Slides in the Language Classroom." In *New Insights into Language Teaching and Learning Practices*, edited by Marek Krawiec, 135–46. Regensburg, Germany: Marek Krawiec. Accessed February 6, 2019. https://eric.ed.gov/?id=ED571538.

[17] Clark, Ruth C., and Richard E. Mayer. 2011. *E-learning and the Science of Instruction: Proven Guidelines for Consumers and Designers of Multimedia Learning*, 3rd ed. Hoboken, NJ: John Wiley & Sons.

[18] Babb, Kimberly A., and Craig Ross. 2009. "The Timing of Online Lecture Slide Availability and Its Effect on Attendance, Participation, and Exam Performance." *Computers & Education* 52, no. 4: 868–81. https://doi.org/10.1016/j.compedu.2008.12.009.

[19] Yilmazel-Sahin, Yesim, and Rebecca L. Oxford. 2010. "Teacher Education Students' Perceptions of the Value of Handouts Accompanying Teacher Educators' Computer-Generated Slide Presentations." *Journal of Technology and Teacher Education* 18, no. 3: 509–35.

[20] Evans, Chris. 2008. "The Effectiveness of m-Learning in the Form of Podcast Revision Lectures in Higher Education." *Computers & Education* 50, no. 2: 491–8. https://doi.org/10.1016/j.compedu.2007.09.016.

[21] Powell, Cynthia B., and Diana S. Mason. 2012. "Effectiveness of Podcasts Delivered on Mobile Devices as a Support for Student Learning during General Chemistry Laboratories." *Journal of Science Education and Technology* 22, no. 2: 148–70. https://doi.org/10.1007/s10956-012-9383-y.

[22] Morris, Neil P. 2010. "Podcasts and Mobile Assessment Enhance Student Learning Experience and Academic Performance." *Bioscience Education* 16, no. 1: 1–7. https://doi.org/10.3108/beej.16.1.

[23] McKinney, Dani, Jennifer L. Dyck, and Elise S. Luber. 2009. "iTunes University and the Classroom: Can Podcasts Replace Professors?" *Computers & Education* 52, no. 3: 617–23. https://doi.org/10.1016/j.compedu.2008.11.004.

[24] Bjork, Robert A., John Dunlosky, and Nate Kornell. 2013. "Self-Regulated Learning: Beliefs, Techniques, and Illusions." *Annual Review of Psychology* 64: 417–44.

[25] Racsmány, Mihály, Agnes Szőllősi, and Dorottya Bencze. 2018. "Retrieval Practice Makes Procedure from Remembering: An Automatization Account of the Testing Effect." *Journal of Experimental Psychology: Learning, Memory, and Cognition* 44, no. 1: 157–66. http://dx.doi.org/10.1037/xlm0000423.

[26] Eglington, Luke G., and Sean H. K. Kang. 2016. "Retrieval Practice Benefits Deductive Inference." *Educational Psychology Review* 30, no. 1: 215–28. https://doi.org/10.1007/s10648-016-9386-y.

[27] Lyle, Keith B., and Nicole A. Crawford. 2011. "Retrieving Essential Material at the End of Lectures Improves Performance on Statistics Exams." *Teaching of Psychology* 38, no. 2: 94–7. https://doi.org/10.1177/0098628311401587.

[28] Roediger, Henry L., Pooja K. Agarwal, Mark A. McDaniel, and Kathleen B. McDermott. 2011. "Test-Enhanced Learning in the Classroom: Long-Term Improvements from Quizzing." *Journal of Experimental Psychology: Applied* 17, no. 4: 382–95. https://doi.org/10.1037/a0026252.

[29] Agarwal, Pooja K., Jeffrey D. Karpicke, Sean H. K. Kang, Henry L. Roediger, and Kathleen B. McDermott. 2008. "Examining the Testing Effect with Open- and Closed-Book Tests." *Applied Cognitive Psychology* 22: 861–76. https://doi.org/10.1002/acp.1391.

[30] Roediger, Henry L., and Jeffrey D. Karpicke. 2006. "Test-Enhanced Learning." *Psychological Science* 17, no. 3: 249–55. https://doi.org/10.1111%2Fj.1467-9280.2006.01693.x.

[31] Ghilic, Irina, Michelle L. Cadieux, Joseph A. Kim, and David I. Shore. 2014. *Assessing the Impact of Interactive Sampling Using Audience Response Systems*. Toronto: Higher Education Quality Council of Ontario.

[32] Heaslip, Graham, Paul Donovan, and John G. Cullen. 2014. "Student Response Systems and Learner Engagement in Large Classes." *Active Learning in Higher Education* 15, no. 1: 11–24. https://doi.org/10.1177/1469787413514648.

[33] Ventola, C. Lee. 2014. "Mobile Devices and Apps for Health Care Professionals: Uses and Benefits." *PT* 39, no. 5: 356–64.

[34] Ozdalga, Errol, Ark Ozdalga, and Neera Ahuja. 2012. "The Smartphone in Medicine: A Review of Current and Potential Use among Physicians and Students." *Journal of Medical Internet Research* 14, no. 5: e128. http://dx.doi.org/10.2196/jmir.1994.

[35] Clay-Williams, Robyn, and Lacey Colligan. 2015. "Back to Basics: Checklists in Aviation and Healthcare." *BMJ Quality & Safety* 24, no. 7: 428–31. http://dx.doi.org/10.1136/bmjqs-2015-003957.

[36] Baeten, Marlies, Filip Dochy, and Katrien Struyven. 2012. "Enhancing Students' Approaches to Learning: The Added Value of Gradually Implementing Case-Based Learning." *European Journal of Psychology of Education* 28, no. 2: 315–36. https://doi.org/10.1007/s10212-012-0116-7.

[37] Al-Shatti, Laila A., and Noura Alhammad. 2014. "The Application of Smartphones and Two-dimensional Barcodes in a Chemistry Laboratory Manual." *Journal of Laboratory Chemical Education* 2, no. 1: 1–3. doi:10.5923.j.jlce.20140201.01.

[38] Stoyanov, Stoyan R., Leanne Hides, David J Kavanagh, Oksana Zelenko, Dian Tjondronegoro, and Madhavan Mani. 2015. "Mobile App Rating Scale: A New Tool for Assessing the Quality of Health Mobile Apps." *JMIR MHealth and UHealth* 3, no. 1. https://doi.org/10.2196/mhealth.3422.

[39] Oppenheimer, Daniel M., and Pam A. Mueller. 2014. "The Pen Is Mightier than the Keyboard: Longhand and Laptop Note-Taking." *PsycEXTRA Dataset*.

[40] McDonald, James E. 2008. "Podcasting a Physics Lecture." *The Physics Teacher* 46, no. 8: 490–3. https://doi.org/10.1119/1.2999066.

[41] Lum, Lydia. 2006. "The Power of Podcasting." *Diverse: Issues in Higher Education* 23, no. 2: 32–5. Accessed February 6, 2019. http://eric.ed.gov/?id=EJ763137.

[42] Plaisant, Catherine, and Ben Shneiderman. 2005. *Show Me! Guidelines for Recorded Demonstration*. Dallas, TX: IEEE Symposium on Visual Languages and Human-Centric Computing. Accessed February 6, 2019. http://hcil2.cs.umd.edu/trs/2005-02/2005-02.pdf.

[43] Chan, Lap K., Nivritti G. Patil, Julie Y. Chen, Jamie C. M. Lam, Chak S. Lau, and Mary S. M. Ip. "Advantages of Video Trigger in Problem-Based Learning." *Medical Teacher* 32, no. 9: 760–5. https://doi.org/10.3109/01421591003686260.

[44] Velegol, Stephanie B., Sarah E. Zappe, and Emily Mahoney. 2005. "The Evolution of a Flipped Classroom: Evidence-Based Recommendations." *Advances in Engineering Education* 4, no. 3: 78.

[45] Vural, Ömer F. 2013. "The Impact of a Question-Embedded Video-based Learning Tool on E-learning." *Educational Sciences: Theory & Practice* 13, no. 2: 1315–23.

[46] Khan, Salman. 2011. "Liberating the Classroom for Creativity." *Edutopia*. Accessed February 6, 2019. http://www.edutopia.org/salman-khan-academy-flipped-classroom-video.

[47] Pickering, James D. 2016. "Measuring Learning Gain: Comparing Anatomy Drawing Screencasts and Paper-Based Resources." *Anatomical Sciences Education* 10, no. 4: 307–16. https://doi.org/10.1002/ase.1666.

[48] Koch, James V. 2006. "An Economic Analysis of Textbook Prices and the Textbook Market." Accessed February 6, 2019. http://www.immagic.com/eLibrary/CBICBT99/FIN_AID/US_ED/A060923K.pdf.

[49] Kingkade, Tyler. 2014, January 27. "A Majority of Students Say the Textbooks Are Too Damn Expensive." *The Huffington Post*. Accessed February 6, 2019. http://www.huffingtonpost.ca/entry/textbooks-prices_n_4675776.

[50] Anderson, Monica. 2015. "Smartphone, Computer or Tablet? 36% of Americans Own All Three." Accessed February 6, 2019. http://www.pewresearch.org/fact-tank/2015/11/25/device-ownership/.

[51] Hendricks, Drew. 2013. "The Complete History of Social Media: Then and Now." Accessed February 6, 2019. http://smallbiztrends.com/2013/05/the-complete-history-of-social-media-infographic.html.

[52] Moran, Mike, Jeff Seaman, and Hester Tinti-Kane. 2011. "Teaching, Learning, and Sharing: How Today's Higher Education Faculty Use Social Media." Babson Survey Research Group. Accessed February 6, 2019. https://eric.ed.gov/?id=ED535130.

[53] Baptiste, Laurelle. 2014. "The Future of Learning: What Today's Stats Mean for Tomorrow's Learners." Accessed February 6, 2019. https://www.marsdd.com/news-and-insights/future-learning-todays-stats-mean-tomorrows-learners/.

[54] Gallego, Jelor. 2016, May 9. "Surprise! Georgia Tech Teaching Assistant Isn't Human, She's a Robot." Accessed February 6, 2019. https://futurism.com/suprise-georgia-tech-teaching-assistant-isnt-human-shes-robot/.

[55] Goel, Ashok. 2016. "A Teaching Assistant Named Jill Watson." TEDxSanFrancisco. Accessed February 6, 2019. https://www.youtube.com/watch?v=WbCguICyfTA&feature=youtu.be.

[56] Warschauer, Mark, and Douglas Grimes. 2008. "Automated Writing Assessment in the Classroom." *Pedagogies* 3, no. 1: 22–36. https://doi.org/10.1080/15544800701771580.

[57] Meziane, Farid, and Sunil Vadera (Eds.). 2010. *AI in Software Engineering: Current Developments and Future Prospects*. Hershey, PA: Information Science Reference.

[58] Wolfram, Conrad. 2014. "Teaching Kids Real Math with Computers" [video]. TED.com. Accessed February 6, 2019. http://www.ted.com/talks/conrad_wolfram_teaching_kids_real_math_with_computers.

[59] Bower, Matt, Cathie Howe, Nerida McCredie, Austin Robinson, and David Grover. 2013. "Augmented Reality in Education: Cases, Places, and Potentials." *2013 IEEE 63rd Annual Conference International Council for Education Media*. https://doi.org/10.1109/cicem.2013.6820176.

[60] Kilteni, Konstantina, Raphaela Groten, and Mel Slater. 2012. "The Sense of Embodiment in Virtual Reality." *Presence: Teleoperators and Virtual Environments* 21, no. 4: 373–87. https://doi.org/10.1162/PRES_a_00124.

[61] Savickiene, Izabela. 2010. "Conception of Learning Outcomes in the Bloom's Taxonomy Affective Domain." *Quality of Higher Education* 7: 37–59. Accessed January 24, 2019. https://eric.ed.gov/?q=EJ900258&id=EJ900258.

Additional Resources

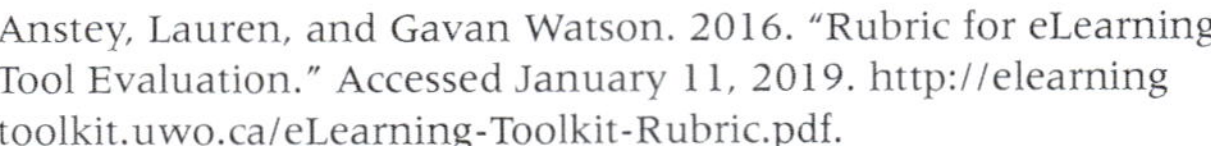

Anstey, Lauren, and Gavan Watson. 2016. "Rubric for eLearning Tool Evaluation." Accessed January 11, 2019. http://elearningtoolkit.uwo.ca/eLearning-Toolkit-Rubric.pdf.

Bailenson, Jeremy. 2018. *Experience on Demand: What Virtual Reality Is, How It Works, and What It Can Do*. New York: W.W. Norton & Company.

Brown, Peter C., Henry L. Roediger, and Mark A. McDaniel. 2014. *Make It Stick: The Science of Successful Learning*. Cambridge, MA: Belknap Press.

Duarte, Nancy. 2008. *Slide:ology The Art and Science of Creating Great Presentations*. Sebastopol, CA: O'Reilly Media.

Lang, James. M. 2016. *Small Teaching: Everyday Lessons from the Science of Learning*. San Francisco: Jossey-Bass.

Paramedic Tutor website. "Learning Resources." https://paramedictutor.net/elearner/.

Reynolds, Garr. 2011. *Presentation Zen: Simple Ideas on Presentation Design and Delivery*. Berkeley, CA: New Riders.

Tegmark, Max. 2017. *Life 3.0: Being Human in the Age of Artificial Intelligence*. Toronto: Alfred A. Knopf.

CHAPTER 17

Tools for Distance Learning

OBJECTIVES

At the conclusion of this chapter, the educator will be able to:

Cognitive Domain

1. List the elements of online learning that make it ideal for student-centered learning.
2. Describe strategies for collaborative online learning.
3. Differentiate between synchronous and asynchronous distance education.
4. Distinguish between benefits and potential barriers of distance learning.
5. Outline the process to design an online emergency medical services (EMS) course.
6. Describe online strategies to assess learning in each domain.

Psychomotor Domain

There are no psychomotor objectives for this chapter.

Affective Domain

1. Respond to the challenges that online education may present to students.
2. Defend the value of student-centered learning at a distance.

"If we teach today's students as we taught yesterday's, we rob them of tomorrow."

~ John Dewey

CHAPTER GOAL This chapter offers insight into the realm of distance education; it describes different model combinations and provides tools to help instructors focus on teaching and learning within the "classroom without walls."

Internet-based learning is widely utilized across the health professions as an accepted and valuable educational delivery system. By removing the constraints associated with time and distance, it provides opportunities for learners to access courses and to build on their education portfolio and professional development. The term **digital learning** refers to instruction that uses various information technologies to deliver educational material to students. In contrast, **distance education (DE)** is a broad term that describes educational activities outside the traditional brick-and-mortar classroom in which the student(s) and instructor(s) are separated by space and/or time.[1]

DE is not a new concept. It offers access for students who otherwise might not enroll into educational programs. For people who lived and worked in rural or remote locations, DE via print materials delivered by the postal service was previously the mainstay of available education. In contrast, students born after roughly 1993 have never known a world without the Internet. The information and technology revolution broke barriers and removed obstacles that previously restricted those who wanted to further their education with formal course work. Geographical distances, scheduling conflicts, work schedules, and family commitments are largely a thing of the past for those who wish to pursue their education. In 2015, almost 6 million students were enrolled in DE at U.S. higher education institutions. Of those, 15% were taking at least one, but not all, of their courses online, and 14% were enrolled exclusively in DE classes.[2]

Technology has mobilized the way humans communicate and has revolutionized the way they work and learn. More than 85% of U.S. homes have a personal computer (PC); PCs are accessible, commonplace, transportable, and affordable.[3] Technology advancements and applications, along with rapid expansion of the Internet, have brought about a proliferation of opportunities for learning at a distance.

Distance Education in Perspective

DE is a system of education whereby students and educators are separated by time and/or distance, so students are not necessarily in the classroom at a scheduled time. DE has several alternate names that aim to capture the classroom without walls philosophy: distance learning, distributed learning, open university, open and distance learning, e-learning, correspondence school, flexible delivery, external study, massive open online courses (MOOCs), and virtual education are some. Many of these terms are interchangeable.

As a delivery system, DE has been around since the beginning of written language! One of the earliest documented attempts was a shorthand correspondence course advertised in the *Boston Gazette* in 1728. In 1858, the University of London offered the first degree via DE, and in 1874 Wesleyan University (Chicago) in the United States offered education via postal service.[4] In Australia, the School of the Air was established in 1944 in an effort to reach children and families in the Outback via two-way pedal-powered radio link, and in 1969 the Open University of the United Kingdom began offering programs that used print and multimedia resources. DE was a popular option in the 1970s and 1980s because it provided an educational opportunity for those who lived too far away from the institutions. During those decades, course material and assignments were posted by mail, and telephone contact was available if required. Technology has played a significant role in the development of all modes of educational material.

Today, courses are developed with the assistance of a wide range of technologies, often in combination, brought together to meet the requirements of the subject. Technological devices have many standard applications (free and paid) that facilitate a range of functions. For example, audio/video recording and editing, presentation software, word processing, and telephone/computer conferencing access all provide excellent means of bringing life to learning. Lectures can incorporate auditory narration, subtitles, 3-D video, interactive quiz questions, digital manipulatives, and animation to deploy a rich learning environment either on their own or in combination with print-based courses. Technologies are available for instructors and students to take advantage of fantastic communication tools—both synchronous (online together at a scheduled time) and asynchronous (the opposite of synchronous, online at different times). Although students participating in a course may be geographically scattered across a city, state, nation, or even the whole world, communication technology

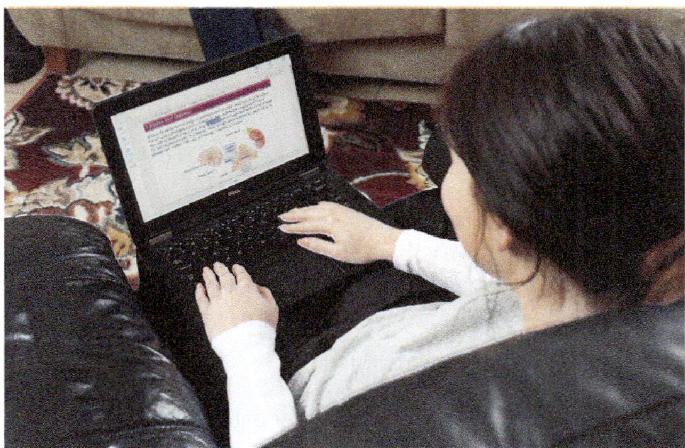

FIGURE 17.1 Geographical barriers to education are eliminated by distance education program delivery.

enables distance learners to meet with the instructor and discuss educational concepts (FIGURE 17.1).

Advances in telecommunications-based technology have allowed DE programs to use methods that were previously regarded as futuristic. Cell phone and wireless (Wi-Fi) communications, coupled with computer conferencing tools, are mainstays in the educator's technology tool bag. From early and rapid expansion into the marketplace, the online distance-learning market grows annually,[5] with more students choosing to enroll and study online.[6] The number of students taking at least one online class has also grown steadily.[7]

The Internet is the most common method of information delivery, and across the globe educational institutions are offering a wide range of programs, with most courses coming from the disciplines of education, business, and humanities—which includes the health sciences.[8] Within the healthcare spectrum, online programs for allied health sciences, EMS, nursing, health education, and health management are common. A quick Internet search for continuing education within any of these allied health specialties will provide many resources to choose from. A similar search will provide information about initial and degree-granting EMS programs. Many other websites can be found through online searches and in journal, newspaper, and magazine advertisements.

Online teaching and learning have demonstrated proven performance with student achievement in the university sector.[9] A multitude of studies has been conducted over the past decade to find out about the effectiveness of online learning as compared with traditional face-to-face (also called F2F and FTF) classroom learning. These studies have also measured student perceptions and satisfaction with level of knowledge and with various delivery modes. Sufficient documentation has shown that no differences in exam scores have been seen between distance learners and traditional classroom learners. In fact, research indicates that the grades of distance learners are at least as good as those of students who undertake face-to-face classroom learning.[10–12] These findings are supported by multiple scientific studies since the mid-1990s.[13]

Learning at a Distance

It is well known that learning is highly individualized and that people learn in a multitude of different ways. It is also well known that instructors must employ various teaching methods and techniques to ensure that students understand what they are learning. Similarly, online teaching and learning have specific features that differ from teaching and learning in the traditional classroom and that require due attention.

Online Learning: Student-Centered Learning

Despite growing evidence regarding the advantages of student-centered learning, the traditional classroom is often teacher-centered; that is, the instructor controls what is to be learned, when it is to be learned, and how it is to be learned. This "sage on the stage" scenario is the way many instructors were taught and how many are most comfortable teaching. It is difficult for many instructors to relinquish direct control over the classroom and transition to a "guide on the side" facilitator. One of the significant differences between learning in the traditional classroom and online learning is a shift in focus between learner and instructor—online learning is student-centered. Students become the controllers of their own learning. Within DE, some general basic themes underpin all student-centered learning.

The Role of the Instructor Changes

The instructor becomes a guide or facilitator; the instructor guides students through their studies. The focus is on the student's needs, interests, and development.

Students Take Responsibility for Their Own Learning

Students must be self-motivated to meet the demands of learning in potential isolation, if they are to adhere to task timelines. Although many distance learners are good independent students, some may need a tremendous amount of encouragement to get their work completed on time. Until students establish good coping skills with regard to independent learning, they may struggle. Transitioning from a classroom environment where an instructor frequently reminds students to complete assignments to an online environment where the student must take on that responsibility can be challenging.

Learning Is Enhanced through Discussion

Much like a face-to-face classroom, distance learning is often a social activity. Technology enhances learning as it provides students with opportunities to discuss lecture content, and to talk, share, and collaborate with other students about the course material and related information even though they might be geographically dispersed. This can be accomplished by many means that allow student–student and student–instructor interaction.

The Instructor Manages Student Learning

The learning process is a shared process; the instructor and the students within the group share information and findings. Learning is ongoing, and students take an active part in the process.

Students Construct Knowledge through Critical Thinking and Problem Solving

One of the advantages of asynchronous discussion is that it offers students more time to think about the question posed by the instructor and how they want to answer it before they respond. Students may also take the time to research the question more thoroughly prior to posting something that their peers (and the instructor) will read and comment on. This may promote deeper critical thinking skills. It also encourages independence and cooperation (appreciating other perspectives), improving understanding, and thinking for oneself.

Teaching and Assessment Are Intertwined

In the classroom setting, teaching is often focused on preparing students for the final test. Online teaching focuses on the learning process. This allows much more opportunity for low-stakes formative assessment and self-checks to ensure long-lasting comprehension of the material rather than short-term rote memorization.

Collaborative Learning

Contrary to what one might think, online learning is ideal for **collaborative learning**—that is, an instructional method in which students work together in small groups toward a common goal. Although this method is a common practice in the face-to-face classroom with small groups who work together, the virtual classroom uses methods such as text messaging, a **discussion board**, a **cloud-based collaborative document**, **video conferencing**, social media, or a **wiki** to foster collaborative learning online. Students can become responsible for each other's learning, and they may nurture mutual success. The collaborative approach to learning stimulates active exchange of ideas, which, in turn, promotes critical thinking. Online collaborative learning often includes students who have not met each other face-to-face; they have not socialized together nor developed social networks together. Thus initially, the personality factor can be absent and the collaborative exercise is bias-free. This includes overcoming some cultural or gender biases because students cannot make biased assumptions based on visual reference about a person who is not sitting next to them in a classroom. Collaborative teaching and learning through written formats can at times be challenging, as contributions to the chat or discussion boards can be void of the individual's true personality and are read and interpreted solely as written. In fact, most people have experienced a text or email being misinterpreted by the recipient. While some online discussion boards contain a sense of formality, many instructors and course designers include a forum for casual discussion between students. It is within this area that students' raw creativeness can explode into an extremely rich learning environment, and social networks can develop.

Asynchronous and Synchronous Learning

Any student enrolled in a Web-based course will find that most of their time spent on coursework is via **asynchronous learning**; that is, it is done independently and without assistance or direct instruction from the educator. The website or lecture materials provide a study guide and comprehensive instructional steps that outline the requirements for course completion.

Because technology has evolved, it is now commonplace for **synchronous learning** to occur online. With this approach, students are in geographically dispersed locations and meet online at a prescheduled time to participate in a Web conference, or they may log on to a website for real-time discussion with the instructor. Instructors may also hold "virtual office hours" during which they are available to students individually or in groups, by appointment or "drop in," via a (web/video/phone) conference. During this time an instructor can help students struggling with difficult concepts

Collaborative Documents

Example 1: Group projects are familiar to most people. However, in an online environment, an instructor cannot simply have a group of students pull their desks together to work on their assignment in class. One of the biggest drawbacks in a group assignment is version control (in other words, "Who has the most recent version of our document?"). If not managed correctly from the start, it is easy for multiple versions to be developed and hours spent figuring out which is most current, or wasting precious time creating duplicate work. With online collaborative documents and presentations, there is only one copy that all group members can access and work on simultaneously. A number of such collaborative platforms exist, such as Google Docs and Google Slides. Collaborative platforms such as these allow students to work together, either in real time or asynchronously; each participant can create, share, discover, and build on the teams' collective knowledge and skills. Participants can also develop a stronger sense of team unity. Assignments may include writing papers and class presentations, but are not limited to these. For instance, teams can be assigned various body systems and create electronic flashcards for the rest of the class to utilize, study from, and learn. In creating materials, students attain deeper learning of the subject and have the opportunity to shine in front of the entire class (some innate competitiveness goes a long way). With a little creativity, virtually any group assignment/project can be effectively facilitated in an online course.

Example 2: *Wiki* is a Polynesian word meaning quick. In modern usage, a wiki refers to a collaborative website (similar in many ways to the collaborative platforms mentioned in Example 1) that allows group members to edit the site and utilize the features of a Web page, including overall appearance, content, links, embedded graphics/video, live newsfeeds/social media, etc. A wiki page can range from simple (text only) to elaborate. The most widely known example of a wiki is Wikipedia. An example of a class assignment using a wiki is for a class to build a "tips for success in our class" wiki (Web page) that they contribute to (edit) throughout the course. Such a document is always up-to-date, and successive course cohorts can build on it. Another example is for students to build an ECG recognition wiki where all could contribute interesting ECGs for the class to attempt to interpret and learn from. Wikis and other collaborative forms of documents usually have privacy settings that either limit access or allow the general public to view, depending on what is desired.

or assignments. This meeting can be accomplished via learning management system (LMS)-associated platforms or with free and widely available communication applications or services such as Skype, Zoom, and Google Meet. Using headsets and microphones, students are able to talk to one another, share documents, and use the whiteboard function to brainstorm ideas or to label/draw on a model. **Chat rooms** are also used for text-based synchronous discussion. Internet-based distance learning is leading to a reduced need for other modes of conferencing technology, such as telephone conferencing and videoconferencing.

Even with a well-designed course, it is good practice to have a back-up plan for distance lessons (synchronous or asynchronous). Many factors, including Mother Nature, can cause system failures by wreaking havoc on crucial infrastructure. Distance instructors should consider what to do if the technology fails before or during a planned Web-conferencing session. The following questions can help an instructor plan how to handle technology failure:

- Is there an alternative platform to utilize?
- Is there another way to notify the class to inform them when and where to meet online, or to let them know that, in the worst case, class is canceled?
- Can the class meet (with presentation of the intended materials) using a telephone conferencing system (audio only)?

The instructor should also plan for contingencies regarding assignments, for example:

- Is there an alternative method to submit an assignment outside of the LMS the class is using?
- Should the student email the assignment as an attachment? (What happens if the file is too large to email?)
- If an assignment must be submitted in the LMS because the system requires in-line grading for student marks, is there a workaround for an emailed submission?

These questions (and many more) need to be answered before the course begins. The technologies used to teach at a distance are in most cases reliable, but failures in software and hardware do happen at the most inconvenient times. Any back-up strategy should also consider issues such as student privacy, which are typically incorporated within an LMS. In the United States, Family Educational Rights and Privacy Act (FERPA) requirements must be considered when choosing alternatives.

CASE in Point

Faced with the dilemma of educating children in a nomadic tribe (frequently moving, no home base) in a West African nation, the innovative solution was to provide lessons via broadcast AM radio and get synchronous questions/feedback from students via text message (SMS) on their flip phones![14] How is this relevant to EMS education? It is a great example of using existing technology and infrastructure to meet a big need. EMS educators face tough choices every day when planning and providing initial and continuing education. One such (related) example is providing continuing education and in-service information to service providers when they are unable to gather at a central location. With a bit of creativity, EMS educators can overcome some significant logistical challenges!

Characteristics of the Distance Learner

Although it is impossible to regard distance learners as a group with the same attributes, many students share demographic and situational similarities from which a profile of the learner can be typified. Their characteristics are varied; however, their commonalities include the following:

- **Age**. The Instructional Technology Council reports that just over half of distance learners are age 18 to 25 years, with about 44% over 26 years of age.[15]
- **Sex**. More female than male students are enrolled in online programs; about 60% of distance learners are women.[15]
- **Geographical distance**. Thompson, Gibson, and Graff report that most distance learners reside less than 100 miles from campus.[16]
- **Life roles**. About 60% of DE students are employed full time.[17]
- **Motivation and autonomy**. Intrinsic motivation and desire for career advancement are significant characteristics of distance learners. Most DE students are self-regulatory; that is, they set aside regular time for study, establish schedules to meet their learning tasks, and do not need regular reminders to get their work completed by the due date. They are autonomous learners.

Essentially, these are characteristics common to adult learners. Therefore, it can be anticipated that the distance learner will most likely have an existing career and may be looking to expand vocational interests or gain qualifications that will facilitate movement into a different career path.

Pros, Cons, and Barriers for Distance Learning

Like any chosen means of delivering content to students, there are justifications that support a given method of delivery and those that do not. Distance learning is no exception. The obvious statement is that a course should never be offered online just because it is possible to do so or because the technology exists. DE is not for everyone (nor is classroom learning). However, multiple studies show that DE (done right) is at least as effective as traditional (face-to-face) instruction.[18] An educator can make inferences both in favor of or against DE. Educators should keep in mind that it is possible to put together a poor classroom experience, too. The next section discusses some factors to consider associated with DE.

Benefits of Distance Learning

Distance learning provides benefits in the areas of travel, cost, time, and productivity; time that would have been spent commuting can be spent doing more productive activities such as studying, spending time with family, or fulfilling other commitments. DE provides access to education, especially for those who have family commitments, need to work to support themselves, or reside a significant distance away from the institution or in rural areas. **TABLE 17.1** summarizes student needs, benefits of DE, and potential barriers.

Travel and Lodging

Generally speaking, offering a course online allows students access to education they could not otherwise attend or afford the time to travel to. These students may live in areas where such offerings simply do not exist (for example, in a rural area) or where travel to attend a face-to-face course is not practical, particularly during inclement weather.

Without the need to travel, the learner can save the cost of a hotel room or other form of housing. It is not hard to envision a number of scenarios in which those costs (whether for a single night once per week or an entire semester or more) quickly add up.

Cost

Some universities offer online courses at a reduced cost. While technological infrastructure is costly, it may still be less than the cost of supporting an aging

TABLE 17.1 Summary of Student Needs, Benefits of DE, and Potential Barriers to DE

Student Needs	Benefits	Potential Barriers
■ Access	■ No travel required	■ Technophobia
■ Media needs	■ Lower cost	■ Unfamiliarity
■ Support	■ No lodging required	■ Lack of computer skills
■ Tech savvy	■ Time savings	■ Lack of access
■ Comfort zone	■ Increased productivity	■ Infrastructure issues
■ Social needs	■ Less infringement on current job	■ Higher cost, additional fees
■ Cultural norms	■ More time for family	■ Age/generational considerations
■ Learning style	■ More time for commitments	■ Cognitive overload
■ Curriculum needs	■ Ideal for nontraditional student	
	■ Personal preference	

physical structure. Some universities offer in-state tuition (lower fees) for any online course regardless of where the student lives. A few large open universities around the world do not have a single physical classroom and yet support the studies of 100,000+ students from dozens of countries. Additionally, massive open online courses (MOOCs) are offered by many universities (and others) at no cost.

What Is a MOOC?

A massive open online course, or MOOC, is an online course with open access to anyone with Internet service. (See Chapter 16, *Using Technology to Enhance Classroom Learning*.) A MOOC can have unlimited (massive) numbers of participants from all over the world. First introduced in 2006, they have become a popular means of learning.

Time and Productivity

For any busy student, parent, or working professional, time is a precious commodity. Not only can online courses solve time and scheduling issues, they can also help gain back time that might be lost in commuting to class. Online courses are often offered in the evening at times more convenient to working adults. Asynchronous courses lend themselves to busy work/family schedules.

Any business major understands the concept of lost productivity. Whether it is your job, family/friends, or studying, time spent commuting is time lost that could have been spent in other activities. It is easy to calculate time lost to a 90-minute one-way commute. The math is simple: 180 minutes × 5 days per week in class = 15 hours per week that could have been spent on more productive endeavors. Busy adult learners could accomplish a lot with an extra 15 hours per week.

Job

A common motivation for adults furthering their education is that it means better pay or a promotion at work. If the needed class is scheduled during normal work hours, the student must take time away from work to take the class. In rare cases, the employer may support this and even still pay the normal salary. Many students are not that fortunate and worry about the effect reduced work hours and pay will have on their ability to meet basic expenses, such as rent. DE can help in this regard.

Family and Other Commitments

The cost to family and friends in terms of lost time is often overlooked. The flexibility and time savings of a DE class can have a huge impact on time with family and friends.

In addition to those listed previously, many other activities compete for a student's time. Social events, school organizations, religious organizations, and hobbies are a few examples.

Nontraditional Students

For reference, consider a "traditional" student as someone who attends higher education (college/university) full time, is between 18 and 22 years of age, is financially dependent on parents, and lives on campus. This is rapidly becoming more the exception than the norm. The consulting firm Stamats suggests as few as 16% of college students fit this description.[19] Nontraditional students may be defined as meeting one of these seven characteristics: delayed enrollment into postsecondary education; attends college part time; works full time; is financially independent for financial aid purposes; has dependents other than a spouse; is a single parent; or does not have a high school diploma.[19] This covers the majority of today's students.

Personal Preference

DE is not for everybody. However, for some people its benefits cannot be ignored, and it is their preferred way to attain a higher education. It accommodates busy lives and commitments, and it offers a way of learning that simply cannot be duplicated in a face-to-face classroom.

Potential Barriers to Distance Learning

Potential barriers to distance learning, whether for the student or the instructor, range from the obvious technological concerns, such as technophobia, or unfamiliarity with or lack of computer skills; to access and infrastructure issues; to perhaps less obvious issues such as high cost, student dissatisfaction, and cognitive overload.

Technophobia

Not everybody is a geek or an information technology (IT) expert. Some instructors and students avoid online courses because they fear the technology involved.

Some outstanding classroom instructors avoid teaching online simply because they are unfamiliar with *how* to teach online. In other words, they are novices to online teaching and fear possible embarrassment.

Lack of Computer Skills

Some students and instructors have never had a reason to acquire solid basic computer skills (i.e., "I've done just fine with a whiteboard and an overhead projector so far . . .") and must overcome this in order to be involved in online education. In addition to needing to access the course online, students may also be required to complete technology-related assignments, such as a small group project to produce short narrated or video presentations. To succeed in this format, students and instructors need to be willing to learn skills they may not have developed before, such as recording and editing video or audio content. Educators and students should know that they are not alone in these efforts.

Age/Generation

Much has been written about generational differences in learning and perspectives. In a nutshell, younger learners tend to look at technology as an enabler.[20] Older learners tend to view it as a novelty that might make things easier or better; however, they may consider it unnecessary, because they grew up without it and did just fine. Many consider Millennials to be experts when it comes to technology. The truth is, although that generation may be good at using an app, often the older students have a better understanding of why and how technology works.

Lack of Access

While some assume that free broadband Wi-Fi service is available everywhere, that is not always the case. The Pew Research Center reports that 89% of American adults use the Internet.[21] However, in 2018 only 65% had home broadband service. There is still a huge disparity in rural/frontier communities regarding Internet access. Some have fiberoptic service to each household, and others have no service at all. When planning to offer an online class, it is important to know what type of access the target audience has. A highly tech/broadband-dependent course (i.e., one that includes a significant amount of high-definition video) will likely lead to a dissatisfying online experience when viewed over a slow Internet connection.[21]

Infrastructure

Related to access issues, if the school's infrastructure is unable to support the content the instructor wants to deliver online (Web-conferencing, video, podcasts, interactivity, etc.), the content and how it is offered will need to be modified. In some cases, infrastructure issues can render the instructor's plans completely infeasible. It is vitally important that the school's IT personnel be involved in course planning early on.

Cost

Cost can be a benefit or barrier. As mentioned earlier, low-cost or free courses may attract large numbers of participants, but they may also increase the sense of isolation a student feels, therefore decreasing their sense of satisfaction with the course and negatively affecting learning outcomes. High-cost courses may make it impossible for many to afford course fees and, therefore, have limited participation. Additionally, high-cost courses may generate certain expectations regarding return on investment and lead to dissatisfaction if they fall short in any way. Technology access fees are common among training institutions (often assessed per course taken rather than as a one-time fee), adding costs on top of tuition.

Cognitive Overload

Online education's potentially media-rich environment and navigational requirements (e.g., where do I submit that assignment?) can lead to cognitive overload for some learners. This can be particularly true for learners who have limited computer skills and those who have little or no experience with online courses (or perhaps only bad experiences). Planning for DE must involve course designers, and potential issues must be mitigated via well-laid-out plans to ensure the course interface and navigation are as simple as possible. Aspects such as question-and-answer discussion threads, knowledge bases, and frequently-asked-question pages can go a long way toward preventing at least some of the overload.

Distance Education within EMS

There is a vast range of undergraduate, graduate, and postgraduate courses conducted throughout universities and community/vocational colleges that prepare their graduates to practice within the allied health spectrum. Nursing, midwifery, physical therapy, occupational health, dietetics, and paramedic programs account for just some of the offerings. Nationally and internationally, many universities and community colleges have developed policies that require all face-to-face courses they offer to have an online presence.[22,23] Training allied health practitioners is a major budget item for governments to support in their endeavors to provide health care to their citizens, and DE is one strategy to address this.

In broad terms, many educational institutions have embraced online delivery of education as a strategy to reach more students utilizing available technologies. In terms of distance, time, and work schedules, the cost of training EMS practitioners is high. When one considers the theoretical perspective of education, the sheer volume of large numbers of students, repeat lectures, and classroom or lecture theatre space, DE provides a valuable alternative.

CASE in Point

Many universities have an online presence for nearly every course topic offered face-to-face at the school. Students who are enrolled in almost all fields of study are able to access a variety of courses entirely online; courses that require clinical skills mastery may require attendance at face-to-face workshops throughout the semester. This can easily be facilitated with a flipped classroom design in which didactic content is covered online (outside classroom time) and face-to-face class time is devoted to psychomotor skills, scenarios/simulation, and guided problem solving. For example, in class, assignments can be completed with the instructor present to assist in working through difficult problems as needed or by collaborating with others.

While DE is instrumental at delivering theoretical content online, courses that are offered completely online may not meet the psychomotor needs of students. The course structure must incorporate face-to-face clinical skills workshops for psychomotor skills practice and clinical experience. For this reason, some would call an EMS distance-learning course a **hybrid course**, rather than a strictly DE course.

Structuring Distance Education for EMS

The structure of DE courses within EMS requires unique conceptualization in accordance with the specific profession of the EMS field. Technology can be incorporated in many ways into models for DE programs. Although the choices are numerous, Internet-based instruction has clearly become the leading DE delivery mechanism. Many factors related to course content and mechanism of delivery must be identified and addressed before a course can be set up. An important early step is to gather together a group of experienced content experts and information technologists to explore suitable possibilities for a particular educational organization. Many universities offer consulting and mentoring assistance for smaller and independent education providers. This can include training in use of the technology, curriculum design, and online instruction for faculty members. With or without this training, instructors should design DE to include commonly agreed-upon elements of quality online education. Appendix A provides the NAEMSE Rubric for Quality Online Education, a resource for EMS educators when planning distance learning.

Determining Course Topics for Distance Delivery

DE is structured to meet the learning objectives of the specific program as determined by the course curriculum. With careful attention to curriculum design, theoretical courses within a program can be readily translated into an online course. There is flexibility for many clinical components to be delivered digitally. For example, topics that relate to anatomy, physiology, and pathophysiology, as well as instruction on significant illnesses (for example, the respiratory illnesses croup, asthma, or pneumonia), lend themselves well to digital media.

Determining the structure of the online course requires input from a number of stakeholders. People who should be at the planning table from the beginning include (but are not limited to) subject matter expert(s) (this may be the instructor and/or other faculty members and/or industry representatives), instructional designer, IT expert, support (help desk) personnel, graphic designer, registrar/registration personnel, assessment personnel, finance personnel, marketing personnel, rules/policies personnel, and administrative personnel. At the planning stage, a conceptual map of the course is drawn, reflecting the following:

- Course content
- Learning outcomes
- Description of the knowledge and the clinical skills required
- Application of the skills in the workplace
- Elements that describe the performance criteria

Deciding the Structure of the Course

Teaching a course online takes more work than its face-to-face counterpart! Deciding how the course is to be structured can be challenging. Various topics must be treated differently with regard to curricular needs, delivery methods, and media. The requirements of the curriculum influence the course design. For example, it might be decided that students will learn the didactic information online, then gather together periodically for practical skills workshops to develop competence in psychomotor skill performance. Bringing students together for in-class work acknowledges the importance of the social nature of learning. However, careful consideration must be made to bring the social aspect of learning to the online portion as well. It is vitally important to plan interactivity.

Decisions must also be made about the use of synchronous and asynchronous communications. Will the course be primarily asynchronous, with some scheduled synchronous (Web-conferencing) meetings, or will it be completely synchronous or completely asynchronous? Each choice has pros and cons, and must align with a number of factors, including course curriculum, goals, content, and learner needs.

Mode of Delivery

The choice of delivery mechanism relies heavily on available resources, administrative support, comfort level with the technology, and level of available technical support. Each of these considerations is important, no matter which modes of delivery are involved. Although Internet-based distribution is exciting, like other forms of educational delivery, it can be done well or poorly. A quality Internet-based program requires that many significant aspects be considered, including the following:

- Are technicians available to set up and maintain the infrastructure for the program?
- Do instructors have appropriate online instructional expertise?
- Is enough administrative support available for the ongoing needs of the course?

When the Internet is the chosen mode of delivery, a number of technical and administrative decisions must be made. Some questions that arise include the following:

- Will the course be located in the public domain?
- Will the course be housed within an LMS?
- If so, which LMS should be used?

It is vital for instructors and administrators to obtain advice from experienced professionals on these important decisions.

NREMT Credit for Online Continuing Education

Most states and the National Registry of EMTs (NREMT) place a limit on the number of hours of EMS continuing education (CE) that is allowed to be received via online education when the content is provided asynchronously.

However, if the content is delivered via live webinar, in which participants have a mechanism or opportunity to interact with the presenter (for example, to ask questions and get answers), this is considered the same as a face-to-face classroom; therefore there is no limit in the number of CE credits obtained by this method. This affords those in rural areas with few CE opportunities the means to obtain their required CE credits from many sources, ranging from local services to institutions/organizations with national and international reach. More and more webinars are available covering current medical topics, practice, and EMS research, making participation both easier and more accessible for all.

Technology for an Online Course

There can be little doubt that online courses have become the preferred method of pursuing DE. As of mid-2018, the Open University of Catalonia (UOC), an entirely online university, had over 70,000 students from over 90 countries.[24] Understanding the available technology, its function, and how to use it to maximize learning are skills that can be readily mastered. While large institutions of education—universities and community colleges—have implemented online teaching and learning, smaller training providers may still be considering the benefits and advantages. The information that follows is provided for the benefit of smaller educational institutions that are curious about the scope of digital learning.

Learning Management Systems

A **learning management system (LMS)** facilitates the creation and implementation of coursework in an online educational environment. An LMS is a system that is used to create online courses, organize the content, deliver the content (online/digitally), and provide interactive tools that supplement courses. LMSs generally also allow students to submit assignments securely, provide for marking/grading those assignments, and allow students to see their progress securely. Numerous LMSs are on the market; many are highly capable, robust, and sophisticated in their components. While some are fairly self-explanatory and easy to use, others are poorly documented and difficult to use. The number of choices and options in setting up a course (meant to add flexibility) can be overwhelming to the novice online instructor. These include commercial (paid) products and open source (free) systems. Organizations are encouraged to find one that best suits their needs. While this may sound simple in theory, it is a complex and difficult choice in practice. A quality LMS performs functions in three key areas:

- **Course structure**. Instructors are able to create course material by uploading lectures, documents, activities, links, and exams onto the system. It is within this structure that the instructional material is contained. It should be reasonably easy to set up and organize this content so that students can easily navigate the course, follow instructions, and find the instructional materials they need for a given lesson.
- **Course tools**. These are used to assist the student in participating in the course. Examples of course tools include announcements, course messaging, threaded discussions, quizzes/exams, document sharing, course calendar, journaling, Web-conferencing, group work areas, help desk/IT support, media gallery, rubrics, grade center, and demographics/profile update.
- **Course management system**. Administrative features are provided for automated grading and quiz/exam results, student tracking (including attendance, student participation in threaded discussions and viewing of content), password authentication, and generation of statistical data related to the course.

Learning Management System Tools

Functional LMS tools are essential with any digital delivery program. A robust LMS includes all aspects of functionality for ease of navigation through the course documentation, information, and delivery. It has the capability to do what the instructional faculty want it to do, and it is simple to use. With that said, "simple to use" is subjective. For example, while the steps for posting a video may be simple, they may be numerous, making it is easy to omit a critical step. When planning an online DE program, the lists that follow in the sections on functional and instructor management tools may help determine which LMS to choose.

Online Course: Functional Tools

A quality LMS offers the following functions:

- **Course content**. This can be subdivided into the following areas:
  - **Topic information**. Description of learning objectives and course/module goals
  - **Assessment items**. Description of assessment requirements and due dates
  - **Assessment criteria**. How the coursework will be assessed (rubrics)
  - **Instructional materials**. A course/module overview, reading assignments, links to additional resources, videos/podcasts, Web-conferencing (and recordings), glossary, and any handouts
- **Announcements**. As in a classroom, these advise students of general announcements made during the progress of the course.
- **Syllabus**. A document that describes teaching and learning methods, course goals, expected learning outcomes, required textbooks, assessments, and grading for successful completion of the course. The instructional details describe what is to be undertaken, how it is to be presented, and what is expected.
- **Assignments**. This function outlines the theme and content of the coursework to be submitted for grading. It provides an outline of the assignment, the inclusions and exclusions, length, and allocated percentage of the grade. Secondary tabs contained in the assignment area contain information that students can view regarding their submitted assignments, graded assignments, and assessment results. More recently, automated plagiarism checkers have

become popular additions to LMS assignment submission. Available as either a built-in, optional, or stand-alone feature, these programs check submitted content against a database and submissions from other students, and produce an originality report expressed in percentage.

- **Discussion board**. Also called threaded discussions, online courses require a portal for students to engage with their peers and tutor. The discussion board provides the means for students to post their responses to tutorial questions, describe their thoughts and opinions, and respond to other students' posts and comments.
- **Wiki**. A wiki is a Web page that can be edited collaboratively directly from a Web browser. Within many commercial LMSs, a wiki tool is available for the entire class or can be limited to individual small groups.
- **Course messaging**. Many LMSs provide a course messaging function within the program. This is much like email; incoming and outgoing messages related to course content are kept separate from general email, thus addressing privacy issues (for example, per FERPA in the United States).
- **Help desk**. Sometimes the FAQs just aren't enough. The help desk area is for students and instructors, who may have operational, technical, or navigational questions about the LMS. Those new to digital learning or who are using a new LMS for the first time appreciate being able to communicate with a knowledgeable person to resolve their problem.
- **Web resources**. In addition to hyperlinks contained within the coursework documents, the Web resources area provides a separate place for course developers to put links to additional informational resources that are an extension of required coursework for students to research.
- **Quizzes and tests**. This area is for **time-released assessment items** and/or **criteria-released assessment items** that are prepared in advance by the instructor. (A *time-released assessment item* refers to an assessment item that is released at a certain time, for example, a certain calendar day. A *criteria-released assessment item* refers to an assessment item that is released once certain criteria, such as completion of homework or assignments, have been met.) These are automatically graded within the capabilities of the LMS. Generally, these are multiple choice questions.
- **Gradebook**. This feature allows students to monitor their progress throughout the course. Feedback is vitally important, and students must be aware of their progress if instructors expect them to meet expected performance criteria.

Instructor Management Tools

Keeping track of student access to the course material, their time on-task, and record keeping of their grades is a key function of the instructor's role. Many LMSs incorporate instructor tools that automatically generate course management functions.

- **Course management**. These functions are generally not seen by students and provide the developer with the ability to control whether tools, modules, and functions are available to students.
- **Gradebook manager**. Grade attempts and grade allocation are automatically fielded within this function. The instructor is also able to create assessment items, choose when items are to be released, make assessment items available to students, and record the student grades.
- **Assignment submission**. As students complete their coursework, the work is submitted and organized in an area where instructors can view the submissions and assign grades.
- **Rubrics**. The developer is able to upload and store grading criteria forms that will be used during the course.
- **Student tracking**. Many instructors have concerns about whether students are attending to their studies. The tracking function generates statistical information from which the instructor can make assumptions. For example, the system can generate a summary of how often a given course item is used or viewed, as well as group or individual student interaction with the course materials.

Although there are a multitude of elements to consider when choosing an LMS, a robust system purchased from a reputable company will include each of these components. Cost often arises as a concern, and many LMSs can be expensive. Open source LMSs are available for little or no cost for the software, but access to a secure server often is needed in order to utilize them. Simplified LMS options are also available at no cost, such as Google Classroom. Such services offer an alternative but have limited functionality when compared to a more robust LMS.

Instructional Design

Instructional design, the most important part of digital education, is a structured and cyclic undertaking. An instructional course must be designed in an organized manner, so that each task is clearly identified within the curriculum and the exact roles and functions of participants are delineated. Schiffman's model provides a clear pathway that identifies each significant design

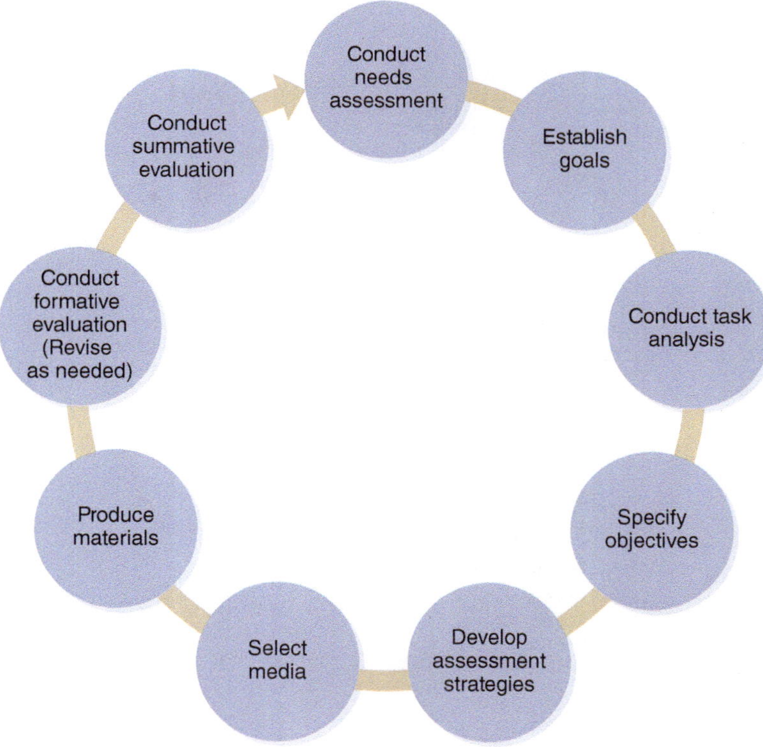

FIGURE 17.2 The instructional design cycle.

Data from Schiffman, Shirl S. 1995. "Instructional Systems Design: Five Views of the Field." In *Instructional Technology: Past, Present, and Future*, 2nd ed., edited by G. J. Anglin, 131–42. Englewood, CO: Libraries Unlimited.

step that must be addressed at preproduction meetings (**FIGURE 17.2**). First, instructors must conduct a needs assessment, establish program goals and objectives, develop an analysis of specific steps needed to design the program, write objectives, and develop assessment strategies. The next steps involve selecting appropriate media to support the course design, developing instructional materials, and conducting formative assessments. Based on the results of the formative assessment, modifications in program design may need to be made prior to conducting the summative program assessment.[25]

Many other instructional design models exist that can easily be adapted for use in a digital environment. One model that is popular and relatively easy to remember is ADDIE: Analysis, Design, Development, Implementation, and Evaluation (**FIGURE 17.3**). This concept is also widely used in instructional systems design and addresses the cyclic nature of good instructional design.

Storyboarding for Instruction

Storyboarding is not a new concept. Filmmakers utilize this tactic to lay out the scenes and sequence for a production. The **storyboard** is the cartoonlike drawings with annotations seen in any "making of . . ." documentary. They help everyone visually conceptualize what is intended for individual activities as well as the overall flow to meet the goal (a well-executed production). Instructional design requires the creation of a similar map of course instruction. The map must include a series of annotations and links that provide an overview of how the instruction will be constructed and presented. Learning outcomes taken from the syllabus guide the development of the map, and each of the learning outcomes must be addressed by the instruction. The storyboard helps developers think through each element and make decisions about how the content will be presented online. Developers determine the mechanism by which learning outcomes are to be distributed. The storyboard is influenced by the type of media selected for delivery of the instructional material and by the resources available to produce the material. Returning to the filmmaking analogy, storyboards help the program development team clearly understand everybody's role and what materials are needed. The process of creating a storyboard can also unearth unanticipated issues, allowing them to then be addressed before course delivery. A large variety of storyboarding templates are available on the Web. A simple search for "storyboard" will produce a rich choice of results, from which educators can choose a template that best fits their individual needs.

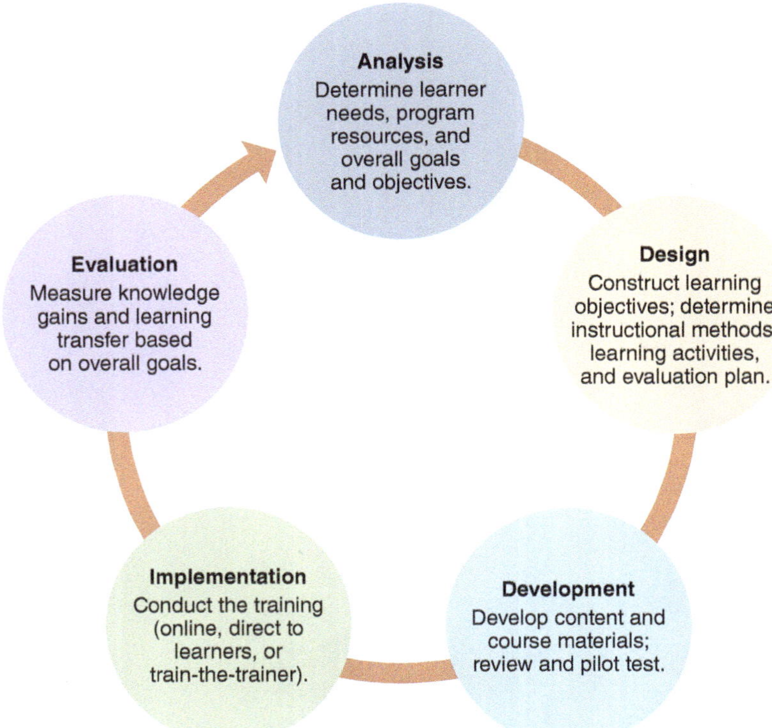

FIGURE 17.3 The ADDIE instructional design model.

Data from Hodell, Chuck. 2010. *The Basics of ISD Revisited*. Alexandria, VA: ASTD Press.

Methods for Assessing Learning Online

Learning is assessed according to the processes of the educational institution, and course content is determined by the curriculum. LMSs have a range of options for built-in tests and quizzes that can be used for formative and summative exams. Most provide options for time-released or criteria-released assessments. The assessment items can be produced well ahead of time, uploaded, and programmed for release at a determined time and/or after a particular module is completed (which is particularly useful for self-paced study). Additionally, assignments can be locked at a specified time when completion criteria have been met, or when a student misses the deadline. Assignments are usually contained within a secured site. Some examples of test types include multiple choice, ordering, true/false, and short-answer questions. When carefully constructed, each of these types of testing methods is capable of evaluating knowledge and comprehension of coursework.

Many instructors choose multiple choice by default for its ease in grading. It should be obvious that a computer system can easily identify whether the correct choice was made by the student and appropriately marked. Short-answer and essay-type questions are more difficult for a computer to grade and often must be manually graded by instructors. Even though it is generally agreed that manual grading offers a more accurate assessment, manual grading can present issues of time and practicality.

Instructors raise concerns around supervision and exam conduct when administering exams online. Institutions must develop policies that state how to best address this. Several mechanisms can be put into place to ensure that the right student is taking the right test.

- **Exam passcodes**. An LMS can provide specific exam passcodes that authenticate the person taking the exam.
- **Timed exams**. An exam can be scheduled to occur within a specified time period. The time period may be anywhere from a narrow time frame (1 to 2 hours) to 1 to 2 days. The time period should be stated at the beginning of the course, so that students are able to schedule the event. Additionally, timed exams are usually of a duration that does not permit the student to look up answers in texts or other sources.
- **Proctored exams**. The student is required to take the exam at a predetermined location such as the school computer lab or library. Instructions are

provided, and arrangements are made with a proctor before the day of the event. Photo identification may be required.

- **Browser lock-down exams**. The student is required to take the exam at a specified time and utilize a specialized browser that prevents the student from opening/utilizing any other programs or windows. Many also require a webcam that allows direct observation and recording of student activity during the exam. Artificial intelligence (AI) algorithms analyze student behaviors (the speed/manner in which questions are answered, looking away from the camera frequently, looking down at their lap, etc.) or the presence of additional persons in the video feed and flag suspicious segments for instructors to review. Photo identification may be required in the form of an official school photo to compare with the exam video (facial recognition).
- **Range of assessment formats**. Coursework assessments can be divided into several sections, each of which accounts for a percentage of the overall grade. Online tests, essays, collaborative work, projects, and online discussions can be incorporated into the student's overall assessment.

Online Assessment of the Domains of Learning

There is a wealth of research from the general education profession that describes learning styles and assessment of each domain of learning: cognitive, psychomotor, and affective. Chapter 5, *Learning Styles: Concepts and Controversies,* details the characteristics of how students learn. In the past there has been anecdotal argument between health educators about how the different domains of learning can be assessed adequately and comprehensively. There is no argument that online learning is well constructed for assessing the cognitive domain of learning, and there is growing evidence that utilization of the right online tools can better assess the affective domain; however, limitations to assessment of the psychomotor domain of learning in the online environment remain.

Assessment of the Cognitive Domain of Learning

The cognitive domain is concerned with the learner's knowledge and information-processing attributes. It involves various mental processes relevant to knowledge acquisition. Once a test bank containing validated questions is developed, online assessments can readily be created, implemented, and graded automatically, without the involvement of the instructor. The assessment items are usually multiple choice questions, and the assessment of knowledge is solely reliant on the student marking the correct response. Careful attention to good test question construction and inclusion of higher-level questions in appropriate ratios improves student assessment accuracy. An analysis of test results should always be performed to determine the reliability of the assessment tool and allow for revision as needed. Tools like computer-adaptive exams can better assess higher-order learning (Bloom's taxonomy) and provide a more accurate assessment of the level of learning the students have attained.

Formative assessment tools can be used to assess preexisting knowledge in online courses. A test with a similar structure to the final exam can be given as the first class assignment. After taking the test, students rate their own knowledge of the exam and then select three questions that they found easiest and three that were most difficult to answer. This helps learners recognize the foundational knowledge they have coming in to the class and helps them anticipate where they will need to be by its conclusion.[26] Other formative assessment tools suitable for DE include concept maps, digital storytelling, synthesis papers designed to summarize ideas from assigned readings, and assigning learners to write editorials about a key topic related to the course content.

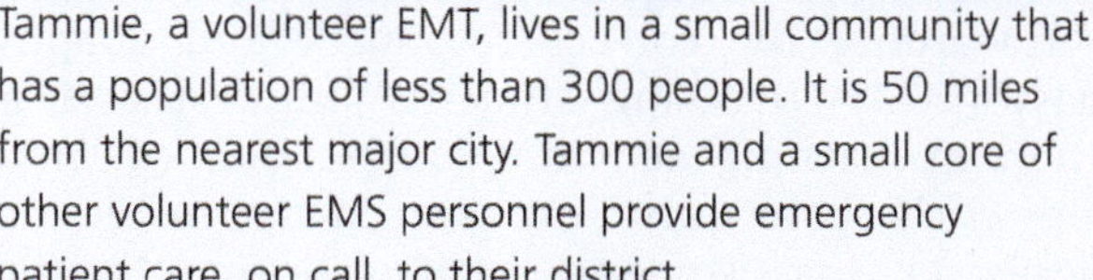

Tammie, a volunteer EMT, lives in a small community that has a population of less than 300 people. It is 50 miles from the nearest major city. Tammie and a small core of other volunteer EMS personnel provide emergency patient care, on call, to their district.

Following completion of initial mandatory coursework, Tammie enrolls in a hybrid paramedic program. She is required to participate in clinical rotations alongside local, paid EMS crews. Throughout her course, Tammie carries out specific learning tasks as determined in the course curriculum and associated with Clinical Development Packages. Study resources include textbooks, worksheets, video, and online resources, which are provided by the university's EMS program.

In order to complete psychomotor skills and demonstrate clinical competency, Tammie joins a core of other students from the region to undertake regular training via weekend skills labs at a central town located 32 miles away.

Assessment of the Psychomotor Domain

Clinical educators argue that it is difficult, but not impossible, to assess the psychomotor domain of learning in an online environment. Emerging technologies such as augmented reality environments, immersive classrooms, 3-D printing, and haptic simulators are increasingly developing usefulness in telemedicine and in online medical education. However most of these techniques are expensive and are limited for EMS.[27–29] In response to this, as mentioned earlier, program construction using a hybrid design has students undertake the didactic parts of the course online and then attend face-to-face clinical lab sessions to learn the motor application of the skill. Clinical lab instructors are free to concentrate on the psychomotor aspects of skills demonstration and can reinforce background knowledge as skills are acquired. Once skills have been mastered, they are incorporated into scenarios (simulations) that allow students to perform and apply skills in the context of emergency care.

Assessment of the Affective Domain

Similar to assessment of the psychomotor domain, there has been debate over the ability to assess the affective domain of learning online. The affective domain is concerned with how student attitudes and values affect performance. It encompasses professional behaviors, emotions, feelings, values, and qualities. As stated by Pattavina, "Affective competencies are related to student learning in the areas of: (1) motivating; (2) rewarding for correct responses and adaptive behavior; (3) involving students' interest and attention in learning activities and school; (4) managing crisis behaviors; (5) perceiving needs and experiences that students exhibit during learning and socialization activities; and (6) demonstrating or modeling optional ways of responding to stress and solving problems."[30] In response to this, many educational organizations have modified the way they assess the affective domain to accommodate online courses. Examples are having students provide short- or long-answer responses to questions that elicit caring behaviors, having students complete open-ended statements, and having students write a patient history and physical interview transcript that incorporates affective behaviors. While these strategies require instructors to spend time grading papers, students are able to respond to coursework that assesses the affective domain of learning. Tools like journaling can also provide assessment of the affective domain by asking students to not only reflect and write about their learning in the course, but also write about what that learning means for their patient care. While students generally may not like to write about "touchy-feely" subjects, journaling is a powerful assessment tool in this regard. Additionally, threaded discussions that ask students to expound on aspects of patient care can produce similar results, as can statements made during live Web-conferencing sessions. Small group work that depends on students working on projects together (literature reviews, class presentations, etc.) can also be revealing in assessing elements of the affective domain. Grading rubrics should include peer review of team member contributions to a group project and specifically seek to identify changes in behavioral competencies over time.

Faculty Administration Matters

Although in many colleges and universities, the institution's student registrar is responsible for general student administration, each instructor's situation may differ, and some administrative matters must be dealt with at the local level. A few examples follow here:

- **Student enrollments must be entered into the LMS**. Student-related policies should mirror the protocol approach used for face-to-face courses. It is prudent for administrators to check the organization's handbook to ensure this has been addressed. If a new online course is planned, the handbook may have to be amended to reflect the change in delivery mode. Depending on the LMS chosen and how it is supported, students may be allowed to self-enroll or the instructor may need to manually enter them into the LMS. In the latter case, every effort should be made to ensure demographic information is complete and accurate. At the end of the course the instructor must be sure grades have been entered into the institution's system so that students receive timely credit for their efforts.
- **Student participation**. When an online program expects student participatory activities, instructors may be concerned about what constitutes a reasonable level of student participation or nonparticipation in the course. When preparing for the course, a decision must be made and clearly communicated to students about how the course instructors will grade student participation. A participation rubric may be developed and a corresponding entry added to the LMS and student handbook.

- **Grading collaborative work.** Students enrolled in the course must know how collaborative work will be graded. Without a clear statement, disputes can arise between students and faculty. A statement within the course instructions that defines how collaborative work will be graded significantly reduces the potential for problems. As previously mentioned, rubrics prevent most of the headache that can go along with this. Effort should be made to inform students that they are being assessed both for individual quality of work and contributing to the group project as a whole. The assignment rubric should reflect this. Additionally, it is important that the instructor create an environment (or culture) in which honest reporting is not only encouraged, but is safe for the student to do and contains inherent reward.

Instructor Skills for Online Teaching and Learning

Many enthusiastic instructors wish to develop their courses using a digital format and are unsure how to go about it. If DE is already established at the instructor's educational institution, then the local faculty-development department usually offers workshops to provide the skills that instructors need to get started. However, the availability of such workshops varies widely between institutions, and many offer no training yet expect faculty to put forth a quality product. It does not take a rocket scientist to realize this is a lose-lose-lose situation—the institution will lose credibility, the instructor will likely be labeled a poor educator, and (most importantly) the student will not receive the education. An LMS might provide a comprehensive guide to assist the instructor in learning the technology, and the help function within the LMS can assist instructors during its use. However, some LMSs are poorly documented or offer little or no training, and the help function can sometimes produce an empty screen (i.e., no information). When purchasing an LMS, the program director should ensure that the vendor includes training as part of the contract. Learning the technology to upload electronic files is not difficult, but it may have a steep learning curve because the placement of "submit" buttons is not always as obvious or intuitive as one might hope. The challenge often lies more in learning the pedagogical framework and the different teaching methods available.

The instructor's experiences from classroom teaching provide a range of skills that are readily adaptable to online teaching. Successful online teaching strategies include the following:

- **Posing real-life scenarios.** Students can relate learning to clinical practice. Real-life scenarios provide sound foundations from which participants can explore a range of "what ifs" on the discussion board or during Web-conferencing. Web-based services are now available that offer video of real patient encounters that adds another dimension (realism) to this learning.
- **Asking students for their opinion.** Adult students bring varied life experiences to the classroom; many will have encountered issues of social and health matters. Students learn from each other. These students must be allowed to share their experiences and insights with each other as it is very relevant to them. The EMS educator should actively plan time and methods for this.
- **Acknowledging good progress.** Prompt feedback given to students through course messaging or the discussion board provides encouragement and allows students to gauge their progress.
- **Maintaining student self-esteem.** Sometimes, the spoken word and the written word are in conflict when nonverbal cues are limited or absent; instructors are encouraged to proofread correspondence sent to students to ensure that student self-esteem is sustained.
- **Engaging students.** Although students may be many miles away, online tasks and activities that require them to reflect on their learning create an environment that is meaningful to them. It is sometimes difficult to accomplish in practice, but efforts aimed at reducing transactional distance and reducing a sense of isolation are well worth the time and thought. Adults often learn in a social setting, so instructors need to provide that sense of community.
- **Creating and maintaining a learning environment.** This is the tenet of teaching principles. Because online learning may not provide the benefit of classroom visual cues, instructors and students alike may be anxious to know if learning in a digital environment can be effective. This is a valid query, and evidence confirms that the learning that results is at least equivalent.[31,32] Instructors can help to mitigate student concerns by creating a vibrant online community that encourages active participation. The challenge for most EMS instructors is "exactly how can this be accomplished?" Many EMS educators have taught a course face-to-face that they then are tasked with teaching online. In a face-to-face course, an instructor uses

a number of strategies, ranging from lecture to small group work to skills labs, to keep students engaged. Instructors have typically developed a comfort level in the physical classroom. Online courses have similar needs in terms of strategies, but require a different approach. For example, instructors want to provide a sense of social interaction in the online offering. To facilitate this in a digital environment, an instructor can create and moderate threaded discussions, hold regular periodic (weekly) synchronous (webinar) sessions, assign projects to small groups, facilitate online (synchronous or asynchronous) student presentations, and allow constructive peer feedback on them. Instructors must challenge their students. People perform best when challenged to go just beyond their comfort zone. The obvious go-to method for challenging students is quizzes (formative assessment), but learning games can make learning both fun and memorable. Educators should seek out learning resources such as podcasts and videos. (See Chapter 16, *Using Technology to Enhance Classroom Learning*.) Information that is valid, relevant, and from an outside source can help keep students engaged and encourages them to dig a little deeper into the subject (these resources often have links to additional similar materials).

Research has generated an influential amount of information about the scope of DE. One study wished to find out whether two different distance-learning techniques were as effective as classroom teaching for training students at a rural location.[33] This study explored a range of technologies, including two-way audio and computers, and it employed synchronous teaching techniques. Study investigators concluded that "no difference was found" between the two types of study, and they promoted distance-learning techniques as an effective way to provide educational opportunities to rural students. Research from general education and allied health disciplines confirms that learning does occur through DE courses.

Issues of Student Learning

Before a student embarks on an online program, several significant concerns must be considered. Basic computer skills are essential. Students who are entering universities or community colleges will have developed computer literacy as part of their schooling (many degree programs require this). Older students, however, might not be as competent as their younger peers. Although keyboard speed may present some limitations, skills for site navigation and basic software applications are required. Many local libraries or community centers offer short courses that teach computer basics. Importantly, potential students require access to a computer with current software and programs to access course material. While similar in many respects, there are significant differences between PC and Mac programs. The instructor should make sure students understand expectations regarding acceptable file format(s) when submitting assignments so that the instructor will be able to view and grade them. For example, some schools require a specific file format so assignments can be run through a plagiarism checker before grading.

Potential students may find it helpful to be informed about course expectations and about how undertaking an online course can affect the home environment. Information packages that contain helpful hints about how to create a home study center and how to plan and attend to learning provide useful information for supporting and optimizing student learning. An orientation session (preferably face-to-face) is helpful both for informing students of needs/expectations and getting past some basic apprehension.

Instructors need to remind students that online learning requires self-discipline, because it is easy to defer course tasks in favor of personal commitments. To overcome this, it is recommended that students schedule specific times during the week to dedicate to course activities and learning so that the benefits

TEACHING TIP

Instructors must consider the way students process information; the learning environment that an instructor creates directly affects student learning. Instructors should do the following:

- Provide opportunities for students to share ideas and experiences.
- Provide opportunities for students to feel both challenged and supported.
- Empower students toward learning on their own by making course objectives clearly defined and accessible.
- Establish relationships with students—relationships are essential if students are to be successful.
- Design teaching to reflect high expectations for the success of all students.
- Provide opportunities for students to collaborate with classmates.

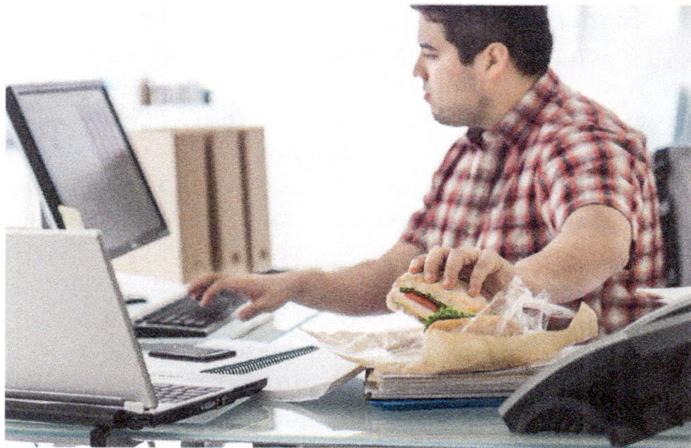

FIGURE 17.4 Students enrolled in distance-learning courses are able to structure their class time around work time.

associated with accessing the online course can be balanced with personal endeavors (FIGURE 17.4).

Challenges for Distance Education in EMS

As with all new initiatives, EMS instructors will face differing personal challenges as they learn to master the skills to deliver online instruction. Some might find the challenges easier than others. Without trying to place stereotypical labels on age groups, younger instructors might have the advantage of developing their digital literacy skills earlier in life and are often referred to as digital natives, whereas older instructors might feel threatened to learn a new paradigm of instructional delivery (referred to as digital immigrants).[34] There are certainly exceptions to these preconceived stereotypes, and one should be careful about making assumptions regarding any group. Older educators that have been lifelong early adopters of technology may in fact have a better skill set than their younger counterparts. Along with the personal challenges, external challenges also exist that are drawn from the educational institution, its guiding policies, and its staff-support resources.

Personal instructor challenges may include the following:

- **The new online instructor as learner**. The instructor who needs to become a learner to master the change from face-to-face instruction has significant benefits. Those new to digital learning may find a certain level of discomfort in once again becoming a novice and must work to master unfamiliar skills needed to be successful. Progressing through this new learning cycle will give the instructor a sense of what the students might experience. Instructors begin to understand their own learning strategies, and this, in turn, will have a follow-on effect into the virtual classroom. Instructors will understand what students are experiencing as a result of the course design, and they will better understand how to plan the online course. While learning a new form of instructional delivery may be a challenge, the outcomes often have a positive result.
- **The individual instructor's challenge of reconceptualizing F2F to DE pedagogy**. Seasoned instructors might face moving from highly interactive face-to-face teaching into an online medium with trepidation. They may need support and mentorship as they learn to master the technology, adapt to accommodate new resources into their teaching practice, and adjust their instructional style to develop and maintain a sense of student community and active participation within the course.

Institutional challenges may include the following:

- **The challenge associated with inclusion of lab, clinical, and field instructors (those who work with students in lab skills and scenarios or one-to-one in patient settings).** The nature of EMS demands mastery of psychomotor skills that are difficult to demonstrate through online classes. To support this, these instructors must be encouraged to participate in DE programs so that education and industry cohesiveness can be maintained. This results in the best outcomes for students and for the patients in their care. Arrangements need to be put into place for these instructors to update their skills, thereby maintaining a strong liaison between educational faculty and lab/clinical/field instructors. Sometimes also referred to as interrater reliability, it keeps everyone "on the same page" and ensures consistency in training and assessment. This may necessitate robust communication mechanisms and frequent workshops for field instructors to allow them to gain sufficient competence in utilizing digital skills prior to taking on a student.
- **The challenge of access and equity**. Vocational and higher-education institutions have policies that include access and equity. DE complements these policies by making education available to people who are unable to attend in the classroom. Given the far-reaching nature of online education, instructors must now appreciate their own cultural biases and be ready to adjust their teaching method/style to accommodate norms outside their own culture. Workshops on cultural sensitivity take on a whole new importance for instructors in this context as significant differences can exist locally, regionally, and across a given country.[35]

Political and professional challenges may include:

- **The challenge for EMS educators to provide optimal educational programs to return competent prehospital healthcare providers to adequately serve their communities.** Many government leaders from different countries state that their healthcare system is in crisis, and solutions to abate the crisis are constantly being reviewed. In fact, the U.S. Bureau of Labor Statistics projects that employment of emergency medical technicians (EMTs) and paramedics will grow by 15% from 2016 to 2026.[36] The idea of extended-practice EMS providers is not new, and initiatives such as mobile integrated healthcare and community paramedicine are growing in popularity in the United States. These specialties present a means to reduce hospital readmission rates and provide patient-centered resources aimed at improved patient outcomes. They also potentially decrease emergency department overcrowding and healthcare costs. These programs require additional training and specific continuing education. A strong argument could be made that DE is ideal to help provide much of that education.

Continuing Education for EMS Providers

While DE is a viable option for a range of courses for undergraduate educational programs within the health sciences, it is also a practical choice for continuing education (CE) and professional development programs, as the students have already developed fundamental skills within their professional practice.

Within U.S. EMS systems, CE is mandatory to maintain certification, licensure, or specialty credentialing. Practitioners have a responsibility to stay up-to-date with current and contemporary practices, incorporate new policies into their practice, and keep abreast of evidence-based medicine that impacts care. DE is uniquely situated to provide timely, up-to-date information and education. Unlike printed media, edits within the online environment involve little or no delay in order to publish. CE can be delivered synchronously (webinars) and asynchronously (recorded materials) to meet the needs of busy healthcare providers. Learning materials can be accessed on or off duty from any location with Internet service, can be tracked by instructors, and allow virtually instant feedback. DE is not just for formalized courses. It can be utilized for scheduled monthly subjects relevant to a particular service area and/or used to provide new, updated, or changed materials in a timely and cost-effective way. In a properly structured CE program, many of the needs of learners (employees) could be addressed via DE.

Accreditation and regulation boards of professional bodies often oversee and administer CE programs. Each state and/or country has different criteria that individual EMS practitioners must meet to retain currency of licensure. EMS accrediting bodies have the expectation that educational programs will reflect contemporary methods by addressing issues of policy, quality of educational program content, access, and equity.[37]

The Commission on Accreditation for Prehospital Continuing Education (CAPCE) is the body that accredits CE courses within the United States, including those offered via DE. This organization can be found at www.cecbems.org; the website provides contact details and information about the process required for newly created online CE programs to gain accreditation approval.

Summary

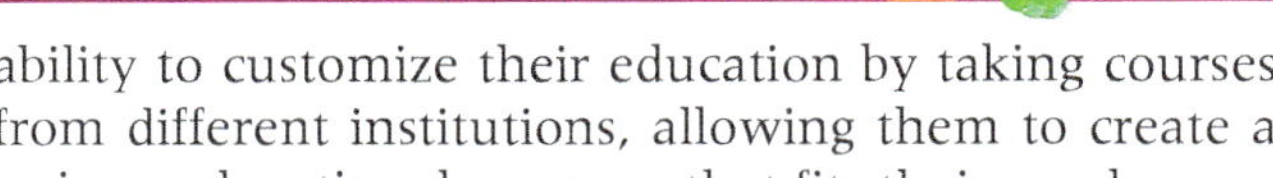

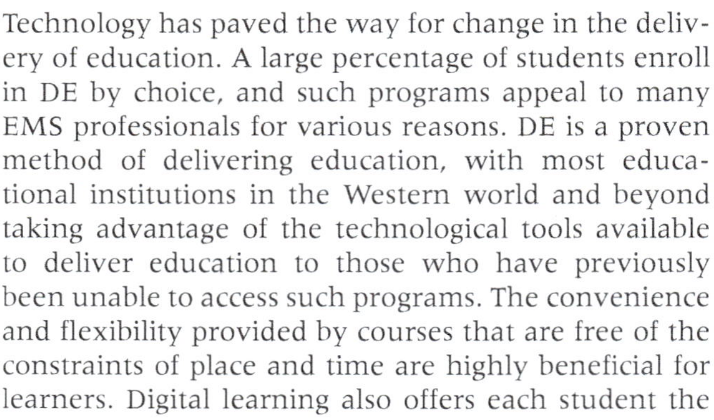

Technology has paved the way for change in the delivery of education. A large percentage of students enroll in DE by choice, and such programs appeal to many EMS professionals for various reasons. DE is a proven method of delivering education, with most educational institutions in the Western world and beyond taking advantage of the technological tools available to deliver education to those who have previously been unable to access such programs. The convenience and flexibility provided by courses that are free of the constraints of place and time are highly beneficial for learners. Digital learning also offers each student the ability to customize their education by taking courses from different institutions, allowing them to create a unique educational program that fits their needs.

Because EMS professions include a significant psychomotor skills component, the use of DE in EMS works best when offered in the form of a hybrid course. In this structure, some portions of the course are delivered online, while other portions such as clinical skills practice and laboratory sessions occur face-to-face.

DE can work particularly well in the context of EMS continuing education.

Glossary

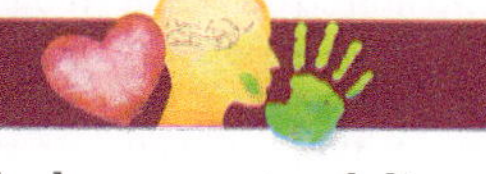

asynchronous learning Student-centered education that utilizes digital/online learning resources to facilitate knowledge sharing independent of time and place.

chat rooms Synchronous electronic text communication system that resembles actual real-time conversations.

cloud-based collaborative document Document accessed through the Internet that can be updated by multiple users at the same time.

collaborative learning Instructional method in which students work together in small groups toward a common goal.

criteria-released assessment items Assessment items that are released once certain parameters, such as completion of homework or assignments, have been met.

digital learning Any type of learning that is facilitated by the effective use of technology. It includes the application of a wide range of educational methodologies including blended/hybrid, online, gamification, and virtual/augmented reality.

discussion board Tool used to facilitate threaded discussions within an online course; it is often accessed through a learning management system.

distance education (DE) System of education whereby students and instructors are separated by time and/or location. It includes learning materials delivered in a variety of formats, from paper-based correspondence courses to online digital materials.

F2F Face-to-face classroom learning; also called FTF.

hybrid course Course that includes aspects of distance (online) education and traditional education, such as clinical experience or laboratory practice of psychomotor skills.

instructional design Process for creating instructional content; key steps include assessing the needs of the learners, writing course objectives, structuring course content, determining assessment strategies, and assessing course effectiveness.

learning management system (LMS) Software application that facilitates the delivery and administration of education courses in an online educational environment.

storyboard Document that outlines detailed plans, frame by frame; for example, for the production of an online course.

synchronous learning Describes forms of teaching and learning that occur at the same time, but not in the same place. In an online environment, this is typically accomplished utilizing a Web-conferencing application.

time-released assessment items Assessment items that are released at a certain point, for example, on a certain calendar day.

video conferencing Meeting that occurs online and that has both visual and audio capability.

wiki Website that allows users to collaboratively modify a Web page using their browser. Can be utilized for group projects. The term comes from the Hawaiian/Polynesian word for quick.

References

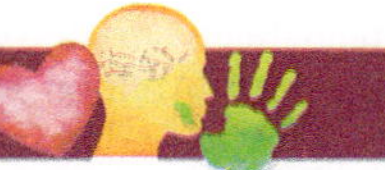

[1] Kaplan, Andreas M., and Michael Haenlein. 2016. "Higher Education and the Digital Revolution: About MOOCs, SPOCs, Social Media, and the Cookie Monster." *Business Horizons* 59, no. 4: 441–50. https://doi.org/10.1016/j.bushor.2016.03.008.

[2] U.S. Department of Education, National Center for Education Statistics. 2018. *Digest of Education Statistics, 2016* (NCES 2017-094), Table 311.15. Accessed December 13, 2018. https://nces.ed.gov/fastfacts/display.asp?id=80.

[3] Leichtman Research Group. 2017. "84% of U.S. Households Get an Internet Service at Home" Accessed February 15, 2019. https://www.leichtmanresearch.com/84-of-u-s-households-get-an-internet-service-at-home/.

[4] Emmerson, Anne M. 2005. "A History of the Changes in Practices of Distance Education in the United States from 1852–2003." Dissertation, Dowling College. Accessed February 15, 2019. https://www.learntechlib.org/p/127019/.

[5] Seaman, Julia E., I. Elaine Allen, and Jeff Seaman. 2018. *Grade Increase: Tracking Distance Education in the United States*. Babson Park, MA: Babson Survey Research Group, Babson College.

[6] Gallagher, Sean. 2003. "The Future of Online Learning: Key Trends and Issues." *The Distance Education and Training Council (DETC) 77th Annual Conference Summary*. Washington, DC: DETC.

[7] *The Chronicle of Higher Education*. 2011, November 6. "6 Online Learning Trends." Accessed February 15, 2019. https://www.chronicle.com/article/Charts-6-Online-Learning/129634.

[8] Ashby, Cornelia M. 2002. "Distance Education: Growth in Distance Education Programs and Implications for Federal Education Policy." GAO-02-1125T. Washington, DC: U.S. General Accounting Office Report.

[9] Redding, Terrence R., and Jack Rotzien. 2001. "Comparative Analysis of Online Learning Versus Classroom Learning." *Journal of Interactive Instruction Development* 13: 3–12.

[10] Smeaton, Alan, and Keogh, Gary. 1999. "An Analysis of the Use of Virtual Delivery of Undergraduate Lectures." *Computers and Education* 32: 83–94.

[11] Wade, William. 1999. "Assessment in Distance Learning." *The Journal* 27: 94–100.

[12] Sener, John, and Mary Liana Stover. 2000. "Integrating ALN into an Independent Study Distance Education Program: NVCC Case Studies." *Journal of Asynchronous Learning Networks* 4, no. 2. Accessed March 6, 2019. https://www.researchgate.net/publication/228606994_Integrating_ALN_into_an_independent_study_distance_education_program_NVCC_case_studies.

[13] Nguyen, Tuan. 2015. "The Effectiveness of Online Learning: Beyond No Significant Difference and Future Horizons." *MERLOT Journal of Online Learning and Teaching* 11, no. 2: 309–19.

[14] Aderinoye, R. A., Ojokheta, K. O., and Olojede, A. A. 2007. "Integrating Mobile Learning into Nomadic Education Programmes in Nigeria: Issues and Perspectives." *The International Review of Research in Open and Distance Learning* 8, no. 2: 1–17.

[15] Instructional Technology Council. 2016. "ITC Annual National eLearning Report." Accessed February 15, 2019. https://www.itcnetwork.org/sites/default/files/content-files/itc_2016_survey_results_infographic.pdf.

[16] Best Colleges.com. "2018 Online Trends in Education Report." Accessed February 6, 2019. https://www.bestcolleges.com/perspectives/annual-trends-in-online-education/.

[17] CollegeAtlas.org. "41 Facts about Online Students." Updated July 28, 2017. Accessed February 7, 2019. https://www.collegeatlas.org/41-surprising-facts-about-online-students.html.

[18] Bernard, Robert M., Philip C. Abrami, Yiping Lou, Evgueni Borokhovski, Anne Wade, Lori Wozney, Peter A. Wallet, Manon Fiset, and Binru Huang. 2004. "How Does Distance Education Compare with Classroom Instruction? A Meta-Analysis of the Empirical Literature." *Review of Educational Research* 74, no. 3: 379–439. https://doi.org/10.3102/00346543074003379.

[19] Pelletier, Stephen G. 2010. "Success for Adult Students." *Public Purpose.* Accessed February 15, 2019. https://www.aascu.org/uploadedFiles/AASCU/Content/Root/MediaAndPublications/PublicPurposeMagazines/Issue/10fall_adultstudents.pdf.

[20] Van Volkom, Michele, Janice C. Stapley, and Vanessa Amaturo. 2014. "Revisiting the Digital Divide: Generational Differences in Technology Use in Everyday Life." *North American Journal of Psychology* 16, no. 3: 557–74.

[21] Pew Research Center. 2018. "Internet/Broadband Fact Sheet." Accessed February 15, 2019. http://www.pewinternet.org/fact-sheet/internet-broadband/.

[22] McDonnell, Andrew, and Dale Edwards. 2000. "From the Classroom by Cyberland: 21st Century Education for Paramedics." *Australasian Journal of Emergency Care* 7: 231–4.

[23] Lord, Bill. 2003. "The Development of a Degree Qualification for Paramedics at Charles Sturt University." *Australasian Journal of Paramedicine* 1, no. 1. http://dx.doi.org/10.33151/ajp.1.1.40.

[24] Universitat Oberta de Catalunya. 2019. "Facts and Figures." Accessed February 7, 2019. https://www.uoc.edu/portal/en/universitat/fets-xifres/index.html.

[25] Schiffman, Shirl S. 1995. "Instructional Systems Design: Five Views of the Field." In *Instructional Technology: Past, Present, and Future*, 2nd ed., edited by G. J. Anglin, 131–42. Englewood, CO: Libraries Unlimited.

[26] Barkley, Elizabeth F., and Claire H. Major. 2016. *Learning Assessment Techniques*. San Francisco: Jossey-Bass.

[27] Maertens, Heidi, Amin Madani, Tara Landry, Frank Vermassen, Isabelle Van Herzeele, and R. Aggarwal. 2016. "Systematic Review of e-Learning for Surgical Training." *The British Journal of Surgery* 103, no. 11: 1428–37. https://doi.org/10.1002/bjs.10236.

[28] Birt, James R., Emma Moore, and Michael Cowling. 2017. "Improving Paramedic Distance Education through Mobile Mixed Reality Simulation." *Australasian Journal of Educational Technology* 33, no. 6: 69–83. https://doi.org/10.14742/ajet.3596.

[29] Kim, Kwangtaek. 2018. "Image-Based Haptic Roughness Estimation and Rendering for Haptic Palpation from In Vivo Skin Image." *Medical & Biological Engineering & Computing* 56, no. 3: 413–20. https://doi.org/10.1007/s11517-017-1700-4.

[30] Pattavina, Paul. 1981. "Generic Affective Competencies: A Description of Applied Teaching Behaviors." ED 238842. Washington, DC: Department of Education. Accessed February 15, 2019. https://eric.ed.gov/?id=ED238842.

[31] Boston, Roger L. 1992. "Remote Delivery of Instruction via the PC and Modem: What Have We Learned?" *American Journal of Distance Education* 6, no. 3: 345–57. https://doi.org/10.1080/08923649209526799.

[32] Simonson, Michael, Sharon E. Smaldino, Michael Albright, and Susan Zvacek. 2011. *Teaching and Learning at a Distance: Foundations of Distance Education,* 5th ed. Boston: Pearson Education.

[33] Hobbs., Gregory D., James F. Moshinskie, Sean K. Roden, and Jeffrey L. Jarvis. 1998. "Education and Practice. A Comparison of Classroom and Distance-Learning Techniques for Rural EMT-I Instruction." *Prehospital Emergency Care* 2, no. 3: 189–91. https://doi.org/10.1080/10903129808958870.

[34] Herther, Nancy. 2009. "Digital Natives and Immigrants: What Brain Research Tells Us." *Online* 33, no. 6: 14–21.

[35] Gunawardena, Charlotte N., and LaPointe, Deborah. 2007. "Cultural Dynamics of Online Learning." In *Handbook of Distance Education,* 2nd ed., edited by Michael G. Moore, 593–607. New York: Routledge.

[36] U.S. Bureau of Labor Statistics. 2018. "Occupational Outlook Handbook: EMTs and Paramedics." Accessed February 15, 2019. https://www.bls.gov/ooh/healthcare/emts-and-paramedics.htm.

[37] Council for Higher Education Accreditation. 2002. "Accreditation and Assuring Quality in Distance Education." CHEA Monograph Series 2002, No. 1. Accessed February 15, 2019. https://www.chea.org/userfiles/CHEA%20Monograph%20Series/mono_1_accred_distance_02.pdf.

Additional Resources

Deil-Amen, Regina. 2011, November. "The "Traditional" College Student: A Smaller and Smaller Minority and Its Implications for Diversity and Access Institutions." In *Mapping Broad-Access Higher Education Conference at Stanford University, Vol. 1*. Stanford, CA: Stanford Center for Education Policy Analysis; 2014.

Halsne, Alana M., and Louis A. Gatta. 2002. "Online Versus Traditionally Delivered Instruction: A Descriptive Study of Learner Characteristics in a Community-College Setting." *Online Journal of Distance Learning Administration* 5, no. 1. https://www.learntechlib.org/p/92518/.

CHAPTER 18

Tools for Simulation

OBJECTIVES

At the conclusion of this chapter, the educator will be able to:

Cognitive Domain

1. Define *simulation*.
2. Outline the benefits of simulation.
3. List elements needed in the preparation phase of simulation, including briefing.
4. Describe the process to develop objectives for the simulation.
5. Discuss considerations of the conditions of the simulation.
6. Outline essential elements of scenario design to achieve learning objectives.
7. Describe the role of standardized patients in simulation.
8. Describe considerations related to equipment used during simulation.
9. Discuss the facilitator role during the simulation.
10. Outline the elements of an effective simulation debriefing process.

Psychomotor Domain

1. Design a simulation experience to achieve specific student learning objectives.

Affective Domain

1. Recognize the need to construct simulation in a manner that achieves desired learning objectives.
2. Engage in effective debriefing techniques that promote student learning in a safe environment.

"Simulation is a technique—not a technology—to replace or amplify real experiences with guided experiences that evoke or replicate substantial aspects of the real world in a fully interactive manner."

~ David M. Gaba

CHAPTER GOAL The goal of this chapter is provide an introductory discussion of the utilization of simulation concepts and techniques in emergency medical services (EMS) education.

Simulation in EMS education can play an essential role in helping students transfer and translate classroom theory into real-world practical application within the relative safety of controlled environments. Implementation of simulation in EMS education should be considered on a continuum—from the isolated and simple to the large and complex.[1]

In the early 16th century, manikins (referred to as "phantoms") were used to teach obstetrical skills to physicians in an attempt to reduce the number of women and infants who died during childbirth. Simulation in EMS education today traces its roots to the aviation industry and draws inspiration from disciplines and fields where expertise is required in responding to low-frequency, high-acuity events.

Often the terms *simulation* and *scenario* are used interchangeably. Both have a wide range of interpretations. In recent years, advances in simulator technology have made the term "simulation" synonymous with the use of **high-fidelity** resuscitation manikins. It is important to recognize, however, as noted in 2004 by Gaba, that "simulation is a technique and not a technology."[2] Many simulation techniques can be effective in EMS education. These simulation techniques include standardized patients, moulage, virtual reality, 3-D interactive computer systems, and gaming, as well as manikins that range from **low-fidelity** task-based manikins to high-fidelity resuscitation manikins. Simulation is an experiential learning practice designed to mimic real-world situations as closely as possible. A simulation experience should invoke emotion and stress in as real a context as possible in a controlled, safe environment, while allowing students to demonstrate skills, knowledge, and affective behaviors with high levels of competency.

Simulation is a pathway through which health care, education, and theater intersect to produce an experiential learning experience. An experiential learning experience is designed to immerse students into real-world situations where their decisions, skills, and behavior can be developed, practiced, and assessed in a controlled and safe environment. Simulation is most powerful when it is based in an education program's curriculum and learning objectives. Comprehensive integration of simulation in the educator's lesson plans allows for reinforcement of student learning and competencies.

As with any teaching technique, EMS educators must strive to utilize simulation appropriately, ensuring its coordination with educational objectives. In the initial phase of psychomotor skills learning, students should practice specific skills on a simple **task trainer** or manikin. As student competency improves, the EMS educator can develop **scenarios** that allow for progressive complexity using a variety of simulation techniques.

There are numerous advantages to the use of simulation in EMS education. The major benefits include the following:

- Allowing students freedom to make mistakes without patient risk or safety consequences
- Providing students with the experience of high-acuity, low-frequency clinical and operational situations in a safe, controlled environment
- Allowing students to practice critical thinking and clinical decision making in a safe, controlled environment
- Providing students the chance to practice teamwork and leadership skills in a safe, controlled environment
- Enabling students to recognize gaps in their knowledge and experience and to identify their own learning needs
- Standardizing learning environments
- Identifying weaknesses or gaps in the curriculum

Preparation

When designing any simulated event, careful consideration of the elements needed for effective student learning is essential. Software packages from the various simulator manufacturers generally provide two options for simulation events. Preprogrammed scenarios transition from situation to situation according to a set algorithm. These algorithm-based scenarios are generally basic and designed to meet a broad standard curriculum or scope of practice. **On-the-fly programming** allows the EMS educator to manipulate the program software in response to student decisions and interventions. As EMS educators become more adept at using these on-the-fly programming options, they can make use of the opportunity to create and catalogue more precise, evidence-based scenarios that align with their program's curriculum, learning objectives, and student needs.

Components of a simulation session include the following:

- Objectives
- Tasks
- Conditions
- Scenario
- Time frame
- Participants
- Equipment and setup
- End points and grading rubrics (if assessment is the goal)
- **Debriefing** topics or questions

Simulation Scenario Planning

In order to realize the greatest benefit from a simulation session, EMS educators must be thoughtful and deliberate when planning the purpose and scope of any scenario or simulated event. The resources (human and material) needed to effectively conduct the simulation must match the size, depth, and complexity needed to achieve the stated educational objectives. The scope of the simulation may be limited to the resources available within the organization or consortium of organizations planning the simulation.

One helpful tool to begin planning and organizing the simulation is to make lists of the tasks for the students to demonstrate, the conditions under which they should be able to perform these tasks, and the minimum standards to measure successful achievement of the desired competencies, outcomes, or objectives.[3] Some educators find it helpful to utilize a template or worksheet that allows them to plan and implement a scenario in a uniform and consistent manner. A wide variety of templates and worksheets are available commercially; however, many educators prefer to create their own.

Objectives

The key to integrating simulation into EMS education is to ensure that the simulations are in solid alignment with the course goals and specific lesson learning objectives. They must also be realistic in content and expectations while ranging from simple to extremely complex.

Factors to consider in the simulation design process are student knowledge, equipment, resources available, and the desired outcomes or learning objectives. A common error in simulation design involves overdramatization and unrealistic expectations. To avoid this simulation design pitfall, educators should ask themselves the following questions:

- Could this be a real EMS response?
- Would an EMS crew with this level of student knowledge and skill be expected to handle this situation with the available resources?

If either answer is "no," the simulation is not realistic in content and expectations, and it should be modified.

One of the best options to avoid this design error is to adapt real EMS cases as simulations. When simulating real EMS cases, it is important to adjust the level of decision making, skills, **branching** (the number of different directions a simulation may take), and the consequences of the interventions performed to the level of the student's knowledge. The objectives the student must demonstrate in order to be successful in the scenario should guide the endpoint and grading or assessment (if that is the purpose of the simulation). Designating an expected **time-in-simulation** (the time the students spend in the simulation activity) is helpful so that simulations are realistic and manageable for both the student and the instructor. This will also help ensure adequate time is allotted for a thorough debriefing.

The first step in creating a simulation is to develop a basic list of the overall goals and objectives for the scenario. It is helpful to identify the overall pedagogical goals of the simulation. Is it for teaching and instruction, or is it a method of assessing student learning, performance, or competency? If it is performance or competency, is it formative or summative? Setting objectives for the simulation session is similar to the process of developing objectives. (See Chapter 9, *Goals and Objectives*.) Objectives can focus on one or more of the three domains of learning (cognitive, psychomotor, and affective) and should be clear, specific, and measurable. For example, an objective such as "The student will perform the five steps involved in bandaging a laceration with active bleeding" is clearer and more measurable than "The student will care for the trauma patient." Tasks and objectives may range from simple skill acquisition to complex integration of cognitive, psychomotor, and affective behaviors. Clear, realistic task goals help guide the development of a simulation plan.[4]

Educators should also consider the stage of learning that the students are in at the time of the simulation.[5,6] During the initial stages of learning, a simulation should be simple and should isolate specific new tasks. At this point in the student's learning, a simulation may consist simply of introducing oneself to a patient or obtaining an accurate set of vital signs. What separates simulation from a simple task exercise is the performance of these tasks in an immersive, realistic setting. During later stages of learning, students should be expected to combine and integrate multiple concepts and tasks, and operate under more realistic conditions. At this point, students may be required to assess and treat a patient with multiple, complex medical issues that require critical thinking, effective communication, and competent procedural care. Summative simulation sessions should be complex and focus on determining whether or not the student is performing at an acceptable level as an entry-level EMS provider. The simulated patient's history, behavior, and acuity should realistically reflect the kind of patients the student will care for in clinical practice.[7]

Because there are limitations to the realism and skills performance in the simulated environment, the EMS educator must ensure that the students are oriented to the simulation process, rules, and limitations. Information regarding what steps a student may verbalize and what skills must be performed on the simulators being used is critical to delivering a realistic immersive simulation. For example, in a simulation it is not enough that students verbalize that they are wearing gloves. Having students locate and apply gloves at the appropriate time during the simulation adds to the realism while demonstrating a best practice of EMS.

The student's orientation to the simulation process must include an awareness of the functionality of the simulators. On some simulators, the pupils of the eyes react to light or medications, while others do not have this feature. Some simulators have a blood pressure that can be auscultated, though it may not sound exactly like the blood pressure of an actual patient.

Instructors must be aware of the dangers of negative transference and identify any skill or procedure that deviates significantly from the way it is performed on a real patient.

TEACHING TIP

A simulator (manikin, standardized patient, task trainer, etc.) should be chosen after defining goals, objectives, learner types, and budget considerations.

Conditions

Key to achieving the desired outcomes and objectives in a simulation session is the realism of the environment and the ability for the students to "suspend their disbelief" as they move and interact in the simulated environment. Creating an immersive learning environment is essential for allowing the students to practice skills and situations that they will encounter in the clinical environment (**FIGURE 18.1**). Many educational programs conduct simulations in a skill lab or classroom environment. While a stand-alone simulation center is desirable, it is not required for EMS educators to conduct realistic simulation sessions. The key is a realistic re-creation of the experience. To do this the simulation needs to capture the visual, auditory, tactile sensations, and even the smells of the actual environment being simulated while keeping the experience safe. The presence of simulated patients or **confederates** (individuals other than the simulated patient, for example, a simulated family member or bystander) to provide a social and environmental context within which the students can operate will add to the realism and allow the students to practice critical thinking and complex-factor decision making while experiencing multiple sensory inputs.

Low light, loud noise, realistic odors, seasonal temperature, tactile sensations, and inclement weather are all factors within the EMS environment. Varying the

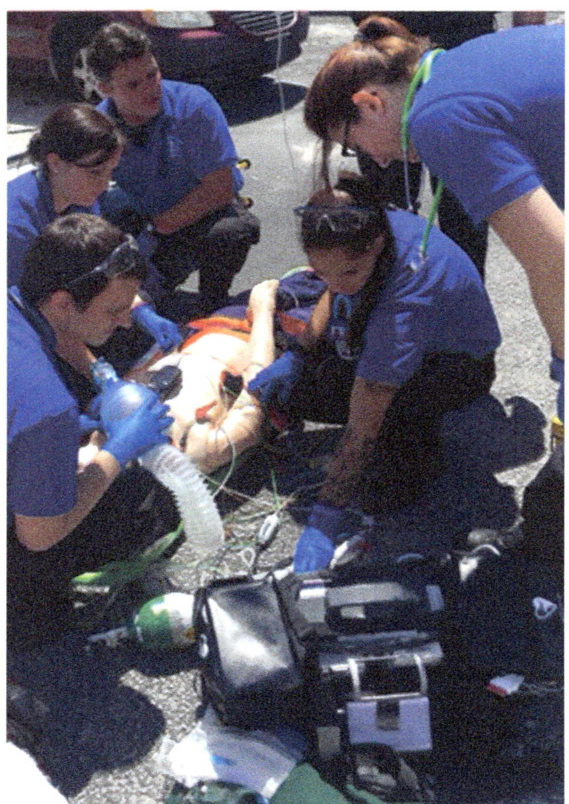

FIGURE 18.1 It is important, when possible, to conduct simulations in an environment similar to the conditions that students will face while on the job.

Courtesy of John Todaro.

conditions of simulation can add extra challenges as well as a greater degree of realism. While there is a risk of overwhelming the new student with the complex sensory inputs, in the final stages of learning the educator should make every attempt to create intricate, complex, and critical simulations that are as realistic as possible. These should be sufficient in depth and variety as to really test the ability of the provider while still providing the layer of safety that cannot be achieved during a real emergency.

The setting of the simulation is an important factor in creating the illusion of realism. While many simulation centers are built to look like hospitals or in-patient clinical settings, the EMS educator should strive to create simulated environments that mimic the prehospital environment. The back of an ambulance is one of the most common simulated environments. Allowing students to practice skills in the relatively confined spaces of an ambulance exposes them to the challenges of this environment. A simulated environment that recreates the motion and the sounds of a moving ambulance adds further realism to the scenarios. Simulations may also take place in a simulated home environment. With a minimum of relatively inexpensive props and furniture, EMS educators can turn a classroom into a home or an apartment. Staging simulations in public spaces allows students the experience of caring for patients and interacting in another type of environment they may be exposed to in clinical practice (**FIGURE 18.2**). In order to avoid confusion and misunderstanding on the part of the general public, it is essential to obtain the appropriate permission for use and to notify the proper authorities and organizations when simulation is taking place outdoors or in a public space. Designating a safety officer (a role that will be discussed in greater detail later) ensures that the public does not mistake a simulated emergency for the real thing.

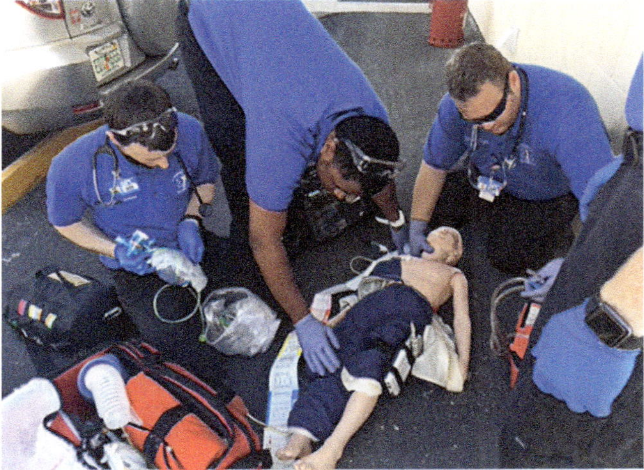

FIGURE 18.2 Simulations can be staged in public spaces, and can allow students to practice skills they will need on real emergency calls such as using a length-based resuscitation tape, shown here.

Courtesy of John Todaro.

Simulations can be staged in parking lots, on the grounds of colleges or hospitals, in firehouse or ambulance living quarters, and in various public spaces. Simulations in real-world environments are easy to stage with the advent of wireless high-fidelity simulators and standardized patients.

While caution must be taken when exposing high-fidelity simulators or standardized patients to extreme environmental conditions, the advantage of utilizing them is that they can be cared for and transported just as if they were real patients, moving from the prehospital to the hospital environment without disrupting the continuity or realism of the simulation.

An alternative to the dedicated indoor simulation lab is the mobile simulation lab. Similar to a stand-alone lab, these mobile classrooms often have a mock emergency department room or the back of an ambulance inside a large vehicle. Mobile simulation labs have the added benefit of portability, allowing EMS educators to take simulation education to areas that might not have the access or financial resources to maintain a simulation lab.

While sometimes introducing more distractions, outdoor events generally provide a greater degree of difficulty, such as uneven terrain and weather. When conducting an outdoor simulation, consideration for the well-being of the participants is paramount. Appropriate attire, equipment, and back-up plans in case the educational experience needs to be relocated are essential. Some degree of discomfort should be expected, but remember Maslow's hierarchy of needs (discussed in Chapter 4, *Principles of Adult Learning*)—if a student is so uncomfortable that they cannot concentrate on the lesson, much of the learning may be lost.

Safety

Safety should be an overarching concern of educators when planning and conducting simulation sessions. Safety of the participants during simulation training is both psychological and physical. The student must feel comfortable enough to attempt to perform skills and receive feedback without risk of humiliation.[8] This means the educator must develop a high trust level with students. Realism and learning are enhanced by the perception, but not necessarily the reality, of risk. Educators must balance that perception of risk with a need for a safe learning environment. If the student perceives that the patient care or the crew safety may suffer if a mistake is made, they will be more motivated and engaged in their learning.

Physical safety is of paramount importance. Every effort should be made to safeguard against the potential injury of a simulated patient or the crew caring for them. Simple precautions, such as the use of inert medications or specialized extrication manikins, are best practices. As simulations become more realistic, it becomes more challenging to keep the risk of injury low. After all, EMS is an inherently dangerous profession, and many of the procedures and devices in EMS practice carry a high risk of injury. The educator should consider and mitigate the risks of more dangerous practices in education. It is essential, however, that EMS students practice under realistic conditions. For example, lifting a stretcher poses risk of a back injury, but graduating EMS providers who cannot perform lifts safely while still caring for patients may be of greater risk to patients and the EMS team.

All simulation sessions should include a technical and safety briefing as a part of the pre-simulation session. Students should be familiar with the equipment and explicitly told what tasks they are expected to perform versus verbalize. Whenever possible, a safety officer should be designated to monitor the simulation and alert participants to potential dangers (**FIGURE 18.3**). Students should also be given clear direction on the lifting and moving of simulated patients and the geographical and temporal boundaries of the simulation session. Whenever possible, radio communication should be performed on an education-designated channel. When education-designated channels are not available, an announcement such as "this is a drill" or similar wording should be repeated periodically throughout the simulation to avoid misunderstanding of monitored radio traffic. As mentioned earlier, it is essential that the appropriate permission be obtained and that the proper authorities and organizations are notified when simulation is taking place outdoors or in public spaces.

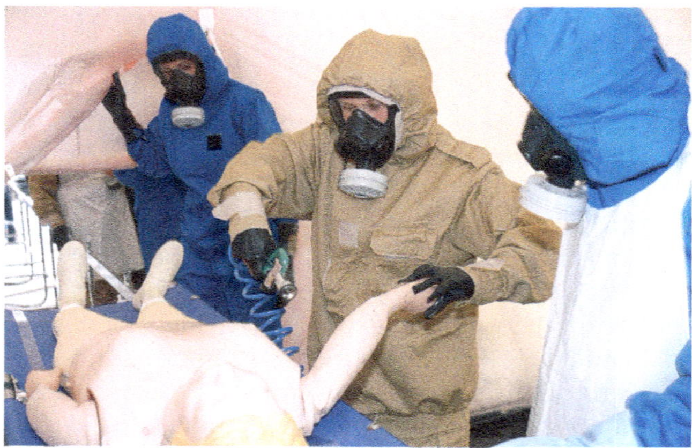

FIGURE 18.3 Every effort should be made to safeguard against potential injury to the simulated patient or to the crew caring for them.

Scenario

The scenario is the narrative or story that lays the foundation for the events that will occur within the simulation. The scenario is a combination of "who, what, where, and when" that allows the learners to establish a context within which they will perform. Often the initial scenario is presented in the form of an EMS dispatch narrative. "Medic 1 respond to 93 Elder Drive for a man down. PD is on scene." Subsequent information, also called **injects**, may be supplied by the simulated dispatcher, a facilitator, or confederates within the simulation to allow the scenario to progress with information that otherwise may not be available to the students (the progression of time, back-up or specialty unit availability).

The Scenario Template

Templates are standardized forms that can provide a framework for scenarios. These help standardize the scenario format and make it easier to quickly find key information during the simulation. Although templates are available from the major simulation companies and a variety of simulation organizations, many EMS educators ultimately adapt or develop a system for planning, delivering, and refining simulation scenarios that works best for their organization and students. At a minimum, templates should include the following elements:

- Simulation goals and objectives
- Learning/debriefing objectives
- Student knowledge/skill level
- Tasks, conditions, and standards
- Expected time in simulation
- Dispatch narrative
- Patient/scenario summary
- Pertinent patient information (i.e., demographics, medical history, etc.)
- Pertinent assessment, history, and exam findings
- Setting or environment
- **Fidelity** ("the degree to which the simulation replicates the real event and/or workplace; this includes physical, psychological, and environmental elements")[9]
- Injects (subsequent information provided as a simulation scenario progresses)
- Required equipment or supplies
- Identified roles, if extra personnel are involved
- Availability of back-up or specialty units

If summative assessment is the purpose of the simulation, the scenario template may include elements needed for assessment, including critical interventions that are expected from the candidate.

Essential to any simulation is the narrative or story line that drives the simulation. Educators must resist the temptation to create a narrative that is too ambitious or tries to do too much in the time allotted. The story line should align with the goals and learning objectives as stated in the simulation flowchart or template. The story line is a combination of dispatch information, patient information, setting, and expected interventions. The story line (sometimes called the "narrative") is a key component to any simulation. Story lines can be modeled after actual events to make them more realistic; however, care must be taken to not create a simulation that is too specific or unusual. With an established story line, anticipated branching or consequences should also be considered. *Branching* refers to the potential choices that the student may make and a preplan for the consequences of those choices. They are the "if-then" statements in a scenario that allow the person running the simulation the flexibility to respond to the actions of the students as they occur. Branching can add a level of complexity to any scenario, depending on the objectives and story line. To help the evaluator, flowcharts, matrices, or other diagrams that offer a visual map of the scenario can be created to help guide the correct pathway for decisions. Finally, the simulation narrative must be realistic and believable. While it is tempting to make a simulation epic in scale and proportion, the educator must consider the physical, material, financial, and human capital limitations that exist within their organization.

While many commercially developed simulation scenarios are available for the EMS educator, there is great value in customizing a simulation to meet the needs of the students as they exist for a specific cohort or group. The creation of a good simulation scenario is a combination of lesson plan, short story, and assessment tool. As a result, developing a customized scenario can be very time consuming. EMS educators should consider incorporating a mixture of commercially available and custom-made simulation scenarios into their curriculum.

Time Frame

The time frame should include the anticipated amount of time that will be spent in simulation and the time that will be needed to conduct a debriefing. If the EMS educator plans to run the same simulation multiple times consecutively, they must also plan time to reset the scenario. This can be a time-consuming process, as equipment must be disassembled and repackaged and computer programs reset. Although there is no rigid rule, an educator can use the guideline of allowing twice as much time for debriefing as will be spent in simulation; for example, a 20-minute simulation session should allow for 40 minutes to debrief. (However, the best approach is to pilot a simulation to get an accurate idea of the amount of time needed.) If adequate personnel exist, the resetting of the simulation can occur simultaneously with the debriefing session. The practice of videotaping simulations can add the opportunity for video debriefing, faculty assessment, and student self-assessment to the simulation education process.

Participants

When matching simulations with students, it is essential that the EMS educator properly identify the target audience. Student knowledge levels, equipment availability, provided resources (back-up and specialty units), desired outcomes or learning objectives, and as mentioned previously, the psychological and physical safety of the participants must always be taken into account.

A simulated chest pain patient created for the EMT student will involve different learner outcomes, tasks, and patient progressions than one created for the paramedic student. In addition to the level of the respondent, it is helpful for the EMS educator to know where in their education process the students are.

The matching process is particularly important when the simulation involves multiple levels of EMS providers or when students from other public safety or healthcare disciplines will participate in interdisciplinary simulations.

Standardized Patients

Often forgotten as EMS educators integrate simulation technology into their teaching is the invaluable role standardized patients play in the simulated environment. A **standardized patient** is an individual who is trained to portray a patient with a specific condition in a realistic, standardized, repeatable way. Standardized patients are ideal for scenarios in which the students need to interact with their patients (for example, scenarios that include performing patient assessment or taking a medical history). In some ways the standardized patient is the ultimate simulator and can be a valuable resource in assessment of the affective domain.

Educators should integrate the use of standardized patients into all aspects of the learning experience. However, just as preparation and organization are key in the use of simulations, they are also essential when using standardized patients in the simulated environment. Standardized patients should be carefully selected, thoroughly trained, and properly briefed on their roles and responsibilities. A script or a series of "if-then" prompts should be provided to the standardized patient so that they may respond in a uniform and consistent manner when interacting with students in the simulated environment.

The simulated scenario dictates the types of standardized patients that are appropriate. Elderly patients, patients with preexisting medical conditions (irregular heartbeat, mastectomy, amputee), and patients representing different ethnic and racial backgrounds provide the students with the ability to interact in a realistic manner with patients who are representative of the diversity of the population as a whole. Former students can greatly enhance the perceived reality, based on their own experiences of managing similar patients or having gone through the simulated scenario before. When attempting a larger scale simulation, such as a mass-casualty incident, reaching out to community groups is a great way to secure patients. The use of children as standardized patients can have a great benefit in that it exposes the students to the pediatric population. When considering the use of children, EMS educators should consider the relevant legal and safety aspects, as these differ from region to region.

Simulation is about creating events that are plausible and realistic in order to give the student the feeling of managing an actual event. An advantage of using standardized patients is that it allows the learner to experience and the educator to assess the affective domain. The real-time interaction and the ability for the student to form a relationship and have meaningful exchanges with the patient are some of the greatest benefits of using a standardized patient in a simulated EMS environment. The chance for students to receive feedback from the standardized patient is another advantage. Prehospital providers rarely receive feedback from patients. When standardized patients give feedback to the student, the student can experience what the patient sees, feels, and understands, thus enabling some insight into the affective domain of learning. Wearable skills devices can enhance the standardized patient experience by allowing clinical skills to be performed safely on the standardized patient and adding to the realism of the simulation. Balancing that, however, is the limitation on the ability to perform certain skills and assessments on the standardized patient. The greatest benefit of the high-fidelity simulator is and probably always will be the ability to perform high-acuity, low-frequency skills in an environment where the errors and mistakes that characterize learning will not have a negative impact on the well-being of the patient.

Research has shown that the use of simulation enhances teamwork and may improve patient and provider safety in the field.[10–12] The importance of this cannot be overstated. Behavior that is modeled in the classroom will result in changes in the field.[13–15] Educators who integrate simulation with a well-designed scenario, balancing high- and low-fidelity simulators with standardized patients, will create in their students a culture of teamwork and collaboration that has been shown to enhance patient safety and reduce errors.

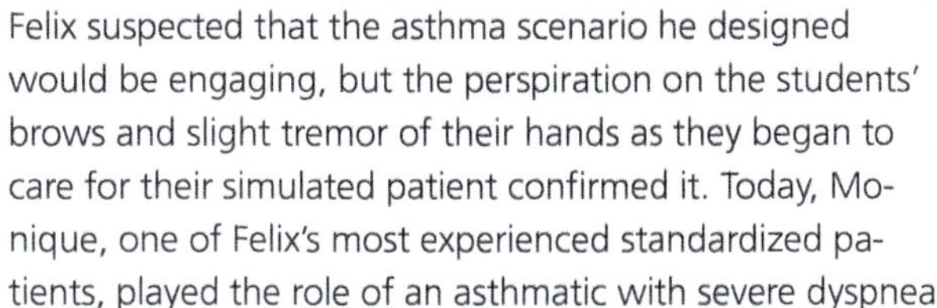

Felix suspected that the asthma scenario he designed would be engaging, but the perspiration on the students' brows and slight tremor of their hands as they began to care for their simulated patient confirmed it. Today, Monique, one of Felix's most experienced standardized patients, played the role of an asthmatic with severe dyspnea.

As the students entered the room, Monique leaned forward with her hands on her knees, clearly struggling to breathe as she answered their questions. The vest Monique wore contained speakers that perfectly conveyed her wheezing when the stethoscope was appropriately placed on her chest. The simulated monitor displayed her vital signs and ECG rhythm as they were assessed during the scenario. The students quickly administered the appropriate simulated medications and started an IV on the task trainer that was strapped to Monique's forearm.

During the debrief, the students related that they got "caught up" in the scenario and felt they were on a real call, stating they felt the pressure to provide care quickly. Monique shared that although the students were polite, as a patient she would have wanted more information about their treatments because not knowing what was happening made her feel somewhat anxious. At the end of the debrief, the students requested more simulations like this one because they felt they had learned so much. Felix knew he had really succeeded when one of the students subsequently ran a similar, real-life ambulance call and said he was able to perform well due to having experienced almost the same situation in a simulation.

TEACHING TIP

A culture of safety in the classroom and laboratory can continue to serve students well in their field practice and should be intertwined throughout the learning objectives. Even the learning objectives can be specifically targeted to safety and teamwork.

Equipment

Equipment Testing

Simulation includes various amounts and types of equipment. When conducting simulation, every effort should be made to provide all the patient care equipment required to work through the simulation. All patient care equipment should be in full working order. Equipment that is not operational can negatively affect the realism of the simulation, and can inadvertently cause a "normalization of deviance" effect, which can be a threat to patient safety.

A few days prior to the scheduled simulation activity, all equipment should be tested to ensure it is in good working order. Instructors should test the equipment in the same manner in which it will be used on lab day.

When preparing for a lab, it is a good idea to plan for as many conceivable issues as possible, but have a back-up plan. Back-up plans can include having additional (or alternate) equipment on standby in case something fails, or having an emergency classroom lesson plan that can be implemented at the last minute. Equipment failures, facility issues, and scheduling conflicts are inevitable; having a back-up plan will greatly reduce participant and instructor anxieties.

Orientation or Familiarization

Setup of the simulation is crucial to delivering a quality scenario. The use of checklists can assist in the consistency of the simulation set-up process. Simulation set-up checklists are particularly important when the simulation needs to be consistent over multiple iterations, such as in assessments. In order to successfully deliver consistent simulations, clear and concise instructions for facilitators, patients, and participants are key. Instructions must guide the facilitator as the simulation evolves and should indicate when facilitator intervention is necessary. When utilizing standardized patients, their orientation and instructions should include limits on what they can and cannot do or say, and they should provide explicit direction on how to react to certain questions, inserts, or treatments, as well as how to interact with the environment during the simulation.

It is important to ensure familiarity with equipment. Facilitators and participants should work through an orientation checklist that identifies the nuances of the scenario. The less the student has to imagine or verbalize, the more realistic the scenario. If parties are not familiarized, the flow of the scenario may be interrupted or halted, decreasing the value of the simulation experience. Ample time should be allowed for the students to familiarize themselves before they work through the scenario. A simple way to avoid unfamiliarity with the equipment is to include time for familiarization in the simulation orientation process. During a simulation **briefing**, instructions and simulation ground rules should be provided to students, including the simulation learning objectives, what is expected, available equipment, safety issues, and specifics on what is and is not permitted.

Simulation ground rules are a component of the set-up process that includes a **fiction contract** and expectations. The fiction contract is an agreement between the educator and the student to make the simulation as real as possible. The fiction contract can be explicit or implicit, but should be clearly communicated and understood by both the educator and student.

Expectations of the simulation and consequences of any assessment also need to be communicated to the students. Students must understand what is expected of them and how they are to perform during the simulation.[17] During a briefing of the students, the expectations can be reviewed and clarified. It is important to note that the briefing should be conducted away from the simulation setting and patient(s). This helps to preserve the "realness" of the simulation.

Normalization of Deviance

Normalization of deviance refers to "the gradual process through which unacceptable practice or standards become acceptable. As the deviant behavior is repeated without catastrophic results, it becomes the social norm for the organization."[16]

The theory of normalization of deviance was developed by Diane Vaughan, PhD, and was published in her book, *The Challenger Launch Decision: Risky Technology, Culture, and Deviance at NASA*.[16]

Moulage

Moulage (from the French word "to mold") supports the sensory perceptions of participants and supports the fidelity of the simulation scenario through the use of makeup, attachable artifacts (e.g., penetrating objects), and smells (**FIGURE 18.4**). Moulage can be created from commercially available kits, or, with a little creativity, many common household and construction-related items can be utilized for moulage.

Moulage is an important component to increase realism in simulation. The use of moulage can be a valuable tool in assessment-related skills and scenarios;

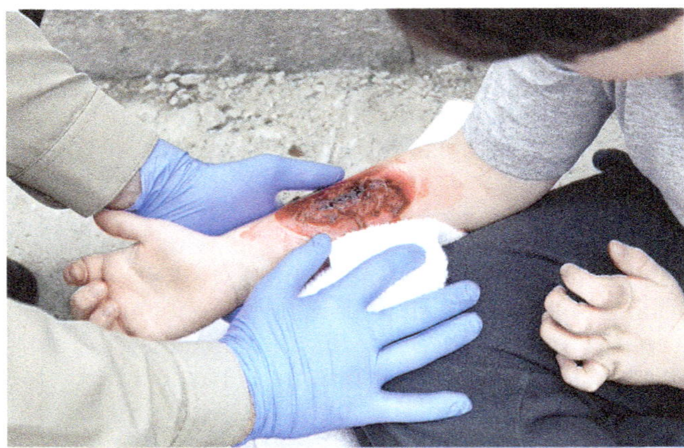

FIGURE 18.4 Moulage is an important component to increasing realism in simulation.

however, if used improperly, moulage can take away from the realism of the event. Accurate simulation of injuries creates a more realistic situation and helps participants familiarize themselves with how injuries look in a real-world situation.[18]

Both standardized patients and manikins can be moulaged to change appearances or show various types of trauma (bruising, open fractures, burns). Moulaging patients and manikins takes time, but it is essential to realism. Moulage can be as simple as applying dirt to a standardized patient or as complicated as creating an actively bleeding multiwound trauma patient. The art and science of moulage are constantly expanding, as evidenced by the numerous textbooks and specialty courses available. As mentioned previously, it is important to avoid the pitfalls of overdramatization and unrealistic expectations in simulation design; thus, balancing the "cool factor" of moulage with the realism effect needed for the simulation is a vital component of the simulation design.

Simulators

High-tech manikins are controlled by computers. They are capable of modeling the wide range of physiological states of adults, children, and infants and of replicating complex disease processes and injury patterns. These capabilities allow students to experience a broad range of patient presentations and practice a wide range of sophisticated and invasive procedures, such as chest decompression, medication administration, and surgical cricothyrotomy without the risks associated with practicing on human patients.[19,20] These high-fidelity simulators can display realistic assessment findings, including heart and lung sounds, cardiac rhythm disturbances, and other vital sign alterations. They are capable of responding to student interventions in a realistic manner, including airway management and medication administration. From the earliest CPR and airway manikins to today's high-fidelity simulators capable of realistic oxygen/carbon dioxide exchange, simulation in health care has progressed enormously. This rapidly evolving industry is developing technology that has been proven highly effective in achieving EMS educational goals.[5,21,22]

Sophisticated simulator technology can be costly.[23] Simulators and task trainers (isolated body parts that allow students to practice specific psychomotor tasks) can run from four to six figures in cost. Task trainers may use mechanical or electronic interfaces to teach and give feedback on manual skills. They generally are used to support procedural skills training; however, they can also be used in conjunction with other learning technologies to create integrated clinical situations.[9] Other costs can include maintenance contracts, parts and rebuild kits, audio/visual equipment, information technology hardware and software, media storage, moulage, props, and infrastructure, as well as training that allows educators to utilize simulation in the appropriate learning environments.

Often one of the most expensive costs is the investment an institution or organization must make in human capital—investing funds and time for the personnel to maintain, create, and facilitate learning experiences in the simulated environment. Unfortunately, the human resources and time required to preprogram and operate simulators are often underestimated. It is not uncommon for simulation programs to suffer serious setbacks when a simulation champion leaves the institution, taking invaluable simulation expertise and knowledge. To make an active simulation lab fully operational, many institutions hire full-time simulation operations specialists or other personnel.[5,23–26]

Equipment Cleaning, Repair, and Maintenance

At the end of each lab session, every piece of equipment should be thoroughly cleaned and inspected for damage or worn parts. It is important to ensure that all cleaning and maintenance practices are in alignment with manufacturer guidelines. Equipment that is damaged to the extent that would potentially prevent its proper functioning should be tagged, reported, and taken out of service.

Many manikin-related and task trainer repairs can be accomplished with simple hand tools and the proper replacement parts. More complex medical equipment such as suction machines, stretchers, ventilators, and cardiac monitors should be repaired only by qualified repair technicians.

Simulation can be hard on manikins, and the importance of proper maintenance cannot be emphasized enough. Common manikin failures from wear-and-tear can be avoided by establishing a regularly scheduled maintenance program and utilizing a standard checklist for simulation set-up. The manufacturers of simulators offer maintenance packages that can help with wear-and-tear issues. These can range from primary purchase warranties to post-warranty maintenance plans.

TEACHING TIP

Whenever learning about simulation methodologies or techniques, the educator should seek guidance from multiple sources (triangulate). Taking one source as gospel will lead an educator to trouble. Triangulate and ground practice in validated standards.

Endpoints and Assessment

During the simulation, the facilitator assumes the role of the silent observer whenever possible. The facilitator's role is to facilitate the natural progression of the simulation by injecting information and coordinating actions with the operations specialist (in the event that the facilitator is not also functioning as the operations specialist) to provide a realistic simulation experience that allows the learners to suspend disbelief and immerse themselves in the simulation environment.

Simulation should move toward a specified endpoint or conclusion. This could be identified as the specified physiological presentation or patient status, or it could be when a certain set of objectives or learner outcomes are (or are not) realized or achieved. Allowing enough time for the student to attempt performance, even if the student seems to struggle, is important, as valuable learning and confidence-building can occur. If the student or team exhibits signs of extreme struggle or frustration, then careful mid-scenario guidance may be appropriate, or ultimately, it may be necessary to stop the simulation in favor of a more productive debriefing.

Prompting during a summative assessment simulation should be kept to a minimum. Some prompting may be needed to continue the evolution. The amount of necessary prompts depends on the type of simulation being conducted (formative vs. summative). Limited prompting is an important part of the learning process, as it forces the student to apply critical-reasoning and problem-solving skills, which is one of the major goals and benefits of simulation.

TEACHING TIP

Whenever an action has the potential to compromise the safety of the participants, standardized patients, or confederates, the educator must intervene.

TEACHING TIP

It is appropriate for the educator to intervene when initially teaching a motor skill. However, during simulation, the educator should avoid intervening during performance, instead opting to discuss later during the debriefing session.

It has been shown that participant performance during a scenario can be enhanced by using checklists during and after the scenario to ensure key points are discussed.[27] Checklists to score scenario performance have been used by the American Heart Association (AHA) for Advanced Cardiac Life Support protocols since 2003. Using the checklists in simulation-based education showed a 40% increase in adherence to AHA protocols after training, and an improvement in performance in simulation and patient care.[28]

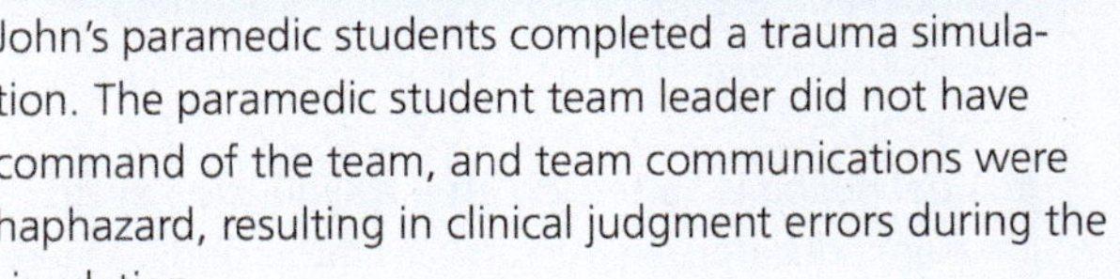

CASE in Point

John's paramedic students completed a trauma simulation. The paramedic student team leader did not have command of the team, and team communications were haphazard, resulting in clinical judgment errors during the simulation.

As John begins the debriefing for the simulation, he knows he will need to address these problems and highlight key elements to help the students understand how these issues occur and what can be done to avoid them in the future.

Utilizing the Debriefing for Meaningful Learning (DML) method,[29] John facilitates a consistent, reflective process. Working through the six phases of DML (engage, explore, explain, elaborate, evaluate, and extend) fosters deep thinking that drives the students and faculty to reflect on the experience as they strive to make sense of the simulation and improve their understanding of the experience. The debriefing leads to increased reasoning and meaningful learning, while preparing the students for future patient experiences.

Debriefing

The debriefing period can be one of the most beneficial components of the simulation experience, for both the student and the educator.[27] During the debriefing session, students are given the opportunity to examine, reflect on, and discuss the simulation experience. Because simulation challenges the students' perspectives or preconceived ideas on how situations should be managed, learning is facilitated. During the debriefing, instructors should promote student reflections on action and inaction, as they are key components of experiential learning. While the simulation itself may have been rich in content and experience, without a thorough and purposeful debriefing, much of the learning may be lost.[28,30] A variety of simulation debriefing models are available for the EMS educator to utilize in debriefing simulations. A few examples of debriefing models include Plus/Delta, Advocacy and Inquiry, Debriefing Assessment for Simulation in Healthcare (DASH), and Debriefing for Meaningful Learning (DML). The use of a particular debriefing model is a choice that each educator should make based on the simulation process, the desired outcomes, and the educator's experience.

Debriefing versus Feedback

Debriefing and feedback are distinguished from each other as follows:

- *Feedback* is an activity in which information is relayed back to a learner. It should be constructive, should address specific aspects of the learner's performance, and be focused on the learning objectives.[9]
- A *debriefing* is "a session after a simulation event where educators/instructors/facilitators and learners reexamine the simulation experience for the purpose of moving toward assimilation and accommodation of learning to future situations."[9,31]

TEACHING TIP

Examples of questions an educator can pose during simulation debriefing include the following:

- How did the learning activity go?
- What did you gain?
- What feedback do other participants have?
- Let's discuss the challenges.

To enhance the debriefing experience, educators may opt to use recording devices to capture some elements or the entirety of the simulation.[32] The use of video, audio, and vital sign display when recording simulation sessions can provide valuable, detailed feedback to students after the simulation. There are times when students may not be able to accurately recall all the events of the simulation, or their perception of what occurred during the simulation may be inaccurate. Therefore, these tools can help facilitate the self-reflection process.

To help students recognize the learning points that arise from the simulation, students should be encouraged to engage in self-reflection of the events of the simulation. Self-reflection provides students with the opportunity to consider their actions and inactions, and how they fit into the overall picture of the simulation.[33] Providing students this opportunity prepares them for events they may encounter in their future work in the field.

Because simulation is about learning to manage and treat actual cases, applying the lessons learned during the simulation to similar events can facilitate student understanding.[34] This practical approach gives the EMS educator the ability to facilitate educational opportunities that can have a direct impact on improving patient safety and care.

Summary

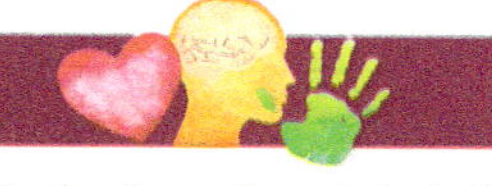

The use of simulation in EMS education can have a positive impact on the student's critical decision-making skills, psychomotor skills, emotions, attitudes, and competency levels. Learning occurs when students are faced with a "crisis," which then forces them to alter their frame of understanding and think critically about their actions.[35–41] These stressors and student responses should be addressed during the debriefing phase of the simulation.

Simulation allows EMS educators to standardize the learning experience with a uniform and consistent method of evaluating competency. While students and health professionals in training are required to meet the same criteria for performance and competence, the variable nature of health care and the unique presentation and dynamic of any patient care interaction or situation make it difficult to measure competence or success based on performance in the clinical environment. Simulation enables educators to gather objective evidence of performance and map the learner's "trajectory"[37] with a great degree of detail and specificity. In a simulated environment, errors can be tracked and the simulation be repeatedly "rewound and restarted"[38] until proficiency is achieved. The ability to standardize the learning experience also enables the educator or institution to evaluate its processes and teaching methodology.[39]

Proper planning, preparation, facilitation, and debriefing are all essential elements of simulation. Each is important to ensure that students have a meaningful and safe learning simulation experience that promotes key learning objectives. Simulation experiences are another tool to advance student learning within the EMS setting.

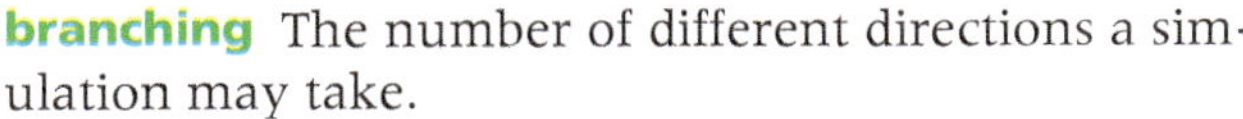

Glossary

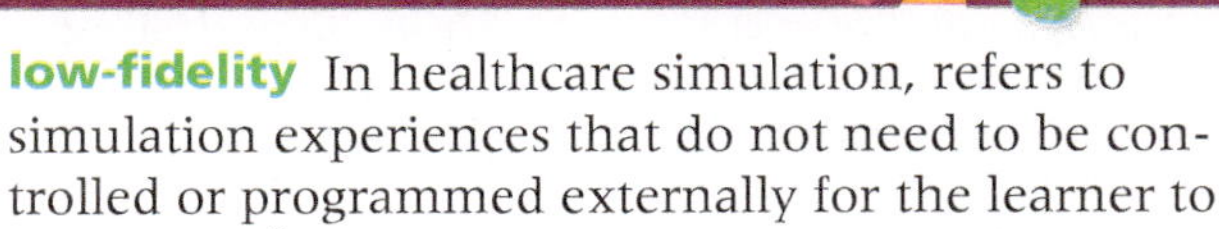

branching The number of different directions a simulation may take.

briefing Activity immediately preceding the start of a simulation activity where the participants receive essential information about the simulation scenario such as background, information, vital signs, instructions, or guidelines.[9]

confederates Individuals other than the patient (for example, a simulated family member or bystander) who are scripted in a simulation to provide realism, additional challenges, or additional information for the learner.[9]

debriefing Session conducted after a simulation event where educators/instructors/facilitators and learners reexamine the simulation experience for the purpose of moving toward assimilation and accommodation of learning to apply in future situations.[9]

fiction contract Agreement between the educator and the student to make the simulation as real as possible.

fidelity Degree to which the simulation replicates the real event and/or workplace; this includes physical, psychological, and environmental elements.[9]

high-fidelity In healthcare simulation, refers to simulation experiences that are extremely realistic and provide a high level of interactivity and realism for the learner.[9]

injects Information provided by a simulated dispatcher, a facilitator, or confederates within a simulation that allows the scenario to progress with information that otherwise may not be available to the students.

low-fidelity In healthcare simulation, refers to simulation experiences that do not need to be controlled or programmed externally for the learner to participate.[9]

moulage Techniques such as use of makeup, attachable artifacts, or smells used to simulate injury, disease, aging, and other physical characteristics specific to a scenario.

on-the-fly programming Simulation programming that allows the educator to manipulate the program software in response to student decisions and interventions.

scenarios In healthcare simulation, descriptions of a simulation that includes the goals, objectives, debriefing points, narrative description of the clinical simulation, staff requirements, simulation room set-up, simulators, props, simulator operation, and instructions for standardized patients.[9]

simulation Technique that creates a situation or environment to allow students to experience a representation of a real event for the purpose of practice, learning, assessment, or testing, or to gain an understanding of systems or human actions.[9]

standardized patient Individual trained to portray a patient with a specific condition in a realistic, standardized, and repeatable way and where portrayal/presentation varies based only on learner performance.[9]

task trainer Model of a part or region of the human body, such as an arm or abdomen, that may use mechanical or electronic interfaces to allow students to practice specific psychomotor tasks such as IV insertion, ultrasound scanning, suturing, etc.[9]

time-in-simulation Amount of time spent in a simulation activity.[9]

References

[1] McGaghie, William C., Saul Barry Issenberg, Emil Petrusa, and Ross J. Scalese. 2010. "A Critical Review of Simulation-Based Medical Education Research: 2003–2009." *Medical Education* 44, no. 1: 50–63. https://doi.org/10.1111/j.1365-2923.2009.03547.x.

[2] Gaba, David M. 2004. "The Future Vision of Simulation in Health and Care." *BMJ Quality and Safety* 13: i2–10. http://dx.doi.org/10.1136/qshc.2004.009878.

[3] DeGiusti, Marisa R., Ariel J. Lira, and Gonzalo L. Villareal. 2008. "Simulation Framework for Teaching in Modeling and Simulation Areas." *European Journal of Engineering Education* 33, no. 5–6: 587–96. https://doi.org/10.1080/03043790802568138.

[4] Schneider Sarver, Patricia A., Elizabeth A. Senczakowicz, and Bernadette M. Slovensky. 2010. "Development of Simulation Scenarios for an Adolescent Patient with Diabetic Ketoacidosis." *Journal of Nursing Education* 49, no. 10: 578–86. https://doi.org/10.3928/01484834-20100630-07.

[5] King, Jason M., and Deanna L. Reising. 2011. "Teaching Advanced Cardiac Life Support Protocols: The Effectiveness of Static versus High-Fidelity Simulation." *Nurse Educator* 36, no. 2: 62–5. http://dx.doi.org/10.1097/NNE.0b013e31820b5012.

[6] Wotton, Karen, Jordana Davis, Didy Button, and Moira Kelton. 2010. "Third-Year Undergraduate Nursing Students' Perceptions of High-Fidelity Simulation." *Journal of Nursing Education* 49, no. 11: 632–9. https://doi.org/10.3928/01484834-20100831-01.

[7] Nehring, Wendy M., and Felissa R. Lashley. 2010. *High-Fidelity Patient Simulation in Nursing Education*. Burlington, MA: Jones and Bartlett Publishers.

[8] Blum, Cynthia A., Susan Borglund, and Dax Parcells. 2010. "High-Fidelity Nursing Simulation: Impact on Student Self-confidence and Clinical Competence." *International Journal of Nursing Education* 7, no. 1: 1–14. https://doi.org/10.2202/1548-923X.2035.

[9] Lopreiato, Joseph O. 2016. *Healthcare Simulation Dictionary*. AHRQ Publications No. 16(17)-0043. Rockville, MD: Agency for Healthcare Research and Quality.

[10] Kozmenko, Valeriy, John T. Paige, and Sheila Chauvin. 2008. "Initial Implementation of Mixed Reality Simulation Targeting Teamwork and Patient Safety." *Studies in Health Technology and Informatics* 132: 216–21.

[11] Herzer, Kurt R., Jose M. Rodriguez-Paz, Peter A. Doyle, Paul W. Flint, David J. Feller-Kopman, Joseph Herman, Robert E. Bristow, Renee Cover, Peter J. Pronovost, Lynette J. Mark. 2009. "A Practical Framework for Patient Care Teams to Prospectively Identify and Mitigate Clinical Hazards." *The Joint Commission Journal on Quality and Patient Safety* 35, no. 2: 72–81. https://doi.org/10.1016/S1553-7250(09)35010-2.

[12] Berkenstadt, Haim, Yael Haviv, Atalia Tuval, Yael Shemesh, Alexander Megrill, Amir Perry, Orit Rubin, and Amitai Ziv. 2008. "Improving Handoff Communications in Critical Care: Utilizing Simulation-Based Training toward Process Improvement in Managing Patient Risk." *Chest* 134, no. 1: 158–62. https://doi.org/10.1378/chest.07-0914.

[13] Wayne, Diane B., John Butter, Viva J. Siddall, Monica J. Fudala, Leonard D. Wade, Joe Feinglass, and William C. McGaghie. 2006. "Mastery Learning of Advanced Cardiac Life Support Skills by Internal Medicine Residents Using Simulation Technology and Deliberate Practice." *Journal General Internal Medicine* 21: 251–6. https://doi.org/10.1111/j.1525-1497.2006.00341.x.

[14] Batchelder, Andrew J., Allan K. Steel, Regina Mackenzie, Anil P Hormis, Taumi S. Daniels, and N. Holding. 2009. "Simulation as a Tool to Improve the Safety of Pre-hospital Anaesthesia: A Pilot Study." *Anaesthesia* 64, no. 9: 978–83. https://doi.org/10.1111/j.1365-2044.2009.05990.x.

[15] Rosenthal, Marnie E., Mari Adachi, Vanessa Ribaudo, J. Tristan Mueck, Roslyn F. Schneider, and Paul H. Mayo. 2006. "Achieving Housestaff Competence in Emergency Airway Management Using Scenario-Based Simulation Training." *Chest* 129: 1453–8. https://doi.org/10.1378/chest.129.6.1453.

[16] Vaughan, Diane. 1996. *The Challenger Launch Decision: Risky Technology, Culture, and Deviance at NASA*. Chicago: University of Chicago Press.

[17] Simones, Joyce, Joan Wilcox, Kim Scott, Darci Goeden, Darlene Copley, Renee Doetkott, and Margaret Kippley. 2010. "Collaborative Simulation Project to Teach Scope of Practice." *Journal of Nursing Education* 49, no. 4: 190–7. https://doi.org/10.3928/01484834-20091217-01.

[18] Ralston, Emerald. 2008, June 5. "Fake Wounds Bring Reality to Training Scenarios through Moulage." *Malmstrom Air Force Base*. https://www.malmstrom.af.mil/News/Features/Display/Article/349844/fake-wounds-bring-reality-to-training-scenarios-through-moulage/.

[19] Chandra, Deven B., Georges L. Savoldelli, Hwan S. Joo, Israel D. Weiss, and Viren N. Naik. 2008. "Fiberoptic Oral Intubation: The Effect of Model Fidelity on Training for Transfer to Patient Care." *Anesthesiology* 109, no. 6: 1007–13. http://dx.doi.org/10.1097/ALN.0b013e31818d6c3c.

[20] Cooper, Jeffrey B., and David Murray. 2010. "Simulation Training and Assessment: A More Efficient Method to Develop Expertise than Apprenticeship." *Anesthesiology* 112, no. 1: 8–9. http://dx.doi.org/10.1097/ALN.0b013e3181c62a1a.

[21] Gillett, Brian, Brad Peckler, Richard Sinert, Cherie Onkst, Spencer Nabors, Steven Issley, Christopher Maguire, Sagar Galwankarm, and Bonnie Arquilla. 2008. "Simulation in a Disaster Drill: Comparison of High-Fidelity Simulators versus Trained Actors." *Academic Emergency Medicine* 15, no. 11: 1144–51. https://doi.org/10.1111/j.1553-2712.2008.00198.x.

[22] Fritz, Peter Z., Tim Gray, and Brendan Flanagan. 2008. "Review of Mannequin-Based High-Fidelity Simulation in Emergency Medicine." *Emergency Medicine Australasia* 20, no. 1: 1–9. https://doi.org/10.1111/j.1742-6723.2007.01022.x.

[23] Weinstock, Peter H., Liana Kappus, Alexander Garden, and Jeffrey Burns. 2009. "Simulation at the Point of Care: Reduced-Cost, In Situ Training via a Mobile Cart." *Pediatric Critical Care Medicine* 10, no. 2: 176–81. http://dx.doi.org/10.1097/PCC.0b013e3181956c6f.

[24] Tuoriniemi, Pamela, and Darlene Schott-Baer. 2008. "Implementing a High-Fidelity Simulation Program in a Community College Setting." *Nursing Education Perspective* 29, no. 2: 105–9.

[25] Parker, Brian C., and Florence Myrick. 2009. "A Critical Examination of High-Fidelity Human Patient Simulation within the Context of Nursing Pedagogy." *Nurse Education Today* 29, no. 3: 322–9. https://doi.org/10.1016/j.nedt.2008.10.012.

[26] McKenna, Kim D., Elliot Carhart, Daniel Bercher, Andrew E. Spain, John Todaro, and Joann Freel. 2015. "Simulation Use in Paramedic Education Research (SUPER): A Descriptive Study." *Prehospital Emergency Care* 19, no. 3: 432–40. https://doi.org/10.3109/10903127.2014.995845.

[27] Andersen, Peter O., Michael K. Jensen, Anne Lippert, Doris Østergaard, and Tobias W. Klausen. 2010. "Development of a

Formative Assessment Tool for Measurement of Performance in Multi-professional Resuscitation Teams." *Resuscitation* 81: 703–11. https://doi.org/10.1016/j.resuscitation.2010.01.034.

[28] Elfrink, Victoria L., Bonnie Kirkpatrick, Jami Nininger, and Carolyn Schubert. 2010. "Using Learning Outcomes to Inform Teaching Practices in Human Patient Simulation." *Nursing Education Perspective* 31, no. 2: 970100.

[29] Dreifurest, Kristina T. 2015. "Getting Started with Debriefing for Meaningful Learning." *Clinical Simulation in Nursing* 11, no. 5: 268–75. https://doi.org/10.1016/j.ecns.2015.01.005.

[30] Carlson, Jim, John Tomkowiak, and Patrick T. Knott. 2010. "Simulation-Based Examinations in Physician Assistant Education: A Comparison of Two Standard Setting Methods." *Journal of Physician Assistant Education* 21, no. 2: 7–14.

[31] Johnson-Russell, Judy, and Catherine Bailey. 2010. "Facilitated Debriefing." In *High-Fidelity Patient Simulation in Nursing Education*, edited by Wendy M. Nehring and Felissa R. Lashley, 369–85. Burlington, MA: Jones and Bartlett Publishers.

[32] Leonard, Brenda, Elaine L. H. Shuhaibar, and Ruth Chen. 2010. "Nursing-Student Perceptions of Intraprofessional Team Education Using High-Fidelity Simulation." *Journal of Nursing Education* 49, no. 11: 628–31. https://doi.org/10.3928/01484834-20100730-06.

[33] Birkhoff, Susan D., and Carol Donner. 2010. "Enhancing Pediatric Clinical Competency with High-Fidelity Simulation." *Journal of Continuing Education in Nursing* 41, no. 9: 418–23. https://doi.org/10.3928/00220124-20100503-03.

[34] Harder, B. Nicole. 2010. "Use of Simulation in Teaching and Learning in Health Sciences: A Systematic Review." *Journal of Nursing Education* 49, no. 1: 23–8. https://doi.org/10.3928/01484834-20090828-08.

[35] McLaughlin, Michael P. 2010. "Medical Simulation in the Community College Health Science Curriculum: A Matrix for Future Implementation." *Community College Journal of Research and Practice* 34, 462–476. https://doi.org/10.1080/10668920903235811.

[36] Parker, Brian N., and Florence Myrick. 2010. "Transformative Learning as a Context for Human Patient Simulation." *Journal of Nursing Education* 49, no. 6: 326–32. https://doi.org/10.3928/01484834-20100224-02.

[37] Kneebone, Roger. 2003. "Simulation in Surgical Training: Educational Issues and Practical Implications." *Medical Education* 37: 267–77. https://doi.org/10.1046/j.1365-2923.2003.01440.x.

[38] Dawson, Steven. 2002. "A Critical Approach to Medical Simulation." *Bulletin of the American College of Surgeons* 87, no. 11: 12–8.

[39] Hammond, Jeffrey, Mordechai Bermann, Bo Chen, Lawrence Kushins. 2002. "Incorporation of a Computerized Human Patient Simulator in Critical Care Training: A Preliminary Report." *Journal of Trauma* 53: 1064–7.

[40] McCarthy, Jennifer, Amar P. Patel, Andrew E. Spain, and Timothy Whitaker. 2017. "A Guide to Integrating Simulation into EMS Education." *Journal of Emergency Medical Services* 42, no 2. http://www.jems.com/articles/print/volume-42/issue-2/departments-columns/successful-simulation/a-guide-to-integrating-simulation-into-ems-education.html.

[41] McKenna, Kim D., Elliot Carhart, Daniel Bercher, Andrew E. Spain, John Todaro, and Joann Freel. 2016. "Interprofessional Simulation in Accredited Paramedic Programs." *The Internet Journal of Allied Health Sciences and Practice* 14, no. 2: Article 6.

Additional Resources

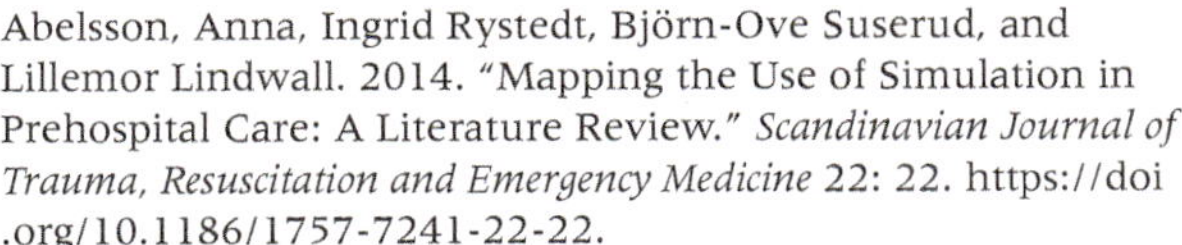

Abelsson, Anna, Ingrid Rystedt, Björn-Ove Suserud, and Lillemor Lindwall. 2014. "Mapping the Use of Simulation in Prehospital Care: A Literature Review." *Scandinavian Journal of Trauma, Resuscitation and Emergency Medicine* 22: 22. https://doi.org/10.1186/1757-7241-22-22.

Adamson, Katie A., and Suzan Kardong-Edgren. 2012. "A Method and Resources for Assessing the Reliability of Simulation Evaluation Instruments." *Nursing Education Perspectives* 33, no. 5: 335–9.

Alexander, Maryann, Carol F. Durham, Janice I. Hooper, Pamela R. Jeffries, Nathan Goldman, Suzan Kardong-Edgren, Karen S. Kesten, et al. 2015. "National Council of State Boards of Nursing (NCSBN) Simulation Guidelines for Prelicensure Nursing Programs." *Journal of Nursing Regulation* 6, no. 3: 39–42.

Association of Standardized Patient Educators (ASPE) website. https://www.aspeducators.org/.

Dalski, Chester L. 2014. "Paramedic Professional and Leadership Development Using High-Fidelity Healthcare Simulation and Audiovisual Feedback: One Michigan Community College Case Study." Dissertation, Andrews University. http://pqdtopen.proquest.com/doc/1647466079.html?FMT=ABS.

Foronda, Cynthia, Siwei Liu, and Eric B. Bauman. 2013. "Evaluation of Simulation in Undergraduate Nurse Education: An Integrative Review." *Clinical Simulation in Nursing* 9, no. 19: e409–16. https://doi.org/10.1016/j.ecns.2012.11.003.

Fraser, Kristin L., Paul Ayres, and John Sweller. 2015. "Cognitive Load Theory for the Design of Medical Simulations." *Simulation in Healthcare* 10, no. 5: 295–307. http://dx.doi.org/10.1097/SIH.0000000000000097.

Hatala, Rose, David A. Cook, Benjamin Zendejas, Stanley J. Hamstra, and Ryan Brydges. 2014. "Feedback for Simulation-Based Procedural Skills Training: A Meta-analysis and Critical Narrative Synthesis." *Advances in Health Science Education* 19: 251–72. https://doi.org/10.1007/s10459-013-9462-8.

Hayden, Jennifer K., Richard A. Smiley, Maryann Alexander, Suzan Kardong-Edgren, and Pamela R. Jeffries. 2014. "The NCSBN National Simulation Study: A Longitudinal, Randomized, Controlled Study Replacing Clinical Hours with Simulation in Prelicensure Nursing Education." *Journal of Nursing Regulation* 5, no. 29 (Suppl): S1–64.

INACSL Standards Committee. 2017. "INACSL Standards of Best Practice: Simulation: Operations." *Clinical Simulation in Nursing* 13, no. 12: 681–7. https://doi.org/10.1016/j.ecns.2017.10.005.

Jeffries, Pamela R. 2005. "A Framework for Designing, Implementing, and Evaluating Simulations Used as Teaching Strategies in Nursing." *Nursing Education Perspectives* 26, no. 2: 96–103.

Jeffries, Pamela R. 2014. *Clinical Simulation in Nursing Education: Advanced Concepts, Trends, and Opportunities*. Philadelphia: Wolters Kluwer, Lippincott Williams & Wilkins.

Jeffries, Pamela R. 2012. *Simulation in Nursing Education from Conceptualization to Evaluation*. Philadelphia: Lippincott Williams & Wilkins.

Kenney, Johanna K. 2014. "The Future of Simulations in Allied Healthcare Education and Training a Modified Delphi Study Identifying Their Instructional and Technical Feasibility." Dissertation, University of Florida. http://ufdc.ufl.edu/UFE0046484/00001.

Leggio, William J., and Kenneth J. D'Alessandro. 2015. "Support for Interdisciplinary Approaches in Emergency Medical Services Education." *Creighton Journal of Interdisciplinary Leadership* 1, no. 1: 60–65.

Lewis, Karen L., Carrie A. Bohnert, Wendy L. Gammon, Henrike Hölzer, Lorraine Lyman, Cathy Smith, Tonya M. Thompson, Amelia Wallace, and Gayle Gliva-McConvey. 2017. "The Association of Standardized Patient Educators (ASPE): Standards of Best Practice (SOBP)." *Advances in Simulation* 2: 10. https://doi.org/10.1186/s41077-017-0043-4.

Lioce, Lori, Clinta Che Reed, Debora Lemon, Michalene A. King, Petra A. Martinez, Ashley E. Franklin, Teri Boese, et al. 2013. "Standards of Best Practice: Simulation Standard III: Participant Objectives." *Clinical Simulation in Nursing* 9, no. 6: S15–8. https://doi.org/10.1016/j.ecns.2013.04.005.

McGaghie, William C., Saul B. Issenberg, Jeffrey H. Barsuk, and Diane B. Wayne. 2014. "A Critical Review of Simulation-Based Mastery Learning with Translational Outcomes." *Medical Education* 48, no. 4: 375–85. https://doi.org/10.1111/medu.12391.

NAEMSE Trading Post. https://naemse.org/default.aspx.

Page, David and Bill Robertson. 2016, February 29. "Applying Cognitive Load Theory to Design Effective Simulation Training." *Journal of Emergency Medical Services* [online]. http://www.jems.com/articles/print/volume-41/issue-3/departments-columns/research-review/applying-cognitive-load-theory-to-design-effective-simulation-training.html.

Palaganas, Janice C., Juli C. Maxworthy, Chad A. Epps, and Mary E. Mancini. 2015. *Defining Excellence in Simulation Programs*. Philadelphia: Wolters Kluwer, Lippincott Williams & Wilkins, and Society for Simulation in Healthcare.

Patel Amar P. 2016, July 1. "How Simulation Can Refine Individual and Team Skills and Competencies." *Journal of Emergency Medical Services* [online]. http://www.jems.com/articles/print/volume-41/issue-7/features/how-simulation-can-refine-individual-and-team-skills-and-competencies.htm.

Patel, Amar P., Donald Garner, and David Crosby. 2015, September 4. "Removing the Barriers That Prohibit Using Simulation in EMS." *Journal of Emergency Medical Services* [online]. http://www.jems.com/articles/print/volume-40/issue-9/features/removing-the-barriers-that-prohibit-using-simulation-in-ems.html.

Pinar, Gul. 2015. "Simulation-Enhanced Interprofessional Education in Health Care." *Creative Education* 6: 1852–9. https://doi.org/10.4236/ce.2015.617189.

National Association of EMS Educators (NAEMSE). 2015, November 18. "Simulation in EMS Education: Charting the Future." https://c.ymcdn.com/sites/naemse.site-ym.com/resource/resmgr/Docs/SimPressRelease15.pdf.

Society for Simulation in Healthcare. 2018. "Certified Healthcare Simulation Educator Examination Blueprint, 2018 Version." https://www.ssih.org/Portals/48/Certification/CHSE_Docs/CHSE_Examination_Blueprint.pdf.

Society for Simulation in Healthcare. 2019. "Certified Healthcare Simulation Operations Specialist." https://www.ssih.org/Certification/CHSOS.

Society for Simulation in Healthcare. n.d. "SSH Accreditation of Healthcare Simulation Programs." https://www.ssih.org/Accreditation.

Studnek, Jonathan R., Antonio R. Fernandez, Brian Shimberg, Melissa Garifo, and Michelle Correll. 2011. "The Association between Emergency Medical Services Field Performance Assessed by High-Fidelity Simulation and the Cognitive Knowledge of Practicing Paramedics." *Academic Emergency Medicine* 18: 1177–85. https://doi.org/10.1111/j.1553-2712.2011.01208.x.

Tavares, Walter, Vicki R. LeBlanc, Justin Mausz, Victor Sun, and Kevin W. Eva, 2013. "Simulation-based Assessment of Paramedics and Performance in Real Clinical Contexts." *Prehospital Emergency Care* 18, no. 1: 116–22. https://doi.org/10.3109/10903127.2013.818178.

Ulrich, Beth, and Mary E. Mancini. 2014. *Mastering Simulation: A Handbook for Success*. Indianapolis: Sigma Theta Tau International Honor Society of Nursing.

Wilhaus, Janet, Janice Palaganas, Jennifer Manos, JoDee Anderson, Alan Cooper, Pamela Jeffries, Mary Anne Rizzolo, Elaine Tagliareni, and Mary Elizabeth Mancini. 2012. "Interprofessional Education and Healthcare Simulation Symposium Report." http://www.nln.org/docs/default-source/professional-development-programs/white-paper-symposium-ipe-in-healthcare-simulation-2013-(pdf).pdf?sfvrsn=0.

CHAPTER 19

Tools for Field and Clinical Learning

OBJECTIVES

At the conclusion of this chapter, the educator will be able to:

Cognitive Domain

1. Describe the role of the clinical educator and field preceptor in the student's experiential learning process.
2. Describe the importance of the clinical educator and field preceptor in the determination of a student's entry-level competency.
3. Explain the importance of the clinical and field experiences to prepare students for the capstone/field internship experience.
4. Explain differences in the clinical and field experiences between emergency medical responder (EMR), emergency medical technician (EMT), advanced EMT (AEMT), and paramedic students.
5. Explain the benefits of experiential learning in the clinical and field settings.
6. Describe the attributes of an effective clinical educator.
7. Identify the job requirements and training for an effective clinical educator and field preceptor.
8. Describe the importance of the roles of the clinical educator and field preceptor in the students' learning process.
9. Compare and contrast clinical teaching strategies that promote critical thinking skills for students in clinical and field experiences.
10. Describe the benefits of preceptor training and how training affects student outcomes.
11. Compare and contrast the roles of the student as a team member versus a team leader in the clinical and field environment.
12. Discuss the challenges and solutions in tracking student experiences in the clinical and field environment.

Psychomotor Domain

There are no psychomotor objectives for this chapter.

Affective Domain

1. Value the clinical educator, preceptor, and student's documentation in relationship to teaching and assessing student competency in the clinical and field environments.
2. Explain the value of timely constructive feedback and how feedback fosters critical thinking and lifelong learning.

"Experience develops all our great flute players, but also unfortunately, all our worst players."

~ Plato

CHAPTER GOAL This chapter explores instructional theory and strategy focusing specifically on clinical education, that is, education that is experiential and involves the student's observing, participating in, or leading patient care activities in actual hospital or field patient care settings.

Clinical education is an essential component of emergency medical services (EMS) education, and the clinical educator may be the most influential teacher an EMS student will ever have.[1–3] The terms used to describe educators who work with students in real patient care environments are diverse: mentors, preceptors, practice educators, and field training officers (FTOs).[4] For the purposes of this chapter, **clinical educator** refers to a patient care practitioner who guides experiential learning during real patient care.

A theory-to-practice gap has been well documented by advances in allied health education research. This gap is described as the difference between "best-practice ideals and values that are taught and those actually encountered in everyday practice."[5,6] The goal of effective clinical educators is to help transition a student from the theoretical environment of the classroom to the real world of patient care delivery.

In addition to being a role model, coach, mentor, assessor, and clinical skills expert, the clinical educator must be able to recognize and take advantage of opportunities for the student to assess patients, make decisions, direct the team of caregivers, and perform skills.[7] The clinical educator helps the learner glean the right lesson from existing circumstances. These are so-called teachable moments that create long-lasting retention of student learning.

Both employers and patients expect graduates of EMS educational programs to be competent healthcare providers.[8] Theoretical knowledge and discrete psychomotor skills, although important, are simply not sufficient to prepare someone to work in the hospital or field environment.[7,9] To achieve entry-level competency and some degree of confidence, EMS students, especially paramedic students, must perform as team members and team leaders during real patient care situations.[10,11]

The previous chapters of this text have focused on more traditional educational models and general instructional methods. These theories and strategies are applicable to all types of instruction, and the clinical educator should take time to become familiar with them.

Clinical Education

Clinical education in EMS is performed in actual patient care environments under the direct supervision of an experienced clinician. This clinical educator is both a care provider and teacher who facilitates learning while remaining responsible for real patient care. The educator must balance the educational needs of the student while still being an advocate for good patient care.

Clinical or patient care experience for the EMS student most often is acquired in a hospital emergency department (ED) and on an emergency ambulance, although certainly nonacute clinical areas can provide excellent learning opportunities as well.

Student participation in real patient care settings generally occurs after theoretical knowledge and laboratory practice is sufficient to ensure the learner is prepared to safely care for patients.

In the 2015 paramedic portfolio, the National Registry of EMTs (NREMT), with support from the Committee on Accreditation of Educational Programs for Emergency Medical Services Professions (CoAEMSP), adopted a concept of learning progression that sequences classroom instruction, discrete laboratory practice, simulation or scenario practice, clinical (hospital or clinic setting) experience, field experience, and a final capstone field internship (**FIGURE 19.1**).

The field experience is performed during formative stages of learning, often simultaneously with other experiences and didactic course work. Students have the opportunity to care for patients in the actual environment they will be working in as graduates. In this phase they are expected to perform skills they have already practiced in simulation and hospital clinicals, begin to apply advanced assessment and differential diagnosis techniques, and perhaps lead uncomplicated basic life support (BLS) cases. These simple cases should be within their scope prior to starting paramedic school, but in many cases a student may have little to no previous field experience.

Early exposure to the clinical and field experience may be beneficial to novice learners without any previous field experience. The clinical educator, in concert with the educational institution, should move students progressively from observation and discrete skill performance (such as simple patient communication, history taking, and focused physical examination) toward stronger understanding of field impressions, differential diagnosis, eventually leading to leadership of cases with basic complaints. This scaffolded learning

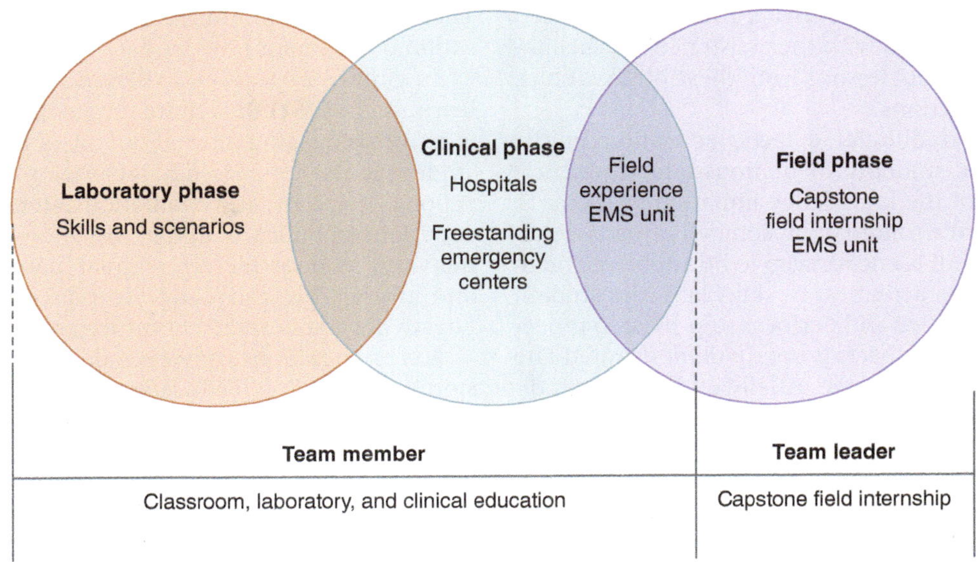

FIGURE 19.1 Psychomotor formative and summative phases noted in the NREMT paramedic portfolio.

Reproduced from Sullivan, Bob. 2017, February 13. "6 Things to Know about the NREMT Paramedic Psychomotor Competency Portfolio." Accessed April 16, 2019. https://www.ems1.com/ems-education/articles/193665048-6-things-to-know-about-the-NREMT-Paramedic-Psychomotor-Competency-Portfolio/.

approach should help decrease cognitive overload and alleviate some of the anxiety and feelings of being overwhelmed that paramedic students report when they are immediately expected to perform in a new and uncontrolled environment.[12–15]

CoAEMSP defines the *field internship* as a capstone event "which must occur after all core didactic, laboratory, and clinical experiences."[16] The expectation of the intern in this summative phase is that they should be able to be in charge of the assessment and care of all encountered patients, particularly those requiring advanced life support (ALS) care. Later in this chapter, concepts around measuring a graduate's achievement of terminal competency and successfully leading the EMS team are further explored.

For the purposes of this chapter, the term **field clinical (field experience)** refers to prehospital or outdoor experiences, which may be primarily observation or performing isolated skills as directed by the EMS personnel on the ambulance; **hospital clinical** refers to experiences in a hospital, clinic, or other indoor setting; **field internship** or *capstone field internship* is a planned, scheduled educational experience on an ALS unit that includes team-leading skills and the management of prehospital patients and scenes. **Preceptors** are individuals who teach in the hospital or field clinical setting. CoAEMSP uses this term frequently in their documents, and the term will be used in this chapter as well.

The type and scope of clinical experiences vary according to the level of education. Clinical education for entry-level EMS providers, such as EMT or EMR students, is usually limited in scope, objectives, and time. EMT clinical experience often involves observation in a hospital ED or a handful of ride-along shifts on an ambulance. At more advanced levels, such as AEMT or paramedic education, students may perform clinical rotations in a wide variety of hospital departments and healthcare settings. Specialized units within hospitals, such as operating rooms, cardiac units, cardiac catheterization labs, psychiatric crisis units, burn care units, obstetric departments, and intensive care units, are common at this level. Advanced field clinical rotations or internships may also involve experiences with critical care transport teams, mobile integrated healthcare paramedics, law enforcement officers, fire or rescue personnel, other EMS-related service providers, and, on some occasions, air ambulance services. Some programs use innovative and nontraditional settings, such as homeless shelters, skilled nursing and geriatric care facilities, pediatric clinics, immunization outreach programs, and morgues, where students can gain a unique perspective (**FIGURE 19.2**).

Experiential Learning

Experiential learning is an educational philosophy that best describes the essence of clinical education. This philosophy is based largely on the original work of John Dewey, with later refinements by the German philosopher Kurt Hahn. At the core of this philosophy of education is the idea that learning begins with an experience. A particular circumstance may require an action on the part of the student, or it may simply be an observation of an action. Once it has been completed or the situation has been resolved, the student reflects on the experience, and with the assistance of a facilitator, draws meaningful lessons from these observations, actions, and reflections.

The goal of traditional didactic education in the classroom is for students to demonstrate a practical understanding of the knowledge imparted to them. In class, the student's role may be somewhat passive, although the student is encouraged to be attentive and to participate in class activities. In skills labs, the student is expected to practice and perform step-by-step procedures after they have been properly demonstrated and rehearsed in a linear manner, usually under ideal conditions.[17–20] Less controlled and sometimes frenetic clinical experiences are often left until the final stages of the educational process. Because the quantity and quality of learning during the clinical phase can be unpredictable, clinical education has been sometimes viewed as less valuable than other methods of instruction.[18]

Several studies have demonstrated that exposure to patient contacts, especially those that involved ALS, increase critical thinking and are directly correlated to successful first time pass rates on the NREMT paramedic cognitive (written) exam.[21–25]

Participation in clinical education in EMS, however, is also an important step toward the development of confident and competent graduates.[26,27]

Unlike the traditional classroom, the "real world" of clinical education requires that students be assertive, take initiative, and eventually, direct others to perform tasks.[19] They must be able to assess patients and circumstances, analyze conflicting information, perform technical skills, apply acquired knowledge, and exhibit professional attributes. This requires that the students perform at higher levels of intellectual functioning.[18] Therefore, the importance of an effective clinical education program for EMS students cannot be overstated.

In clinical education, experience is the catalyst for learning. In the course of treating patients, the student is actively engaging most, if not all, of their senses. The student is also immersed in a complex set of thoughts, actions, reactions, and evaluations. Reflecting on these experiences builds a library of knowledge that will help the student identify similar patterns of disease and injury. This knowledge will aid EMS students to effectively assess and treat future patients.[26]

Experience alone, however, does not necessarily inspire learning. To be educationally sound, experiences should be carefully structured around specific learning goals and should include appropriate orientation, preparation, and critical evaluation.[28] It is the role of the clinical educator to provide background information, to ensure that experiences are put into context, to answer questions, and to direct further learning or review. A proper foundation, combined with timely communication, helps the student to organize learning and makes the student aware of the fact that learning has just taken place.[19]

The Effective Clinical Educator

The clinical educator or preceptor, beyond playing a central role during experience-based learning,[29,30] is a role model for students and is seen as an expert in the field.

Above all, clinical educators must create positive and professional interpersonal relationships with students (**FIGURE 19.3**). They must lead by example and

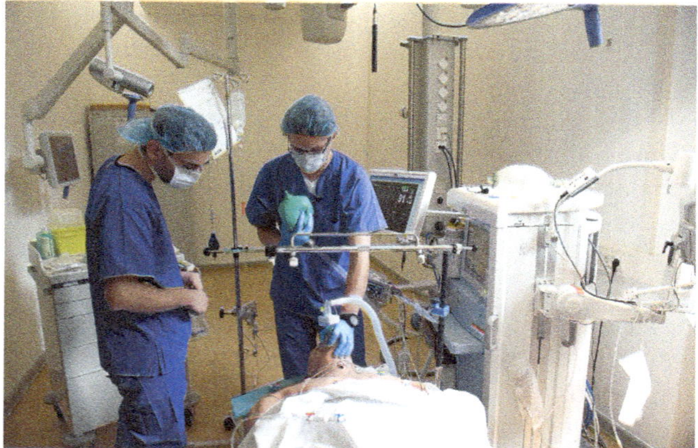

FIGURE 19.2 Some programs use innovative and nontraditional settings for clinical experience where students can gain a unique perspective.

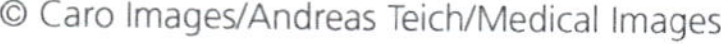

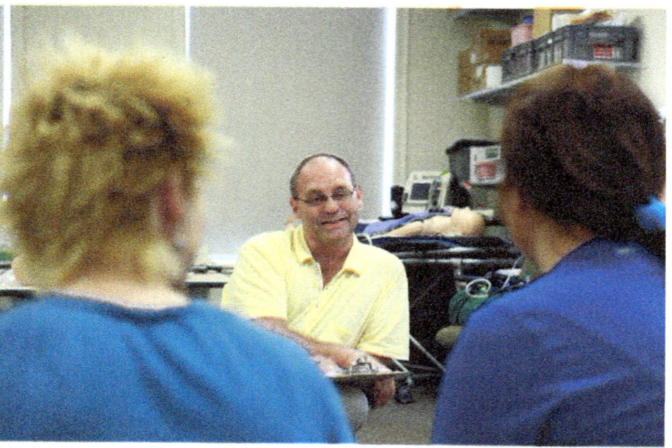

FIGURE 19.3 Clinical educators must create positive and professional interpersonal relationships with students.

Tips for Effective Communication with Students in the Clinical Setting

- Introduce yourself, and use your name.
- Use your students' names.
- Make and maintain eye contact.
- Listen actively, providing verbal and nonverbal cues that you are following the conversation.
- Clarify what is being said by paraphrasing key points and checking to make sure that you understand the communication.
- Do not assume that you understand the student's words or actions until you have heard all of the facts or asked questions that confirm your understanding.
- Watch for context: Most communication is paraverbal (tone, pitch, pace, and power) and nonverbal (behavior, gestures, and actions).
- Do not try to solve problems or give advice; instead, help students explore options to help themselves.
- If you feel that your own feelings are clouding your ability to stay calm and communicate effectively, then take a break and return to the interaction when you are prepared to place students' needs above your own.

respect students, display confidence in them, show genuine interest in what they do, and encourage mutual respect. The personal attributes of an educator that promote learning include enthusiasm, patience, friendliness, a sense of humor, flexibility in the clinical setting, and a willingness to honestly admit limitations or mistakes.

Research shows that student learning is enhanced significantly when clinical educators are skilled at using teaching objectives, able to ask appropriate questions, and willing to provide specific and timely feedback. Additionally, formal preparation and instruction for clinical educators on how to teach in the clinical setting have proved to correlate with better student achievement.[30]

Attributes of Effective Clinical Teachers[29,30]

Effective clinical teachers demonstrate the following attributes:

1. Create an environment that is conducive to learning with the following:
   - Knowledge of the practice area
   - Clinical competency
   - Desire to teach
2. Are supportive of learners, which requires the following:
   - Knowledge of the learners; explore what has been learned before
   - Knowledge of the practice area
   - Mutual respect
3. Possess teaching skills that maximize student learning; this requires the following abilities:
   - Diagnose student needs; set short- and longer-term learning goals
   - Learn about students as individuals, including their needs, personalities, and capabilities
4. Foster independence so that students learn how to learn.
5. Encourage exploration and questions without penalty.
6. Accept differences among students.
7. Relate how clinical experiences facilitate the development of clinical competency.
8. Practice effective communication and questioning skills.
9. Serve as a role model with excellent clinical skills.
10. Enjoy practice and teaching.
11. Are friendly, approachable, understanding, enthusiastic, and confident about teaching.
12. Are knowledgeable about the subject matter and able to convey that knowledge to students in their practice areas.
13. Exhibit fairness and objectivity in evaluation.
14. Provide frequent feedback and positive reinforcement.

Field Preceptor Job Requirements and Training

For the purposes of this section, the *preceptor* is the clinical educator in the field setting who is working directly with EMS students. Although all levels of EMS students can benefit from clinical and field preceptors, most of the emphasis in EMS clinical education is placed on the AEMT- or paramedic-level provider. In fact, the presumption is that if a preceptor can facilitate education for paramedic students, the preceptor is also qualified to teach EMT students. This may seem logical, but it remains one of the enduring myths of EMS. Providers such as EMRs and EMTs have needs and expectations that are different from those of advanced-level providers. Paramedic preceptors who usually provide training to entry-level students may not be aware of the needs of providers who practice at the EMR or EMT level. This phenomenon diminishes the advanced provider's oversight value, unless the preceptor is first tutored in the training needs and protocols of EMR or EMT caregivers in the area.

Many EMS programs are measured by the capabilities of their preceptors. Just as with any other educational setting, high standards in both clinical skills and teaching strategies are to be expected. Programs should regularly evaluate performance and develop the skills of preceptors.

Preceptor Job Requirements

A clinical educator for any type of EMS student acts as a role model, and a preceptor's clinical knowledge and patient care skills—including the ability to establish patient rapport—should be carefully screened and evaluated. A preceptor candidate who will be overseeing interns new to ALS should probably have at least 1 to 2 years of concentrated field experience at the level they are precepting. Preceptor candidates who will be evaluating interns with previous ALS field experience should probably have at least 3 to 4 years of concentrated field experience. It should not be assumed that an expert in ALS or the best-liked employee would make a good clinical educator. The preceptor candidate must be able to deal constructively with adult learners. The preceptor needs to view interns as active learners with whom the instructor will collaborate to solve problems; they must be seen as students who will require guidance regarding actions of human beings during a crisis, and who will need help to understand how to apply ALS protocols to specific situations.

The following is a list of qualifications exhibited by strong candidates for preceptor-training programs:

- Significant field experience (measured by numbers of emergency patients seen, as well as time spent at the provider level)
- Demonstrated ability to work with people who are learning (not the same skill as caring for patients)
- Experience with teaching or planning educational events
- Supervisory/leadership and/or critical incident stress management training
- Experience or training in conflict management, negotiations, quality improvement, and similar subjects
- Awareness of current EMS research literature and of the value of clinical and educational research (candidate reads current journals and literature, participates in an EMS journal club, attends regional or national conferences, values continuing education)

The medical director should approve preceptors after a review of their personnel file and track record.

If available potential preceptor candidates do not possess any of these qualifications, then a different approach should be used for evaluation. For example, a teaching or role-playing demonstration in front of a select panel or an appropriate audience might prove to be a useful evaluation tool. The candidate should also be observed while providing patient care and interacting with other responders and the public. Potential preceptors should be evaluated on calls rather than by talking with them about responses. Informal and formal interviews should focus on the candidate's attitudes toward and expectations regarding the role of the clinical educator.

Role of the Clinical Educator

Through effective hospital and field clinical instruction, didactic knowledge and practical skills are reinforced by experience, which helps to prepare the student to become a competent entry-level clinician.[26,31,32]

In general, the role of the clinical educator or preceptor is to do the following:

- Size up the needs of the student.
- Assist the student in creating a plan to facilitate learning.
- Help the student put theoretical knowledge into practice.
- Extend knowledge and learning by relating experience to general theory.
- Promote skills development.
- Promote professionalism.
- Provide feedback to learners about progress toward goals and objectives in the clinical area.
- Be responsive to the needs and concerns of other clinical staff.
- Evaluate, document, and report student progress and achievement.[18]
- Promptly report concerns to the program if significant performance or behavior issues occur.

The clinical educator has a particularly challenging role in EMS education. In addition to regular patient care duties, either in the hospital or in the field, the clinical educator must balance the needs of

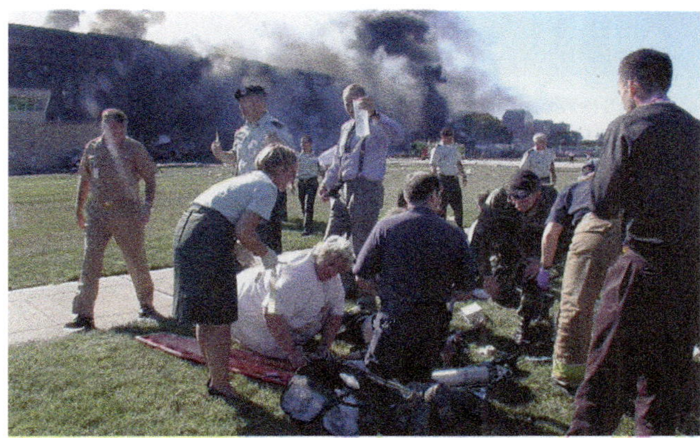

FIGURE 19.4 The clinical educator must balance the instructional needs of the student with the needs of the patient, bystanders, family members, support staff, and coworkers.

Courtesy of Journalist 1st Class Mark D. Faram/U.S. Navy.

the student with the needs of the patient, bystanders, family members, support staff, and coworkers (**FIGURE 19.4**).

By definition, students are not as skilled or competent as the clinical staff with whom they are working. The clinical educator must be willing to allow a student to attempt procedures and other patient care duties. This requires the ability to recognize any opportunity to do so and to perform a quick analysis of the risks to the patient versus the benefits to the student. An effective clinical educator can turn a call with a patient who has a nonemergent, superficial dog bite into a fascinating description of the mandated reporting requirements, importance of infection control, proper wound irrigation and dressing, the mechanism of healing, recognition of rabies or sepsis, and variations in animal and human bites.

More importantly, clinical educators must have enough seniority and trust from coworkers to transfer patient care authority to the student. Eager and well-meaning staff members or EMTs wanting to perform rapid and efficient care can present an unintended barrier to student learning. Experienced clinical educators know to discuss the educational plan with other staff members, whenever possible, before a patient encounter. Students should be identified by a school badge, a distinctive uniform, or a patch reading "EMT Student" or "Paramedic Intern" to minimize confusion, particularly when advanced procedures are being performed.

The clinical educator should try to remain in the background as much as possible, seeming to carry on a casual social conversation, or quietly getting a private report from EMTs, family members, and other interested parties for the purpose of creating some space and time for the student to function. At the same time, a seasoned clinical educator should be able to keep an ear and a watchful eye on the student's performance. However, at times, education must be sacrificed in favor of patient care. Then, the role of the clinical educator is to help students reflect on events to find valuable learning points in their observations and in the actions of others.

It is recommended that students make the transition from the role of observer to practitioner, and finally, in the field to team leader.[26] Clinical educators must seek out opportunities for students to function at the level of their current abilities and to develop higher-level abilities. In some cases, students may be able to lead uncomplicated patient encounters, but they may function only as team members in situations that are more complex. The clinical educator must be keenly aware of students' strengths, weaknesses, current capabilities, previous successes, and ongoing challenges.

The clinical educator also plays a key role in reducing high levels of student stress. Evidence suggests that students experience significant stress and anxiety during clinical education.[18,30,33,34] Performance anxiety can be a serious barrier to achievement when students are unable to concentrate or receive and process information. Although stress and anxiety are common in emergency health care, the clinical educator should be able to recognize when a student's fear is actually preventing learning or inhibiting performance. Once this

TEACHING TIP

In the early stages of a clinical education, a student's performance may be unpredictable when the student is attempting new skills. In this stage, the clinical educator should be directive in giving guidance and feedback, and should ask the student to focus on specific objectives before the student encounters them in the next patient. For example, if a student is having difficulty obtaining a patient history, the instructor should try to have the student focus solely on creating a conversation with the next patient. An objective should be introduced for the student to simply introduce themself, then to elicit the patient's name, chief complaint, and history. As the student successfully completes this task with the first patient, the instructor can add additional objectives for the next patient contact, such as obtaining a history from a family member or bystander. Giving feedback and building on small successes increase the student's level of confidence.

Steps to Help Reduce Student Anxiety[33]

1. Establish a safe relationship.
   - Be empathetic.
   - Deal with mistakes calmly.
   - Emphasize positives.
   - Remember that a trusting relationship takes time to build.
   - Be honest.
2. Build self-esteem.
3. Confront the problem (talk about the anxiety).
4. Draw from the student's past coping mechanisms.
5. If the student appears blocked, give specific direction.
6. Set strict limitations (insist that the student attempt or try to perform).
7. Divide tasks into smaller parts.
8. Set realistic expectations.

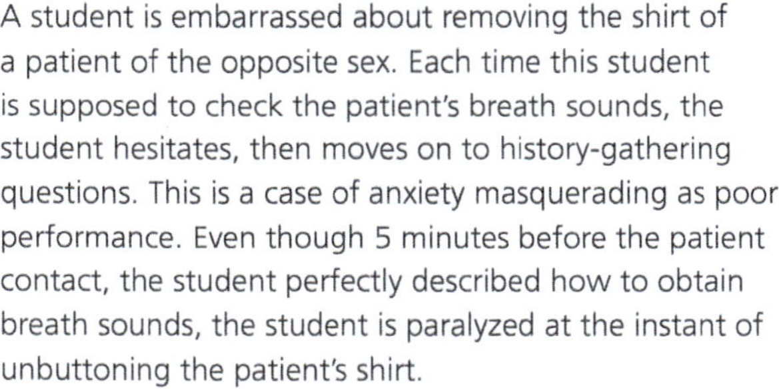

A student is embarrassed about removing the shirt of a patient of the opposite sex. Each time this student is supposed to check the patient's breath sounds, the student hesitates, then moves on to history-gathering questions. This is a case of anxiety masquerading as poor performance. Even though 5 minutes before the patient contact, the student perfectly described how to obtain breath sounds, the student is paralyzed at the instant of unbuttoning the patient's shirt.

The clinical educator is the best person to help the student get past the overwhelming feelings that are paralyzing them. The clinical educator should assist the student by first identifying the fear, then rehearsing what the student will say and do with a mock patient, such as a classmate or a patient who is not threatening. A good strategy is to take "baby steps." The student can be coached to listen to breath sounds through the shirt at first, then coached to raise the back of the shirt only; finally, once the student is more comfortable, the student can begin removing the shirt altogether while taking steps to preserve the patient's modesty.

is recognized, the clinical educator should take steps to create a less-threatening environment and should focus the student on specific tasks that will serve to build self-confidence.

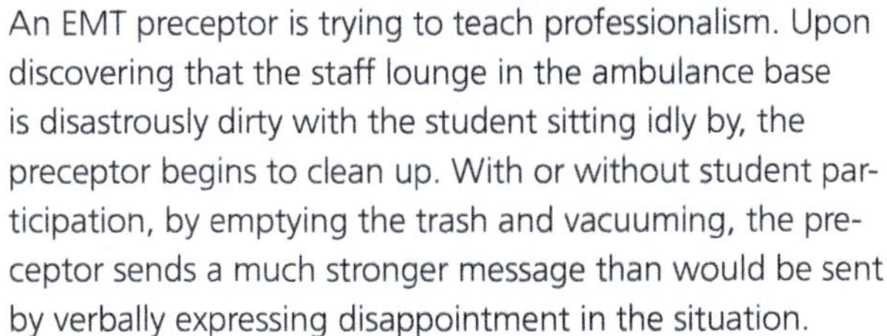

An EMT preceptor is trying to teach professionalism. Upon discovering that the staff lounge in the ambulance base is disastrously dirty with the student sitting idly by, the preceptor begins to clean up. With or without student participation, by emptying the trash and vacuuming, the preceptor sends a much stronger message than would be sent by verbally expressing disappointment in the situation.

Clinical Teaching Strategies

Performance expectations of students at the end of their EMS clinical experiences are high, particularly for paramedic students. In a relatively short amount of time—as little as 1 to 6 months—students are expected to observe, practice, and direct field emergency care. Entry-level competency requires that the student master the building blocks of assessment, recognize pathophysiology in actual patients, demonstrate motor skills in adverse circumstances, and exhibit professional behavior in stressful situations. The clinical educator should help students move quickly through the learning process without overwhelming them. The following sections focus on strategies that are specific to clinical teaching and that complement previously discussed teaching techniques.

Do as I Do: Actions Speak Louder than Words

One of the most effective clinical teaching techniques is the consistent modeling of the behavior or skill that is being asked of the student.[18] When the instructor demonstrates the professionalism, technical aptitude, and leadership that are expected, a student learns by observing and emulating behavior. An educator should remember that a student is carefully observing the educator's actions before, during, and after patient care activities.

Even if some clinical or operational steps seem redundant and unnecessary to the expert provider, clinical educators should practice all the good habits they would like to see in their students. For example, spending time at the beginning of a shift doing equipment checks and inventory may seem boring and routine to an expert, but it teaches the student that it is important to be thorough and prepared, and to have all equipment in working order. The instructor who arrives on time and is well groomed, ready for duty, and wearing a smile teaches the student that the instructor takes pride in the work.

When a choice exists between explaining and doing, the clinical educator should choose to *do*. Performing an action or exhibiting a behavior that demonstrates a point will make a more lasting impression on a student than will a simple explanation. The best teaching method is to involve the student in actively demonstrating, practicing, or researching the topic.

Ask Questions

An instructor's effective questioning and answering of questions lead to improved student learning.[35] This reflection on observation and action is an essential element of learning by experience.[36] Clinical educators should encourage an atmosphere where it is safe to ask questions so that no detail is missed; also, the sophistication of the student's inquiries can be a good clue to the instructor about the student's level of progress. Simple questions can be especially important because hospital, EMS operations, protocols, and culture vary dramatically, and it is easy for misunderstanding to occur. Educators can also use questions to help students filter information and focus on the most important issues in patient care.[37]

Questions can be broadly categorized as convergent, where students are asked to analyze or synthesize information, or divergent, where students are asked to extrapolate on a concept. **Convergent questions** seek specific information, whereas **divergent questions** do not have a single right answer.[37]

Research shows that clinical educators have a tendency to pose low-level questions that ask the student to recall memorized facts.[30,37] The clinical educator should be careful not to fall into this common trap. More effective questioning revolves around asking the student to apply information, think critically, and make decisions. Higher-level questions improve reasoning and eventually lead to improved clinical performance.[37]

The following are some tips on asking effective questions:

- *Slow down*. The slower the question and the longer the wait time for a response, the more time the student has to carefully consider possible answers; thus, higher cognitive levels can be expected.
- *Have students compare their actual experience with general theoretical expectations*. This helps bridge the conflict between the classroom (general didactic expectations) and the reality of actual practice. (Examples: Was the patient exhibiting classic signs and symptoms? Is it possible for a patient to have pulmonary edema and bronchospasm at the same time?)
- *Have students provide alternative solutions*. Encouraging students to think creatively about situations will improve their problem-solving abilities. These situations may involve real difficulties that they have encountered or hypothetical scenarios, but they should always be realistic.[17]
- *Have students predict and anticipate changes in patient condition or reaction to treatment*. In addition, have students propose possible plans to address these changes. (Example: What symptoms would you expect of this patient if her condition worsens? Improves? What will you do if there is no improvement after the first medication administration?)
- *Avoid "yes or no" questions*. These types of questions do not provide information about how the student is thinking or arriving at decisions.[38]
- Limit each question to one main thought, and make sure that the question is understandable. Vague questions force students to guess what the preceptor is asking.

Examples of Questions Used to Evaluate the Cognitive Domain[29]

Knowledge (lower-level cognition)

Define ________.

List the five principles for ________.

Based on your assignment, what do you recall about ________?

Comprehension

Explain the meaning of ________.

Tell me in your own words what is meant by ________.

Which of the examples demonstrates ________?

Application

What is a new example of ________?

How could ________ be used to ________?

Show how this information could be graphed.

Analysis

What are the implications of ________? What is the meaning of ________?

What are the key components of ________?

Synthesis of Ideas

What are some possible solutions to the problem of ________?

From this information, create your own model of ________.

Suppose you could ________. How would you approach ________?

Evaluation

Explain the effectiveness of this approach. Which solution would you choose? Justify your opinion.

What are the consequences of ________?

TEACHING TIP

Clinical educators should create an environment that welcomes questions and encourages curiosity. This does not mean that educators must know the answers to all questions. It is best to teach students to "fish for themselves" by showing them where and how to look up reference information. Modeling this continued quest for knowledge encourages lifelong learning that will serve the students well past the day of certification.

Pairing Students with Preceptors

Unfortunately many EMS services have adopted a policy that "everyone" is a preceptor. Students are often paired with crews based on schedules. This "luck of the draw" method of pairing students can be inconsistent at best, and may result in poor educational experiences as unwilling, untrained, and low-performing clinicians are drafted into a teaching role. EMS clinicians who are interested in teaching need training to become effective preceptors. The common EMS perception that exposing students to a diverse set of clinicians teaches the student many different "styles of care" has not been scientifically tested or proven as a best practice. On the contrary, in early formative stages of learning the student needs consistency, accurate feedback, and gradual skill development. Having too many preceptors may make that consistent feedback very difficult to attain. At least one study has demonstrated that pairing paramedic students with fewer preceptors (the fewer the better) results in a greater number of successful student-team leads.[39]

In one study, paramedic students who spent 90% to 100% of the internship with one preceptor were able to achieve competency in an average of 35 patients contacts, compared to an average of 65 patients with multiple preceptors.[40]

Care should be given to maintaining impartiality and avoiding conflicts of interest by pairing students with preceptors who can be objective and fair, even if they have had previous working relationships with the student. Cases in which personal relationships between a student and their preceptor are already present should be avoided at all cost. A student requesting a specific preceptor should raise instructor concern, and further evaluation is necessary.

Pairing a student with the right preceptor can be challenging. Ideally, pairings should be thoughtful, deliberate, and well coordinated. Teaching and learning styles as well as personalities are key components of the pairing.[4,15,31] Clinical program coordinators should consider each pairing as an opportunity to develop both the student and the preceptor. Adopting a long-range view of preceptor development in this manner can continuously improve the communication and teaching skills of the preceptor.

Preceptor Training

A combination of innate skills and proper training helps ensure success for preceptor candidates and prepares them for the challenges of teaching adults under stressful circumstances. There is currently no national standard curriculum recommended for EMS preceptors. While various states recommend a minimum number of training hours or topics, no formal EMS research exists on this topic.

The following is a suggested outline of topics that should be included in a preceptor-training program:

- Preceptor roles and responsibilities, program faculty roles and responsibilities
- Legal and ethical issues: confidentiality, harassment, discrimination, potential exposure and injury reporting, and subsequent follow-up
- Principles of adult learning
- Setting goals and objectives
- Effective learning environments
- Teaching methods: communication skills, teaching aids, and questioning techniques
- Purposes of evaluation
- Evaluation criteria and forms, and appropriate use
- Effective feedback methods
- Conflict resolution, mediation, and advocacy for education
- Roles of the team member and team leader
- Effective coaching techniques
- Familiarity with the curriculum and student schedules

CoAEMSP standards require that paramedic field preceptors receive training. Program coordinators should keep logs of successful training completion and topics covered. This training can best be provided in a partnership between the educational institution and the EMS agency. One acceptable option is to provide some of the training in a distributed format. This can be accomplished with Internet technology, video, or self-study packets, along with a method to have preceptor questions answered. Clinicians can complete the training at their own pace while at work. This helps cut down on the expense of paying providers to attend training outside their shifts.

CoAEMSP standards interpretations specifically mention that training must include the following elements:

- Purposes of the student rotation (minimum competencies, skills, and behaviors)
- Evaluation tools used by the program
- Criteria of evaluation for grading students
- Contact information for the program
- Program's definition of team lead
- Program's required minimum number of team leads
- Coaching and mentorship techniques

Assessment System

In addition to a preceptor-training module, the field education program must have a well-defined, written assessment system for documenting the clinical progress of students. A rating system that removes as much ambiguity as possible from subjective assessments is valuable. Understanding how one is to be graded can provide a great boost in confidence for the student and can provide a frame of reference for use as the student moves through the educational process. Having a defendable assessment tool also makes it easier for students who are seeking a change of preceptor, or who challenge the fairness of their evaluation. (See Chapter 22, *Other Assessment Tools*, for additional information.)

Preceptors benefit from receiving program reference materials, such as a job description that includes reasonable expectations, limits on the numbers of interns (depending on the system, usually one to three per year with a break in between), and communication with the supervisor and school representative to whom they will report.

Feedback and continuing education for the preceptor are highly desirable and should be based on the actual experiences of the preceptor, so as to fine-tune the preceptor's skills and provide information on which the preceptor can base improvements. If possible, the preceptor program and other clinical education opportunities should be integrated into the provider organization's career ladder. A well-defined training, educational, and feedback system will improve the retention rate of quality clinical educators and will increase the educator's level of job satisfaction.

A Model for Teaching Team Leadership

The ability of the paramedic intern to successfully lead a field encounter is in many ways as much of a capstone to the student's academic career as successful completion of certification and licensure exams. Beginning in 1998, the successful completion of *team leads* became part of the EMT-intermediate and EMT-paramedic curriculum.[a,b] The assessment of ability to lead teams is not unique to EMS and is seen routinely in the education of medical students and residents.

As each individual is not necessarily born with leadership traits or may not have the life experiences that provide an opportunity to develop leadership skills, these skills should be experienced and practiced in the classroom prior to clinical rotations. A long academic study in the facets of leadership is not what is needed. The focus of the EMS classroom prepares the student to lead the patient care encounter. The educator has flexibility in how the students will demonstrate leadership, but a foundation is necessary to provide a strong, initial framework from which to work.

Definition

Team leader—Someone who leads the call and provides guidance and direction for setting priorities, scene and patient assessment, and management. The team leader may not actually perform all the interventions, but may assign others to do so.[c]

One option for teaching a leadership framework comes from the Agency for Healthcare Research and Quality (AHRQ). The AHRQ is the lead federal agency charged with improving the quality, safety, efficiency, and effectiveness of health care. In 2007, AHRQ released the TeamSTEPPS curriculum, which is the first research-based curriculum on crew resource management that is directed at healthcare settings.[d] Hospitals and other healthcare organizations across the United States have adopted this curriculum. TeamSTEPPS identified six topics that make team leaders effective. In 2012, TEAMSTEPPS 2.0 was released and the numbers of topics under leadership was increased to 10. In many cases these topics were drawn from the expectations that teams had of their leaders.

Organize the Team

In most situations, team membership is based on the resources assigned to an incident by dispatch protocols and system polices. The purpose of the team leader is to take the incoming resources and choreograph the EMS response.[a,b] The primary task associated with team organization is role identification.

(continues)

A Model for Teaching Team Leadership (*Continued*)

The team leader should identify themself to the patient and other responders on scene. If the leader is unfamiliar with other personnel on scene, the leader may take the opportunity to identify caregivers and their roles and determine what they have done for the patient so far. Successful role identification will assist the team leader assigning tasks, managing resources, and developing a plan for managing the patient or incident.

Identify and Articulate Clear Goals

In a protocol and algorithm-dominated field, the articulation of clear goals may seem trivial; however, it is the key to a functioning team. The leader will assess the situation, make a plan, and then share the plan so that all team members know what is going to happen. The expectation is that everyone is on the same page. In the world of crew resource management (CRM), this is often referred to as the shared mental model.[e] Examples of this would include working with the rescue group at a motor vehicle collision to determine how the patient will be accessed and extricated, or advising the team of the plan for splinting a complicated fracture. (A video on crew resource managmeent is available from Jones & Bartlett Learning here: https://www.youtube.com/watch?v=2AtyMuYEk9M.)

Assign Tasks and Responsibilities

In this phase of leadership, the leader assigns tasks, which is referred to as *delegation*. Often in the healthcare environment this seems inconsistent, because hospital-based code teams tend to fill necessary roles based on provider type, while fire-based services tend to assign roles based on seat assignments in the apparatus. One way for the EMS provider to think about this task assignment difference is to consider that in many cases, the EMS crew will receive assistance from other agencies. For example, delegation becomes more like integration as first responders move from a BLS role with cardiopulmonary resuscitation (CPR) and an automated external defibrillator (AED) to assisting in an ALS code.

Monitor and Modify the Plan: Communicate Changes

The team leader needs to maintain a high level of situational awareness. As tasks are being completed, reassessment of the situation must occur and the plan must be changed and communicated to the team if needed. For example, in the cardiac arrest patient, perhaps an anti-arrhythmic medication was ordered, but at the rhythm check the patient is found to be in asystole. At this point it is appropriate for the leader to ask for the medication to be set aside and a new set of orders given.

Review the Team's Performance and Provide Feedback

A crucial part of team leading is to ensure whether or not the leader's instructions have been understood and carried out, along with the results. By engaging in monitoring, the leader will ensure that future decisions are not based on faulty assumptions.[f] One practical example of this includes the request for intravenous (IV) epinephrine to be administered during a code, but being unaware that IV access has not yet been achieved.

Manage and Allocate Resources

Patient care events can be dynamic in nature. It is important for the leader to request additional assistance as needed, but also to know when to release personnel from the scene.

Facilitate Information Sharing

Since the landmark *To Err Is Human*[g] report, a growing recognition exists in health care that the team leader, whether paramedic, nurse, or physician, is not an island. As a recent change in the healthcare culture, students should be aware that asking for input from the team is not a sign of weakness. Likewise, it is important for preceptors to understand that, in many cases, the paramedic intern who asks for input about treatment should not be regarded as incompetent. The preceptor should model team collaboration and ensure the most beneficial treatment plan for the patient is generated.

Also important to note is that because most patients seen by EMS are responsive and alert, they are part of the team as well, which is in many ways the ultimate informed-consent process. As Thom Dick et al. said in *People Care*,[h] patients have the right to understand what is being done to them, including the right to consent to or refuse treatment without coercion through intimidation, subterfuge, or outright dishonesty.

Encourage Team Members to Assist One Another

Since 2000, there has been an increasing realization that errors occur in medicine. Often errors are the result of a sequence of poor decisions and the inability to recognize them early and correct them.[f] One of the primary ways to mitigate this process is to ensure that team members are watching out for each other. The team leader should create a safe environment where team members can feel free to speak up when they see something wrong. This occurs in the surgical theater, where it is accomplished in part by a verbal cue made by the surgeon during the preoperative brief. Although the precall brief is usually not possible in emergency situations, the team leader should incorporate the verbal cue into the call. A common way to invite the team to participate is to say, "Does anyone have any concerns or does anyone have any suggestions?" The leader should also be aware that body language and verbal responses to feedback and suggestions also serve to communicate how seriously the leader takes the input of others.

Facilitate Conflict Resolution

Training for conflict resolution in health care is often centered on issues that occur with patients and family members. Additionally, conflict may arise between team members for a variety of reasons. Listening is the primary tool at the leader's disposal in conflict resolution. Although no one methodology will solve every conflict,[f] the leader can offer the following guidelines:

- Tackle the problem, not your counterpart.
- The patient needs to be the primary focus.
- Clarify where there may be areas of agreement.
- Acknowledge feelings.
- Treat everyone with respect

Model Effective Teamwork

A tremendous percentage of the team leader's responsibilities involve communication, which is the primary way to model effective teamwork.

An effective communication tool that should be used to facilitate good teamwork is the briefing. The primary purpose of briefing team members is to ensure that they are focused on the goals and have a shared mental model; this also has the benefit of creating space for inquiry, concerns, and suggestions.[f] To accomplish this, the team leader should check in with different parts of the team and allow them the chance to share their findings. Another method for briefing is called "recapping," where the leader starts at the beginning and covers everything that has been done to date. In many ways this resembles handoff communication that normally occurs at the transfer of care. During cardiac arrest management, recapping can easily be done during the two-minute phase in between interventions, when the primary concern is effective compressions and ventilations and no other interventions are being performed.

Conclusion

In practice, these 10 leadership activities are not a hierarchy; rather, they are used as often as needed during an episode of care for the betterment of the patient. The common thread in the TeamSTEPPS of team organization, articulating clear goals, decision making, team member empowerment, teamwork promotion, and conflict resolution is communication. Consider that these skills can be taught to all EMS provider levels. Ideally, students should learn these skills early in their EMS education so they can practice them throughout their time in class and clinical. A little bit of practice with some feedback will dramatically increase a student's confidence in leading teams.

Courtesy of Todd M. Cage, MEd, NRP, FAEMS.

[a] U.S. Department of Transportation: National Highway Traffic Safety Administration. *1998 Emergency Medical Technician-Intermediate: National Standard Curriculum.*

[b] U.S. Department of Transportation: National Highway Traffic Safety Administration. *1998 Emergency Medical Technician-Paramedic: National Standard Curriculum.*

[c] U.S. Department of Transportation: National Highway Traffic Safety Administration. 2009. *National Emergency Medical Services Education Standards.*

[d] Agency for Healthcare Research and Quality. 2007. *TeamSTEPPS Instructor Guide.* Accessed August 25, 2011. http://www.ahrq.gov/teamsteppstools/instructor/index.html.

[e] Leonard, Michael W. 2005, October 27. Personal communication.

[f] St. Pierre, Michael, Gesine Hofinger, and Cornelius Buerschaper. 2008. *Crisis Management in Acute Care Settings: Human Factors and Team Psychology in a High Stakes Environment.* New York: Springer.

[g] Institute of Medicine. 2000. *To Err Is Human. Building a Safer Health Care System.* Washington, DC: National Academy Press.

[h] Dick, Thom, Steve Berry, Jeff Forster, and Mike Smith. 2005. *People Care: Career-Friendly Practices for Professional Caregivers.* Van Nuys, CA: Cygnus Business Media.

Cultivating Preceptors: Developing a Culture of Preceptorship

Introduction

Paramedic education has placed an emphasis on experiential, competency-based learning during the field internship. This emphasis provides students with the opportunity to apply classroom theory and skill lab sessions in the real-world classroom of the back of an ambulance under the watchful eye of a preceptor. The key to the success of this learning affirmation is the importance of the preceptor's role. Preceptors are tasked not only with the responsibility for patient care but also the role of clinical teachers, motivators, professional role models, and evaluators of student performance. With this in mind, it should be no surprise that there is a supply-and-demand problem with preceptors. This is due in part to paramedic programs steadily increasing the number of accepted students while the availability of preceptors is decreasing, causing paramedics to feel the effects of increased workloads and added responsibilities. To maintain the value of field internships and overall high standards of paramedic education, educators need to consider potential shortfalls in the preceptorship model and develop strategies that emphasize the development and sustainability of preceptorship programs focusing on establishing a culture of preceptorship.

The six Rs of developing a culture of preceptorship identify the key areas. These areas focus on: recognizing professional responsibilities, finding the right people for the job, providing them with essential skills, avoiding their burnout, providing ongoing support, and recognizing their contribution.

The six Rs of establishing a culture of preceptorship:

- Responsibility
- Recruitment
- Readiness
- Retention
- Reassurance
- Recognition

Responsibility

As with other health professionals, there is a professional responsibility to participate in clinical education of new practitioners. For paramedics, this provides an opportunity to "give back" to the profession. Experienced paramedics have so much to offer students, not just in terms of skill performance but also in sharing of their experiences and clinical judgment. Educational programs should place heavy emphasis on this aspect of professional responsibility when discussing the roles and responsibilities of the paramedic and throughout the course.

Recruitment

The next step in establishing a culture of preceptorship is to increase the number of preceptors. Right now the most significant challenge facing the preceptorship model is preceptor availability and fatigue. Educational programs are often competing with other programs for preceptors; often this constant stream of students leads to burnout of preceptors. To avoid preceptor fatigue and to increase the numbers of available preceptors, programs should consider developing a preceptor recruitment strategy in response to these challenges. The strategy would focus on attracting new preceptors who exemplify excellence in clinical and professional competency, along with an interest in clinical teaching. This strategy would do the following: set standards for preceptor qualifications, establishing minimum years of service and certification level; develop a role description that defines expectations; get the word out that preceptors are needed by posting notices in stations and hospitals and holding information sessions; and develop a selection process, where potential preceptors could be interviewed.

The following characteristics are what educators are looking for in a preceptor:

- Willingness
- Experience
- Above-average skills
- Knowledgeability
- Excellent communication skills
- Professional deportment
- Responsibility
- Caring and empathetic nature
- Patience
- Commitment

Readiness

Once the right people are recruited for the job, the next step is to prepare them for their new responsibilities. The goal is to provide new preceptors with skills and knowledge to ensure they are confident and competent to precept students with a focus on roles and responsibilities, facilitating clinical learning and student evaluation. Most programs provide some sort of preceptor preparation, usually in the form of a workshop. These workshops provide an excellent opportunity for faculty to meet the preceptors and discuss preceptorship issues. The disadvantage of workshops is that it is often a challenge to fill classrooms due to scheduling or getting people to give up a day off to attend unpaid training. Perhaps one solution to increasing participation would be to put preceptor training online, just as many medical schools have done.

Some topics covered in preceptor workshops are the following:

- Roles and responsibilities
- Principles of adult learning
- Motivating students
- Providing feedback
- Conflict resolution
- Evaluating student performance
- Practicum policies and procedures

Retention

Once an investment has been made in a recruitment and training program and a highly trained and committed pool of preceptors has been established, the biggest challenge is to keep them. To achieve this, programs must provide opportunities to keep preceptors involved and interested in the program, such as serving as adjunct faculty or guest lecturers, or participating on advisory committees. Programs must also be aware of the dangers of student overload and its effects on preceptors. If preceptors are constantly bombarded with students, they will steadily get tired of precepting. Some ways to avoid preceptor fatigue include rotating preceptors or limiting numbers of students going to a site. Educators should consider expanding their preceptor pool by establishing new sites and having a recruitment drive.

Reassurance

One of the most common complaints from preceptors is that they feel that, other than the occasional site visit or telephone conversation when a problem arises, they do not get the level of support they expect from program faculty. Remaining in constant contact and providing ongoing support is critical to keeping preceptors. Some ways to achieve this include increasing frequency of site visits, starting a preceptor newsletter or website, establishing a faculty–preceptor committee, and developing a mentoring system where experienced preceptors can provide support to new preceptors.

Recognition

Most preceptors go above and beyond expectations when precepting students. While some preceptors are paid, most are volunteers, receiving nothing more than a thank you. Whether they are paid or not, preceptors make a significant contribution to the development of their students, so it is important for programs to recognize their efforts and commitment. Programs would be wise to consider implementing preceptor recognition programs to acknowledge the great work that preceptors do. A small token or gesture goes a long way in letting preceptors know that they are valued.

Preceptor recognition ideas can include the following:

- Thank you letters
- Preceptor time as continuing education credit
- Preceptor awards
- Prize draws
- Free continuing medical education courses
- Gift certificates
- Teaching opportunities
- Invitation to graduation
- Preceptor recognition pins, patches, or other uniform insignias
- Trinkets

Conclusion

The field internship is an essential component in the development of competent, "job ready" prehospital providers. The key ingredient to the success of this component is the availability of effective preceptors who are committed to clinical teaching. Paramedic programs need to be aware that, as the need for preceptors increases, so too does the demand placed on existing preceptor pools, and preceptor interest may drop due to the added demands. To avoid this scenario and to ensure sustainability of the preceptorship model, programs need to cultivate preceptors and look at ways to emphasize professional responsibility to new preceptors, attract new preceptors, train them, provide ongoing support, keep them interested, and recognize their contribution to paramedic education.

Courtesy of Dean Vokey, MAdEd, BEd, ACP.

CASE in Point

As an instructor, you have been assigned to evaluate a student who becomes quiet and withdrawn on select calls. After reviewing a report of the student's past clinical experiences, you note that when a psychiatric patient is encountered, the student steps back into the role of observer. Armed with this information, you investigate the cause of this particular problem and develop a plan to overcome it. The solution might be as simple as providing more time in a hospital psychiatric unit. Review of different types of psychiatric complaints and questions that would help the student assess these patients and defuse aggressive behavior might also be helpful.

You might discover that this student is shy and afraid, or has a family history of mental illness, which makes the student uncomfortable about talking with this patient. Working with the student one-on-one to discover this and to arrange for the student's personalized help with a counselor could be a life-changing strategy that will help the student grow as a caregiver and as a person.

Preparation and Debriefing

Coming to a clinical experience properly prepared is as important for the educator as it is for the student. If the clinical educator is using a facility with a predictable pattern of patient complaints, volume, or population, much work can take place to maximize learning opportunities when students are present. Careful planning of goals, objectives, and specific activities can focus students, create a productive learning environment, and make the experience more valuable. For example, a cardiac care unit with a predictable flow of patients with myocardial infarction or angiography is the ideal site for a student to practice cardiac assessments.

Preclinical and postclinical conferences have been found to be useful in the clinical setting.[41,42] In the preclinical conference, the educator can guide students through a goal-setting process that focuses student efforts for the day and sets the stage for later analysis of the experience. Focusing students' activities into concrete steps and assignments also helps to reduce anxiety, wasted time, and misdirection.[33] In the postclinical debriefing, students analyze their experiences, clarify relationships between theory and practice, and reflect on their actions and feelings, patient conditions, and the learning process. **TABLE 19.1** provides useful guidelines for clinical educators.

Measuring Student Progress and Competency in the Clinical Environment

Currently, little research in EMS education definitively proves the value of clinical learning or explains the best way to track and measure it; however, it seems that something magical occurs when students get hands-on clinical experience. The transition from classroom theory to practical, lifesaving skills can quickly transform students into functional EMS practitioners. Field experience is the setting in which some students and instructors discover that they may not be well suited for a career in EMS, and look for an alternate pathway or an exit strategy. The educator's ability to manage and predict the quantity and quality of clinical experiences needed by the student directly correlates with the success of the clinical training program. But how does an educator manage and predict what will be needed? Once goals are created, how do educators track student achievement in the field?

The logistics of scheduling, creating documentation, evaluating progress, and keeping records during EMS clinical education can be overwhelming. Scheduling alone can become a logistical challenge depending on how many accommodations are made for clinical sites, preceptors, other classes, and student work commitments. More importantly, tracking the development of student learning and performance in an unpredictable setting can be time consuming and too expensive to do with any accuracy or depth. Some programs have a single individual deal with clinical schedules and other clinical logistics and have the class instructor(s) deal with student performance issues. This assists in having a single person consistently control where students are and how they are assigned, especially if more than one class is in clinical at one time. Terminal objectives, such as graduating competent entry-level EMS practitioners, are often not easily measured, and patient census or run volume can vary greatly. Indeed, tracking student progress during clinical rotations is a challenging but essential task for the EMS educator. The educator must create a plan for student learning that is based on realistic expectations, focuses on developing competency, and includes measurable terminal goals and objectives. Students and preceptors should focus on the development of assessment, decision making, and team leadership skills. Progress throughout the internship must be tracked, and accomplishments must be rewarded in the areas of emphasis.

TABLE 19.1 Guidelines for Clinical Educators

Before the Clinical Session	During the Clinical Session	After the Clinical Session
■ Bring references: • Drug handbook • Medical dictionary • Pocket preferences or apps • Current standard operating procedures (SOPs) • Point-of-care resources ■ Set goals for the day. • Review and address students' past weakness. • List current successes that should continue. • If possible, visit the site or department, and determine patient census, patient and staff willingness to work with students, and potential learning opportunities. ■ Come prepared with activities that can complement patient experiences or serve as guided tutorials when patient census or call volume is low. Examples of this include the following: • Bringing real electrocardiogram (ECG) strips that you have collected over time to practice interpretation and verbalize treatment plans • Going through the medication cart or ambulance drug box and randomly selecting medications and quizzing the student on indications, contraindications, dosage, route, mechanism of action, and antidotes or reversal agents • Role-playing past patient encounters and having students ask interview questions and verbalize assessment impressions and treatment plans • Practicing map reading by listening to other ambulance calls or selecting random addresses • Performing an ambulance inventory and having students attempt to verbalize three uses for each piece of equipment	■ Do not be afraid to look up reference information and ask questions of experts in the presence of students. ■ Look for windows of opportunity (sometimes referred to as "teachable moments") to give students a chance to practice skills and direct the team. ■ Smartphones are used to store extensive reference material, such as drug reference materials, diagnostic aids, SOPs, and other useful point-of-care material.	■ Start by discussing positive aspects of student performances. ■ Make the transition to areas that could be improved. ■ Discuss whether the patient presented with typical signs and symptoms; ask about what could have been done sooner. ■ Where possible, and without violating privacy, follow up on patient outcomes. ■ Discuss some of the emotions noted in the patient and staff members, along with strategies to address those behaviors. ■ Ask students to describe alternate methods for assessing and treating patients who were just encountered.

The Challenges

Measuring progress during EMS clinical experiences can often take the form of the easiest, most objective measurement available—time on task, also described as "seat time" in more traditional educational settings. Hour-based clinical experiences from past EMS curricula were much simpler to schedule and track. Once the student completed a predetermined number of hours, the student's clinical experience was deemed completed, regardless of performance or ability. However, simply completing hour requirements does not necessarily translate to competency in EMS-provider graduates.

Newer educational standards now recommend that students perform multiple successful assessments and demonstrate team leadership skills during patient contacts. Often, as is the case with the paramedic didactic curriculum, the student is required to perform more than a dozen assessments and treatments for a particular complaint before the student is considered competent. Because patients often present with multiple complaints at the same time and must be simultaneously treated for several differential diagnoses, documentation of student learning may be very complex.

Performance-rating criteria must be straightforward and easy to use because interrater reliability can also present a challenge. Many programs find that it can be logistically impossible to keep one student working with the same preceptor over time. As the student moves from preceptor to preceptor, coaching and evaluations may become inconsistent. Likewise, what constitutes a required team leader or a patient contact at the ALS level may vary greatly from one clinical education site to another.

The Solutions

When tracking student progress during clinical training, educators should focus on the following areas:

- Confirming that the student attended the clinical, arrived on time, dressed in appropriate attire, and prepared to work (assess professionalism)
- Keeping accurate counts of the quantity of experiences the student has accumulated and has yet to finish, measured both in time and in number of patient encounters
- Identifying the nature of the illness or injury of patients with whom the student is coming in contact
- Identifying skills that the student has observed and performed during patient encounters
- Documenting instructor evaluation of the student and coaching the student on issues to address
- Continually assessing the student's progress toward completion of the goals stated in the clinical learning plan

Tracking and Documentation

Both students and clinical educators must document learning activities thoroughly. Because so many variables are at play and so much information is managed simultaneously, a searchable electronic database is one of the best ways of managing all the data being collected. Although these data have to be backed up and safeguarded, it is usually easier to do this than it is to store hard copy forms (paper and pen) in a secure location for a specified time. Although paper forms may be necessary to confirm attendance and document preceptor evaluations, they are not so helpful in analyzing student clinical experiences. Using the power of the Internet to share and manage schedules has become much less cumbersome, but it may require expert advice to prevent data loss and to preserve patient and student privacy. Computerized clinical scheduling and skill tracking enable students and faculty to readily assess student progress. These systems provide reporting information to ensure students have met program and accreditation requirements.

All records, whether hard copy or electronic, must be maintained in a manner consistent with the privacy practices of every public agency, corporation, and/or educational institution involved. At a minimum, the student should complete a summary of the complaints and field impressions of the patients they have encountered, skills that have been observed and performed both successfully and unsuccessfully, standard patient care reports, and attempts at team leadership. Doing so is vitally important to the field education process as it actively reinforces learning and teaches the student the importance of keeping detailed records in future practice.

Clinical educators should confirm the accuracy of the student's documentation and should provide a written review of learning activities and performance. The process of reviewing the student's documentation allows the educator to identify patterns in student performance both good and bad, and to record the successful completion of learning objectives.

When possible, students and educators should go beyond the minimum data-tracking and patient documentation requirements. Students can benefit greatly from a more detailed log of their activity and performance. By tracking detailed information over time, students can also identify patterns in their performance, or lack thereof. A review of the student's experiences will help the educator to monitor the student's progress and anticipate needed learning opportunities or the need for more aggressive coaching.

Additional written work that is helpful in maximizing reflection and learning from experience includes the following activities for the student:

- Keeping a journal of learning activities, lessons learned, emotions, and specific milestones or accomplishments
- Creating a running log of prescription medications encountered (This log can include the indications for use, typical dosages and side effects, and a brief description of the diseases the medications are used to treat.)
- Documenting sources of references used to obtain additional information about a patient's disease, injury, or behavior
- Writing patient care reports in prose with the appropriate use of abbreviations (In some locations, patient care reports require only the completion of check boxes and short words. Students who must synthesize and compose full sentences on a relatively blank section of paper with the use of, for instance, the Subjective Objective Assessment Plan [SOAP] method, the Chief complaint or concern, History, Assessment, Treatment, Transport [CHART] method, or other method, will be intellectually stimulated.)

- After critical events, answering, in writing, a few questions regarding the nature of the experience (This exercise can spark critical thinking and pattern recognition.)

Eureka Graphs

In 1991, Dr. Wilson proposed a novel graphical method of tracking motor learning in IV and endotracheal intubation skills. He arbitrarily defined the moment of competence for IV cannulation as achieving a success rate of 80% over 20 attempts.[43] By having his anesthesia students mark, on graph paper, a downward mark for a miss, and an upward mark for success, Wilson was able to visually identify a period of trial and error, followed by a dramatic and sustained upward swing of the graph representing sustained successful performance. This study was later reproduced with more than 800 paramedic students with the same results.[44] Competency in this context is not just a single moment, but rather a history sustained performance that might reliably indicate a person has achieved consistent positive performance.

In the 2015 NREMT portfolio, experts recommended paramedic students reach an average 90% success rate over 20 team leadership attempts.[1] Using Wilson's graphing method, Cage et al. in 2012 were able to validate that 87% of paramedic students who achieved 90% success rate over 20 attempts (18 of the last 20 leads) would maintain that level of competency moving forward.[45,46]

Team Leadership

In the 2015 Paramedic Psychomotor Competency Portfolio, the NREMT advanced the following definition of team leadership:

> The student has successfully led the team if he or she has conducted a comprehensive assessment (not necessarily performed the entire interview or physical exam, but rather been in charge of the assessment), as well as formulated and implemented a treatment plan for the patient. This means that most (if not all) of the decisions have been made by the student, especially formulating a field impression, directing the treatment, determining patient acuity, disposition and packaging/moving the patient (if applicable). Minimal to no prompting was needed by the preceptor. No action was initiated/performed that endangered the physical or psychological safety of the patient, bystanders, other responders or crew. (Preceptors should not agree to a "successful" rating unless it is truly deserved. As a general rule, more unsuccessful attempts indicate willingness to try and are better than no attempt at all.)[47(p.2)]

While educational programs can edit or adapt this definition, they should do so with caution as this definition was derived based on information from several formal expert panels, two research projects using a nominal group process, and hundreds of paramedic programs piloting the definition to validate the accompanying rating system.[1,11,31]

The NREMT evaluation system (FIGURE 19.5) describes four possible ratings:

> NA = Not applicable, not needed or expected. This is a neutral rating. (Example: Student expected to only observe, or the patient did not need intervention.)
>
> 0 = Unsuccessful, required excessive or critical prompting; includes "Not attempted" when student was expected to try. This is an unsatisfactory rating.
>
> 1 = Marginal inconsistent, not yet competent. This includes partial attempts.
>
> 2 = Successful/competent no prompting.[47(p.1)]

Rater	Objectives						
	Pt Interview + HX gathering	Physical Exam	Field Impression Tx Plan	Skill Performance	Communication	Professional Behavior (Affect)	Team Leadership

FIGURE 19.5 Appendix K of the NREMT *Paramedic Psychomotor Competency Portfolio Manual* is the Capstone Field Internship Shift Evaluation Worksheet, which contains a rating system and objectives to be evaluated shown here. The full worksheet can be found at NREMT.org within the Psychomotor Competency Portfolio Manual.

Reproduced from National Registry of Emergency Medical Technicians. 2015. "Appendix K: Capstone Field Internship Shift Evaluation Worksheet." In 2015 *Paramedic Psychomotor Competency Portfolio (PPCP)*. Columbus, OH: National Registry of Emergency Medical Technicians. The form/information can change without notice.

Using this system, the student should first rate themselves. A cornerstone of professionalism is the clinician's ability to assess themselves, recognize gaps, and seek out new learning to remediate that gap. By having the student self-assess, the preceptor not only encourages reflection on action and critical review, they also teach a lifelong skill of personal accountability. It is only after the student has articulated and perhaps even advocated for the validity of the rating they have assigned themselves, that the preceptor should reveal their rating and reconcile any differences.[1,48,49]

For a sample paramedic internship evaluation tool, see the NREMT Capstone Field Internship Shift Evaluation Worksheet.

Assessment and Feedback

Educators must provide support and feedback throughout a student's clinical experience because this is a vital part of formative evaluation.[50] Students must have the opportunity to safely attempt, fail, regroup, and try again under the conscientious oversight of their instructor. Constructive feedback should lead to changes in style and habits and to experimentation by the student, all of which should be encouraged. Resultant positive achievements should be highlighted, no matter how minimal or small the progress might be. Educators may feel personally challenged and even frustrated when students are not progressing quickly or steadily. Discussions with peers and frequent breaks can alleviate some of the impatience and self-blame that an educator may feel.

Feedback can be given in many formats. One successful feedback tool that educators find helpful is called SMART. SMART provides educators with the following five guidelines for formatting feedback:[51]

S *Specific*. Focus on behavior and performance. Give examples.

M *Meaningful*. Focus on important issues and events. Avoid trivial events.

A *Appropriate*. Provide balanced and fair review, keeping in mind that students respond best to positive feedback. Choose the right moment to praise improvement. The student must be receptive, and the educator has to stay professional.

R *Reality-based*. Give concrete examples that are based on actual behavior and performance.

T *Time*. The closer to the event that feedback is given, the more helpful it is.

See Chapter 22, *Other Assessment Tools*, for more information on evaluation of field and clinical experiences.

Summary

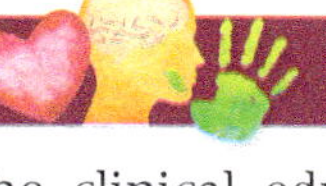

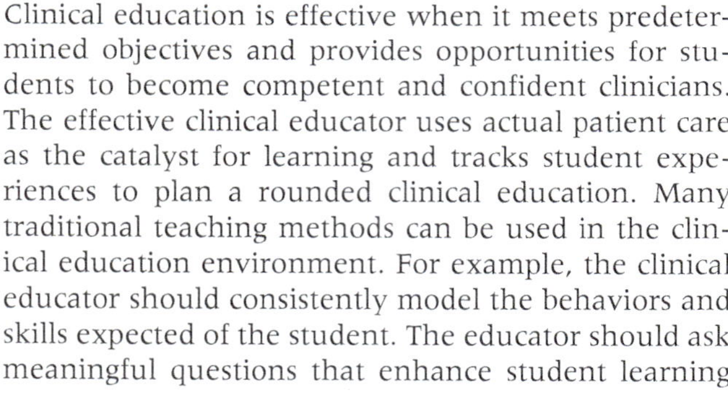

Clinical education is effective when it meets predetermined objectives and provides opportunities for students to become competent and confident clinicians. The effective clinical educator uses actual patient care as the catalyst for learning and tracks student experiences to plan a rounded clinical education. Many traditional teaching methods can be used in the clinical education environment. For example, the clinical educator should consistently model the behaviors and skills expected of the student. The educator should ask meaningful questions that enhance student learning and promote critical thinking. The clinical educator must prepare for the clinical student just as in the traditional classroom environment. The educator must also evaluate a student's clinical performance. However, a clinical educator must plan for the unique challenges of educating a student in a busy patient care environment and must work hard to take advantage of a student's teachable moments. Being an effective clinical educator can be vastly rewarding and can make a difference in a student's readiness for a real work experience.

Glossary

clinical educator Patient care practitioner who guides experiential learning during real patient care.

convergent questions Questions that seek specific information.

divergent questions Questions that do not have a single correct answer.

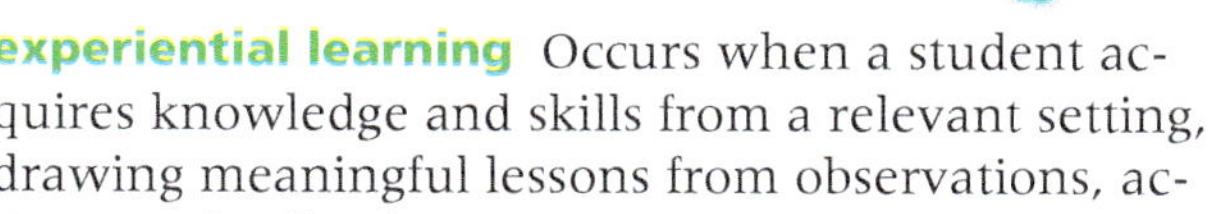

experiential learning Occurs when a student acquires knowledge and skills from a relevant setting, drawing meaningful lessons from observations, actions, and reflections.

field clinical (field experience) Prehospital or outdoor experiences, which may be primarily observation or performing isolated skills as directed by the EMS personnel on the ambulance.

field internship Planned, scheduled educational experience on an advanced life support unit that includes team-leading skills and the management of prehospital patients and scenes. Also, a capstone event in which the student leads the assessment and care, particularly of patients requiring advanced life support care.

hospital clinical Experiences in a hospital, clinic, or other indoor setting.

preceptors Individuals who teach in the hospital or field clinical setting.

References

[1] National Registry of Emergency Medical Technicians. 2019. "National Registry of Emergency Medical Technicians." Accessed May 2, 2019. https://www.nremt.org/rwd/public.

[2] Michau, Rebecca, Samantha Roberts, Brett Williams, and Malcolm Boyle. 2009. "An Investigation of Theory-Practice Gap in Undergraduate Paramedic Education." *BMC Medical Education* 9, no. 1. https://doi.org/10.1186/1472-6920-9-23.

[3] Mulholland, Susan, and Michele Derdall. 2007. "An Early Fieldwork Experience: Student and Preceptor Perspectives." *Canadian Journal of Occupational Therapy* 74, no. 3: 161–71. https://doi.org/10.1177/000841740707400304.

[4] College of Paramedics. May 2017. *Practice Educator Guidance Handbook*. Bridgewater, UK: College of Paramedics.

[5] Maben, Jill, Sue Latter, and J. M. Clark. 2006. "The Theory–Practice Gap: Impact of Professional–Bureaucratic Work Conflict on Newly-Qualified Nurses" *JAN* 55, no. 4: 465–77. https://doi.org/10.1111/j.1365-2648.2006.03939.x.

[6] Cook, Stephen H. 1991. "Mind the Theory/Practice Gap in Nursing." *Journal of Advanced Nursing* 16, no. 120: 1462–9. https://doi.org/10.1111/j.1365-2648.1991.tb01594.x.

[7] Tavares, Walter, and Sylvain Boet. 2015. "On the Assessment of Paramedic Competence: A Narrative Review with Practice Implications." *Prehospital Disaster Medicine* 31, no. 1: 64–73. https://doi.org/10.1017/S1049023X15005166.

[8] Crowe, Remle P., Roger Levine, Severo Rodriguez, Ashley D. Larrimore, and Ronald G. Pirrallo. 2016. "Public Perception of Emergency Medical Services in the United States." *Prehospital Disaster Medicine* 31, Suppl 1: S112–7. https://doi.org/10.1017/S1049023X16001126.

[9] Tavares, Walter, and Justin Mausz. 2015. "Assessment of Non-clinical Attributes in Paramedicine Using Multiple Mini-interviews." *Emergency Medicine Journal* 32, no. 1: 70–5. http://dx.doi.org/10.1136/emermed-2013-202964.

[10] Walker, Mary, Jan L. Jensen, and Andrew H. Travers. 2010. "Paramedic Confidence in Clinical Care." *Canadian Journal of Emergency Medicine* 12, no. 3: 248–9. https://doi.org/10.1017/S1481803500012318.

[11] Crowe, Remle P., Robert L. Wagoner, Severo A. Rodriguez, Melissa A. Bentley, and David R. Page. 2017. "Defining Components of Team Leadership and Membership in Prehospital Emergency Medical Services." *Prehospital Emergency Care* 21, no. 5: 645–51. https://doi.org/10.1080/10903127.2017.1315200.

[12] Fraser, Kristin L., Paul Ayres, and John Sweller. 2015. "Cognitive Load Theory for the Design of Medical Simulations." *Simulation in Healthcare* 10, no. 5: 295–307. http://dx.doi.org/10.1097/SIH.0000000000000097.

[13] Devenish, Anothony S. 2014. "Experiences in Becoming a Paramedic: A Qualitative Study Examining the Professional Socialisation of University Qualified Paramedics." PhD dissertation, Queensland University of Technology. Accessed March 9, 2019. https://eprints.qut.edu.au/78442/1/Anthony_Devenish_Thesis.pdf.

[14] Lane, Matthew. 2014. "Student Perceptions in Relation to Paramedic Educator (PEd) Roles." *Journal of Paramedic Practice* 6: 200–2. https://doi.org/10.12968/jpar.2014.6.4.194.

[15] Williamson, Graham R., Lynn Callaghan, Emma Whittlesea, Lauren Mutton, and Val Heath. 2011. "Longitudinal Evaluation of the Impact of Placement Development Teams on Student Support in Clinical Practice." *Open Nursing Journal* 5: 14–23. http://dx.doi.org/10.2174/1874434601105010014.

[16] Committee on Accreditation of Educational Programs for Emergency Medical Services Professions (CoAEMSP). 2015. "CoAEMSP Interpretations of the CAAHEP 2015 Standards and Guidelines for the Accreditation of Educational Programs in the EMS Professions." Accessed February 13, 2019. https://coaemsp.org/Documents/2015%20CoAEMSP%20Interpretations%20of%20the%202015%20CAAHEP%20Standards%202018.07.28.pdf.

[17] Carpenito, Linda J., and T. Audean Duespohl. 1985. *A Guide for Effective Clinical Instruction*, 2nd ed. Rockville, MD: Aspen Systems Corporation.

[18] Stengelhofen, Jackie. 1996. *Teaching Students in Clinical Settings*. London: Chapman & Hall.

[19] Hunt, Jasper. 1981. "Dewey's Philosophical Method and Its Influence on his Philosophy of Education." *Journal of Experiential Education* 4: 29–34. https://doi.org/10.1177/105382598100400106.

[20] Shuttenberg, Ernest M., and Brent W. Poppenhagen. 1980. "Current Theory and Research in Experiential Learning for Adults." *Journal of Experiential Education* 3: 27–31. https://doi.org/10.1177/105382598000300106.

[21] Lawler, Ron, and Kyle Chambers. 2010. "Right Dose? An Examination of a Prescription to Enhance Critical Thinking in Paramedic Students." [Oral and poster abstract]. Presented at the National Association of EMS Educators Symposium.

[22] Ricketts, Kathi, Rob Gurliacci, Sara Houston, Tim Howey, Barry Jensen, Liz Neerland, and Ian Young. 2010. "The Effect of Clinical and Field Experience on Critical-Thinking Performance for Emergency Medical Technician Students Taking the EMT Readiness Exam." [Oral and poster abstract]. Presented at the National Association of EMS Educators Symposium.

[23] Bercher, Daniel, Denise A. Wilfong, Debi M. Workman, Kim McKenna, John B. Gosford, Timothey Howey, Brian C. Peterson, and Louise E. Briguglio. 2009. "Predictors of Paramedic Program Success on the National Registry Written Examination." [Poster abstract]. Presented at the National Association of EMS Educators Symposium.

[24] Briguglio, Louise, Charles Soucheray, Ian Young, and Anne Eaton. 2009. "Paramedic Student Internship Experience, Critical Thinking, and NREMTCE Success—Phase Two: Are Paramedic Students Who Perform Well on Critical-Thinking Test Questions More Likely to Pass the NREMT Cognitive Examination?" [Oral and poster abstract]. Presented at the National Association of EMS Educators Symposium.

[25] Salzman, Josh, Justin Dillingham, Jenny Kobersteen, Koren Kaye, and David Page. 2008. "Effect of Paramedic Student Internship Experience on Performance on the National Registry Written Exam." *Prehospital Emergency Care* 12, no. 2: 212–6.

[26] National Highway Traffic Safety Administration. 2009. *National Emergency Medical Services Education Standards*. Washington DC:

U.S. Department of Transportation/National Highway Traffic Safety Administration.

[27] Cherry, Richard A. 1998. *EMT Teaching: A Common Sense Approach.* Upper Saddle River, NJ: Prentice Hall.

[28] Davis, Barbara G. 2001. *Tools for Teaching.* San Francisco: Jossey-Bass; 167.

[29] Billings, Diane M., and Judith A. Halstead. 1998. *Teaching in Nursing: A Guide for Faculty.* Philadelphia: W. B. Saunders; 286.

[30] Oermann, Marilyn H. 1996. "Research on Teaching in the Clinical Setting." In *Review of Research in Nursing Education*, edited by Kathleen R. Stevens, 91–126. New York: National League for Nursing.

[31] Bentley, Melissa A., Jennifer J. Eggerichs-Purcell, William E. Brown, Robert Wagoner, Gregory C. Gibson, and Ritu Sahni. 2013. "A National Assessment of the Roles and Responsibilities of Training Officers." *Prehospital Emergency Care* 17, no. 3: 373–8. https://doi.org/10.3109/10903127.2013.785618.

[32] Allan, Helen T., Carin Magnusson, Karen Evans, Khim Horton, Kathy Curtis, Elaine Ball, and Martin Johnson. 2017. "Putting Knowledge to Work in Clinical Practice: Understanding Experiences of Preceptorship as Outcomes of Interconnected Domains of Learning." *Journal of Clinical Nursing* 27, no. 1–2: 123–31. https://doi.org/10.1111/jocn.13855.

[33] Meisenhelder, Janice B. 1987. "Anxiety: A Block to Clinical Teaching." *Nurse Educator* 12: 27–30.

[34] Kleehammer, Kelly, A. Louise Hart, and Juanita F. Keck. 1990. "Nursing Students' Perception of Anxiety-Producing Situations in the Clinical Setting." *Journal of Nursing Education* 29: 183–7. https://doi.org/10.3928/0148-4834-19900401-10.

[35] Reese, Andy C. 1998. "Implications of Results from Cognitive Science Research for Medical Education." *Medical Education Online* 3: 4295. https://doi.org/10.3402/meo.v3i.4295.

[36] Kolb, David A., Irwin A. Kolb, and James M. McIntyre. 1971. *Organizational Psychology: An Experiential Approach.* Upper Saddle River, NJ: Prentice-Hall.

[37] Wink, Diane M. 1993. "Using Questioning as a Teaching Strategy." *Nurse Education* 18, no. 5: 11–15.

[38] Parvensky, Catherine A. 1995. *Teaching EMS: An Educator's Guide to Improved EMS Instruction.* St. Louis, MO: Mosby Lifeline.

[39] Page, David I., Baxter Larmon, and Timothy Howey. 2007. "A Chance to Lead: Does Having Fewer Paramedic Preceptors Result in More Student Leadership?" [Oral and poster abstract]. Presented at the National Association of EMS Educators Symposium.

[40] Cage, Todd M., James Dinsch, Mike Mayne, Steve Asche, and David Page. 2014. "Fewer Preceptors Leads to Faster Attainment of Team Leadership Competency during Paramedic Student Internships." [Poster abstract]. Presented at the NAEMSP Scientific Meeting, Tucson, AZ.

[41] Worlf, Z. R., and O'Driscoll, R. W. 1979. "How Useful is the Preclinical Conference?" *Nursing Outlook* 27, 455–7.

[42] Matheney, Ruth V. 1969. "Pre- and Post-conferences for Students." *American Journal of Nursing* 69: 286–9. http://dx.doi.org/10.2307/3453961.

[43] Wilson, M. E. 1991. "Assessing Intravenous Cannulation and Tracheal Intubation Training." *Anaesthesia* 46: 578–9. https://doi.org/10.1111/j.1365-2044.1991.tb09662.x.

[44] Howey, Timothy, and David Page. 2005. "Eureka! Measuring Competency in Intravenous (IV) Cannulation by Paramedic Students." [Oral abstract]. Presented at the National Association of EMS Educators Symposium: Prehospital Care Research Forum.

[45] Widmeier, Keith, Marshall Washick, James Dinsch, Todd M. Cage, Mike Mayne, and Steve Asche. 2012. "When Is a Paramedic Student a Competent Team Leader?" Presented at the National Association of EMS Educators Symposium: Prehospital Care Research Forum.

[46] Page, David I., Tom Brazelton, Gordon Kokx, and Michael Johnson. 2015. "How Good Is Good Enough? Predicting Team Leadership Competency in Graduating Paramedic Students." [Poster abstract]. Presented at the 2015 Symposium: Prehospital Care Research Forum.

[47] National Registry of Emergency Medical Technicians. 2015. "Appendix K: Capstone Field Internship Shift Evaluation Worksheet." In *2015 Paramedic Psychomotor Competency Portfolio (PPCP).* Columbus, OH: National Registry of Emergency Medical Technicians.

[48] Epstein, Ronald M., and Edward M. Hundert. 2002. "Defining and Assessing Professional Competence." *Journal of the American Medical Association* 287, no. 2: 226–35. http://dx.doi.org/10.1001/jama.287.2.226.

[49] Bloor, Lindsey E., Katherine A. Kitchen Andren, and Cathy J. Strader Donnell. 2018. "Preparing to Be a Clinical Supervisor: Avoiding a 'Trial by Fire' and Using Reflection." *Psychology* 9, no. 4: 809–19. http://dx.doi.org/10.4236/psych.2018.94052.

[50] Joplin, Laura. 1997. *On Defining Experiential Education: The Theory of Experiential Education*, 2nd ed. Boulder, CO: Association for Experiential Education.

[51] Rubin, Robert S. 2002. "Will the Real SMART Goals Please Stand Up?" *The Industrial-Organizational Psychologist* 39, no. 4. Accessed April 30, 2019. http://www.siop.org/tip/backissues/tipapr02/03rubin.aspx.

Additional Resources

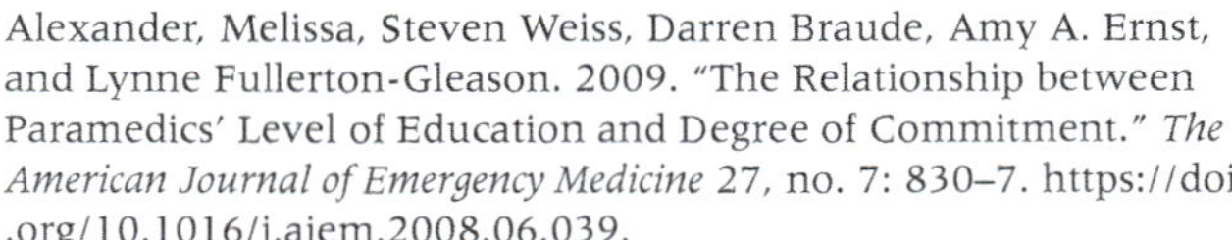

Alexander, Melissa, Steven Weiss, Darren Braude, Amy A. Ernst, and Lynne Fullerton-Gleason. 2009. "The Relationship between Paramedics' Level of Education and Degree of Commitment." *The American Journal of Emergency Medicine* 27, no. 7: 830–7. https://doi.org/10.1016/j.ajem.2008.06.039.

Baxter, Pamela, and Geoff Norman. 2011. "Self-Assessment or Self Deception? A Lack of Association between Nursing Students' Self-Assessment and Performance." *Journal of Advanced Nursing*, 2406–13. https://doi.org/10.1111/j.1365-2648.2011.05658.x.

Belur, Jyoti, Winifred Agnew-Pauley, and Lisa Tompson. 2018. "Designing a Graduate Entry Route for Police Recruits: Lessons from a Rapid Evidence Assessment of Other Professions." *Police Practice and Research* 1–18. https://doi.org/10.1080/15614263.2018.1526685.

Boney, Jo, and Jacqueline D. Baker, J. 1997. "Strategies for Teaching Clinical Decision Making." *Nurse Education Today* 17: 16–21. https://doi.org/10.1016/S0260-6917(97)80074-3.

Bourn, S., and M. Smith. 1995. "Reliability of EMS Instructors as Evaluators of Practical Skills Stations. Prehospital Care Research Forum." *Journal of Emergency Medical Services* 20: 113.

Boyle, Malcolm, and Lisa McKenna. 2017. "Paramedic Student Exposure to Workplace Violence during Clinical Placements—A Cross-sectional Study." *Nurse Education in Practice* 22: 93–7. https://doi.org/10.1016/j.nepr.2017.01.001.

Boyle, Malcolm J., Brett Williams, Jennifer Cooper, Bridget Adams, and Kassie Alford. 2008. "Ambulance Clinical Placement—A Pilot

Study of Students' Experience." *BMC Medical Education* 8, no. 1: 19. https://doi.org/10.1186/1472-6920-8-19.

Brenner, Judith, Jeffrey Bird, Samara B. Ginzburg, Thomas Kwiatkowski, Vincent Papasodero, William Rennie, Elisabeth Schlegel, Olle Ten Cate, and Joanne M. Willey. 2018. "Trusting Early Learners with Critical Professional Activities through Emergency Medical Technician Certification." *Medical Teacher* 40, no. 6: 561–68. https://doi.org/10.1080/0142159X.2018.1444745.

Buis, Caroline A. M., Marina A. W. Eckenhausen, and Olle ten Cate. 2018. "Processing Multisource Feedback during Residency under the Guidance of a Non-medical Coach." *International Journal of Medical Education* 9: 48–54. https://dx.doi.org/10.5116/ijme.5a7f.169d.

Carlson, Jestin N., and Henry E. Wang. 2017. "Paramedic Intubation: Does Practice Make Perfect?" *Annals of Emergency Medicine* 70, no. 3: 391–3. https://doi.org/10.1016/j.annemergmed.2017.03.024.

Clements, R., and R. Mackenzie. 2005. "Competence in Prehospital Care: Evolving Concepts." *Emergency Medicine Journal* 22: 516–9. http://dx.doi.org/10.1136/emj.2005.026237

Criss, Elizabeth A. 1998. "EMS Research: Obstacles of the Past, Opportunities in the Present, Models for the Future. Prehospital Care Research Forum." *Journal of Emergency Medical Services* (Suppl). https://www.cpc.mednet.ucla.edu/sites/default/files/pcrf_attached_files/pdf1.pdf.

Dowd, S. B. 1994. "Clock Hours or Competencies?" *Radiology Technology* 65: 325–6.

Duke, Maxine. 1996. "Clinical Evaluation: Difficulties Experienced by Sessional Clinical Teachers of Nursing: A Qualitative Study." *Journal of Advanced Nursing* 23: 408–14. https://doi.org/10.1111/j.1365-2648.1996.tb02685.x.

Dyson, Kylie, Janet E. Bray, Karen Smith, Stephen Bernard, Lahn Straney, Resmi Nair, and Judith Finn. 2017. "Paramedic Intubation Experience Is Associated with Successful Tube Placement but Not Cardiac Arrest Survival." *Annals of Emergency Medicine* 70, no. 3: 282–390. https://doi.org/10.1016/j.annemergmed.2017.02.002.

Edwards, Dale. 2011 "Paramedic Preceptor: Work Readiness in Graduate Paramedics." *The Clinical Teacher* 8, no. 2: 79–82. https://doi.org/10.1111/j.1743-498X.2011.00435.x.

Edwards, Deborah, Clare Hawker, Judith Carrier, and Colin Rees. 2015. "A Systematic Review of the Effectiveness of Strategies and Interventions to Improve the Transition from Student to Newly Qualified Nurse." *International Journal of Nursing Studies* 52, no. 7: 1254–268. https://doi.org/10.1016/j.ijnurstu.2015.03.007.

Epstein, Ronald M., Daniel J. Siegel, and Jordan Silberman. 2008. "Self-Monitoring in Clinical Practice: A Challenge for Medical Educators." *Journal of Continuing Education in the Health Professions* 28, no. 1: 5–13. http://dx.doi.org/10.1002/chp.149.

Gardner, Elaine A. C. 2006. "Instruction in Mastery Goal Orientation: Developing Problem Solving and Persistence for Clinical Settings." *The Journal of Nursing Education* 45, no. 9: 343–7.

Goodwin, Tress, B. Elizabeth Delasobera, Matthew Strehlow, Jolyn Camacho, Mary Koskovich, Peter D'Souza, Gregory Gilbert, and S. V. Mahadevan. 2012. "Indian and United States Paramedic Students: Comparison of Examination Performance for the American Heart Association Advanced Cardiovascular Life Support (ACLS) Training." *The Journal of Emergency Medicine* 43, no. 2: 298–302. https://doi.org/10.1016/j.jemermed.2011.05.096.

Hilding, Hanna, Zoe Jordan, and Micah D. J. Peters. 2018. "Experiences of Learning, Development and Preparedness for Clinical Practice among Undergraduate Paramedicine Students, Graduate/Intern Paramedics and Their Preceptors." *JBI Database of Systematic Reviews and Implementation Reports* 16, no. 12: 2253–9. http://dx.doi.org/10.11124/jbisrir-2017-003618.

Innes, Tiana, and Pauline Calleja. 2018. "Transition Support for New Graduate and Novice Nurses in Critical Care Settings: An Integrative Review of the Literature." *Nurse Education in Practice* 30: 62–72. https://doi.org/10.1016/j.nepr.2018.03.001.

Irwin, Carole, Julie Bliss, and Karen Poole. 2018. "Does Preceptorship Improve Confidence and Competence in Newly Qualified Nurses: A Systematic Literature Review." *Nurse Education Today* 60: 35–46. https://doi.org/10.1016/j.nedt.2017.09.011.

Jensen, J. L., Bienkowski, A., Travers, A. H., Calder, L. A., Walker, M., Tavares, W., and Croskerry, P. 2016. "A Survey to Determine Decision-Making Styles of Working Paramedics and Student Paramedics." *Canadian Journal of Emergency Medicine* 18, no. 3, 213–22. https://doi.org/10.1017/cem.2015.95.

Jensen, Jan L., Pat Croskerry, and Andrew H. Travers. 2015. "Consensus on Paramedic Clinical Decisions during High-Acuity Emergency Calls: Results of a Canadian Delphi Study." *Canadian Journal of Emergency Medicine* 13, no. 5: 310–8. https://doi.org/10.2310/8000.2011.110405

Kassirer, Jerome P. 2010. "Teaching Clinical Reasoning: Case-Based and Coached." *Academic Emergency Medicine* 85, no. 7: 1118–24. http://dx.doi.org/10.1097/ACM.0b013e3181d5dd0d

Kennedy, Sean, Amanda Kenny, and Peter O'Meara. 2015. "Student Paramedic Experience of Transition into the Workforce: A Scoping Review." *Nurse Education Today* 35, no. 10: 1037–43. https://doi.org/10.1016/j.nedt.2015.04.015.

Klein, Gloria J. 2000. "The Relationships among Anxiety, Self-Concept, the Impostor Phenomenon, and Generic Senior Baccalaureate Nursing Students' Perceptions of Clinical Competency." D.N.Sc. doctoral dissertation research, Widener University.

Konrad, Christoph, Guido Schupfer, Markus Wietlisbach, and Helmut Gerber. 1998. "Learning Manual Skills in Anesthesiology: Is There a Recommended Number of Cases for Anesthetic Procedures?" *Anesthesia and Analgesia* 86: 635–9. http://dx.doi.org/10.1213/00000539-199803000-00037.

Kowlowitz, Vicki, Peter Curtis, and Philip Sloane. 1990. "The Procedural Skills of Medical Students: Expectations and Experiences." *Academic Medicine* 65: 656–8. http:// http://dx.doi.org/10.1097/00001888-199010000-00016.

Kuiper, RuthAnne. 2002. "Enhancing Metacognition through the Reflective Use of Self-Regulated Learning Strategies." *The Journal of Continuing Education in Nursing* 33, no. 2: 78–87.

Lambert, Jim. 2018. "The Impact of Emotional Intelligence and Affective Behavior on Paramedic Student Field Internship Success." PhD dissertation, Brandman University. https://digitalcommons.brandman.edu/edd_dissertations/215.

Lenson, Shane, and Jason Mills. 2018. "Undergraduate Paramedic Student Psychomotor Skills in an Obstetric Setting: An Evaluation." *Nurse Education in Practice* 28: 13–19. https://doi.org/10.1016/j.nepr.2017.08.004

Marchigiano, Gail A., Nina Eduljee, and Kimberly Harvey. 2011. "Developing Critical Thinking Skills from Clinical Assignments: A Pilot Study on Nursing Students' Self-Reported Perceptions." *Journal of Nursing Management* 19, no. 1: 143–52. https://doi.org/10.1111/j.1365-2834.2010.01191.x.

Margolis, Gregg, and Stoy, Walt. 1998, March. "The Length of Paramedic-Education Programs in the United States. Prehospital Care Research Forum." *Journal of Emergency Medical Services* (Suppl): S-21.

McGuire, Christine H., and David Babbott. 1997. "Simulation Technique in the Measurement of Problem-Solving Skills. *Journal of Educational Measurement,* 4. https://doi.org/10.1111/j.1745-3984.1967.tb00562.x.

National Highway Traffic Safety Administration. 2009. "*National Emergency Medical Services Education Standards.*" [DOT HS 811 077A]. https://www.ems.gov/pdf/National-EMS-Education-Standards-FINAL-Jan-2009.pdf.

O'Meara, Peter, Brett Williams, and Helen Hickson. 2015. "Paramedic Instructor Perspectives on the Quality of Clinical and Field Placements for University Educated Paramedicine Students." *Nurse Education Today* 35, no. 11: 1080–4. https://doi.org/10.1016/j.nedt.2015.06.002.

Page, David. 2016, September 28. "Medication Safety: Medication Cross-Check Procedure." *EMS Reference/Fisdap*. https://emsreference.com/articles/article/medication-safety-0.

Pascoe, Jennifer M., James Nixon, and Valerie J. Lang. 2015. "Maximizing Teaching on the Wards: Review and Application of the One-Minute Preceptor and SNAPPS Models." *Journal of Hospital Medicine* 10, no. 2: 125–30. http://dx.doi.org/10.1002/jhm.2302.

Pasila, Katariina, Satu Elo, and Maria Kääriäinen. 2017. "Newly Graduated Nurses' Orientation Experiences: A Systematic Review of Qualitative Studies." *International Journal of Nursing Studies* 71: 17–27. https://doi.org/10.1016/j.ijnurstu.2017.02.021.

Pitt, Victoria, David Powis, Tracy Levett-Jones, and Sharyn Hunter. 2012. "Factors Influencing Nursing Students' Academic and Clinical Performance and Attrition: An Integrative Literature Review." *Nurse Education Today* 32, no. 8: 903–13. https://doi.org/10.1016/j.nedt.2012.04.011.

Rush, Kathy L., Monica Adamack, Jason Gordon, Meredith Lilly, and Robert Janke. 2013. "Best Practices of Formal New Graduate Nurse Transition Programs: An Integrative Review." *International Journal of Nursing Studies*, 50, no. 3: 345–56. https://doi.org/10.1016/j.ijnurstu.2012.06.009.

Sloboda, John A., Jane W. Davidson, Michael J. A. Howe, and Derek G. Moore. 1996. "The Role of Practice in the Development of Performing Musicians." *British Journal of Psychology* 87: 287–309. https://doi.org/10.1111/j.2044-8295.1996.tb02591.x.

Smith, Michael W., Melissa A. Bentley, Antonio R. Fernandez, Gregory Gibson, Sharon B. Schweikhart, and David D. Woods. 2013. "Performance of Experienced versus Less Experienced Paramedics in Managing Challenging Scenarios: A Cognitive Task Analysis Study." *Annals of Emergency Medicine* 62, no. 4: 367–79. https://doi.org/10.1016/j.annemergmed.2013.04.026.

Snyder, Wayne, and Steve Smit. 1998. "Evaluating the Evaluators: Inter-Rater Reliability on EMT-Licensing Examinations." *Prehospital Emergency Care* 2: 37–46. https://doi.org/10.1080/10903129808958838.

Tavares, Walter, Vicki R. LeBlanc, Justin Mausz, Victor Sun, and Kevin W. Eva. 2013. "Simulation-Based Assessment of Paramedics and Performance in Real Clinical Contexts." *Prehospital Emergency Care* 18, no. 1: 116–22. https://doi.org/10.3109/10903127.2013.818178.

van Houten-Schat, Maaike A., Joris J. Berkhout, Nynke Van Dijk, Maaike D. Endedijk, A. Debbie C Jaarsma, and Agnes D. Diemers. 2018. "Self-Regulated Learning in the Clinical Context: A Systematic Review." *Medical Education* 52, no. 10: 1008–15. https://doi.org/10.1111/medu.13615.

Waldo, Narisa, and Melina Hermanns. 2009. "Journaling Unlocks Fears in Clinical Practice." *RN* 72, no. 5: 26–31.

Williams, Angela. 2013. "The Strategies Used to Deal with Emotion Work in Student Paramedic Practice." *Nurse Education in Practice* 13, no. 3: 207–12. https://doi.org/10.1016/j.nepr.2012.09.010.

Williams, Brett, Chris Fielder, Gary Strong, Joe Acker, and Sean Thompson. 2015. "Are Paramedic Students Ready to Be Professional? An International Comparison Study." *International Emergency Nursing* 23, no. 2: 120–26. https://doi.org/10.1016/j.ienj.2014.07.004.

PART V

Student Assessment and Remediation

In previous chapters, the emergency medical services (EMS) educator has been portrayed as a coach who works closely with students to bring out their best performance and help them achieve learning success. However, the instructor must play another key role—that of evaluator. Just as a coach assesses players at the end of the preseason, the EMS instructor must carefully assess whether the student is prepared to play in the "big leagues" of managing real-world patients in real-world environments.

This vital aspect of the teaching process is often overlooked or "thrown together" at the last minute. Assessment is a challenging task that requires collaboration and careful planning. A well-crafted testing strategy can both assess and enhance learning. To measure learning effectively, instructors must know how to develop or select the proper type of assessment—one that measures objectives and desired attributes, and provides a reliable manner for test delivery and a mechanism to interpret results properly.

Without a solid evaluation system that assesses students in all domains, instructors will fail at their goal to graduate EMS providers who are competent in their knowledge, skills, and behaviors/attitudes. When students begin to move down a failing path in any of the three domains of learning, the instructor must know how to develop a remediation strategy and, in some cases, a formal learning contract, to attempt to guide them to success. This part of the text is designed to jump-start instructors by describing general principles of assessment, written and other types of assessment tools, and implementation of the remediation process.

CHAPTER 20

Assessing Learning

OBJECTIVES

At the conclusion of this chapter, the educator will be able to:

Cognitive Domain

1. Discuss how to assess student learning.
2. Describe how student assessment results may be used.
3. List types of assessments of learning.
4. Distinguish between formative (low-stakes) and summative (high-stakes) assessments.
5. Define *reliability* and *interrater reliability*.
6. Outline measures to increase assessment reliability.
7. Define *validity* and its constituent aspects.
8. Outline strategies to ensure assessment validity.
9. List the steps to design a valid and reliable assessment.

Psychomotor Domain

There are no psychomotor objectives for this chapter.

Affective Domain

1. Defend the need for valid and reliable student assessment.

"Good people are good because they've come to wisdom through failure. We get very little wisdom from success, you know."

~ William Saroyan

CHAPTER GOAL This chapter introduces the concepts of purpose, reliability, and validity and applies them to the development of a strategy to assess learning.

Assessing student performance is a task that is often seen as especially daunting. Creating appropriate tools for use in evaluating student performance requires knowledge of the core concepts of purpose, reliability, and validity.

Assessment is an important component of student learning. Although the most common use of student assessment is to assign a grade, it has other important purposes for students and instructors. Additionally, although the types of assessment are numerous, in all cases the process of student assessment should be carefully considered and planned.

Assessment

The act of teaching involves facilitating student acquisition of new knowledge, skills, and attitudes. The process of determining whether a student has successfully acquired new capabilities is referred to as *assessment* (although some sources may refer to this process using other terms, such as *evaluation*). The program administrator and instructors evaluate many aspects of the educational process during program evaluation. This chapter focuses on the principles involved in assessing student mastery.

Multiple Messages of Assessment

The results of assessments contain information that enables the instructor to make judgments. To make appropriate judgments on the basis of an assessment, the instructor must understand several core concepts. First and foremost, the instructor must be aware that all assessments combine evaluation of the student's acquisition of knowledge and the effectiveness of teaching. Thus, two messages are contained within each assessment: how well the student is performing and how well the instructor is enabling learning. The effective instructor carefully considers each assessment to look for *both* messages. Barbara Davis writes in her book, *Tools for Teaching*:

> Testing is an integral part of instruction, and well-designed tests serve four principal functions. First, tests can motivate students and help them structure their academic efforts. . . . Second, tests give students an indication of which topics or skills they have not yet mastered and should concentrate on. Third, tests help instructors identify students' errors and misconceptions and adjust instruction to improve learning. Fourth, tests help instructors document whether students are learning what they are expected to learn.[1(p362)]

Importance of Different Tools

The effective instructor does not rely solely on any single assessment tool. Instructors assess student knowledge through formal methods such as written examinations, research projects, practical examinations, and observational reports. Instructors also use informal methods, such as questions delivered in class and homework assignments. Typically, formal assessments are used to determine a "grade" for each student, while informal assessments may not be part of the grading system. Informal assessments are particularly valuable for providing immediate feedback regarding instructional effectiveness. On the other hand, informal assessments lack the rigor necessary to justify decisions regarding student competency or pass/fail status. Although formal systems inform sound judgment regarding the student's mastery of objectives, formal systems may not be useful in providing feedback for modifying the teaching strategy unless the feedback is provided in a timely manner. The combination of these different formal and informal assessments provides a complete view of student performance.

TEACHING TIP

The effective instructor uses more than one tool to assess learning.

Importance of a System for Constructing Assessment Tools

Properly constructing appropriate assessment tools from scratch can be a challenging task that is generally beyond the scope of a novice instructor. Constructing assessment tools often requires systems and processes. Even a seasoned instructor may be unable to complete the task alone. When courses are taught and coordinated by individual instructors, an informal network of instructors can accomplish the same tasks as institutional systems that design tools for assessment. Individual instructors can and should work together for the improvement of each instructor's assessment strategies and tools. Although the processes described in this section for design of assessment strategy, creation of tools for assessment, and analysis of the effectiveness of these tools may be beyond the capability of a single instructor, they can be effectively implemented by networks of instructors who are working for the common good. Professional associations such as the National Association of EMS Educators (NAEMSE) can encourage these networks. Individual instructors have the responsibility of actively participating in these networks, whether they are formed within a single institution, in collaboration with multiple institutions, or in a cooperative effort between independent instructors.

Assessing student performance is a core competency for all those who have a role in instruction. For instance, while preceptors in the clinical environment are unlikely to develop written tests, they definitely conduct observational reports and make assessments of candidates' knowledge. Similarly, all instructors use techniques such as informal questioning to evaluate student understanding. Instructors in all settings, from the classroom, lab, or clinical site, should understand the core concepts of assessment, and must appreciate the implications of these concepts for their particular setting. Although specific tools may vary, the core concepts of assessment are applicable to all instructor roles.

The Purposes of Assessment

The first step in designing a tool is to decide on the purpose of the assessment. Appropriate design of evaluation instruments begins with consideration of the judgment that will be made from that assessment. Significant differences can be found when instruments and tools used to provide feedback to the student are compared with assessments used to determine whether the student is prepared to graduate from an educational program. Differences in design follow from differences in intended purpose.

Formative versus Summative Assessment

Formative assessment is the ongoing evaluation of student performance throughout a course. Formative assessment is important for instructors to gain insight early in the course, while the instructor can adapt teaching methods. Examples of formative assessments include audience feedback systems or oral questions asked in class, having students write out questions for the instructor's consideration during a break, frequent short quizzes, practical drills, and homework assignments. The intent of these strategies is to provide feedback to students and instructors regarding progress made toward achieving the course objectives. By using formative assessment, the instructor can modify course structure, adapt presentation strategies, or provide remediation during the course. Students use information from formative assessment to modify study habits and develop an idea of the relative importance of different concepts.

CASE in Point

An instructor in an EMT program is teaching the airway and ventilation portion of a course. During the early phases of the section, the instructor wishes to gain an understanding of how well students are absorbing the information and skills. The instructor decides to give a daily quiz and intends to use the information to adapt her teaching strategy for the next class period. Quiz results will provide feedback to students so they can adjust study strategies and to the instructor, so that she can modify her teaching strategy before the time of the unit exam. This is a formative assessment.

Summative assessment is the evaluation given to students at the end of a course or at the end of a unit within a course. Summative assessment is used to determine whether the terminal goals and objectives of the course or unit were met. Examples of summative assessments include final written examinations, major projects conducted near the end of a unit, final practical examinations, and end-of-course survey instruments. Summative tools provide valuable information on student performance, instructor and preceptor performance, and effectiveness of clinical and field rotations to determine whether course objectives have been met. Unfortunately, feedback from summative assessments can be used only in future courses to inform education strategies.

Most evaluation tools represent a mix of formative and summative assessment. An example of a mixed tool includes the unit examination. A unit exam is summative in the sense that it is used to assess student mastery of a complete block of instructional material. The instructor may require students to pass a unit exam to proceed to the next block of material. There may be little or no time allowed for remediation. The same unit examination may be considered formative in the sense that students will complete several units

CASE in Point

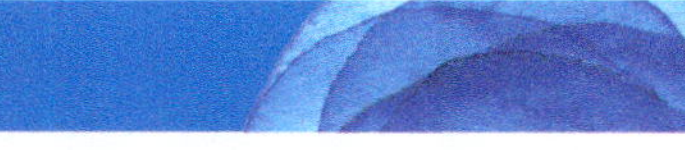

An emergency medical responder (EMR) instructor is approaching the conclusion of the course. Before sending students to sit for certification examinations, he knows he must verify that each student has mastered the knowledge and skills of the curriculum. He administers a final written and skills exam that each student must pass to qualify to take the certification exam. This is a summative assessment.

before they have successfully completed an entire program. Evaluation of each unit gives students feedback on the effectiveness of their strategies for study. Completion of each unit may give the instructor feedback on the integration of different types of material by the students. These formative assessments occur while the unit exams fulfill the summative role of evaluating student mastery of that particular block of content.

High-Stakes Assessments

Instructors should consider the stakes of the assessment before they actually design the instrument (**FIGURE 20.1**). A **high-stakes assessment** is one in which the student's continuation in the program depends on successful completion of (passing) the examination. An example of a high-stakes assessment is a unit or final exam that the student must pass if the student is to pass the overall course. High-stakes examinations are usually summative in nature, with little possibility that feedback can be used to modify learning strategies. Students taking high-stakes examinations often experience significant stress. Also, a high-stakes examination typically raises concerns regarding how well the examination was designed and whether a proper analysis was conducted. With higher stakes come higher standards to defend the examination. In emergency medical services (EMS), the assessment with the highest-stakes is a certification or licensure examination. Thus, these examinations are subject to the highest levels of scrutiny. High-stakes summative assessments require more careful construction than do low-stakes formative assessments.

CASE in Point

An EMS instructor is asked to prepare a written examination to be used as part of the screening process for candidates for employment. If a candidate scores poorly on the examination, the candidate will not be hired, and no opportunity for retest will be provided. The instructor knows that the exam is a high-stakes assessment; therefore, it will need careful analysis and construction.

TEACHING TIP

High-stakes examinations must be created and analyzed with rigor so that they can withstand scrutiny.

Low-Stakes Assessments

A **low-stakes assessment** has relatively little effect on whether a student passes a particular course. Typically, low-stakes assessments are used for formative evaluations. Examples include classroom quizzes and homework assignments. Although each individual assessment carries relatively low stakes, a number of these assessments may collectively have a significant impact on the final grade. Low-stakes examinations are typically subjected to less scrutiny. If the instructor has questions about the quality of the assessment tool, the safest strategy is to reduce the stakes associated with those instruments while their quality is tested and improved as necessary. However, instructors should not consider low-stakes assessments unimportant. Low-stakes formative assessments serve the critical purpose of preparing students for higher-stakes examinations. If an instructor uses only poorly constructed items for low-stakes formative assessments, students will not be prepared for high-stakes exams that use properly constructed items. The instructor should exercise care when selecting items for low-stakes formative assessments so that these experiences will adequately prepare students for final summative assessments.

CASE in Point

An instructor at a community college is using daily quizzes for formative assessment. All quizzes in the course together count for 10% of the final grade. This is an example of low-stakes assessment. The instructor uses these low-stakes quizzes to pilot test items for future use. If an item is shown to be reliable and valid, then the item is used for unit examinations. This allows for items to be evaluated in low-stakes uses and ensures the use of proven items for high-stakes examinations.

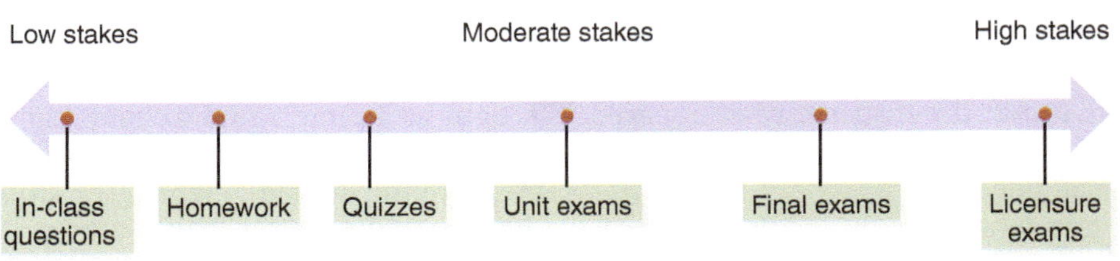

FIGURE 20.1 Comparison of the stakes of assessment tools.

Basis for Assessment

The basis for the assessment relates to consideration of purpose. A curriculum-based assessment is built on the objectives of the educational program. Alignment is the matching of the terminal goals for the course with lesson objectives, presentation of material, and assessments used. In a well-designed and well-conducted course, the examinations match the presented material, which is derived from the lesson objectives. In this way, assessment helps students to attain terminal course goals. Mismatch between goals, objectives, presentation, and assessment leads to difficulties. One symptom of lack of performance agreement is general complaints from students about the examinations. When a performance agreement exists, the examination is a natural and readily accepted component of the learning process.

Assessments designed to verify the competency of the EMS provider, such as examinations administered by the National Registry of Emergency Medical Technicians (NREMT), are designed in a slightly different manner from those based on a prepared curriculum. Competency evaluations are derived from a practice analysis. The practice analysis is a formal evaluation of specific knowledge, skills, and abilities that are needed for acceptable entry into the role of a provider. The distinction between an evaluation designed to verify competency, based on a practice analysis, and a curriculum-based evaluation is especially important for instructors who serve as training officers for an EMS organization. These instructors are occasionally called on to design an assessment strategy that accurately verifies or reverifies the competency of EMS providers. The specific competencies needed within that particular EMS organization may or may not accurately match course objectives, particularly if the initial training was conducted by a different organization. In a perfect world, there would be agreement between curriculum objectives and practice analysis; however, perfect agreement rarely exists. For example, a delay is typically noted between the implementation of new treatment modalities and the inclusion of new treatment modalities in initial training programs for EMS providers. Another example involves competencies specific to a particular area of practice. These are critical to the success of the provider, yet are unlikely to be included in a general EMS initial training program. This makes it essential that the instructor be prepared and willing to modify education standards or standard curricula to meet local needs.

These concepts form the basis of decisions regarding the purpose of an evaluation tool. It is frequently helpful to begin with the question of what will be done with the results (low stakes vs. high stakes). This allows the distinction between formative and summative assessments. Summative assessments used to verify the competency of students as field providers should be based on formal practice analysis in the expected area of application.

Test-Enhanced Learning

Along with the advantages of assessment for instructors, frequent assessment of learning has been found to have substantial benefits for student learning. Researchers have found that the use of **test-enhanced learning** strategies (sometimes known as *retrieval practice*) with frequent formative assessments, in which learners are asked to recall and retain concepts and facts, may have more benefit than traditional studying or rereading strategies.[2–4] While studying using traditional memorization methods may demonstrate more benefit when short-term recall is desirable, test-enhanced learning appears to have greater impact on long-term retention.[5] This benefit appears to be enhanced when tests are repeated over time and feedback is provided after (rather than during) completion of the assessments.[6]

Concerns have been raised regarding the benefit of test-enhanced learning to improve higher cognitive levels as compared to rote learning. Smith and Karpicke found that student ability to answer questions related to both facts and inferences increased when a test-enhanced approach was used.[7]

Reliability of Assessment

For an examination to be an appropriate assessment tool, it must measure consistently. This property is referred to as **reliability**. In other words, an exam with high reliability would produce a consistent result if repeated. If a person weighs in at 150 pounds, a highly reliable scale would produce the same result when the same person is weighed again. Similarly, a reliable exam produces similar results if it is retaken by the same student later. A reliable exam would also produce similar results in different students who have mastered the material to the same degree. Another example can be drawn from target shooting, in that reliability measures the grouping of shots on the target. A tight grouping is said to have high reliability. When an instructor gives an exam, the instructor is aiming to measure the degree to which the student has mastered the material (aiming at the same point on the target). The reliability of the exam is dependent on the variation in results caused by extraneous factors unrelated to student mastery of course information. The impact of these extraneous factors is sometimes referred to as **measurement error**.

One area of reliability that can be particularly troublesome for EMS instructors is **interrater reliability**. This is the consistency in scores that different people assign while grading a particular exam. Concern for interrater reliability is especially high when the instructor is considering the use of practical examinations and other exams that consist of some degree of subjective evaluation, such as tests containing essay questions. Instructors must exercise special care to ensure consistency between evaluators when these types of exams are used. Interrater reliability is analyzed through comparison of scores from different evaluators who are scoring the same examination. Several techniques can be employed to ensure interrater reliability. In general, it is preferable to reduce the subjectivity of the examination by focusing on behaviors or steps that were or were not observed, rather than use of a rating scale to grade parts of the performance. When rating scales are necessary, clearly worded behavioral anchors can enhance consistency among items that are scored according to a rating scale. (A *behavioral anchor* is a description of observable behaviors that is linked to

CASE in Point

A program director is concerned with interrater reliability among part-time EMT lab instructors. The director reviews the skills evaluation forms used to assess student performance to ensure that clear criteria and behavioral descriptions are provided for each skill rating. The director uses a spreadsheet to compare the scores of each instructor. The scores for each instructor are consistent, demonstrating interrater reliability.

Testing Exam Reliability

In the ideal world, the instructor could test reliability by administering the same exam to the same students at a later time. Exams that produce consistent results are said to exhibit stability over time. This test of reliability is called *test-retest reliability*. Although stability over time is important, this approach to testing reliability has a number of drawbacks. Test-retest is expensive and time consuming. If the time interval between tests is short, students will remember some questions and their responses. If the time interval is longer, students will have learned more in the intervening time, in a sense representing a different group of students.

A different and probably better method of testing the reliability of an examination is to assess the same content using different forms of the test and then compare the results. Exams that demonstrate consistent results according to this method have demonstrated *form equivalence*, or *alternate form reliability*. A drawback to this method of testing reliability is that there will invariably be some differences in content or difficulty between forms of the exam, making apples-to-apples comparison difficult.

Constructing different versions (or forms) of the same exam is common with larger classes. The formal procedure to ensure the form equivalence between versions of the same exam is called *equating*. For example, after a new unit exam has been developed for a specific topic such as pediatrics, the instructor can compare the new examination scores with the scores of quizzes that were previously administered. The quizzes contained different items from those in the examination. If scores on the examination roughly match scores on the quizzes, alternate form reliability is demonstrated.

A different method of assessing reliability is to look for internal consistency among examination items. If a survey containing multiple questions is administered, respondents who agree with the statement, "I am comfortable dealing with pediatric patients," should also agree with the statement, "I am comfortable taking care of kids." Examinations can be evaluated according to the same principle.

The **split-half method** of testing internal consistency consists of dividing the exam into halves (commonly odd and even questions), then comparing the percentage of correct answers between the two groups of items. The response pattern should be consistent. Of course, the instructor must exercise care to ensure that the two groups of items are comparable in terms of content and difficulty. One drawback of the split-half method is that results of the analysis will change according to how the data are grouped. To correct this weakness, more complex methods of assessing internal consistency, such as **Cronbach's alpha** and the **Kuder–Richardson** formulas (KR20 and KR21), can be used. These statistical measures assess internal consistency by comparing results for a particular item with all possible combinations of similar items. The Cronbach and Kuder–Richardson methods are typically completed using specialized statistical software.

For example, an instructor in a certification course is using an examination of 40 items without access to statistical software. She assesses the reliability of the examination by comparing scores on the even-numbered items with scores on the odd-numbered items. The scores are roughly equivalent. This is an assessment of reliability performed by the split-half method.

specific ratings in an evaluation.) Interrater reliability can generally be improved by the use of a greater number of evaluators, although without behavioral anchors, these improvements may be obscured by measurement error. One technique is to have a panel of evaluators grade the same student performance. Another would be to have the student performance repeated for multiple evaluators. Some instructors average the scores among evaluators; others eliminate outlying (highest and lowest) scores. Formally quantifying and controlling for interrater reliability can be challenging, but it is necessary to ensure the comparisons are not affected by variations from different observations or performances.

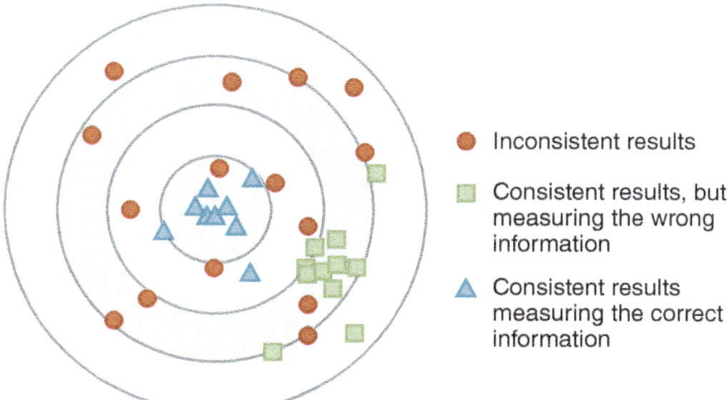

FIGURE 20.2 A target analogy for examination validity and reliability. The red dots represent a low-reliability examination; the examination results are not consistent, therefore, comparison with the objectives (the target) is meaningless. The green squares represent an examination with high reliability and low validity; although preferable to a low-reliability examination, this exam is consistently measuring the wrong material. The blue triangles represent an examination with high reliability and high validity; this tool is measuring knowledge consistently and appropriately.

TEACHING TIP

Instructors must exercise special care to ensure consistency between evaluators when practical exams that consist of some degree of subjectivity are used.

Validity of Assessment

Reliability of the examination tool is critical, but it is not sufficient by itself. An exam must also measure the knowledge, skills, or abilities that it is intended to evaluate. This property is referred to as **validity**. Students with more knowledge of a particular subject area would score better on a valid exam than would students without the requisite knowledge. To return to the analogy of the scale, consistent performance of the scale is necessary for that scale to be accurate, but consistency is not enough. A scale can deliver results that are consistently 10 pounds too low and thus not be accurate. Returning to the analogy of target shooting, a tight grouping is necessary for a consistent bull's eye, and once the shooter can produce reliable groups of shots, the aim is adjusted relative to the target. A tight grouping centered on the bull's-eye would be considered both reliable and valid (**FIGURE 20.2**). Consideration of reliability is the appropriate first step, but direct consideration of validity is also important.

CASE in Point

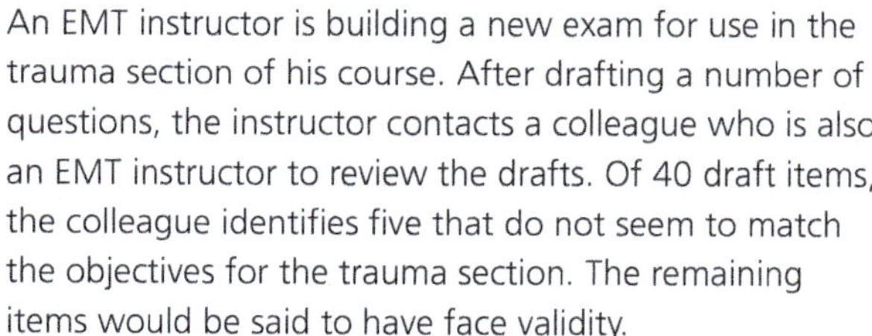

An EMT instructor is building a new exam for use in the trauma section of his course. After drafting a number of questions, the instructor contacts a colleague who is also an EMT instructor to review the drafts. Of 40 draft items, the colleague identifies five that do not seem to match the objectives for the trauma section. The remaining items would be said to have face validity.

There are many aspects to consider when evaluating validity of assessments. The most important is whether the test measures what it is intended to measure so it will be appropriate and useful for the specific purpose of the evaluation.

The simplest aspect of validity is sometimes referred to as **face validity**, or commonsense validity. Although the concept is considered to be a simplistic assessment of content validity, it may be useful for the EMS instructor. Review of an examination by colleagues, with their agreement that the test items "make sense," establishes face validity. Assessment of face validity is useful in the initial stages of examination analysis.

Content validity refers to the extent to which examination items accurately represent the wider body of knowledge that is being tested. Examination items should collectively form a reasonably representative sample of the body of knowledge. The depth of material covered in the course should be equal to the depth of items on the exam. For instance, testing advanced life support (ALS) knowledge by including only items related to basic life support (BLS) procedures would not provide sufficient depth. Also, the breadth of material on the exam should match the breadth covered in that portion of the class. For example, a test with a medical emergencies section that includes only questions related to cardiology would not provide sufficient breadth. The level of thinking required

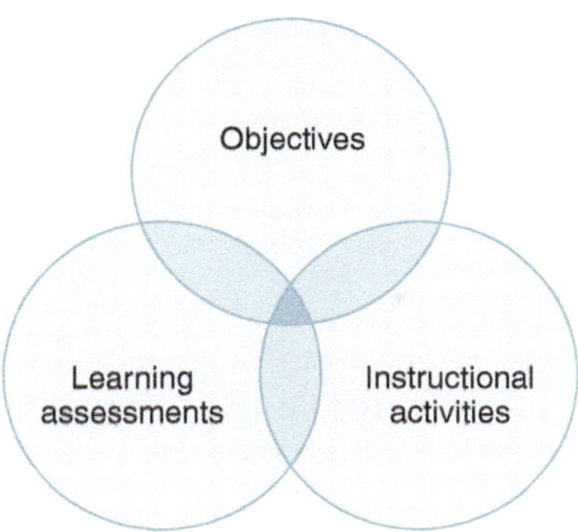

FIGURE 20.3 When learning objectives, activities, and assessment tools align, there is performance agreement (alignment of instructional design), which ensures content validity.

by examination items should match the level of thinking required for actual practice. High-level critical thinking cannot be effectively assessed through recall-level items. Examination items must also be technically correct. In other words, the correct answer must be supported by course content, expert opinion, or science. Basic content validity can be achieved when performance agreement (alignment) between course objectives and assessment instruments is ensured (**FIGURE 20.3**). Assessments and objectives should agree in terms of breadth, depth, and level of thinking required. Mismatch in any of these areas could cause problems with validity.

It is now generally agreed that validity is actually a description of one's interpretation of examination results, rather than a description of characteristics of the test itself. All examination items test something. The important question is: What conclusions can be drawn from the results? To assess validity appropriately, the instructor must have defined the purpose of the assessment at the start of the assessment creation process.

CASE in Point

An emergency medical technician (EMT) instructor is tasked with building a summative assessment for a unit on oxygen delivery. To ensure appropriate breadth, the instructor constructs an examination blueprint based on the objectives of the unit. (For more on blueprints, see Chapter 21, *Written Assessment*.) To achieve appropriate depth, the instructor also includes criteria for each cognitive level of objectives in the blueprint. These efforts help to ensure content validity.

Predictive Validity

Predictive validity (an aspect of a property known as *criterion validity*) refers to the ability of an examination to predict performance under other conditions. For example, a unit exam is administered, and results match the results of observational reports in the clinical setting. This examination would have high predictive validity for performance in this particular clinical setting. In other words, a high score on the exam predicts high scores on observational reports. The measurement of this can be achieved through use of a statistical procedure called *regression analysis*. In the example cited previously, the score on the unit exam would be the predictor variable, and the score on the observational reports would be the criterion variable. The calculated correlation coefficient would describe the strength of the predictive relationship.

Without a clear statement of purpose, the evaluation of validity becomes needlessly complex. For instance, in constructing a low-stakes, formative evaluation, ensuring face validity is usually sufficient. If the instructor is constructing a curriculum-based evaluation, checking content validity by comparing it with learning objectives is important. Consideration of predictive validity is key when one is constructing examinations designed to verify competency.

As noted, validity is the degree to which an assessment measures what it intends to measure. The degree of validity is the strength of the evidence linking the assessment to the conclusion. This relies on assumptions and a series of logical conclusions. The higher the stakes for an assessment, the stronger the evidence must be to support its conclusions. The score must prove to be an accurate reflection of performance on the assessment. The assessment must be reliable, only measuring intended aspects and under consistent conditions. There must be a proven link between the assessment and the conclusions—whether that link be content-based or predictive.[8,9]

Constructing an Assessment Strategy

The concepts of purpose, reliability, and validity are central to the construction and administration of appropriate assessment instruments. Explicit discussion of purpose dramatically improves the chance that stated purpose will be achieved. Analysis and improvement of reliability reduce the chance that results may be due to error rather than representing a true measure of knowledge. Careful consideration of validity ensures that the evaluation matches the expected outcome, with clear linkage to learning objectives. Alignment among learning objectives, course presentation, and assessment tools is a core concept to which all instructors must adhere if quality instruction is to be achieved. Even though not all instructors will be called on to construct an assessment strategy, the major steps required to construct one should be understood to maximize the quality of implementation.

Step 1: Decide on a Purpose

The instructor must make a careful and explicit decision about the purpose of the assessment. The key is to avoid leaving the purpose assumed, which can lead to confusion. Novice instructors sometimes assume that a test is an end in itself. Each test is nothing more (or less) than an assessment of student knowledge and/or performance. Assessing a patient's condition can be considered as an analogy. For example, appropriate interpretation of a patient assessment finding requires that the EMT understand why the assessment is being conducted. If an EMT student is unclear about the purpose of a particular step in patient assessment, it is unlikely that the student will respond to a patient need with the appropriate action. Just as with any research problem, the first step in constructing a tool for student assessment is to have a clear question that the tool is seeking to answer. Possibilities include the following:

1. Does the student have the needed skills and knowledge to move into the clinical environment?
2. Has the student mastered the objectives of a particular educational unit?
3. Does the student have more knowledge of the subject than when they started the course?
4. Which students have the best mastery of the material in comparison with other students?
5. Is the student competent to work independently as a provider?
6. Is the student progressing toward mastery of the material?

The instructor must remember that each assessment will reflect both student performance and the quality of instruction. Each of the purposes provided as examples earlier in this discussion will lead to dramatically different tools for assessment, as well as to different ways of using the results. Examples are as follows:

- Does the student have the needed skills and knowledge to move into the clinical environment? This purpose leads to a summative tool with high stakes. It includes aspects of competency verification, which results in the need for assessments with predictive validity.
- Has the student mastered the objectives of a particular educational unit? This purpose also implies the use of a summative tool. Comparison with the stated objectives of the program is needed.
- Does the student have more knowledge of the subject than when they started the course? This purpose can be accomplished with the use of a pretest and a post-test. Comparison of results before and after course administration will answer this question, without the need for grades or even determination of a passing score.
- Which students have the best mastery of the material in comparison with other students? This purpose leads to the use of a normative grading strategy. (See Chapter 21, *Written Assessment*, for explanation of normative grading.) To answer this question, the instructor could grade on a curve, comparing each student's performance with that of other individual students. This purpose leads the instructor away from establishing pass/fail criteria, or even issuing grades. A ranking of student performance is all that is required to meet this purpose.
- Is the student competent to work independently as a provider? This purpose requires that the test be based on a practice analysis instead of on course objectives.
- Is the student progressing toward mastery of the material? This question implies a formative strategy, with greater emphasis on providing feedback to the student than on grades.

The purpose of each assessment should be clearly communicated to students and to everyone involved in administration of the test. This helps to prevent misinterpretation of the results. Use of a tool designed for formative purposes to draw summative conclusions can lead to dramatic misinterpretation of test results.

Step 2: Specify What Will Be Done with the Results

After the purpose has been specified, the instructor must consider the meaning and impact of the results. This follows naturally from a clearly stated purpose. To illustrate this, examples from earlier in the chapter are used here (the purpose is italicized):

- Does the student have the needed skills and knowledge to move into the clinical environment?

Achieving a passing score on the examination is necessary before clinical rotations can begin.

- Has the student mastered the objectives of a particular educational unit? *Achieving a passing score on the exam is necessary if the student is to move on to the next unit.*
- Does the student have more knowledge of the subject than when they started the course? *Comparison of knowledge before and after administration of the course (or lesson) is conducted.*
- Which students have the best mastery of the material in comparison with other students? *Example: students with the top three scores on the examination qualify for preferential selection of their shift schedules.*
- Is the student competent to work independently as a provider? *Achieving a passing score on the field evaluation is necessary for the employee to be taken off probation and work independently.*
- Is the student progressing toward mastery of the material? *Graded quizzes are returned to the student and collectively will count for 10% of the final grade.* (Note: Because some students will regard assignments without grade impact as unimportant, it may be helpful for the instructor to assign small grade impact to formative assignments.)

Decisions regarding what will be done with results account for the potential stakes of an examination. The importance of these decisions determines the care with which the instructor must ensure reliability and validity. The higher the stakes, the more diligent the instructor must be in constructing and using the exam.

Step 3: Select Assessment Tools

Once the purpose and impact have been specified, assessment tools are selected. In the ideal world, the instructor would simply select from a bank of valid and reliable tools. Unfortunately, this situation rarely exists. Test-item banks and other tools available from publishers can provide valuable starting points, but these generally require modification before they are used. The instructor should consider the objectives to be evaluated and should select tools that match the domain and level of performance specified by the objectives. For example, high-level psychomotor skills should be evaluated by skills performance in a monitored or simulated setting; whereas, cognitive objectives can be evaluated by a written examination.

Specific techniques for the construction, use, and analysis of different types of evaluation tools are contained in Chapter 21, *Written Assessment,* and Chapter 22, *Other Assessment Tools.*

Step 4: Specify How Reliability Will Be Ensured

After examination items have been selected, the instructor must next address the monitoring of reliability. The simplest method for ensuring reliability is to reduce reliance on any single test and look for agreement among multiple tests. In essence, this is a variation on alternate form reliability. This approach to monitoring reliability is relatively easy and is almost always indicated. Assessment of internal reliability is generally indicated for high-stakes examinations. For examinations that involve subjective evaluation by more than one grader, such as practical examinations, essay questions, and oral examinations, the instructor monitors interrater reliability.

Step 5: Specify How Validity Will Be Ensured

Face validity and content validity should be checked throughout the item selection and editing processes. As examination items are selected, the instructor and at least one other colleague should review the items for face validity. Referencing the examination key to the stated course objectives can help demonstrate content validity. Alignment and content validity are reinforced when each item is referenced to a specific course objective or reference.

Predictive validity requires the piloting of examination items to test the predictive value of each item. To test predictive value, the instructor must have access to good evaluations of actual performance data, as well as to examination item pilot results. Because most EMS instructors do not have ready access to actual performance data, the applicability of predictive testing is limited for most EMS educational programs. However, some test vendors have assessed their exams for predictive value as compared to the certification examination.

Because examinations or examination items are commonly reused over multiple courses, it is

TEACHING TIP

A key to validity includes careful item review by one or more colleagues and referencing of each item according to a specific course objective.

important that their validity be tested periodically. A regular review process of the examination and key is essential to maintain current content validity. Testing students on outdated treatment modalities is useless.

Case Studies in Construction of Assessment Strategy

Many examples exist in EMS education to illustrate how to construct an assessment strategy. These cases identify each step of the strategy.

Case 1: A Preceptor Seeks to Confirm Progress

The instructor is a paramedic preceptor with a local ambulance service. She seeks to confirm that an intern is making progress throughout the internship and is incorporating lessons learned from previous shifts into development of patient assessment skills.

Purpose

The instructor believes she needs to confirm the student's knowledge of patient assessment and the lessons from previous shifts before beginning the next level of instruction. She decides to assess the intern's knowledge at the beginning of each shift to track the intern's development and guide that shift's activities. The instructor decides that the purpose of these evaluations is fundamentally formative and that the assessments will not be graded.

Impact

The preceptor decides that providing feedback to the intern is the point of this assessment. She will use this feedback to assess the effectiveness of the intern's work to date. She will provide the feedback to the intern to focus the work for that shift and correct any misconceptions. After a short conversation with the program's clinical coordinator, the preceptor decides not to record the results, but to approach this as an informal assessment.

Select Tools

The preceptor elects to use an oral quiz of three to five questions at the beginning of each shift. At the end of each shift, she creates three to five questions, based on that day's calls, to ask the intern at the beginning of the next shift.

Reliability

Because the preceptor is the only grader, no problems will occur with interrater reliability. She talks with the clinical coordinator about reliability; and together, they decide to review the situation if the intern does poorly on two days of oral quizzes; then they will compare quiz results with the intern's evaluations in class (checking consistency with other evaluations).

Validity

The preceptor and clinical coordinator agree that if there are questions about a correct answer, the preceptor will check with the coordinator. The clinical coordinator gives the preceptor a copy of the program learning objectives to be used for reference purposes. The preceptor agrees to base the questions on the objectives provided.

Case 2: An Instructor Seeks to Confirm Mastery

The instructor is teaching a paramedic course held at a community college. He is teaching at a remote satellite location and works with several adjunct lab instructors to teach the classes. He began teaching last year and does not have the tests used by previous instructors. He is preparing to begin the section on airway management and is considering what to use as a unit examination at the end of the section.

Purpose

In the course syllabus, the instructor told the students that there would be an exam for each unit and that successful completion of the unit exam is necessary if students are to progress to the next unit. The instructor decides that he is aiming for a summative strategy based on the course objectives.

Impact

The instructor has already decided that passing the exam will be required if students are to progress to the next unit. This is a high-stakes examination, which requires increased vigilance. The exam will have a significant grade impact. To lower the stakes, the instructor could allow more than one attempt at the exam.

Select Tools

The instructor decides to use a combination of a written exam and practical exams for each skill. He bases the examination on the airway management unit objectives and related education standards. Written exam items are drawn from a publisher's test bank and revised by the instructor to improve applicability.

Practical examination check sheets are taken from the publisher's instructor resource kit. The instructor proceeds to construct the written examination, along with a key that references specific course objectives.

Reliability

The instructor divides the written exam into content sections so that he can assess internal consistency. He has been using daily quizzes and expects to compare the results of the examination with those of the quizzes. He knows that he must monitor interrater reliability for the practical component, so he makes sure that students repeat each practical station so that different lab instructors can check for consistency. This allows him to assess the consistency of evaluation between practical stations. The instructor prepares lab examiners by meeting with them as a group before the time of the exam for a discussion regarding specific descriptions of acceptable and unacceptable performance.

Validity

The instructor uses an examination blueprint (described in Chapter 21, *Written Assessment*) to ensure that the breadth of the exam is representative of the entire unit. The instructor edits each item, checking for face validity. He asks a colleague to review the exam for validity as well. He knows that this colleague will ask him to return the favor in the future. He then prepares the examination key, noting the objective and textbook reference that correspond to each item. After final preparation, he sends the exam to his medical director for final review.

Case 3: A Training Officer Seeks to Verify Competency

The instructor in this case is the training officer for an ambulance service. The service has just added a new advanced airway device. The service director asks the training officer to verify the competency of all providers for the device before implementation.

Purpose

The instructor is verifying competency in the use of a new airway device. He realizes that although materials are available from the manufacturer, some aspects of the skill may not be well covered by these materials. This is a summative evaluation that should be based on a practice analysis.

Impact

The service director has made it clear that all providers must pass this test before use of the devices will be implemented. In a conversation with the service director, the training officer confirms that this will have no impact on performance appraisals, but that each provider must pass the test. Remediation and retest will be allowed until all have successfully completed the exam.

Select Tools

The instructor starts by meeting with the medical director, a representative from the manufacturer, and a field paramedic. This group outlines the specific skills and knowledge necessary for use of the new device. The training officer uses this rudimentary practice analysis to decide that a practical examination is needed. The training officer then has the manufacturer's representative demonstrate the skill, while he identifies the steps required to complete the skill. From this, the practical check sheet will be constructed.

Reliability

The training officer decides to conduct each assessment on his own, thereby minimizing problems with interrater reliability. To help achieve stability of the test over many uses, the training officer uses the check sheet that he created, with critical criteria identified. The training officer arranges for the medical director to monitor a random selection of the examinations to ensure reliability.

Validity

The training officer forwards the completed check sheet to participants in the practice analysis meeting to check for content validity. He and the medical director decide to review the first 25 real-life uses to assess the criterion (predictive) validity of the practical examination.

Summary

An understanding of the principles of assessing student performance assists the instructor in the selection and development of evaluation tools. The effective instructor uses both formal and informal systems to assess student performance. Assessments provide information regarding student performance; they are also one tool to help the instructor assess the effectiveness of teaching strategies. Formative assessments provide feedback to the instructor and the student. Results of the formative assessments lead to changes in instructional and learning strategies. Summative assessments contain information regarding student mastery of the objectives, but they do not allow modification of learning strategies for the current students.

Reliability and validity are characteristics of assessments. Reliability refers to the ability of the exam to produce consistent results. A reliable exam maximizes the true measurement of knowledge and skills and minimizes the impact of measurement error due to irrelevant details. Validity refers to the applicability of the examination and confirms that the exam actually measures what it purports to measure. A valid examination is technically correct; contains content that is an accurate, representative sample of the wider body of knowledge; and, in some cases, can predict future performance. Validity and reliability are important characteristics of evaluation tools. The instructor must be prepared to monitor and improve examination reliability and validity.

As the instructor constructs an assessment strategy and tools to support that strategy, the most important step is to explicitly identify the purpose of the evaluation. An explicit description of purpose is needed to enable the instructor to select or create the appropriate tool, accurately interpret the results of the evaluation, and decide on best actions to take, as indicated by the results. Instructors who assume that everyone involved understands the intended purpose of an examination are likely to encounter problems. Explicit description of purpose is the foundation upon which successful assessment is built.

Glossary

assessment Process of evaluating whether a student has successfully acquired knowledge, skills, and attitudes.

content validity Extent to which exam items accurately represent the wider body of knowledge being tested.

Cronbach's alpha Complex statistical method of assessing internal consistency.

face validity Commonsense validity; when an assessment appears to evaluate what it is intended to evaluate.

formative assessment Ongoing evaluation of student performance throughout a course.

high-stakes assessment Assessment in which the student's continuation in the program depends on successful completion of the exam.

interrater reliability Consistency in scores that different people assign when grading a particular exam.

Kuder–Richardson Statistical formula to evaluate internal consistency.

low-stakes assessment Assessment that has relatively little effect on whether a student passes a course.

measurement error Variation of an exam score due to factors not related to the knowledge the exam intends to measure.

predictive validity Ability of an exam to predict performance under other conditions.

reliability Ability of an assessment tool to measure consistently.

split-half method Test of internal consistency that divides the exam into halves (commonly odd and even questions), then compares the percentage of correct answers between the two groups of items.

summative assessment Evaluation of student performance given to students at the end of a course or unit of learning.

test-enhanced learning Teaching strategy in which frequent formative assessment occurs, in which learners are asked to recall and retain concepts and facts; also called *retrieval practice*.

validity Measuring the knowledge, skills, or abilities that an assessment is intended to evaluate.

References

[1] Davis, Barbara G. 2009. *Tools for Teaching*, 2nd ed., 362–74. San Francisco: Jossey-Bass.

[2] Green, Michael L., Jeremy J. Moeller, and Judy M. Spak. 2018. "Test-Enhanced Learning in Health Professions Education: A Systematic Review: BEME Guide No. 48." *Medical Teacher* 40, no. 4: 337–50. https://doi.org/10.1080/0142159X.2018.1430354.

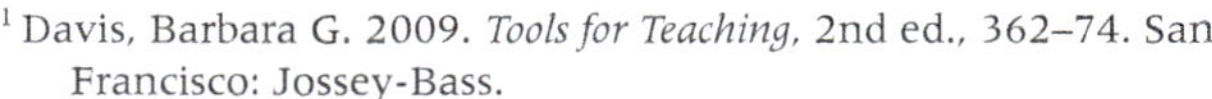

[3] Roediger III, Henry L., and Andrew C. Butler. 2011. "The Critical Role of Retrieval Practice in Long-Term Retention." *Trends in Cognitive Sciences* 15: 20–7. https://doi.org/10.1016/j.tics.2010.09.003.

[4] Roediger III, Henry L., and Mary A. Pyc. 2012. "Inexpensive Techniques to Improve Education: Applying Cognitive Psychology to Enhance Educational Practice." *Journal of Applied Research in Memory and Cognition* 1: 242–8. https://doi.org/10.1016/j.jarmac.2012.09.002.

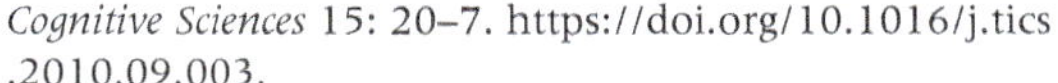

[5] Roediger III, Henry L., and Jeffrey D. Karpicke. 2006. "Test-Enhanced Learning: Taking Memory Tests Improves Long-Term

Retention." *Psychological Science* 17: 249–55. https://doi.org/10.1111/j.1467-9280.2006.01693.x.

[6] Butler, Andrew C., and Henry L. Roediger III. 2008. "Feedback Enhances the Positive Effects and Reduces the Negative Effects of Multiple-Choice Testing." *Memory and Cognition* 36: 604–16. https://doi.org/10.3758/MC.36.3.604.

[7] Smith, Megan A., and Jeffrey D. Karpicke. 2014. "Retrieval Practice with Short-Answer, Multiple-Choice, and Hybrid Tests." *Memory* 22: 784–802. https://doi.org/10.1080/09658211.2013.831454.

[8] Kane, Michael T. 1992. "An Argument-Based Approach to Validity." *Psychological Bulletin* 112, no. 3: 527–35. http://dx.doi.org/10.1037/0033-2909.112.3.527.

[9] Kane, Michael T. 2006. "Validation." In *Educational Measurement*, 4th ed., edited by Robert L. Brennan, 17–64. Westport, CT: Praeger.

Additional Resources

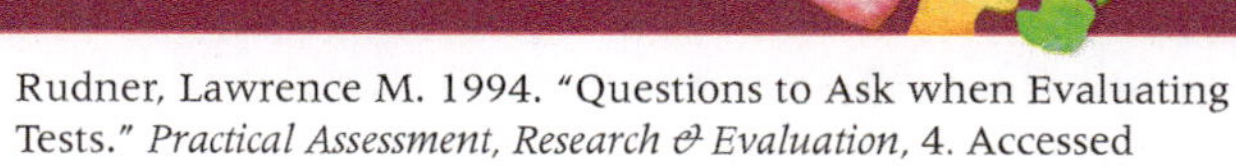

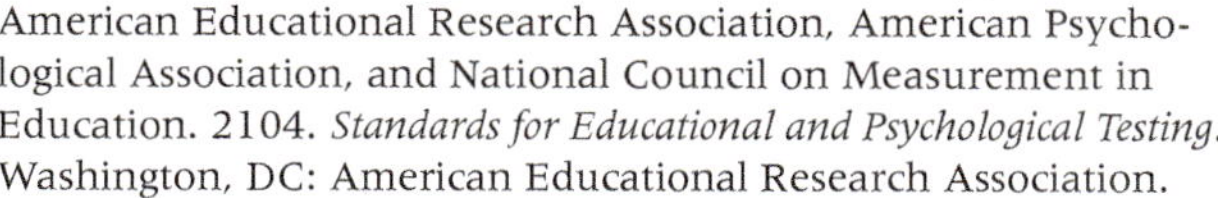

American Educational Research Association, American Psychological Association, and National Council on Measurement in Education. 2104. *Standards for Educational and Psychological Testing*. Washington, DC: American Educational Research Association.

Jacobs, Lucy C., and Clinton I. Chase. 1992. *Developing and Using Tests Effectively: A Guide for Faculty*. San Francisco: Jossey-Bass.

National Highway Traffic Safety Administration. 2002. *National Guidelines for Educating EMS Instructors*. Accessed February 18, 2019. http://www.nhtsa.gov/people/injury/ems/Instructor/TableofContents.htm.

Rudner, Lawrence M. 1994. "Questions to Ask when Evaluating Tests." *Practical Assessment, Research & Evaluation*, 4. Accessed February 18, 2019. http://pareonline.net/getvn.asp?v=4&n=2.

Rudner, Lawrence M., and William D. Schafer. 2001. "Reliability." College Park, MD: ERIC Clearinghouse on Assessment and Evaluation. Accessed February 18, 2019. http://www.ericdigests.org/2002-2/reliability.htm.

Yu, Chong H. n.d. "Reliability and Validity." Accessed February 18, 2019. http://www.creative-wisdom.com/teaching/assessment/reliability.html.

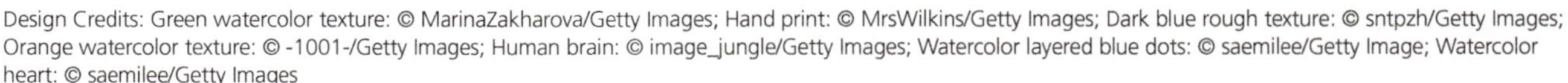

CHAPTER 21

Written Assessment

OBJECTIVES

At the conclusion of this chapter, the educator will be able to:

Cognitive Domain

1. Describe benefits and limitations of using written assessment tools in each domain of learning.
2. List steps to enhance reliability of written examinations.
3. Describe measures to improve written assessment validity.
4. Outline the steps to blueprint an examination.
5. Describe how to select appropriate items for an examination.
6. List effective test construction measures.
7. Distinguish between limited response and open (constructed) response items.
8. Explain the principles of constructing effective limited response items.
9. Given an example of a poorly selected (limited) response test item, edit it to improve its measurement precision.
10. Describe strategies to construct effective distractors for multiple choice questions.
11. Differentiate advantages and disadvantages of short-answer, essay, and fill-in-the-blank question types.
12. Describe advantages of formative assessments.
13. Outline effective test administration strategies.
14. Describe strategies to analyze examinations during a post-test review.
15. Distinguish between norm-referenced and criterion-referenced grading.
16. Describe methods to set a cut score for an examination.
17. Describe how item-response theory is used to establish passing criteria for computer adaptive testing.

Psychomotor Domain

There are no psychomotor objectives for this chapter.

Affective Domain

1. Defend the need to establish procedures that establish test validity and reliability.
2. Value the need to maintain test security.

"To those of you who received honors, awards, and distinctions, I say well done. And to the 'C' students, I say you too may one day become President of the United States."

~ George W. Bush

CHAPTER GOAL This chapter presents information on the construction, use, and analysis of written assessments.

Assessing students' knowledge is a key task for instructors. This is usually done through the use of written assignments and examinations. Each type of written assessment has its strengths, weaknesses, and implications for use.

The Written Assessment

One of the most common formal assessments of student performance is the written examination. The instructor can determine whether a written examination is the appropriate assessment instrument by considering the purpose of the assessment. Written examinations provide insight on student knowledge, but provide little information about a student's ability to perform a skill or consistently demonstrate a given attitude. Thus, written examinations are most useful for evaluating the cognitive domain. Written exams are not useful tools to evaluate psychomotor objectives. They can evaluate only lower levels within the affective domain. Grading, validating, or compiling results of written examinations is typically easier than other types of assessments. Because of this, written examinations are easily used with large numbers of students in a single class setting or across multiple classes. Written examinations that rely largely on multiple choice, true/false, and matching items are especially easy to grade; thus they are very useful with large classes. Students should also be exposed to testing strategies that mimic certification examinations to ensure they are prepared. As state and national examinations all have a multiple choice examination component (typically conducted using a computer system), the instructor should include that testing strategy in the emergency medical services (EMS) classroom—including the use of computer-based testing.

Appropriate selection of an assessment tool always depends on the proposed purpose of the assessment. Written examinations are best suited to answer questions such as the following:

- What does the student know about the subject?
- Which of the cognitive objectives has the student mastered?
- Does the student have the necessary knowledge to progress to more advanced material or complete the course of instruction?
- Have scheduled materials been presented adequately?

Properly constructed written exams can operate with high levels of reliability (an examination's ability to measure consistently). Because each student is being asked the same questions in the same way during the exam, consistent administration of the test is ensured. Most written examinations provide for consistent scoring, although there are challenges to ensuring grading reliability with some types of short-answer and essay questions. Because written examinations by nature are usually consistent in administration, reliability is mostly related to the quality of the individual items and scoring practices. This eases the processes of checking and monitoring reliability. Of course, poorly constructed items can, and usually do, have low reliability. Monitoring and improving reliability by evaluating and editing examination items promotes the appropriate function of these easy-to-use tools.

Similarly, high levels of validity (the ability of the exam to measure what it purports to measure) can be ensured by the use of carefully designed and written questions. Written exams generally encounter difficulties in this area. It is relatively easy to write examination items that assess low-level cognitive objectives, such as recall of key facts. Assessing higher-level thinking, such as problem solving or analysis, is more difficult with written examinations. Because of this, a common error for novice instructors is to assume that students have mastered higher-level objectives simply because they scored well on an examination filled with recall items. Efforts to ensure validity should include consideration of (1) the level of difficulty of required thinking (e.g., recall versus synthesis), (2) the breadth of the material covered (making sure the sampling of items is reasonable), and (3) the depth of the knowledge assessed by test items. The planning process to do this is referred to as **blueprinting**.

Each type of written examination item has its strengths, weaknesses, and implications for use. Proper use of written examinations requires an understanding of these strengths and weaknesses. Just as the selection of an assessment strategy is based on an understanding of the purpose of the assessment, the construction of a written examination requires the instructor to apply knowledge of test-item types to the objectives that the instructor is attempting to assess.

Construction of a Written Examination

Constructing well-written examination items from scratch is difficult, but can be learned and refined. Entry-level instructors should initially focus their efforts on using and improving existing examination items from their educational institutions and other instructors. Textbook publishers and others are sources of exam items; however, many are low-level recall items and will need to be edited by the instructor. Using existing examination items still presents challenges for the instructor. Just because examination items are available does not mean that those items are valid or reliable, especially if they are used for several classes in a row. The instructor must always review and edit examination items for each class.

Some examination item banks and sources have been pretested for reliability. In these cases, the instructor can have more confidence in the items after reviewing the technical reports for item performance. The instructor should still exercise caution to ensure that the examination blueprint is a valid assessment for the material presented. The pilot population may be representative of the students being assessed, but those students may not be similar to students in any given instructor's class, which poses another potential problem. Still, pretested items are a valuable commodity to the instructor; it is much easier to begin with questions to modify than to create an entire exam from scratch.

Construction of a written examination consists of several key steps before the test can be put together. A flowchart of the examination construction process is shown in **FIGURE 21.1**. The first step is to carefully consider the purpose of the examination. The second step is to blueprint the examination, relating the breadth and depth of the examination to the stated objectives for the course. The third step is to develop or select draft examination items. Draft examination items are then reviewed by others and edited as needed (**FIGURE 21.2**). Reviewing exam items with other instructors or paramedics, and with the program medical director is important to verify the relationship of items to the objectives, to ensure their proper construction, to confirm the correct answer, and to discuss their relevance to practice. This review should be documented in some way to provide evidence that steps to ensure exam validity were taken.

For high-stakes exams, test items should be piloted to ensure items perform as expected.

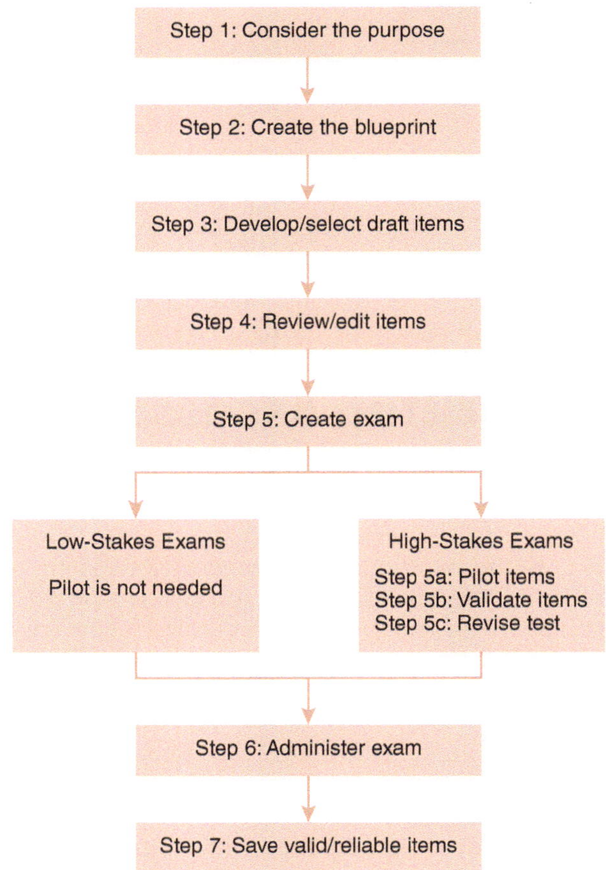

FIGURE 21.1 The examination construction process.

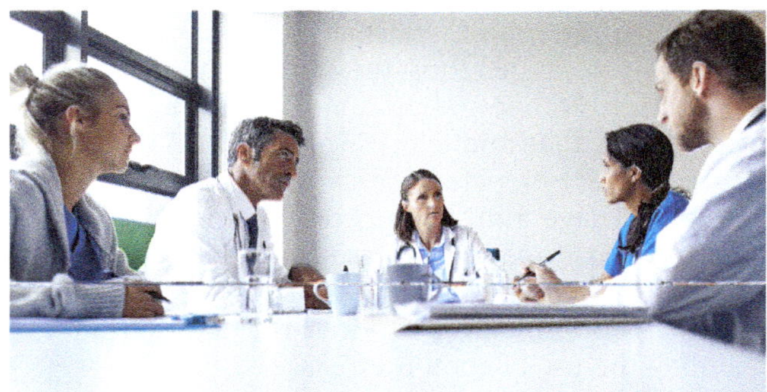

FIGURE 21.2 It is important that the instructor review exam items with knowledgeable sources (such as other instructors, paramedics, or the medical director) to verify that they are constructed properly and are relevant to the objectives and the practice.

Carefully Consider the Purpose of the Written Examination

The types of written examination items and the content of those items depend on the purpose of the assessment. Clear differences exist between the breadth of material used for formative exams and that used for summative exams. Elements to consider for purpose include the following:

- Are the subjects cumulative? In other words, should material from previous units be included? Including some material from previous units is a good method to make sure students keep up with all material.
- What section(s) of the educational standards or course curriculum is being evaluated? To which objectives will the exam be tied? Ensuring the breadth

of the educational standards is well represented helps to prepare students for national certification examinations as well as for clinical practice.

- Are there limiting factors within the course design that affect assessment strategy? Examples might include available class time, need for immediate grading and feedback to students, or a large number of students with only one instructor to grade exams.

Blueprint the Examination

Once the purpose has been established, the next step is to blueprint the examination. The blueprinting process is conducted using the following steps:

1. The instructor lists the course objectives to be evaluated by the examination.
2. The instructor assigns a percentage of total questions (or points, if varying numbers of points are to be assigned to each question) written to cover each objective. If necessary, objectives can be grouped together and percentages assigned to each group.
3. The instructor selects the exam length. In general, use of more questions increases reliability, but very long tests (with more than approximately 150 multiple choice items) are much more difficult to develop and administer, and their use does not significantly improve reliability. Fatigue associated with very long examinations can reduce reliability and offset gains from the increased number of items. Conversely, examinations of less than 50 items frequently have difficulty proving reliability.
4. The instructor multiplies each section's percentage by the total exam length to determine the number of questions needed for each section.

Using the same strategy, the instructor should also construct a blueprint of the level of difficulty, based on the level of cognitive material that is being tested (i.e., recall versus synthesis). Instructors may wish to group objectives into categories so that the blueprint does not become overly complex. The instructor should balance the specificity of the blueprint with the complexity. It is rarely useful to specify item selection down to the individual item. If there are several categories in the blueprint with a single item, consolidation of the blueprint is usually indicated. For example, blueprints should indicate categories of items rather than specific items (for example, airway adjuncts rather than oral or nasal airway devices specifically).

Certification examinations usually publish the blueprint, also referred to as the test plan. Consulting the blueprint for certification examinations can provide an idea of the level of detail required for an effective blueprint.

Generalizing

Instructors are sometimes tempted to assure themselves that students are prepared for examinations by emphasizing the content that is on the test. An example would be the instructor who knocks on the desk when a lecture point is covered on the exam. If students face items that are randomly selected from a large body of knowledge, it is more likely that one can generalize their knowledge of the entire body by their performance on the random sample. The ability to generalize is lost if the students know the sample ahead of time. For instance, if an instructor is trying to evaluate a body of 300 objectives, the instructor might select a random sample of 100 to include on the test. If the students do not know which 100 are on the test, the instructor can be assured that the students are preparing to address all 300. However, if the students know which 100 the instructor chose for the test, the instructor can only be assured that the students prepared for the 100 they knew would be on the test, not the wider body of knowledge. Test preparation should include all objectives in a module, not just those selected for the exam.

Develop or Select Draft Examination Items

From the blueprint, the process moves to the selection or drafting of items for use in the examination. The number of draft items collected should equal at least two times the number of items called for by the blueprint. Having more draft items than are called for in each area of the blueprint allows the editing process to select the most promising items to be refined. Some draft items will need extensive editing. If substantially more draft items are included than needed, items that require considerable rework can be eliminated if time becomes an issue.

Once an adequate number of draft items has been created or collected, the instructor can begin the review and editing stage. Only those items that have previously been validated can bypass this stage. The instructor should have colleagues and the medical director review the items and assist in the editing process.

Items taken from any commercially available test bank must also be reviewed and edited by the instructor before they are used. When possible, it is preferable for the instructor to employ unbiased editors who have not drafted the selected examination items or presented the material to students. These editors should consider the following questions for each exam item:

- Are any grammatical or spelling corrections needed?
- Is the item clearly related to a stated course objective? A common mistake is to base items on instructors' presentation materials instead of on the course curriculum. One method to help counter this tendency is to have those providing draft selections also provide an annotated key that references each item to a course objective.
- Has the information/material been presented to the class in a lecture, reading assignment, or other means? Although it is appropriate to ask questions from reading assignments or nonclass content, care should be taken to ensure that the content is relevant to core objectives of the course. Some instructors also reference test items to a specific textbook reference to assist with later review and consideration. While this technique is useful to justify a correct answer, it is rarely helpful in justifying why a **distractor** (an incorrect answer option, also referred to as a foil) is incorrect. Additionally, higher-level cognitive or problem-solving items are rarely tied to specific reference in the text and may require more clinical judgment than is available in the text. Overreliance on textbook content can lead to an excessive number of recall-level items, particularly if textbook passages are used in the item.
- Is the item constructed appropriately? (See the following sections of this chapter on technical considerations for specific types of items.)
- What is the correct answer that is being sought? If it is a multiple choice item, is there only one correct (or clearly best) answer?
- Are the distractors clearly incorrect or substantially less correct than the key? The difficulty and reliability of an examination item frequently depends on the distractors, so these should receive the most attention.
- Are there any inadvertent hints to the correct answer?
- Is the level of difficulty of the question appropriate?

TEACHING TIP

Working cooperatively with other educators facilitates item development and editing. This could be as simple as a test-item exchange program between educators. A more complex approach would be for instructors to jointly host an item-writing workshop, inviting participation from a number of educational programs, and allowing all participants to use the results of a day's worth of item writing and editing.

Question Levels

Sometimes a simplified version of Bloom's taxonomy that includes three levels of test questions is used.

1. Recall questions assess understanding or memorization of facts.
2. Application questions require learners to categorize or apply their knowledge to new situations.
3. Problem-solving questions test the learner's ability to prioritize or make judgments using their knowledge of rules or principles in situations that vary from previously encountered situations.

CASE in Point

Blueprinting

An instructor is preparing a written examination to serve as a summative assessment of the cognitive material for a trauma unit that covers bleeding, soft-tissue trauma, burns, and chest trauma. The instructor prepares a blueprint of the exam.

The first step performed by the instructor is to gather information on the emphasis to be placed on each content area. The instructor begins by consulting the National Registry of EMTs' (NREMT) practice analysis, while using three parameters (risk of harm, frequency, and difficulty). The instructor assesses each area for the risk of harm to the patient, assigning the greatest value to the riskiest, a lower value to the next riskiest, and so on. (Results are shown in **TABLE A**.) The instructor then does the same for frequency and perceived difficulty. Next, the instructor assesses the objectives of the particular course being evaluated. Counting objectives, the instructor notes that 30% of the module objectives are related to bleeding, 25% to soft-tissue trauma, 25% to burns, and 20% to chest trauma. The amount of

TABLE A NREMT Practice Analysis Example

	NREMT Practice Analysis			Curriculum Review		Expert Opinion		
Area	**Risk of Harm**	**Frequency**	**Difficulty**	**Number of Objectives**	**Class Time Spent**	**Medical Director**	**Program Director**	**Adjusted Average**
Bleeding	30	35	15	30	30	40	35	31
Soft-tissue trauma	25	50	10	25	30	30	35	29
Burns	20	10	35	25	20	10	15	19
Chest trauma	25	5	40	20	20	20	15	21
Total	**100**	**100**	**100**	**100**	**100**	**100**	**100**	**100**

class time spent on each content area is considered next, with the use of percentage allocation. The instructor also asks the medical director and the program coordinator to provide their opinions on the emphasis to be placed in each area, in terms of percentages. Results are averaged, and the totals are slightly adjusted by the instructor so the percentages add up to 100%. Table A shows the results.

The instructor next considers the level of thinking required for the objectives. The instructor assesses objectives written for the module and determines the percentage of objectives for each content area that is provided for each cognitive level. **TABLE B** shows the results.

The instructor next combines Tables A and B to determine the percentage of items that will be needed for each area and each level. This is calculated by multiplying the percentages assigned to each content area (Adjusted Average column from Table A) and the percentage of each level shown on Table B. The results are shown in **TABLE C**.

The instructor had previously decided that the examination would consist of 100 items of equal weight (each item worth one point). The number of questions required is determined by multiplying the percentage in each column by 100 (the total number of items on the examination). **TABLE D** shows the number of items needed for each level within each area.

The instructor now knows how many questions of each level and content area are needed for creation of a valid assessment of the student's knowledge of the content for this module of the course. The instructor can now select appropriate items from a test bank and proceed to the editing stage.

TABLE B Assessment of Course's Cognitive Objectives

Area	Remember (C1)	Apply (C3)	Evaluate (C5)
Bleeding	20%	30%	50%
Soft-tissue trauma	25%	30%	45%
Burns	25%	35%	40%
Chest trauma	25%	35%	40%

(continues)

CASE in Point (*Continued*)

TABLE C Percentage of Items Needed for Each Content Area and Level

Area	Total	Remember (C1)	Apply (C3)	Evaluate (C5)
Bleeding	31%	6%	9%	16%
Soft-tissue trauma	29%	7%	9%	13%
Burns	19%	5%	7%	7%
Chest trauma	21%	5%	7%	9%

TABLE D Assignment of the Number of Problems for Each Level per Content Area

Area	Remember Items	Apply Items	Evaluate Items
Bleeding	6	9	16
Soft-tissue trauma	7	9	13
Burns	5	7	7
Chest trauma	5	7	9

Editing Multiple Choice Test Items

Many instructors find editing multiple choice test items particularly difficult. Collecting a group of instructors to jointly edit draft items can ease the task. This strategy is commonly used by large educational programs and those charged with certification examinations. Invited instructors are asked to bring a number of draft items as specified by the blueprint. The group then works together to edit the items, projecting the items so that all participants can see the editing process. Sharing editing tasks can improve the questions for a number of reasons:

- The bias and familiarity of the writer does not influence the revisions, as editing is shared between people who did not initially write the item. A single examination contributor introduces a significant challenge to reliability, as the interests and knowledge of that contributor becomes a major factor in the exam.
- Different options can be rapidly introduced and considered. Having multiple editors approach the task at the same time greatly reduces the cycle time of changes.
- Discussion of types of problems leads to more rapid solution when a number of items are edited together. The editing process speeds up over time.
- Frankly, more heads are better than one. The creativity of solutions builds as more editors are introduced.
- Local or regional bias or terminology is eliminated when individuals from a cross-section of the country work together on a national exam.
- Transparency of references and resources is ensured. For example, which textbooks or standards are appropriate to the exam?

Of course, there are limits to the benefits based on the number of editors and the time frame. Predetermined criteria for items can be established beforehand to clarify personal preferences and avoid arguments (such as those suggested in the following section). While a small group of editors is useful, a large group has difficulty reaching consensus. Fatigue limits creativity; so long editing sessions may be counterproductive. It is usually apparent when an editing team has "hit the wall" and fatigue sets into the group.

The Examination Construction Process

After items have been edited, the instructor can construct the examination. Instructors should consider the following guidelines regarding test construction:

- Be consistent in the use of punctuation and abbreviations. For example, periods are used at the end of the distractors if they complete a sentence, but not used if they are incomplete sentences.
- Use a consistent strategy to draw attention to material in the test (underline, bold, italics, or a combination).
- Use capital and lowercase formatting consistently for multiple choice items and for the first word of each option.
- If a separate answer sheet is to be used, ensure that the answer sheet and the test use consistent identification of options (e.g., 1, 2, 3, 4; A, B, C, D; or a, b, c, d).
- Provide clear and complete instructions for the examination—for example, whether the student can write on the test, whether there is a time limit, whether breaks are allowed, and (specifically for multiple choice items) whether there is only one correct answer versus whether students should select the *best* answer.
- For short-answer questions, students will commonly perceive the amount of space provided for the response as a suggestion for the length of the answer.
- The exam should be organized in a logical manner, with items from a similar content area grouped together. Some instructors believe that, similarly, the examination should begin with the easiest items, moving to harder items. The instructor should note that while these suggestions are intended to improve student satisfaction with the "flow" of the exam, certification examinations are often randomized. The use of greater randomization for summative examinations can help prepare students for certification examinations.
- If several items are related to a single scenario, then those items should follow a logical sequence. Care should be taken to ensure that a single incorrect answer does not jeopardize students' ability to answer the next question correctly. In other words, although a single scenario can be used to set up a number of questions, each question should be capable of standing alone. Additionally, items linked to a single scenario should appear on the same page to avoid confusion.

Pilot use and validation should be conducted before an item is included in a high-stakes examination.[1] Items that demonstrate reliability and validity can be included in future exams, and items that fail can be returned to the editing process for improvement. A common mistake made by instructors is to pilot examination items using a single source that may not be representative of the intended audience. An example would be asking only other instructors their opinions on items for an entry-level examination. Although this may be useful to check content validity, other instructors are clearly not the same population that will be evaluated by the examination items. It is more useful in this situation to pilot the items using a population of other entry-level students.

For low- and moderate-stakes examinations, grading of the exams can be coupled with analysis. Two useful characteristics that can be identified in the analysis are difficulty level and item discrimination. **Difficulty level**, or difficulty index, is the percentage of students who answer each item correctly. **Item discrimination** is the degree to which a correct answer for a particular item is associated with high overall scores on the exam. Item discrimination is essentially a test of reliability. More on the analysis of written examinations is included later in this chapter.

One critical area for consideration with test items is the level of cognition and difficulty of the items that are used. Certification examinations, such as the NREMT, use items that test high-level problem solving. If lower levels such as recall and comprehension are the dominant form of test item within the educational program, then student performance on certification examinations will suffer. In identifying characteristics of educational programs that had high NREMT pass rates, Margolis noted three characteristics directly relating to written testing:

- Create and administer valid examinations that have been through a review process (such as qualitative analysis).
- Incorporate critical thinking and problem solving into all testing.
- Deploy predictive testing with analysis prior to certification.[2]

Items that test lower levels of cognitive objectives, such as recall, are relatively easy to construct. Therefore, there is a general tendency to choose items that evaluate lower levels of thinking than is intended by the writer. Instructors who are editing and reviewing items should be aware of this tendency and attempt to compensate by consistently ensuring that items evaluate problem solving and critical thinking.

Well-constructed and validated examination items are extremely valuable to the instructor and to the assessment process. This value is effectively destroyed if the security of items is compromised by the items being distributed to students in advance of the test. At the very least, such action converts an item that potentially evaluated high-level cognitive thinking into a simple memorization question. As such, validated items should be secured to the highest degree possible to preserve their usefulness.

Examination security can be breached in subtle ways. Letting students know which specific items are to be covered on a written examination is counterproductive in that students may then display false mastery of the material, which is not representative of their true abilities. A written assessment typically comprises a sample or "biopsy" of the objectives included in the course content. For this reason, if the student knows which specific knowledge areas are contained within the sample from which a broader conclusion is drawn, then the validity of the conclusion is challenged. In this case, the conclusion that the student has mastered the necessary material can extend only to what is directly assessed, and the conclusion that the student has mastered the broader areas from which the sample is drawn cannot be made. Although it is unavoidable that the instructor has previous knowledge of the test items, care must be exercised to not focus greater attention on specific content or items that will be covered in a future examination. An instructor does not *need* to know what specific items are covered on an examination, such as a licensure examination; the instructor needs to know only the objectives on which the examination is based. The idea of "teaching to the test" is often considered controversial. Instead of teaching directly to a test, both the teaching and test should be based on a common blueprint. When the examination and course are both derived from a common set of objectives, alignment is ensured.

Using Limited Response Items

The instructor may choose several different types of written examination items. Each offers its own advantages and disadvantages. Like other areas of evaluation of student performance, no single tool works for all situations. A combination of different types of examination items provides the strongest validity and reliability. Limited response (selected response) items contain a question or stem and require the student to select from answer options that are provided.

True/False Items

True/false items offer a complete statement with two possible choices: the statement is entirely true, or it is entirely false. True/false questions can present complex ideas to be evaluated, and they can be easily scored. Additionally, because students can complete them quickly, much more content can be tested in the allotted examination time with true/false questions

Examples of True/False Items of Various Cognitive Levels

Recall Item

T/F Positive-pressure ventilation is used for patients with inadequate spontaneous ventilation.

Note that this item is derived from a list of indications. Recall that "inadequate spontaneous ventilation" is a listed indication that enables the student to answer correctly.

Application Item

T/F A patient with cyanosis and a respiratory rate of 10 breaths per minute has adequate spontaneous ventilation.

Note that this item explores whether a situation fits within the category of adequate ventilation. The novelty of the description is important. If a study guide listed this situation as inadequate ventilation, the item would be testing recall. A higher level of cognition is tested by evaluating whether the student can correctly sort novel situations into the appropriate category.

Problem-Solving Item

T/F The head-tilt chin-lift maneuver is the preferred initial method of opening the airway for a child who is unresponsive and is not breathing after being struck in the head by a baseball.

Note that this item goes further than categorization. The student is given a novel situation and asked to evaluate a solution by applying several categories to the situation. First the student must categorize the situation into inadequate ventilation and recognize a need for spinal motion restriction. The student must then apply the indications and contraindications of the head-tilt chin-lift maneuver to the situation. Again, the novelty of the situation is important to preserve the assessment of higher levels of cognition. If a study guide said, "being struck in the head is a contraindication of the head-tilt chin-lift maneuver," the item would test only recall.

Examples of How to Edit True/False Items

Poor

T/F Effective splinting always immobilizes the joints above and below the injury.

Better

T/F Effective splinting of long bone fractures immobilizes the joints above and below the injury.
(*Avoid absolutes.*)

Poor

T/F Oral airways are not used in responsive patients.

Better

T/F Oral airways are contraindicated in responsive patients.
(*Use positive statements to avoid confusion. Students taking a test will sometimes miss a single word in reading the item, and this presents a source for incorrect answers other than lack of knowledge.*)

than with other types of questions. One difficulty is that with only true or false as options, the statement must be either completely true or completely false. For example, if a statement is almost always true, the student is forced to guess whether the person writing the exam was thinking of the 99% of the time that the statement is true, or the 1% of the time that the statement is false. Another difficulty is that the chance of a random correct answer is 50%. In general, true/false questions tend to be very easy or very difficult. The result is that they do not always work well in discriminating between students of varying cognitive abilities. True/false items can be effectively combined with a short-answer format by asking students to justify their response. This can be used to assess higher levels of cognition and provide a framework that is slightly more directive than an open short answer.

True/false items should be written in the positive voice, avoiding negatively worded statements such as "is not." It is also important to avoid absolute statements such as "always" or "never." Very few absolute statements are entirely true, and students know this. The practice of taking statements directly out of the text should be avoided, as these are recall items of low difficulty. If a test is being taken by hand, to help eliminate problems in deciphering handwriting, instructors should have students indicate true or false by circling or otherwise marking among provided selections, rather than having students write "T" or "F."

Matching Items

Matching items typically present two columns of information with the intent that the test taker will select items from one column and match them to items in the second column to form correct statements or direct relationships. This strategy works best with terms and definitions, or with simple concepts and obvious relationships. However, this type of item can be confusing for the student unless clear instructions are provided.

This item does not work well when attempting to assess higher levels of cognitive learning, such as synthesis or evaluation.

Items to be matched should bear some similarity to each other to avoid making the correct response obvious. In other words, the list of responses should be homogeneous (e.g., do not mix doses with administration routes). With matching items, it is important for the instructor to provide clear instructions such as whether students will use each of the provided possible responses, whether one term can be used once or multiple times, or whether multiple answers are needed to complete a match. Poorly designed matching items are rather simple logic exercises, allowing students to use the process of elimination to greatly improve their chances of selecting the correct answer. The longer and more involved responses should be in the **stem** (the part of the item that is first offered, which may be written as a question or as an incomplete statement), keeping the responses short and simple. During construction, the instructor should take care to avoid giving grammatical cues to the correct answer. Matching sets should not exceed 15 items and should not break across pages. If the instructor is using scannable forms as answer sheets, the number of possible responses may be limited by the form used. This can be a significant limitation to the use of matching items.

Multiple Choice Items

Multiple choice items are commonly used in national and state certification examinations. Although multiple choice items are extremely easy to grade and demonstrate high interrater reliability (which is why these items are used for certification exams), they are difficult to properly construct. Multiple choice items consist of three main components: the stem, the distractors, and the key. The stem, as noted previously, is the part of the item that is first offered and can be written as a question or as an incomplete statement. The distractor is an incorrect answer designed to be a

Examples of How to Edit Matching Items

Poor

1. Cyanosis
2. Nasal cannula
3. Oral airway
4. Bag-valve-mask
5. Nasopharyngeal airway

a. Used for unresponsive patients
b. Used for airway control in responsive patients
c. Delivers low-flow oxygen
d. A sign of poor oxygenation
e. Used to assist ventilation

Better

1. Provides high-flow supplemental oxygen
2. Provides low-flow supplemental oxygen
3. Provides precise concentrations of oxygen

a. Bag-valve-mask
b. Venturi mask
c. Nonrebreather mask
d. Nasal cannula

plausible alternative to the correct answer. The key is the correct (or best) answer to the stem.

Multiple choice items can be used to test both low and high levels of cognitive thinking, although constructing multiple choice items that evaluate high-level thinking is challenging. Multiple choice items are extremely easy to grade, and they allow for computer scoring of examinations. This makes it possible for a relatively large number of items to be used, thus increasing the reliability of the assessment instrument. On the other hand, because valid and reliable multiple choice items are difficult to construct, the instructor is not able to rapidly develop these items. Constructing the examination items the night before the examination is simply not possible. Because a limited number of responses are allowed with multiple choice items, these items are unable to evaluate the thinking behind the selection of an answer. One variation on multiple choice items designed to overcome this limitation is to provide space within which the student can explain a selection, if the student believes that the provided information is not sufficient for a clear choice.

Suggested strategies for the proper construction of multiple choice items are as follows:

- Be on the watch for bias cueing (leading students to the correct answer by the way the stem is worded or from grammar choices).
- Avoid negatively worded stems. It is easy for students to misread negatively worded stems. Some educators propose that it is okay to use negatively worded stems when the concept tested is an important exception such as when *not* to do something. Medication contraindications are one example of this, such as "Nitroglycerin should *not* be administered to a patient with a systolic blood pressure of less than 90 mm Hg." Where negative stems are needed, the negative word, such as "not" or "except," should be italicized or boldfaced to draw attention.

In general, items should not build on previous items. Exceptions to this occur when the sequencing of steps is being assessed, or when a number of multiple choice items are related to a single, provided scenario. When a single scenario is used as the basis for several multiple choice items, the related items should be grouped together, should not break across pages, and may have a box drawn around the scenario and all related questions to ensure that students understand which questions belong to each scenario (**FIGURE 21.3**). Additional strategies include the following:

- Avoid questions written with a fill-in-the-blank segment in the middle of the stem; these are difficult to read.

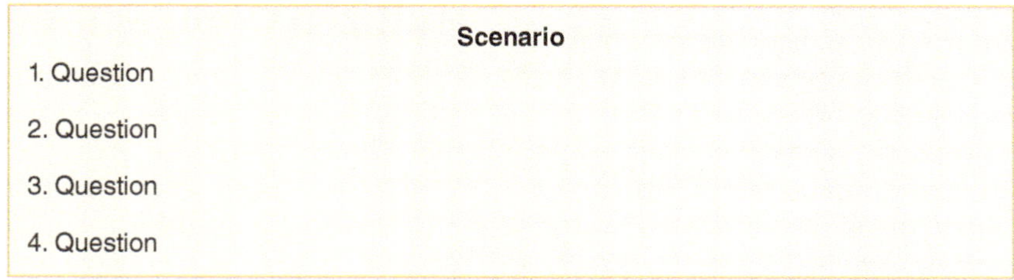

FIGURE 21.3 When a single scenario is used as the basis for several multiple choice items, related items should be grouped together, should not break across pages, and may have a box drawn around them, along with the scenario, to ensure that students understand which questions relate to each scenario.

- Avoid the use of "all of the above" or "none of the above" as an option. Recognition of one incorrect distractor immediately eliminates "all of the above" as the key. Recognition of more than one distractor as correct immediately indicates "all of the above" as the correct answer. Although "none of the above" presents less of a problem, it still presents the student with the ability to use simple logic instead of content knowledge to derive the correct answer. Often, rewriting the stem can prevent the use of "all of the above" and "none of the above" as choices. Additionally, if the instructions for the examination are to select the "best" answer, then use of "none of the above" is inappropriate, as one of the choices will be the best of those provided.
- Avoid the use of "multiple multiple choice" items—questions that provide a list of possible components to the answer, with distractors and keys containing different combinations of components (for example, a question that includes answer options A–D, and then includes a list of options 1–4, along the lines of "1. A and B; 2. A, B, and C; etc."). This type of item can be solved with basic knowledge, and these items are actually nothing more than a series of true/false questions. Instructors can easily convert "multiple multiple choice" items to a series of true/false items, thus correcting the deficiency.
- Avoid overlapping responses. Overlapping responses present unnecessary difficulty to students. If the stem asks for a range and a distractor offers a single number, this can be immediately eliminated. Overlap of distractors into the correct range can be confusing for the student.
- Ensure that all distractors are approximately the same length. Common wisdom is that the longest option is usually the correct choice. This is because the writer of the item typically spends the most time with the wording of the correct option (to ensure that it is completely correct) and spends less time with the distractors.
- Ensure that all distractors make grammatical sense. Frequent issues include problems with agreement of plural/singular and a/an. One way to easily avoid grammatical cueing is to use complete sentences as the stem.
- Ensure that the correct answer is randomly distributed. A general tendency is for instructors to predominantly use (b) and (c) as the key.
- Be aware that in constructing a multiple choice question, instructors tend to distribute the distractors so that two of the three are at the extreme positions, leaving the correct choice among the two middle answers (e.g., if the correct answer is 4, options would typically be 1, 3, 4, and 7). Students are aware of this tendency as well.
- Place responses in a logical order. If the responses are assigned a numeric value, place the lowest numeric response as the first choice, the next highest as the second, and so forth.

Examples of Multiple Choice Items That Test Different Cognitive Levels

Recall

Which of the following parameters is included in the primary patient assessment?

a. Blood pressure
b. Level of consciousness
c. Movement of distal extremities
d. Bowel sounds

Application

Which of the following assessment findings is most helpful for determining the adequacy of ventilation?

a. Skin color
b. Heart rate
c. Blood pressure
d. Respiratory rate

Problem Solving

A patient from a motor vehicle collision presents with decreased level of consciousness, blood pressure of 170/100 mm Hg, heart rate of 60 beats per minute, and a respiratory rate of 10 breaths per minute. The skin is pale, cool, and moist. How should you administer oxygen to this patient?

a. Bag-valve-mask
b. Nasal cannula
c. Nonrebreather face mask
d. Venturi mask

Examples of Bias Cueing

Poor

A patient presents as unresponsive, with no spontaneous respirations, after being hit in the head with a baseball bat. Which of the following would be the most appropriate device to use to secure the airway?

a. Recovery position
b. Oral airway
c. Nasal airway
d. Head-tilt chin-lift

(The term "device" in this example immediately eliminates choices a and d.)

Better

A patient presents as unresponsive, with no spontaneous respirations, after being hit in the head with a baseball bat. Which of the following would be the most appropriate means of securing the airway?

a. Recovery position
b. Oral airway
c. Nasal airway
d. Head-tilt chin-lift

(Bias cueing is removed by rewording the stem to remove the clue.)

Example of Multiple Choice with Fill-in-the-Blank

Poor

You have initiated CPR on a patient in cardiac arrest. As soon as the equipment arrives, connecting ___ would be the next appropriate step.

a. Oxygen
b. Automatic external defibrillator
c. Supraglottic airway
d. Automatic transport ventilator

Better

You have initiated CPR on a patient in cardiac arrest. As soon as the equipment arrives, which of the following would be the next appropriate step?

a. Oxygen
b. Automatic external defibrillator
c. Supraglottic airway
d. Automatic transport ventilator

(The blank in the middle of the statement can present unnecessary confusion and is easily removed by rewording the stem.)

Example of Removing "All of the Above" as an Answer Choice

Poor

Which of the following would be appropriate care for the patient with a serious chest injury from a motor vehicle collision?

a. High-flow oxygen
b. Spinal motion restriction
c. Rapid transport
d. All of the above

Better

Which of the following would **NOT** be appropriate care for the patient with a serious chest injury from a motor vehicle collision?

a. High-flow oxygen
b. Spinal motion restriction
c. Rapid transport to the nearest trauma center
d. Application of sandbags to the chest

(The easiest way to remove the "all of the above" option is to convert the stem into a negative phrase. In this case, the negative "not" is in boldface and is capitalized to minimize confusion. Also, in the revised example, one of the distractors is lengthened, so the key is not the longest phrase among the choices.) The instructor should recognize that negative stems commonly have reliability problems as mistakes in reading produce measurable rates of error. Although it is easier to change to a negative stem, this may not be the best solution. Creative editing can correct this problem.

Better (without the Negative Stem)

Which of the following would be contraindicated in the patient with a serious chest injury from a motor vehicle collision?

a. High-flow oxygen
b. Spinal motion restriction
c. Rapid transport to the nearest trauma center
d. Application of sandbags to the chest

- Do not create words or abbreviations just to fill a response.
- Do not create humorous or ridiculous options just to fill space. The use of humor can create problems with reliability in addition to the fact that it may be perceived negatively by many students. As humor is culturally and often regionally based, the use of humor is a source of potential bias in the examination.
- All answers should be plausible to students. On later analysis, distractors that no students have selected should be edited to improve the plausibility. Implausible distractors improve the odds of guessing the correct answer without the necessary knowledge.

Example of Removing Multiple Multiples

Poor

Which of the following assessment findings is consistent with a patient who is suffering from hypoperfusion due to internal bleeding?

1. Warm and flushed skin
2. Rapid pulse rate
3. Low blood pressure
4. Anxiety
   - a. 1, 2, and 3
   - b. 1, 3, and 4
   - c. 1 and 3
   - d. 2, 3, and 4

Better

Which of the following assessment findings is **NOT** consistent with a patient who is suffering from hypoperfusion due to internal bleeding?

- a. Warm and flushed skin
- b. Rapid pulse rate
- c. Low blood pressure
- d. Anxiety

Another Option

Questions 12–15 refer to the following statement:
The following assessment findings are consistent with a patient who is suffering from hypoperfusion due to internal bleeding. Circle true or false for each assessment finding.

12.	Warm and flushed skin	True	False
13.	Rapid pulse rate	True	False
14.	Low blood pressure	True	False
15.	Anxiety	True	False

Example of Fixing Overlapping Ranges

Poor

Which of the following is a normal respiratory rate for a patient who is 4 years old?

- a. 8–16
- b. 12–20
- c. 15–30
- d. 20–40

Better

Which of the following is a normal respiratory rate for a patient who is 4 years old?

- a. 10–15
- b. 16–30
- c. 31–50
- d. 80–100

(The overlapping ranges present an unnecessary difficulty. The situation is best avoided, even with the addition of a distractor that is far outside the range.)

Example of Ensuring Comparable Length of Answer Choices

Poor

A patient with severe respiratory distress should be transported in which of the following positions?

- a. Sitting, if the patient has a normal level of consciousness
- b. Supine
- c. Prone
- d. Recovery position

Better

A conscious patient with severe respiratory distress should be transported in which of the following positions?

- a. Sitting
- b. Supine
- c. Prone
- d. Recovery position

(Any necessary conditions for the key to be correct are moved to the stem, removing the obvious clue to the correct answer.)

Example of Removing Grammar Cues

Poor

A patient has an injury to the leg with severe pain and bone fragments protruding from the site of injury. This patient has an:

- **a.** closed fracture.
- **b.** open fracture.
- **c.** dislocation.
- **d.** sprain.

Better

A patient has an injury to the leg with severe pain and bone fragments protruding from the site of injury. This patient has a(n):

- **a.** closed fracture.
- **b.** open fracture.
- **c.** dislocation.
- **d.** sprain.

(Grammatical cueing, or grammar cueing, is easily avoided by using a complete sentence as the stem.)

Example of the Middle Value

Poor

Which of the following best expresses the range of respiratory rates considered normal for an infant?

- **a.** 12–20
- **b.** 15–30
- **c.** 25–50
- **d.** 50–70

Better

Which of the following best expresses the range of respiratory rates considered normal for an infant?

- **a.** 8–12
- **b.** 12–16
- **c.** 18–30
- **d.** 30–60

(Although all cases of the middle value being the correct choice do not need to be changed, the instructor should be aware of the tendency and take care to avoid patterns. Occasional use of an extreme value as the correct choice is appropriate. Although overlapping ranges are seen in this example, the student is being clearly asked to identify which range best describes normal, and the ranges in this case are taken directly from the 2011 AHA PALS provider manual: 12–16 normal for adolescents, 18–30 normal for school-age children, and 30–60 normal for infants.)

Challenges of Using the Full Sentence Stem

The examples in this chapter have used full sentence stems. While this practice easily eliminates grammar and bias cues when compared to blanks and incomplete sentences, use of full sentences as a stem also introduces challenges. Full sentences are longer than stems using incomplete sentences. The added length increases the time needed for examinations due to increased reading time. The added length also introduces a source of reliability problems from the unnecessary words. Writing stems as a full sentence is a reasonable practice for novice item writers, but experience with editing should enable more experienced writers to significantly shorten items through the use of incomplete sentences as stems. An example is provided:

A patient presents as unresponsive, with no spontaneous respirations, after being hit in the head with a baseball bat. Which of the following would be the most appropriate means of opening the airway? *(33 words, 167 characters)*

- **a.** Recovery position
- **b.** Oral airway
- **c.** Nasal airway
- **d.** Head-tilt chin-lift

(Editing to shorten the stem would produce a significantly shorter stem that is much easier to read and comprehend. Easy comprehension of key information in the stem is necessary for reliability.)

A patient struck on the head with a baseball bat presents as unresponsive and apneic. You should open the airway by using: *(22 words, 100 characters)*

- **a.** the recovery position.
- **b.** an oral airway.
- **c.** a nasal airway.
- **d.** the head-tilt chin-lift.

TEACHING TIP

One method of ensuring random distribution of the correct answer involves the use of a deck of cards. With each item, a card is selected:

- If the suit is hearts, A is used as the key.
- If the suit is clubs, B is used.
- If the suit is spades, C is used.
- If the suit is diamonds, D is used.

One must be sure to shuffle the deck before cards are chosen.

Using Open Response Items

Open-ended response items (constructed response items) can also offer advantages and disadvantages. In these question types the student must construct their own answer. A combination of different types of examination items provides the strongest validity and reliability.

Completion Items

Completion (also known as fill-in-the-blank) items are statements from which part of the information has been omitted; students must complete the statement. Enough information must be included for students to glean the intent of the statement without being led to the answer. One issue with open-response items arises when the meaning of the incomplete statement is unclear and several student responses emerge as correct, presenting a problem for the test grader. Items with unclear statements present a challenge for maintaining interrater reliability if more than one person is grading the exam. Completion items are not capable of evaluating higher-order thinking such as problem solving. These items are best used to evaluate recall, especially for key phrases that should be known verbatim or for definitions of key terms.

The provided answer space may present a problem for completion items. If one blank is used for each word of the correct response, the student is presented with a significant clue as to the answer. If only one blank is provided, students frequently assume that the answer consists of one word when multiple words are necessary. Either interpretation lowers reliability of the item.

Tips for writing completion items include the following:

- Omit significant words from the statement, but not so many that it is difficult for the student to determine the intent. For example, "An automated external defibrillator is used to treat ventricular _____." is better than "A _____ is used to treat _____ fibrillation." One method of ensuring this is to allow only one blank per completion item.
- Place the blank at the end of the sentence. This shortens the reading time and allows the student to derive the intent of the item before encountering the blank. For example, "_____ is used to assess the percentage of hemoglobin that is oxygenated." should be converted to "The percentage of hemoglobin that is oxygenated is assessed by _____."
- As with other item types, avoid taking statements verbatim from textbooks or workbooks. It is particularly tempting to construct completion items by copying a statement from the text and omitting key words. There are two problems with this practice. First, it ensures that the item evaluates only recall. Second, statements in texts are heavily dependent on context for the correct interpretation. Without that context, a single sentence frequently becomes ambiguous and difficult to complete the missing words.
- As with multiple choice items, be aware of possible cues from the grammar and sentence construction.
- Ambiguity of grading can be difficult with any open-response item. Because completion items require a short answer, it is difficult to evaluate the student's thinking behind a particular response. This challenges the reliability of grading. For instance, consider the stem "Pulse oximetry is used to measure _____." While the instructor may intend the answer to be "oxygen saturation," reasonable responses may include circulation, shock, distal perfusion, oxygenation, and so on. It is difficult for an instructor to predetermine possible interpretations of an item without piloting the item or using reviewers.

Essay Items

Essay items pose a question or situation for which students are required to provide a relatively long, prose-style answer. Essay items are capable of assessing higher levels of cognitive thinking, but they also require that the student be capable of expressing this knowledge in coherent, written fashion. Essays can be used to effectively assess lower and middle levels within the affective domain. These questions also have the advantage of not being as easily susceptible to student guessing, although students may try to bluff. Because essay items are time consuming for students to complete and for instructors to grade, it is seldom practical to include more than a couple of essay items during a classroom assessment.

The sole use of essay questions on an examination presents a challenge to validity; this results from obvious problems with the breadth of material. Ensuring reliability during grading is difficult, as many factors other than knowledge can influence the assigned grade. In general, essay questions should be reserved for those objectives that cannot be effectively evaluated with limited response items.

The instructor should give their students advice for and practice with writing essays. This practice can be part of the formative assessment strategies. The instructor should not give students a choice of questions to answer during examinations. It will be difficult to match the exam blueprint if different students answer different questions. Also, because some questions will be more difficult than others, the test could be unfair. When this choice is presented, each student is actually taking a different examination. Each essay question should be linked to a single objective; the student should avoid attempting to evaluate several objectives with one item.

Tips for writing essay items include the following:

- Avoid using essay items to evaluate recall of facts. Recall items, such as lists and definitions, are better evaluated using items that have fewer problems with grading reliability such as limited response items.
- Be clear in the task expected of students. For instance, "Discuss shock." is much less clear than "Describe the various compensation mechanisms for shock."
- In order to assess different levels of cognition, one useful strategy is to match the verbs used in the objective to the verbs used in the essay assignment.

Short-Answer Items

Between the essay question and the completion item lies the short-answer question. Short-answer questions are similar to essay questions, except that essay questions typically require multipage responses, and short-answer questions rarely exceed a full page. Depending on the stated objectives, it may also be desirable to avoid requiring the use of full sentences to respond to short-answer questions. Allowing students to use bulleted lists or outline forms may provide enough insight for the instructor to effectively assess knowledge, while not relying heavily on writing skills. Because they take less time and fewer writing skills for students to complete, more questions can be included. The strengths, weaknesses, and implications for short-answer questions are otherwise the same as for essay questions. In most cases, essay questions have little use in the EMS classroom compared with short-answer questions.

Writing essay items can be similar to writing short-answer items. It is important when writing a short-answer question to limit the scope of the question. When limiting the scope, the following may be helpful to convert essay items into short-answer items:

- Use a subset of clinical conditions; for example, "Describe compensatory mechanisms for *neurogenic* shock."
- Describe the circumstances in more detail; for example, "The patient fell from a height of 20 feet. Describe the implications of selecting an appropriate destination for this patient."
- Target the response by providing more detail about the expected response; for example, "Describe the pathophysiology of frostbite, paying particular attention to the role of vasoconstriction."

TEACHING TIP

Both limited response items and short-answer items can assess higher levels within the cognitive domain. A simple rule regarding which type the instructor should choose is that short-answer or essay questions should be used when the time to prepare the examination is short and the time to grade the examination is long. When the time to prepare the examination is long and the time to grade the examination is short, limited response items (such as multiple choice) are the preferred tool.

Alternate Item Formats

Alternate item format may be seen on some exams. These question types are frequently used to assess learners' ability to interpret information at higher levels. Alternate item formats include multiple response, drag-and-drop (ordered response), and media-enhanced items. Media-enhanced items, including hot-spot, chart/exhibit, audio item format, and graphic distractor options are variations on the traditional multiple choice question (**TABLE 21.1**).[3,4] These question types are particularly difficult if the students have not previously encountered them.

Homework and Research Projects

A variety of homework and research projects can also add to formative and summative student assessment. Some options are discussed here.

Homework

One tool that can be useful as a formative assessment is the routine assignment of homework to be completed by students. Homework should be spread out relatively evenly across the course. Each assignment need not be graded, but many students will interpret the lack of grade impact as lack of importance. Assigning a nominal grade impact to a random selection of homework assignments can counter this tendency. The instructor should review homework assignments for level of difficulty and should include a mix of easy and difficult items. Encouraging students to collaborate on homework can be a useful practice that helps to build teamwork and peer learning. Frequent assignments, which help to build regular study habits in students, provide the instructor with regular, formative feedback on student progress.

Examples of homework assignments for the EMS classroom include assignments from workbooks, completion and definition worksheets, short research projects, case studies, concept maps, targeted discussion in an online forum (discussion board or blog), writing a summary of key points from lecture, and description of care for a supplied scenario. Electronic homework assignments can include questions embedded in narrated lectures, online quizzes, and virtual simulations. Homework assignments also provide students with examples of what types of problems they will be expected to solve for summative

TABLE 21.1 Alternate Item Types

Alternate Item Type	Description	Example
Multiple response items	Student must select all of the options that are correct. It is possible to have a single correct response, more than one correct response, or all responses are correct. Note that these items allow varied grading strategies for partial credit, which the instructor should make clear in the exam instructions.	A 72-year-old female has abdominal pain after a motor vehicle crash. Which signs and symptoms would you anticipate if she is developing shock? Select all that apply: [ ] Anxious appearance [ ] Increased respirations [ ] Pale skin color [ ] Slowing heart rate
Hot-spot items	Test taker selects a specific area on a figure, graph, or diagram to illustrate the correct answer. Note that these items may also allow multiple responses.	Select the J point on the electrocardiogram below. © Jones & Bartlett Learning
Drag-and-drop (ordered response)	Candidate selects and moves items into a specified order or sequence.	A 22-year-old male with an apparent opiate overdose is unresponsive, with a respiratory rate of 6 breaths per minute. Arrange the following steps in the order the EMT should perform them. **Unordered Options** / **Ordered Response (Answer)** Administer intranasal naloxone / Insert an oropharyngeal airway Begin bag-mask ventilation / Begin bag-mask ventilation Insert an oropharyngeal airway / Administer intranasal naloxone
Audio item	Test taker listens to a sound clip using headphones and selects the correct option.	A 65-year-old female complains of sudden onset difficulty breathing. Her breath sounds are as follows (audio clip of crackles is played). Which intervention is indicated? **a.** Albuterol updraft **b.** Epinephrine IM **c.** Magnesium sulfate IV **d.** Nitroglycerin SL

Alternate Item Type	Description	Example
Graphic option items	Item distractors are images rather than words.	A 65-year-old has fever and tachypnea. Which rash would indicate the need for rescuers to don an N-95 mask? **a.** 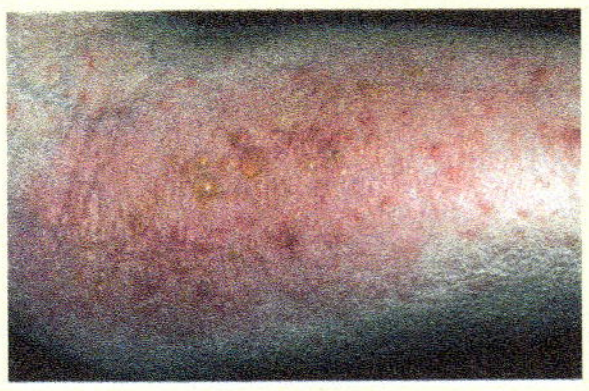 © Joel zatz/Alamy Stock Photo **b.** 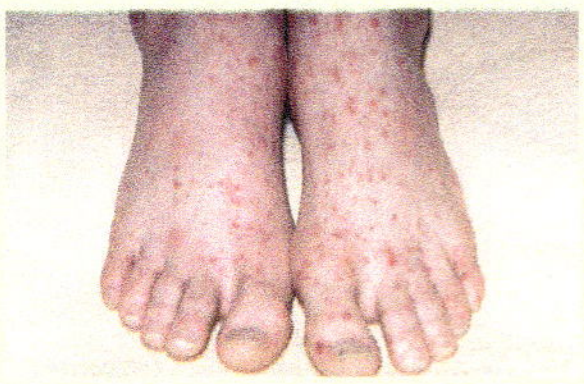 © Mediscan/Alamy Stock Photo **c.** 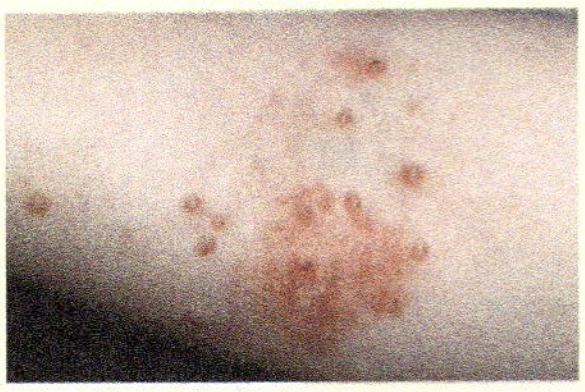 © Allan Harris/Medical Images **d.** 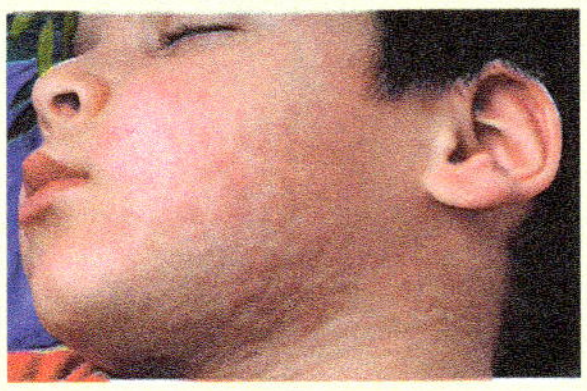 © LeventKonuk/iStockphoto
Chart/exhibit	The candidate interprets information within a chart or exhibit to solve a problem.	The paramedic receives a patient from an urgent care center who complains of weakness, weight gain, and strong-smelling urine. The lab report shows serum: Sodium: 145 mEq/L Potassium: 6.2 mEq/L Hemoglobin: 14 g/dL Leukocytes: 10,000/mm^3 Which should the paramedic assess first? **a.** Capnography **b.** Electrocardiogram **c.** Pupil response **d.** Temperature
Video items	A question is asked based on a video clip of a situation or procedure that is played.	A video illustrating defibrillation with an automated external defibrillator (AED) is played and the candidate is asked: Which action in this sequence was incorrect? **a.** CPR continued during analysis. **b.** Pads applied before AED turned on. **c.** Pulse was checked after defibrillation. **d.** Rescuer touched patient as shock delivered.

assessments. To be effective as formative assessments, homework assignments must be graded and returned to students in a timely manner.

Research Project Assignments

Project assignments based on students' own research are another means of assessing the ability of students to synthesize information. These assignments are a tool for assessing higher-level cognitive learning. Individual projects allow students to use their own specific learning preferences to complete the assignment. Research projects promote student autonomy, enhance student confidence, and encourage independent learning.

Assignment or choice of topic is an important, yet commonly overlooked, component of the project assignment. Allowing students to choose a topic that appeals to them is appropriate, but the instructor must be an active part of the topic selection and determination of project scope. Students should not waste valuable time on consideration of topics. One way of avoiding this scenario is to prepare a list of potential topics from which students can choose. Controlling the project scope is necessary to ensure that projects assigned to different students are roughly equivalent in terms of difficulty. Many instructors require that students obtain approval on project scope early in the process.

Another option is to prepare a rubric that clearly outlines guidelines for determination of grades based on the amount of work that students complete. For example, "To earn a C, the student will complete a written paper of at least 10 pages and a classroom presentation; to earn a B, the student will also complete at least one optional activity; and to earn an A, the student will complete at least two additional optional activities. Optional activities include reporting on an interview of a local medical director, creating a project-related website, completing a survey of at least 20 local EMS providers, and creating and demonstrating a working mechanical model related to a particular topic."

A measure of negotiation between the instructor and the student is appropriate in determining scope while still allowing students to express their own talents and learning preferences. It is also helpful for the instructor to reinforce relevance by creating realistic writing scenarios, such as, "Your medical director has asked you to submit a new protocol for the treatment of anaphylaxis. Please submit your protocol, which should include both assessment and treatment sections. Provide at least five sources from peer-reviewed medical journals that support the care you propose." One problem with project assignments is the tendency of instructors to base the grade on product rather than on process. In most cases, the process used by students to prepare a project is just as important as the product itself. One way that instructors can avoid this trap is by requiring students to submit intermediate steps for consideration and possible impact on grade. An example is to have a check-in for the following steps: (1) description of title, purpose, and major points; (2) sources, data, and references; (3) outline; (4) first draft; and (5) final version.

The process of grading project assignments is essentially the same as that used to grade essay items on written exams. Recommendations provided in the section *Grading Essays* later in this chapter can be applied to written components of the project. Criteria for grading projects should be clearly communicated to students, as noted in the section, *Grading Strategies*. The grade may contain components that measure the quality of the product, as well as the effectiveness of the process.

Project assignments are best viewed as a combination of a learning tool and an assessment tool. As a learning tool, project assignments result in learning that is customized to the individual student's talents and preferences. Project assignments emphasize critical thinking, independent learning, and use of research skills. As an assessment tool, project assignments permit assessment of high-level cognitive objectives and, in some cases, affective objectives.

Administering Written Examinations

The administration of written exams requires careful attention. An inappropriate environment or ineffective method of administration can significantly impact exam validity.

Environmental Considerations

The classroom set-up for a written examination is essentially the same as that used for a traditional lecture format, with the students seated in rows (**FIGURE 21.4**). Students should be seated far enough apart to discourage them from looking at each others' papers. Exam proctors should walk the room from time to time so that they are able to see students' faces as well as observe students' space and activity. Appropriate temperature and lighting should be ensured. Special attention should be given to providing a quiet environment.

For examinations that last longer than an hour, the instructor should set clear rules for restroom breaks. It is helpful to have extra copies of the examination and answer sheets, scratch paper, and pencils readily available.

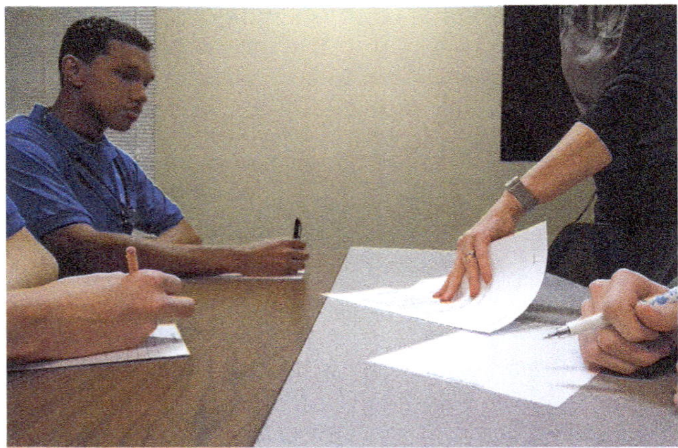

FIGURE 21.4 Answer sheets and test booklets (facedown) can be placed at student seats before the examination. Student notebooks and backpacks should be placed at the back or side of the room.

Courtesy of St. Charles County Ambulance District.

Proctoring

An instructor should supervise written examinations to discourage cheating and to address problems or process questions as they arise. Lead instructors communicate the importance of examinations by **proctoring** the examination themselves. Proctors should arrive early and should be prepared to leave late. During the examination, the proctor should monitor the room without hovering over students. The proctor should have a strategy for addressing questions asked by students during the exam. One common strategy is to allow the proctor to answer only questions regarding examination process—not questions related to examination content. Proctors should be cognizant that any communication of content to a student who asks a question gives an advantage to that student over those who did not ask or attempt to fish for clues. The proctor should keep students apprised as to the time by having a clock in the room, writing (and updating) the time on a whiteboard, or periodically announcing the time remaining for the test.

Appropriate proctoring helps to ensure the integrity of the examination. Cheating can flourish in an unsupervised environment. The proctor must maintain security of testing materials. The ability to look at other students' answers can be prevented by proper seating arrangements. Cell phones, smartwatches, and other recording devices should be prohibited in the testing environment. Any notes or calculations during the examination should not leave the testing environment. Silence during examinations discourages covert communications. Use of multiple versions of an exam, with differing arrangements of item sequence and distractors, discourages organized efforts by groups of students to each memorize parts of an examination and later reconstruct the examination. Another means to defeat that form of cheating is to revise examinations after each administration. Test development software can make creation of multiple randomized versions easier. Diligent observation by the instructor, combined with clear expectations of integrity, are key to preventing cheating.

Computer-Based Testing

Technological developments have enabled more widespread use of computer-based testing in educational settings. Once reserved for high-stakes examinations, these techniques are increasingly available for classroom instructors to incorporate. Testing centers in community colleges and other environments can offer secured, computer-based testing environments, which may be appropriate for high-stakes summative examinations. Other variations exist for use within the classroom. Use of a learning management system (LMS), such as Moodle, Canvas, or Blackboard, may include testing modules. This allows for distributed methods of formative assessments and quizzes. Within the classroom, small, remote, polling devices or audience response systems can connect to a presentation system. This system can allow an additional layer of interaction within the classroom discussion that can blend a tracked, formative assessment with an informal discussion.

A major advantage of computer-based testing systems is that these systems remove a potential source for error in grading and item analysis. By direct entry into the system, grading and analysis are more efficient. With varying degrees of security, tests can be offered in multiple locations—even in the student's home at a convenient time. Computer systems also allow a greater variety of media to be attached to test items such as pictures, audio, and video. Different versions of the test can be offered to students, increasing security. Using different versions of the examination is enabled by the substantial increases in efficiency of grading. Feedback can be offered instantaneously, which is particularly valuable for formative assessments.[5]

These systems typically favor limited response items. This limits the range of items available to instructors. If large numbers of versions are used, an extensive item bank may be required. Item security may be difficult to maintain, particularly in formative exams linked to an LMS. Cheating may be difficult to monitor if the examination is delivered in a distributed mode, although several varieties of exam security and verification of identity may be used in formal testing centers. Some vendors offer examinations that include online remote proctoring in which the examination proctors monitor the student remotely through the use of technology, such as webcams. The examination process that uses computer-based testing can be subject to a variety of technical difficulties that are not present in paper-and-pencil versions, such as network outages.

Some self-directed educational programs build computer-based assessment directly into the learning algorithms. Assessments and performance in electronic simulations guide content. These programs, such as the American Heart Association Heartcode Advanced Cardiovascular Life Support (ACLS) and Pediatric Advanced Life Support (PALS), combine assessment and learning activities into computer-based simulations. This can effectively combine formative assessment, learning, and summative assessment into a blended set of activities that are seamless to the learner and yet contain sophisticated recorded evaluations of learner abilities.

The NREMT and other certification bodies use computer testing systems to deliver certification examinations. Although most computer-based exams use traditional testing theory and are linear, NREMT actually uses a different testing format called **item-response theory (IRT)**. This exam format allows more precise measurement with fewer items. More information on IRT is presented later in this chapter. Although IRT is not usually an option for use in EMS classrooms, it seems reasonable that instructors preparing students for NREMT certification would build a degree of computer-based assessment into their programs. The rapid pace of change in technological environments ensures that developments in technology-assisted assessments will outpace the ability of any text to adequately describe current capabilities.

Time Limits

Each student will take a different amount of time to complete the examination. To exert some measure of control over the time spent on the examination, the instructor must set some limits on time. Setting time limits for examinations is a legitimate strategy for (1) preparing students for certifying examinations and (2) evaluating students' ability to think quickly. The drawback to setting time limits is that some students struggle to complete the examination in the time allowed. In estimating the amount of time a student is given to complete an examination, the instructor can give students four times as long as it takes the instructor to complete the test. As an alternative, Barbara Gross Davis, in *Tools for Teaching,*[6] suggests the following timing strategies:

- Allow half a minute per true/false item.
- Allow 1 minute per multiple choice item.
- Allow 2 minutes per short-answer item.
- Allow 10 to 15 minutes per limited essay item.
- Allow 30 minutes per broader essay item.
- Allow 5 to 10 minutes for students to review their work.
- Factor in time to distribute and collect tests.

It is critical to note that the examination should be designed and administered to assess only those abilities necessary and not inadvertently depend on unrelated abilities. This is particularly important when considering learning disabilities. Examinations can be unreasonably dependent on reading abilities. One strategy to accommodate documented learning disabilities would be to extend the time allowed for an examination. In some cases, a reader would be appropriate for a written examination. The evaluation of disabilities and compliance with the Americans with Disabilities Act (ADA) is beyond the scope of this text. Expert evaluation of the situation may be necessary, in which case the instructor should consult with available experts in the educational setting.

Analysis of Written Examinations

The analysis and potential revision of written exams are important steps in improving student assessment. The type of evaluation depends on the examination stakes as well as available resources.

Post-Test Review

A useful strategy after an examination has been administered is to allow class time for students to review the examination as a group with the instructor. This review highlights areas of weakness for individual students, as well as for the class as a whole. Review can also help the instructor to identify areas where the presentation of material did not adequately prepare students for mastery of the stated objectives. It can serve to alleviate concerns about bias when students see what items other students missed. A climate of fairness is promoted when students can discuss questions, answers, or the wording of a question. Although some instructors allow students to retain the examination after classroom discussion, this practice greatly reduces the validity of test items that are reused. Even on low-stakes examinations, students who have access to the previous classes' exams can develop a false sense of security, thinking they are familiar with the content when in fact they are only recognizing items they have seen on previous exams. Teachers may be misled about the students' understanding of material based on answers obtained on previous exams. Additionally, it is neither time nor cost effective to develop new exams for each class, even for low-stakes exams. Conducting a classroom discussion breaches examination security, but the breach is less significant than when students are allowed to retain copies of the examination.

Pilot use and previous validation may not be possible for all examinations, but they should be conducted before an item is included in a high-stakes examination. One possible strategy for pilot use is to present pilot items for formative assessments, such as quizzes. Another is to have an examination include several (generally not more than 10%) pilot items that do not count toward the exam score. These should be interspersed among regular items. Pilot items that demonstrate reliability and validity can then be included in future examinations. Pilot items that fail validation can be returned to the editing process for revision, guided by pilot data.

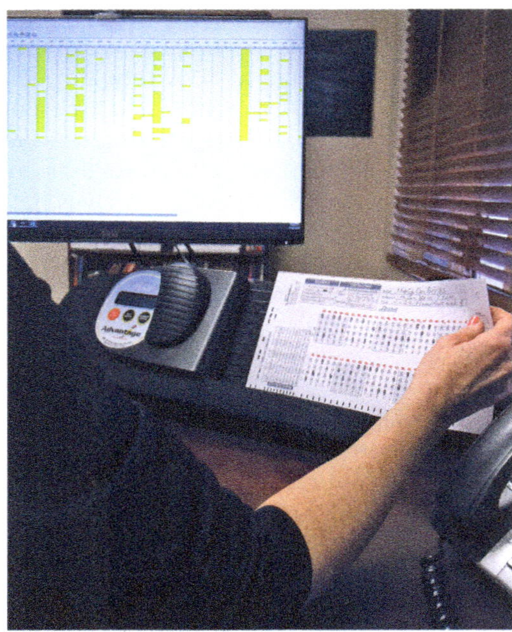

FIGURE 21.5 Scannable answer sheets and grading software can facilitate quick scoring of multiple choice exams and provide a means of performing item analysis.

Courtesy of St. Charles County Ambulance District.

Difficulty Level and Discrimination Index

For low- or moderate-stakes examinations, grading of the examination is coupled with validation of test items. Validation is particularly applicable to limited response items such as true/false, multiple choice, and matching questions. As mentioned earlier, the two characteristics of tests that are useful in validation are difficulty level and item discrimination index (also called the discrimination ratio). (Recall that the difficulty level is the percentage of students who answer each item correctly; the item discrimination index compares the performance of those who scored well on the exam with the performance of those who did not score well on each exam item.) Computerized programs will perform the necessary calculations (**FIGURE 21.5**), but the same measurements can be easily calculated manually, which means the instructor can validate items even when not administering examinations by computer.

Students may find an item difficult for numerous reasons, including that the item may be poorly worded. Adding the discrimination index into the analysis for potential revision of items separates those items that have questionable reliability and validity from those that are appropriately constructed, yet challenging. Items that have extreme difficulty levels (either high or low) will not discriminate as well as those with a difficulty level near 50%. As a result, different thresholds are used to indicate the need for revision depending on the difficulty level of the item. When the difficulty level and the discrimination index are used, the process shown in **FIGURE 21.6** can help identify items that need revision.[6]

Negative discrimination indices indicate that students who scored well overall did worse on those

Calculating the Difficulty Level

The following procedure can be used to calculate the difficulty level and the discrimination index for limited response items, such as multiple choice or true/false questions.

To calculate the item difficulty, the instructor should calculate the percentage of students who had correct responses. The formula for this is:

$$ID = (C/T) \times 100$$

where ID is the item difficulty, C is the number of correct responses, and T is the total number of students who took the examination.

For example, if 30 students took the exam and 20 answered the item correctly, the difficulty level/index would be 67%. The goal is to use only a few items that more than 90% or less than 30% of students answer correctly.[6]

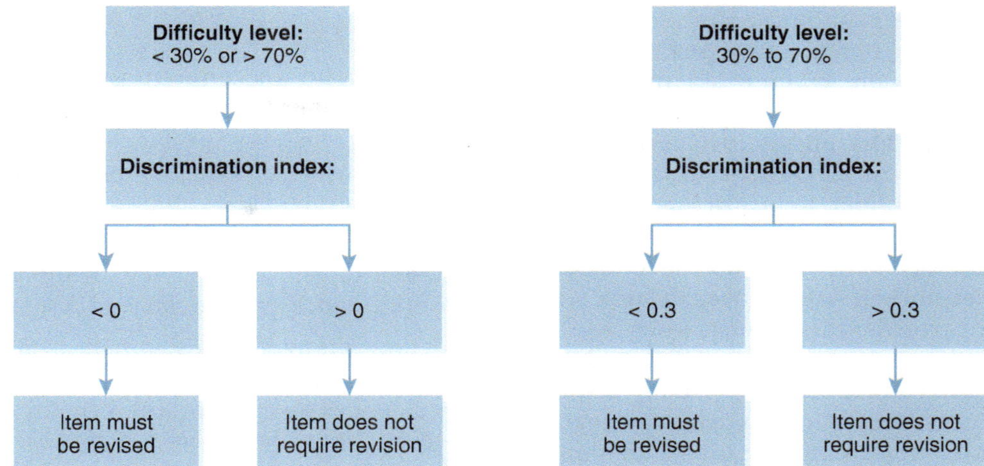

FIGURE 21.6 The difficulty level and the discrimination index can help the instructor identify test items that need revision.

Data from Davis, Barbara G. 2001. *Tools for Teaching*. San Francisco: Jossey-Bass.

particular questions than did students who did not score well overall. Items with a negative discrimination index should be reviewed for validity and revised before they are used again. A common cause of a strongly negative item discrimination index (near to −1.0) is an incorrectly keyed item. Editing of examination items should extend to a check of the answer key as well.

When analyzing items, there are several components of the item that should be considered. Problems with the stem are the most obvious and common to

Calculating the Item Discrimination

The purpose of calculating the item discrimination is to compare the response of the high exam performers on each item to the response of the low exam performers. If an item is constructed correctly, the instructor can expect the high scorers to get the item correct and the low scorers to miss the item. This would be referred to as a *positive discrimination value*. The higher the number, the higher and better the discrimination. If, for some reason, more individuals from the lowest-scoring group than from the highest-scoring group select the correct answer, the result would be a *negative discrimination value*. In general, items with a low (or negative) discrimination value should be reviewed and probably edited. A negative discrimination is most likely a miskeyed item. Negative discrimination could also indicate that the item was tricky and that high performers read into the item and missed it, whereas the low performers got it correct. Other common reasons for negative discrimination include multiple correct answers, and distractors that are actually lesser known, special case situations. As with calculating item difficulty, calculating item discrimination can be accomplished through the application of simple mathematical skills.

The item discrimination is calculated (in a simplified manner) by completing the following steps:[6]

1. The instructor identifies the exams with the 10 highest scores and the 10 lowest scores.
2. For each question, the instructor records the number of students in the top group of 10 who answered the question correctly. The instructor does the same for the bottom group of 10 students.
3. The instructor then computes the discrimination index by subtracting the number of students in the bottom group who answered correctly from the number of students in the top group who answered correctly, and dividing by the number of students in each group (in this case 10). For example, if 8 student from the top group answered correctly, and 4 students from the bottom group answered correctly, the discrimination index would be 0.4.

The discrimination index will fall between −1.0 and +1.0. The closer the index is to +1.0, the more effectively the item distinguishes students who know the material (the top group) from those who do not (the bottom group).

all item types. The stem should be carefully considered to assess for length, ambiguity, and other possible sources for confusion. When evaluating multiple choice items, consideration should also be extended to examine the distractors. Ideally, incorrect responses should be spread across all possible distractors. The instructor should consider item discrimination and the proportion of each distractor chosen to determine next steps. Distractors that are never selected may not be plausible. If knowledgeable test takers are drawn to a particular distractor (shown by a low or negative discrimination), then that distractor may present a possibly correct answer—usually a special case that only advanced students would recognize. Test analysis software can analyze discrimination for each distractor, greatly easing the task of distractor analysis.[7]

It is important for the instructor to note that the item can have an appropriate difficulty level and discrimination index, but if it does not follow the principles of exam item development and construction, it may not be valid and should not be used.

Point Biserial Value

Some test-item analysis programs will report a *point biserial* value for each test item. This statistic is very similar to a discrimination index. However, rather than calculating an index of high overall performance to low overall performance, the point biserial value calculates the statistical correlation between an individual item and the overall score on the exam. Calculation of a correlation coefficient is beyond the scope of this text, but the value is returned by several test analysis programs. Like the item discrimination, the higher the point biserial, the better that item differentiates between those with high overall knowledge and those with low knowledge. Also like the item discrimination, this statistic tends to be low when an item is not very difficult. If an instructor has access to point biserial, it should be used in place of the item discrimination to select those items that require further editing.

Grading Strategies

Appropriate grading strategies are just as important to validity and reliability as the appropriate exam administration and exam content.

Grading Essays

Grading essays and written assignments can be particularly difficult. Because grading essays is inherently subjective, reliability is difficult to ensure. Some suggested strategies that help to improve reliability in the grading of essays are as follows:

- Skim all writing assignments quickly before grading them, to gain an overview of the general level of performance and the range of responses.[8]
- Before the writing assignment is given or the test is administered, the instructor should decide on guidelines for full or partial credit. This is referred to as the *analytic method of grading*. The instructor assigns a number of points to each designated content area. The instructor decides on partial credit for each area and totals the points for an easy grade calculation. It may be useful for the instructor to anchor these points to specific words, phrases, or concepts to help ensure reliability.[9]
- Develop a rubric for scoring essay items, including the characteristics of a correct response and the value of each parameter.[10]
- Choose examples of student responses to serve as anchors for different levels of performance. The instructor chooses one student response as an example of a good essay, one as an example of middle performance, and one as a poor example. This approach is referred to as the *global method* of grading. It is generally helpful for instructors to also compare responses with those on an "ideal" paper prepared before the assignment.[9] Instructors should note that this can be a normative grading scale (discussed in the next section) rather than the more common form of criterion-referenced examination in which performance is compared to an objective standard.
- Grade essay items question-by-question rather than student-by-student. This allows more meaningful comparison of responses between students. Instructors should shuffle the exams between questions to avoid bias in grading caused by student performance on the previous question.[8] Previous warnings about normative grading also apply to this strategy.
- Avoid judging assignments on the basis of extraneous factors such as illegible handwriting and the use of pen versus pencil. Judge essays on the intellectual quality of the response. Instructors must remember the purpose of the essay question when they are grading.[6]
- If possible, repeat the grading process a couple of days later. Another option is to use multiple graders. Agreement in grades across independent grading sessions supports reliability.[9]

CASE in Point

An instructor includes an essay item relating to the pathophysiology of shock on a module examination. Five points are assigned to the item. She constructs the following rubric to assist her in grading:

- (5 points) Clear description of hypovolemic, distributive, cardiogenic, and obstructive shock with at least two examples of conditions that would cause each
- (4 points) Clear descriptions but missing clearly relevant clinical conditions for some types
- (3 points) Descriptions lack clarity, missing key mechanisms of how perfusion is limited in that type of shock
- (2 points) Descriptions or examples provided for only three of the four types
- (1 point) Descriptions or examples provided for fewer than three of the four types

Norm-Referenced Grading

Normative grading (norm-referenced grading) strategies are those that compare student performance with the performance of other students for assignment of a grade. This is commonly referred to as "grading on the curve." The result of this strategy is that a set percentage of students receives an "A," a second group gets a "B," another group receives a "C," and some are given a "D" or an "F." Each student's grade is determined by the group's performance—not by comparison with objectives. This method of grading is commonly attacked because it is based on class performance rather than on comparison of performance with objectives. On the other hand, an advantage of normative grading strategies is that the grading strategy automatically compensates for poorly constructed examinations. If a test is very easy, the curve automatically shifts to require a higher passing score. If a test is very difficult, the passing score shifts lower to compensate. This occurs without additional calculation or analysis by the instructor. A number of variations of normative grading strategies include setting a percentage of students that will receive each grade, assigning grade levels based on natural breaks in the distribution, and assigning grade levels based on a normal statistical distribution. Although purely normative strategies are generally considered inappropriate for summative assessment in EMS courses, normative strategies are useful for assigning grades to formative assessments with minimal impact on final grade. Normative approaches, such as grading on the curve, may be useful as an interim method when using new items in formative assessments such as quizzes.

Criterion-Referenced Grading

Criterion-referenced grading strategies base grade assignment on mastery of course objectives. This approach requires the presence of relatively specific course objectives on which assessments can be based. According to a criterion-referenced strategy, the assessment is drawn from the blueprint, and setting grades is guided by the degree to which objectives are mastered. One example would be that 90% mastery is assigned an "A," 80% is assigned a "B," and so forth. This can be based on depth of mastery (90% knowledge of each objective) or breadth of mastery (complete knowledge of 90% of the objectives). A criterion-referenced strategy requires the use of valid and reliable items to ensure fairness in the assessment process. Because the setting of grades does not automatically adjust for difficulty, the instructor must perform additional analysis to set an appropriate passing score.

Setting a Cut Score

The **cut score** is the score required in order to pass a test; it is the passing score. In general, the instructor has two strategies from which to choose when determining the cut score. In the first, the instructor can build the assessments, analyze exam items, and set the passing score based on the difficulty of the exam. In the second, the instructor can first set a passing score, then analyze draft items and construct an examination with difficulty appropriate for the preset passing score. In other words, the instructor can either set the passing score to fit the exam or engineer the exam to fit the passing score. Either option is appropriate. It is inappropriate for students to consider a course with an 80% passing score harder than a course with a 60% passing score, without consideration of the relative difficulty of the examinations.

Many educational institutions set the grade levels and passing scores as part of institutional policy. This fits with a common expectation that 90% = A, 80% = B, 70% = C, 60% = D, and below 60% is failing. Another common expectation is that 70% is passing, with grades interspersed. If instructors are teaching with preset passing scores and grading levels, then they must construct examinations of appropriate difficulty to match this preset passing score. The instructor does this by predicting the difficulty level for each item and computing the average difficulty index for all items on the examination. The instructor can then adjust the examination to match the computed difficulty with the preset passing score.

Setting the Standard: The Angoff Method

An instructor can use a number of methods to predict item difficulty. The most common is the **Angoff method**. This method is commonly used for high-stakes examinations in educational, certification, and licensure settings. The procedure is to first establish a panel of experts. The panel considers the concept of the "minimally competent candidate," or, in other words, the minimum acceptable level of knowledge. This is not the ideal or average candidate, but the candidate who is barely acceptable. The experts are then asked to estimate the percentage of minimally competent candidates who would answer that item correctly. This is done first with practice items, where the experts' estimates can be compared with actual performance of the item. As the experts rate the items, the consensus that is reached by the experts' estimates forms the Angoff rating. By computing the mean of the Angoff ratings for all items to be included in the exam, the instructor can determine a cut score. Conversion of this predicted cut score into a passing score is a matter of professional judgment for the instructor.

CASE in Point

Setting a Cut Score

An instructor who is teaching a paramedic course at a community college is preparing a module examination for medical emergencies. After collecting and editing a number of examination items, the instructor prepares to predict the difficulty by using the Angoff method. The instructor plans to use the information to set an appropriate passing score.

The instructor contacts four preceptors and three lab assistants who will serve as the expert panel. She starts the process by initiating a discussion on the concept of entry-level competency. She describes the concept in this manner: "The idea is to describe the provider who is barely competent. Not a great paramedic, or even a good paramedic, but instead, the paramedic who has just the amount of knowledge to be considered competent." She asks panel members to describe in their own words the depth of knowledge required for entry-level competency related to medical emergencies. The discussion continues for a short time until the instructor believes that the panel has reached consensus on the concept.

Next, the instructor distributes a set of examination items that have been used for past courses and for which the actual difficulty level is known. The instructor projects the item, without the answer indicated, and asks the panel, "What percentage of entry-level providers would get this question correct?" After panel members have given their thoughts, she shares with the group the answer to the item. Panel members are then allowed to reconsider their rating. The instructor then shows the group how the item actually performed (the difficulty level of each item from previous administrations), and the results of each panel member are shown to the group. The panel has a short discussion on the difference between their estimates and the actual performance of the item. This exercise is repeated several times.

After reviewing these practice items, the instructor distributes the ones she will be using for the examination, without an answer key. Each panel member then rates each item as to the percentage of entry-level providers who would answer the item correctly. The answer key is then provided, and panel members are allowed to reconsider their estimate. The instructor collects and averages the results, as shown in **TABLE E**.

The panel of experts has recommended a cut score (minimum passing score) of 70% for this examination. The instructor takes this into consideration as she determines the passing score for the examination. She takes into account that during the practice session, the panel consistently predicted rates of correct responses that were slightly higher than the actual values (in other words, during the practice session, the panel slightly underestimated the difficulty of items). She also considers the potential for error and decides to set the cut score for this examination at 60%.

(Note: In this case, had the instructor been in an institution that mandated by policy a set passing score, the instructor could just as easily use this procedure to predict the item difficulty for each item, then could base item selection on the predicted difficulty to construct an examination of appropriate difficulty for the mandated minimum passing score.)

TABLE E Example of Expert Panel Ratings Used to Determine Cut Score

Item	Panel Member 1	Panel Member 2	Panel Member 3	Panel Member 4	Panel Member 5	Panel Member 6	Panel Member 7	Average
1	70%	80%	80%	80%	70%	80%	75%	76%
2	85%	80%	85%	90%	90%	85%	75%	84%
3	60%	75%	55%	60%	65%	55%	45%	59%
4	75%	70%	70%	80%	85%	65%	80%	75%
5	55%	50%	50%	80%	50%	45%	45%	54%
6	80%	90%	90%	85%	95%	90%	95%	89%
7	50%	50%	60%	70%	55%	50%	40%	54%
8	70%	80%	70%	75%	80%	70%	75%	74%
9	50%	40%	50%	50%	45%	50%	55%	49%
10	80%	80%	80%	80%	90%	85%	85%	83%
(etc.)								
Total (column average)	71%	69%	70%	76%	69%	69%	66%	**70%**

The Cut Score

The difficulty of the tests an institution uses makes the cut score meaningful. For instance, consider the following two training programs. Program A requires an 80% score to pass the final examination. Program B requires 60% to pass. Program A uses only examination items with an Angoff rating of at least 90%, with an average Angoff rating of 95%. Program B uses a range of Angoff scores from 40% to 90%, with the average Angoff rating of 60%. Program B is thus a much more challenging program, despite the lower cut score, because it uses much more difficult examinations.

Item-Response Theory

Instead of using a set minimum passing score, the NREMT determines whether a candidate passes the examination by directly assessing the difficulty of the items answered correctly by the candidate. Traditional examinations give all candidates a set number of items of comparable difficulty and compare performance of candidates by the percentage of items answered correctly. This approach is referred to as a *linear test* and uses classical test theory.

Computer-adaptive testing allows the use of a more precise tool called item-response theory (IRT). Using this approach, a large test bank is established with items of identified difficulty. IRT and the Angoff method are used to identify item difficulty. The computer adjusts the difficulty of items for the candidate based on the candidate's responses. If a hard item is missed, the next question is slightly easier. If an item is answered correctly, the next is slightly harder. And so on. Each question answered correctly is an indication of the candidate's ability. Once enough items are correctly answered to place the candidate's ability with certainty, the test ends. The more items that are answered, the less the error of measurement. The further the candidate's ability from the competency line, the more measurement error is allowable to determine with statistical certainty that the candidate is competent (or not competent). Therefore, candidates who are far above or below the competency line will have relatively few questions. Candidates who are near the competency line require many more items to accurately determine whether they meet minimum standards of competence.

For this reason, discussions of scores or test length for computer-adaptive examinations that use IRT are not meaningful.

Summary

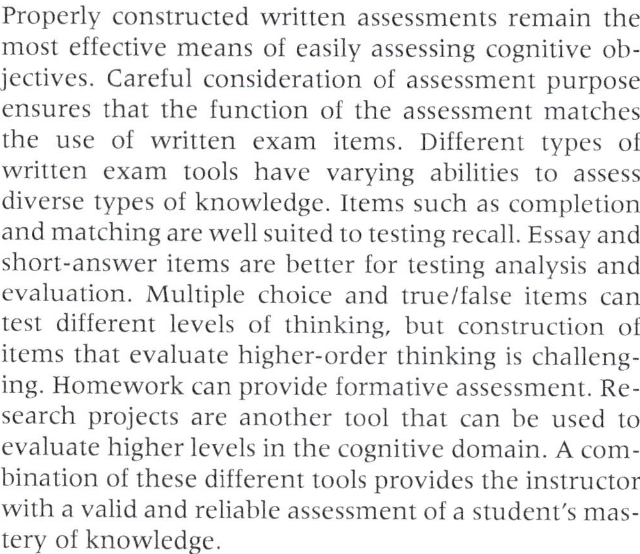

Properly constructed written assessments remain the most effective means of easily assessing cognitive objectives. Careful consideration of assessment purpose ensures that the function of the assessment matches the use of written exam items. Different types of written exam tools have varying abilities to assess diverse types of knowledge. Items such as completion and matching are well suited to testing recall. Essay and short-answer items are better for testing analysis and evaluation. Multiple choice and true/false items can test different levels of thinking, but construction of items that evaluate higher-order thinking is challenging. Homework can provide formative assessment. Research projects are another tool that can be used to evaluate higher levels in the cognitive domain. A combination of these different tools provides the instructor with a valid and reliable assessment of a student's mastery of knowledge.

Security of examination materials is important for limited response tools that prove to be valid and reliable assessments of higher levels within the cognitive domain. Security is not an issue for homework and project assignments, and it is less critical for essay items. Because of the extensive effort needed to properly construct and analyze limited response items, it is necessary that the security of these items be protected. If security is compromised, items that would otherwise test high-end knowledge become items that test only recall. In addition, compromises of examination security may dramatically change the difficulty level and discrimination index of the compromised items.

Limited response items are extremely valuable for the EMS instructor. Testing a large number of cognitive objectives with acceptable reliability and validity requires the use of many more limited response items than essay and short-answer items. This also serves to prepare EMS students for licensure examinations, which use limited response items almost exclusively. Unfortunately, these items become nearly worthless if security is compromised.

Glossary

Angoff method Expert group consensus process to assign item difficulty, in which the group considers the minimum level of acceptable knowledge, then estimates the percentage of minimally competent candidates who would answer the item correctly.

blueprinting Planning the exam to facilitate validity with appropriate level of required thinking, content depth, and breadth.

computer-adaptive testing Type of testing that is able to adjust the difficulty of items for the candidate based on the candidate's responses.

criterion-referenced grading Grading strategies that assign a grade based on mastery of course objectives.

cut score Score required to pass a test; the passing score.

difficulty level Percentage of students who answer each item correctly.

distractor Incorrect answer designed to be a plausible alternative to the correct answer.

item discrimination Degree to which a correct answer for a particular item is associated with high overall scores on the exam; this is essentially a test of reliability.

item-response theory (IRT) Strategy of measuring a test taker's underlying traits or abilities using performance on different test items, which enables computer-adaptive testing to measure ability much more efficiently than classic tests.

negative discrimination Index that indicates that students who scored well overall did worse on those particular questions than did students who did not score well overall.

normative grading (norm-referenced grading) Grading strategies that compare student performance with the performance of other students; grading on the curve.

proctoring Act of monitoring the test-taking environment; helps to ensure security of testing materials and to prevent cheating.

stem Part of the item that is first offered, which may be written as a question or as an incomplete statement.

References

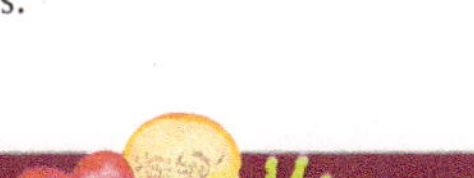

[1] Hertz, Norman R., and Roberta N. Chinn. 2000. *Licensure Examinations.* Lexington, KY: Council on Licensure, Enforcement, and Regulation.

[2] Margolis, Gregg S., Gabriel A. Romero, Antonio R. Fernandez, and Jonathan R. Studnek. 2009. "Strategies of High-Performing Paramedic Educational Programs." *Prehospital Emergency Care* 13: 505–11. https://doi.org/10.1080/10903120902993396.

[3] Oermann, Marilyn H., and Kathleen B. Gaberson. 2009. *Evaluation and Testing in Nursing Education,* 3rd ed. New York: Springer Publishing.

[4] National Council for State Boards of Nursing. 2018. "NCLEX & Other Exams: What the Exam Looks Like." Accessed December 29, 2018. https://www.ncsbn.org/9010.htm.

[5] Cantillon, Peter. 2010. *ABC of Learning and Teaching in Medicine.* Oxford, UK: John Wiley & Sons.

[6] Davis, Barbara G. 2001. *Tools for Teaching.* San Francisco: Jossey-Bass.

[7] Gierl, Mark J., Okan Bulut, Qi Guo, and Xinxin Zhang. 2017. "Developing, Analyzing, and Using Distractors for Multiple-Choice Tests in Education: A Comprehensive Review." *Review of Educational Research* 87, no. 6: 1082–116. https://doi.org/10.3102/0034654317726529.

[8] Jacobs, Lucy C., and Clinton L. Chase. 1992. *Developing and Using Tests Effectively: A Guide for Faculty.* San Francisco: Jossey-Bass.

[9] Cashin, William E. 1987. "Improving Essay Tests." *IDEA Paper* no. 17. Manhattan, KS: Kansas State University Center for Faculty Evaluation and Development.

[10] Johnson, Robert L., James A. Penny, and Belita Gordon. 2008. *Assessing Performance: Designing, Scoring, and Validating Performance Tasks.* New York: Guilford Press.

Additional Resources

Cantillon, Peter, William Irish, and David Sales. 2004. "Using Computers for Assessment in Medicine." *British Medical Journal* 329, no. 7466: 606–9. https://doi.org/10.1136/bmj.329.7466.606.

Case, Susan M., and David B. Swanson. 2001. *Constructing Written Test Questions for the Basic and Clinical Sciences,* 3rd ed. Philadelphia: National Board of Medical Examiners. Accessed March 1, 2019. https://www.nbme.org/pdf/itemwriting_2003/2003iwgwhole.pdf.

Clegg, Victoria L., and William E. Cashin. 1986. "Improving Multiple-Choice Tests." *IDEA Paper* no. 16. Manhattan, KS: Kansas State University Center for Faculty Evaluation and Development.

Frary, Robert B. 1995. *More Multiple-Choice Item Writing Do's and Don'ts.* Washington, DC: ERIC Clearinghouse on Assessment and Evaluation.

Haladyna, Thomas M., and Michael C. Rodriguez. 2013. *Developing and Validating Test Items.* New York: Routledge.

Royal, Kenneth, Marian-Wells Hedgpeth, Jamie Mulkey, and John Fremer. 2016. "The 10 Most Wanted Test Cheaters in Medical Education." *Medical Education* 50, no. 12: 1241–4. https://doi.org/10.1111/medu.13096.

Wendt, Anne, and Lorraine E. Kenny. 2009. "Alternate Item Types: Continuing the Quest for Authentic Testing." *The Journal of Nursing Education* 48, no. 3: 150–6. https://doi.org/10.3928/01484834-20090301-11.

Withers, Graeme. 2005. "Item Writing for Tests and Examinations." UNESCO International Institute for Educational Planning. Accessed March 1, 2019. https://unesdoc.unesco.org/ark:/48223/pf0000214552.

CHAPTER 22

Other Assessment Tools

OBJECTIVES

At the conclusion of this chapter, the educator will be able to:

Cognitive Domain

1. Describe how to assess elements of multiple intelligences during simulation.
2. List principles of constructing a sound oral examination.
3. Distinguish between skills assessment and situational assessment.
4. Outline the process to develop an effective performance checklist for a psychomotor assessment.
5. Describe best practices for developing and conducting an objective structured clinical examination (OSCE).
6. List strategies to improve reliability and validity of performance examinations.
7. Describe how to construct and use rubrics for affective domain assessment.
8. Outline the benefits of using a portfolio to assess student progress.
9. List advantages and disadvantages of global rating scales and other tools to assess student clinical performance.

Psychomotor Domain

There are no psychomotor objectives for this chapter.

Affective Domain

1. Value the need to assess the psychomotor domain using valid and reliable techniques.
2. Integrate sound tools for affective assessment within the curriculum.

"There are no mistakes, save one: the failure to learn from a mistake."

~ Robert Fripp

CHAPTER GOAL This chapter explores the use of oral examinations, practical examinations, attitudinal assessments, portfolios, and assessment of student performance in the setting of actual patient care during clinical and field internships.

Selection of the appropriate assessment is guided by the domain of learning that is described by the objective. Written assessments were discussed in the previous chapter; this chapter describes several other assessments appropriate for use by the emergency medical services (EMS) instructor.

The practice of prehospital emergency medical care requires more than knowledge. Psychomotor skills and appropriate behaviors and attitudes are also essential if EMS students are to successfully perform. In addition to written examinations, other assessments are needed to properly evaluate student performance.

Varied Types of Assessment

Different students exhibit preferences for different learning styles. Learning styles are described in detail in Chapter 5, *Learning Styles: Concepts and Controversies*. Howard Gardner takes this observation further when he asserts that different students actually have different levels of intelligence in various areas, a theory known as *multiple intelligences*."[1,2] Gardner describes the areas of intelligence as verbal/linguistic, logical/mathematical, visual/spatial, bodily/kinesthetic, musical/rhythmic, interpersonal/intrapersonal, and naturalistic.[3] (This is discussed further in Chapter 3, *Brain-Based Learning*.) Assessments can be administered in different ways to allow students to express their mastery of objectives in a manner that is comfortable for them.

An important part of examination validity is standardization so that test takers have a fair and unbiased opportunity to demonstrate their knowledge, skills, and abilities. Although learning preferences may have an impact on the assessment of knowledge, skills, and abilities, studies have not shown this. Empirical studies have failed to demonstrate the impact of learning preferences on comprehension or assessment.[4,5]

Written tests strongly favor those students with preferences and abilities in the verbal and logical areas. Similarly, kinesthetic learners may favor the use of performance examinations. Many instructors describe situations in which the student who does poorly on written tests actually performs very well in the field. Allowing some assessments to vary significantly in form of presentation according to student preference is desirable. This provides the effective instructor with another view of the student's acquisition of new knowledge, skills, and abilities.[6]

Additionally, using various methods of assessment helps to ensure that all needed competencies are verified. In a review of different methods to assess competency in medical evaluation, Gaur and Skochelak noted: "These studies suggest that there is no single standard with which to evaluate medical students and the results of curricular innovations in medicine. None of these tests can be discounted, however, as each may measure a different parameter of competence." Where assessments agree, we can be sure that the student has mastered a broad range of abilities. Where assessments disagree, the students' strengths in different skills become evident.[7]

Assessing All Domains of Learning

Bloom's taxonomy describes learning as divided into three domains: cognitive, psychomotor, and affective. Bloom's taxonomy is described in detail in Chapter 8, *Domains of Learning*. While lacking in empirical evidence,[8] most instructors are familiar with Bloom's taxonomy and it remains a useful model. Knowledge (the cognitive domain) is routinely assessed through written examinations and writing assignments in a variety of educational settings, including the EMS classroom. (See Chapter 21, *Written Assessment*, for further discussion.) The psychomotor domain, or practical skills, is better evaluated by observing the student performance of skills in a controlled environment. Attitudes and behaviors (the affective domain) are dependent on the context. Therefore, assessment of the affective domain is best done over time and in the applied setting. Attempting to evaluate the psychomotor domain through the use of a written examination is ineffective.

Many of the tools described in this chapter require that multiple instructors be involved in performing evaluations. Effective assessments of student performance across the domains of learning require more than a single instructor; they require a system. This does not mean that instructors who teach courses individually cannot perform meaningful assessments, but individual class instructors must work together to create tools for evaluation. When the instructor works with the support of others to construct, use, and analyze assessments within a system, quality assessment is possible. A study of high-performing paramedic education programs clarified the need for systems of assessment. Focus groups conducted among programs with several years of high first-time pass rates on national certification examinations emphasized the need to "provide students with frequent, detailed feedback regarding their performance" in "all aspects of the program (classroom, laboratory, clinical, and field) and in all domains (cognitive, psychomotor, and affective)."[9]

Oral Examinations

Oral examinations are assessments in which the questions and answers are given verbally in an exchange between a student and an instructor or group of instructors. Oral examinations are used to assess the cognitive domain and can extend to the affective domain. They may be used to gain insight through the speed and confidence of response, although the reliability of this assessment is highly variable. The oral exam can assess the student's thought process and the thinking behind a particular answer. Oral examinations are similar in purpose to essay questions. Oral exams have the advantage of allowing assessment by a group of instructors simultaneously. Another advantage is that, unlike essay questions, responding to oral questions does not require a high degree of compositional skill. Consequently, oral examinations can more closely approximate the expectations of the entry-level EMS professional in the job market.

For an oral exam to be fairly administered, a great deal of concentration is required by the student and the examiners. Any unexpected distractions can affect the test and may have a disparate impact on the student who is being examined when the distraction occurs. Instructors conducting an oral examination must exert strong control over the environment to minimize the potential for such distractions. This extends to ensuring that students and examiners minimize the potential for disturbance by having everyone turn off electronic devices. Additionally, the scheduling of examiners can present difficulties in that they may be expected to evaluate a large number of candidates with little opportunity for breaks. This can lead to uneven assessment over time. Another potential problem is the identification of trends, leading to unfair emphasis on those who repeat mistakes made by previously examined students. For example, early in the day, the instructor who is testing may consider a mistake somewhat minor. However, as subsequent students repeat a seemingly minor mistake, it may take on greater significance as an error to the examiner, and expectations may change over the day.

Oral exam items should be blueprinted, drafted, and edited in a similar manner as written essay questions. Oral exam items should be scripted and clear instructions given to the examiners to minimize any variation from the script. Without scripting, oral examinations are impossible to standardize. Examiners must be cognizant of any clues they might inadvertently give to candidates, such as body language, comments, or gestures. By nature, grading of oral examinations is subjective. Ensuring reliability of scoring is a clear challenge. Two or more examiners with independent scoring are needed to assess and ensure reliability. These scores are later combined into a single composite grade.[10]

Clear behavioral anchors help to minimize subjectivity. It is helpful to use a rubric to aid with grading oral examinations. More information on the construction and use of rubrics is contained later in this chapter.

Oral examinations are time consuming and labor intensive. Efforts to address the disadvantages of being able to examine only one student at a time are countered by concerns about reliability. Running parallel stations with different examiners, although more efficient, would have a negative impact on exam reliability. Nonetheless, oral examination remains a valuable tool for use in a comprehensive assessment strategy.

Practical Examinations

Practical skills assessment is conducted through the use of two major types of examination: the simple skills examination and the situational assessment (**FIGURE 22.1**).

Assessment of a rote mechanical skill is conducted through a simple **task analysis**. This is the easiest skills examination to administer. Simple skills examinations test at middle levels of the psychomotor domain, such as precision, and do not provide significant context for the skills. Situational assessment requires more elaborate simulation and is capable of assessing higher levels within the psychomotor domain, such as articulation, and elements of the cognitive and affective domains. For more information on setting up scenarios or simulations, see Chapter 18, *Tools for Simulation*.

Skills Evaluation

When a skills evaluation is conducted, the skill is first defined and the expected degree of proficiency is determined. Checklists may be available for some skills, such as National Registry Practical Skills Examination sheets

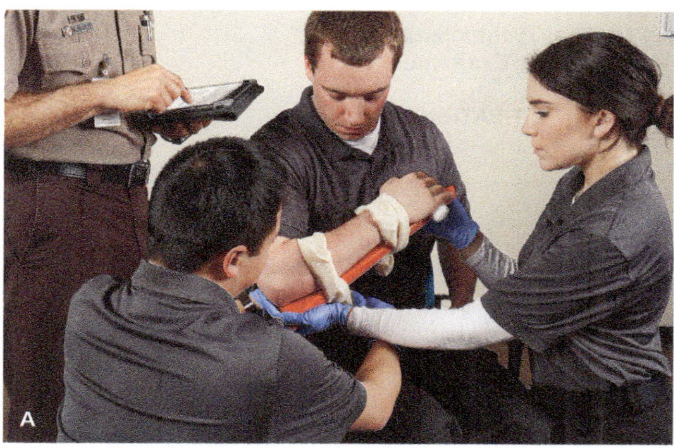
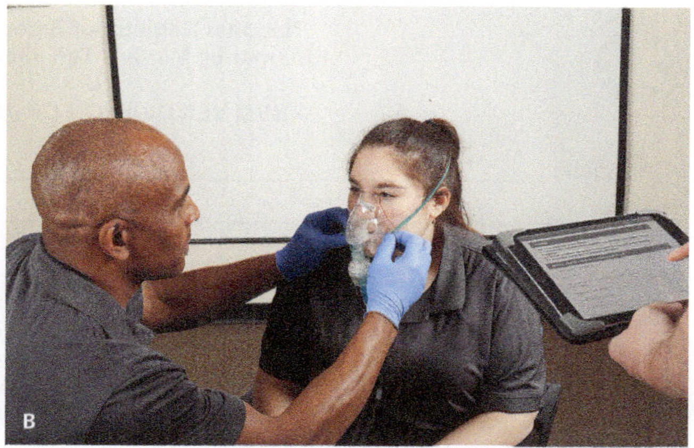

FIGURE 22.1 Practical skills evaluation includes the simple isolated skills exam (**A**) and the situational assessment that evaluates all three domains of learning (**B**).

and commercially available products (**FIGURE 22.2**). Just as written examination materials require review and revision prior to effective use, so do skills checklists. A performance checklist is developed from a task analysis, which provides a list of the steps to be performed. Each step should include objective criteria, so that different examiners can agree on the criteria for successful completion of the step. It is usually best for instructors to keep the number of steps on the checklist to a minimum. This reduces errors in assessment by allowing the examiner to observe the task as it is performed. The checklist should prioritize steps and list them in sequence. Critical steps can be identified, and important aspects should be weighted appropriately. Failure to properly perform any critical step may result in failure of the exam. Whenever possible, the examiner should avoid qualifying or writing out the behavior; instead, the examiner should use the checklist to indicate whether a step was performed or not. The checklist should also provide any information that the examiner would need to give to the candidate. The more closely the examiner sticks to the script, the more reliable the evaluation is likely to be with various students and examiners.

Checklists should use **dichotomous scoring**, in which the observable action is either performed or not, to the greatest extent possible. **Polytomous scoring**, in which the examiner chooses a number of points indicating how well the step was performed, is frequently less reliable and more difficult to standardize.

Identification of critical criteria with high scoring impact can complicate the assessment of skills performance. Critical criteria that automatically result in failure of the entire station are sometimes referred to as "trapdoor scoring." If this is used, a single omission (such as verbalizing standard precautions) may present a scoring impact out of proportion to the error (such as an automatic failure). These should be included with caution to ensure the impact is proportional to the error. Additionally, elements of judgment by the skills examiner (such as "failure to manage the patient as a competent EMT") present variations in scoring by the examiner. This may prove a challenge to assess, monitor, and administer in a valid and reliable manner. Care must be exercised by the instructor in subjective elements included as critical criteria. Independent review by an additional examiner of recorded performance is one way to manage this variation in scoring (see section, *Interrater Reliability*).

To assess performance at the precision level of skills acquisition, context need not be provided and simple skills examinations can be used. Before the skill is tested in context, it is appropriate for the instructor to conduct simple skills evaluations to ensure that the student can perform the skill perfectly in isolation. Testing in context is done through the use of situational assessments. Situational assessments present the student with simulated scenarios; instructors assess the responses and judgments of the candidates in these specific situations. Situational assessments are more difficult to develop and deliver than are simple skills examinations. It is important that the situation and responses be simulated as accurately as possible.

The use of a standardized patient (also known as a programmed patient) is useful in conducting situational assessments. A *standardized patient* is an actor who plays the part of the patient. (See Chapter 18, *Tools for Simulation*.) Standardized patients are provided with descriptions of what responses they should give

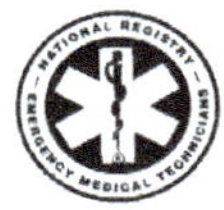

National Registry of Emergency Medical Technicians®
Emergency Medical Technician Psychomotor Examination

BVM VENTILATION OF AN APNEIC ADULT PATIENT

Candidate: ______________________ Examiner: ______________________

Date: ______________________ Signature: ______________________

Actual Time Started: __________	**Possible Points**	**Points Awarded**
Takes or verbalizes appropriate PPE precautions	1	
Checks responsiveness	1	
Requests additional EMS assistance	1	
Checks breathing and pulse simultaneously	1	
NOTE: After checking responsiveness, then checking breathing and pulse for no more than 10 seconds, examiner informs candidate, "The patient is unresponsive, apneic and has a weak pulse of 60."		
Opens airway properly	1	
NOTE: The examiner must now inform the candidate, "The mouth is full of secretions and vomitus."		
Prepares rigid suction catheter	1	
Turns on power to suction device or retrieves manual suction device	1	
Inserts rigid suction catheter without applying suction	1	
Suctions the mouth and oropharynx	1	
NOTE: The examiner must now inform the candidate, "The mouth and oropharynx are clear."		
Opens the airway manually	1	
Inserts oropharyngeal airway	1	
NOTE: The examiner must now inform the candidate, "No gag reflex is present and the patient accepts the airway adjunct."		
Ventilates the patient immediately using a BVM device unattached to oxygen [Award this point if candidate elects to ventilate initially with BVM attached to reservoir and oxygen so long as first ventilation is delivered within 30 seconds.]	1	
NOTE: The examiner must now inform the candidate that ventilation is being properly performed without difficulty.		
Re-checks pulse for no more than 10 seconds	1	
Attaches the BVM assembly [mask, bag, reservoir] to oxygen [15 L/minute]	1	
Ventilates the patient adequately -Proper volume to cause visible chest rise (1 point) -Proper rate [10 – 12/minute (1 ventilation every 5 – 6 seconds)] (1 point)	2	
Note: The examiner must now ask the candidate, "How would you know if you are delivering appropriate volumes with each ventilation?"		
Actual Time Ended: __________ **TOTAL**	16	

CRITICAL CRITERIA

____ After suctioning the patient, failure to initiate ventilations within 30 seconds or interrupts ventilations for greater than 30 seconds at any time
____ Failure to take or verbalize appropriate PPE precautions
____ Failure to suction airway **before** ventilating the patient
____ Suctions the patient for an excessive and prolonged time
____ Failure to check responsiveness, then check breathing and pulse simultaneously for no more than 10 seconds
____ Failure to voice and ultimately provide high oxygen concentration [at least 85%]
____ Failure to ventilate the patient at a rate of 10 – 12/minute (1 ventilation every 5 – 6 seconds)
____ Failure to provide adequate volumes per breath [maximum 2 errors/minute permissible]
____ Insertion or use of any adjunct in a manner dangerous to the patient
____ Failure to manage the patient as a competent EMT
____ Exhibits unacceptable affect with patient or other personnel
____ Uses or orders a dangerous or inappropriate intervention

You must factually document your rationale for checking any of the above critical items on the reverse side of this form.

FIGURE 22.2 The National Registry of Emergency Medical Technicians (NREMT) *BVM Ventilation of an Apneic Adult Patient* skill sheet is an example of a skills checklist.

Objective Structured Clinical Examination[11]

One tool that is commonly used in medical education is the objective structured clinical examination (OSCE). The OSCE is a combination of a situational assessment and a subsequent oral (or written) examination. Students are exposed to a scripted clinical situation. For instance, students could encounter a situation in which a history is provided and they are told to assess the patient. Examiners use a standard checklist to record which assessments were conducted. Each student is then given an oral or written examination regarding different elements of the scenario. Because the interaction is scripted and later questions standardized, cueing by instructors is minimized. Reliability increases with scripting and the use of objective criteria.

to candidates when patient assessment is conducted. *Moulage* is the simulation of injuries with the use of makeup and special effects. Additional actors may be used to play the part of family members and bystanders. The environment of the situation should be as realistic as possible. This may require that simulations be conducted in office areas, restrooms, and outdoors rather than in the typical classroom.

A common problem with skills assessments (both simple skills assessments and situational assessments) is the tendency for examiners to allow candidates to verbalize elements of the skill. This can occur for a variety of reasons, including lack of appropriate equipment for the candidates to use. When candidates are allowed to verbalize components of a skills evaluation, validity is destroyed by the conversion of what would have assessed the psychomotor domain into a cognitive examination. This problem can magnify when the student internalizes these classroom shortcuts into actual performance that is later reflected in actual practice.

Another frequent issue is the consistency of administration of the examination. Unless carefully controlled, each scenario is likely to be presented in slightly different ways, leading to problems with reliability. This is countered by the careful attention of examiners in presenting information consistently. An instructor can help to improve reliability by providing a script to examiners and insisting on compliance with the script.

Maintaining consistency of the administration of an examination is but one part of maintaining reliability. The cautions in the earlier section on oral examinations apply to performance examinations as well. Rater bias, either conscious or unconscious, can influence ratings. Unexpected distractions influence both ratings and student performance. Scheduling and sequencing of the students can introduce elements that cause ratings from a single rater to vary over time. This inconsistency in scoring over time from a single rater is sometimes referred to as *intra-rater reliability*. Complex scenarios and scoring tools may complicate this by challenging mental workloads.[12–14] Avoiding unnecessary complexity and monitoring reliability over time is an important step. Additional considerations are needed for managing reliability among multiple raters.

Interrater Reliability

Assessing interrater reliability is an important part of ensuring reliable examination scores. Maintaining interrater reliability is a significant challenge with practical examinations. A well-constructed performance checklist can help reduce problems by not allowing examiners to qualify observations; instead, they must report and record whether a step was performed according to established criteria. Even with excellent checklists, reliability is invariably a problem when a single examiner observes the student's performance. A panel of examiners can address reliability concerns, but presents challenges when examiners disagree. Some instructors have used multiple iterations for a set type of skills being evaluated (e.g., successfully managing four of five trauma scenarios, each assessed by a different examiner).[15] However, this technique does not fully address interrater reliability because each student performance is unique and scenarios usually vary. More than one examiner observing performance is needed to fully measure and ensure interrater reliability. A third technique for improving interrater reliability is to use a norming process to make sure evaluators are assessing performance in the same manner. In a norming process, multiple evaluators grade the same performance and compare evaluations in order to minimize differences. While not adjusting the test, adding video or audio recording of performance can help to ensure reliability by introducing a mechanism that allows for later review of performance to ensure fair grading, although different angles of video recording are necessary to fully capture the interaction.

It is critically important to train examiners. Examiner training will help to clarify the key points of the assessment and emphasize the importance of standardized presentation. Instructors should provide familiarization to the scenarios and check sheets as a part of examiner training.

High-Fidelity Simulations

Extremely realistic situational assessments (also known as *high-fidelity simulations*) have the capability of assessing all three domains of learning in context. As such, these types of assessments are powerful tools for verifying mastery of objectives. These assessments present a rare opportunity for the instructor to evaluate the student's integration of needed knowledge, skills, and attitudes. Many courses use these assessments as a component of summative evaluations.

Impact of Scenarios on Skills Performance

The scenario used for a situational assessment is a key component for assessment and improvement by the instructor. The scenario contains many points of information on which the student will base decisions. Modification of the scenario may lead students to different decisions and judgments. As a result, the instructor should critically evaluate and modify scenarios to ensure a valid and reliable situational assessment. This may include modifying vital signs for a clearer presentation, eliminating confounding variables, or changing the scripts for standardized patients to present a clearer clinical picture. Just as modifying the stem of a multiple choice item can improve a written examination, modifying the scenario parameters of a situational assessment can improve reliability and validity.

Reliability and Validity of Performance Examinations

As noted in examples provided, conducting valid and reliable performance examinations of skills and abilities is extremely difficult. Consistency of administration, independence of examiners, and interrater reliability are unavoidable challenges. Valid and reliable assessment tools such as check sheets are difficult to construct. Emergency care scenarios present many different variations—which are very difficult to control. Nonetheless, assessment of skills and abilities is clearly necessary to evaluate the readiness and competency of EMS professionals.

As with any assessment of uncertain reliability, one method available to the instructor is to reduce the stakes of a single assessment. Allowing retests and grouping assessments are simple ways to reduce the stakes of a single assessment while providing important evaluation of performance. Consistency of results across multiple forms of assessment helps to increase the confidence in the examinations.

Another important note is that different skills and scenarios have differing difficulties. Ensuring that students have the same probability of success, which is an important part of fair examination, is known as **equating**. Equating procedures used to control for differing difficulties among performance examinations is beyond the scope of this text. To avoid this difficult process, instructors should ensure consistent use of scenarios, rather than using a random selection, which can lead to some students receiving easier scenarios than others.

Affective Evaluations

Assessing the affective domain can be challenging for instructors; however, it is an important component of student assessment. The National EMS Education Standards state that students should be evaluated in all domains, including the affective domain. Some high performing programs allocate one third of the final grade to achieving the affective objectives.

There are several ways to incorporate assessment of the affective domain into classroom assessments. For example, written examinations can incorporate items on therapeutic communications. Situational assessments can include interactions with patients and family members, such as notification of a death. Scenarios can include emergencies with behavioral components, such as psychological presentations. Classroom exercises can include role-play interactions that reinforce professional communications.

Rubrics

A useful tool for affective assessments is the **rubric**. Rubrics are helpful assessment tools anytime there are multiple facets to the evaluation, because each component part can be broken down. In addition to student affective evaluations, rubrics can facilitate the assessment of presentations, oral examinations, or scenarios. The rubric converts a list of characteristics into a graded set of observable criteria to be completed by the examiner. Construction of the rubric consists of first identifying the characteristics to be evaluated. For instance, the following characteristics have been drawn from the 2009 National Emergency Medical Services Education Standards:[16] integrity, empathy, self-motivation, appearance/personal hygiene, self-confidence, communications, time management, teamwork/diplomacy, respect, patient advocacy, and careful delivery

TEACHING TIP

A common rating system is 0 = unacceptable, 1 = acceptable, and 2 = excellent. An alternative is to simply indicate that performance meets or does not meet the stated objective.

TEACHING TIP

To prevent clustering of scores at the middle value of a rating system, the instructor can use an even number of choices.

of service. A rating scale is then selected. A common rating system is 5 = excellent, 4 = above average, 3 = average, 2 = below average, and 1 = unacceptable. A National Academy of Sciences review found: "The weight of evidence suggests that the reliability of ratings drops if there are fewer than three, or more than nine, rating categories. Recent work indicates that there is little to be gained from having more than five response categories. Within that range (three to five), there is no evidence that there is one best number of scale points in terms of scale quality."[17]

When the rubric is completed, observable behaviors are provided for each level of performance. The 2002 National Guidelines for Educating EMS Instructors[18] provides a rubric for the characteristic of appearance/personal hygiene (**TABLE 22.1**). The rubric can be completed by a number of evaluators. By providing relatively detailed descriptions of affective characteristics, different evaluators can conduct assessments with some degree of interrater reliability. These tools should be provided to the student at or near the beginning of the course. Rubrics can be used for formative evaluation, and they provide valuable feedback to the student. Concrete examples of unacceptable conduct should be provided to the student. Because affective behaviors are situation dependent, these examples should provide as much context as possible. When the discussion is framed in terms of observable behaviors rather than vaguely worded "attitudes," student resistance to feedback can be minimized. The more concrete and objective the feedback, the better it will be received. For instance, challenging a student that "he is sloppy" is likely to produce a defensive reaction from the student that the evaluation is an opinion. On the other hand, noting three dates in which the student reported to a clinical site unshaven with a wrinkled uniform is more likely perceived as a clear standard instead of a personal opinion. In some cases, the instructor may also wish to have students fill out rubrics on each other and themselves, a technique known as **360-degree evaluation**. This is particularly valuable when group projects are assigned to class members. Group members can provide valuable feedback to each other regarding teamwork skills. Of course, summative assessments of affective characteristics should also be conducted. The same rubrics can serve as summative tools.

Rubrics can be converted to surveys that the student can use for self-assessment. Self-assessment is a useful formative strategy. Affective assessments should be completed by the lead instructor and can also be completed by secondary and lab instructors who spend appreciable amounts of time with the student. The instructor who uses these affective rubrics in the clinical setting and internship can assess the degree to which a particular behavior is consistently exhibited in the applied-care setting. These assessments provide valuable feedback to the student and can be significant

TABLE 22.1 Sample Rubric

Point Value	Criteria
1	Inappropriate uniform or clothing worn to class or clinical settings. Poor hygiene or grooming.
2	Appropriate clothing or uniform selected most of the time, but the uniform may be unkempt (wrinkled), mildly soiled, or in need of minor repairs; appropriate personal hygiene is common, but occasionally, the individual is unkempt or disheveled.
3	Clothing and uniform are appropriate, neat, clean, and well maintained; good personal hygiene and grooming.
4	Clothing and uniform are above average. Uniform is pressed, and business casual is chosen when uniform is not worn. Grooming and hygiene are good or above average.
5	Uniform is always above average. Nonuniform clothing is business-like. Grooming and hygiene are impeccable. Hair is worn in an appropriate manner for the environment, and student is free of excessive jewelry. Makeup and perfume or cologne usage is discreet and tasteful.

National Highway Traffic Safety Administration. 2002. "National Guidelines for Educating EMS Instructors." Accessed March 2, 2019. http://www.nhtsa.dot.gov/people/injury/EMS/Instructor/Tableofcontents.htm.

indicators of future behavior. A 2004 study of medical students found that records of unprofessional conduct in medical school were correlated with future disciplinary actions by a state medical boards.[19] Evidence of predictive validity such as this makes assessment of the affective domain a critical part of ensuring future professional conduct.

Impact on Grades

Converting rubric scores to grades is relatively easy. The degree of grade impact of affective evaluations is a matter of professional judgment for the instructor to decide. The following excerpt is from the 2015 CoAEMSP (Committee on Accreditation of Educational Programs for the Emergency Medical Services Professions) Interpretations of the CAAHEP (Commission on Accreditation of Allied Health Education Programs) Standards and Guidelines: "As important as the cognitive and psychomotor domains, the program must teach, monitor, and evaluate (i.e., grade) the attitudes and behaviors of the students, including interpersonal interactions."[20]

An acceptable affective evaluation should be required for each student to pass the class. Some programs will also use affective assessments as a part of course grades. The use of rubrics ensures a criterion-referenced strategy. Averaging scores from multiple evaluators may be useful to minimize bias of the rater. Content validity can be assessed through expert review, in a manner similar to written evaluations. Use of rubrics helps the instructor convert a subjective assessment of the affective domain, with poor reliability, to a more objective and reliable assessment. It is important to note that the student must achieve the minimum expected standard in each domain of competency. Ratings for poor behavior and excellent knowledge should not average into a passing grade, just as a student with excellent behavior and substandard knowledge should not pass.

Surveys

Another tool that is used to assess the affective domain is the completion of surveys by students. This tool is especially useful if the course is relatively short and the purpose of the assessment is to look for a change in behavior from precourse evaluation to postcourse evaluation. Surveys can be constructed as a series of statements for which students indicate the degree to which they agree with the statement. A Likert-rating scale is useful to indicate varying levels of agreement, for example, 5 = strongly agree, 4 = agree, 3 = neutral, 2 = disagree, and 1 = strongly disagree. By assessing the same objective with a number of different statements, the reliability of each statement can be measured through a variety of statistical tests, such as **Cronbach's alpha**. (See Chapter 20, *Assessing Learning*, for further explanation of reliability tests.) Surveys can also be used to assess the mastery of affective objectives related to the comfort level of the provider, such as "I am comfortable providing care for pediatric patients." Surveys are better than behavior-based rubrics for assessing objectives that relate to confidence and comfort level because abstract characteristics like confidence are not easily observed. Thus, for affective objectives that are easily translated into observable behaviors, the rubric is a preferred tool; student surveys are more accurate for assessing internal characteristics.

Projects with Varied Activities

Research projects were discussed in the previous chapter. A variation on the traditional research paper is the use of a portfolio project (which differs from a psychomotor skills competency portfolio, discussed in the next section). Portfolio projects are a collection of documents that provide evidence that the student has achieved the desired objectives. Grading strategies used for portfolios vary considerably, depending on the specific forms of presentation used. Grading intermediate steps provides important feedback and an opportunity to provide formative evaluation. Basing a portion of the grade on the results of the intermediate assessments is recommended. Guidelines for grading the written components are provided in the previous chapter. Other formats for presentation of information should have separate grading criteria. In grading written work, it is important to look past the writing style to evaluate the content. Similarly, in assessing other formats, it is important to look past the stylistic elements to assess the content of the presentation. It is helpful to use rubrics to assess alternative presentation formats. Instead of trying to create brand new rubrics, the instructor can modify rubrics through commonly available sources such as RubiStar.[21] Building the rubric with the student or group helps to ensure that the grading criteria are well known to the student. The student can then use the rubrics as a self-assessment tool when working through the final stages of the project. If students are working together in a group to complete the project, the instructor should assess the interpersonal skills used. This can be done with the use of rubrics constructed for this purpose. The instructor who directly observes the group working together can assess teamwork. A combination of self-assessment and 360-degree evaluation can also be used.

CASE in Point

An EMS instructor is tasked with designing a summative affective assessment for paramedic students. The list of characteristics is drawn from the National Emergency Medical Services Education standards list of characteristics of professionalism in the clinical behavior/judgment section. The instructor then consults the interpretation of program accreditation standards, and notes that there should be at least one comprehensive affective assessment for each student, separate from affective components of clinical/field assessments. Keeping this in mind, the instructor decides to use a three-point rating system, with categories of "unacceptable," "average," and "exemplary." In the interest of including advisory committee members in the process, the instructor schedules a meeting for the representatives of EMS services and hospitals on the advisory committee to anchor the rating system with observable behaviors.

The instructor begins the meeting by leading a discussion of the list of characteristics to develop consensus on the specific affective objectives to be assessed. She follows with a discussion of the rating levels, describing the following elements:

- "Unacceptable" as needing improvement before a student can successfully complete the program
- "Average" as the minimum level required for entry-level competency
- "Exemplary" as performance that makes the student a role model for that affective characteristic

The instructor begins with the area of integrity. The instructor starts by discussing the average category, minimum entry-level competency. She reminds everyone that this is the same level used for standard setting for a written exam. The instructor asks the group what behaviors or examples they can cite for students they believe are in this category. Working on a whiteboard, she consolidates these ideas into a few statements of observable behaviors. The group works to achieve consensus on that list. As the group works, they realize that several had slightly different ideas of how integrity applied to EMS. The list of observable behaviors created a shared, common understanding of how to apply the imprecise concept of integrity to the specific actions of the EMS student.

Working from the discussion of minimum acceptable competency, the instructor leads the group to describe characteristics for the unacceptable category. They recognize that most statements would be less than the average category in terms of degree or consistency of behavior. For instance, the minimum standard included the statement: "always tells the truth." The group then developed "sometimes doesn't tell the truth" as a less consistent performance in the same area. Some concepts are expressed only in the unacceptable category. For example, cheating was described by the group as unacceptable, even though that concept was not expressly listed in the minimum acceptable statements.

The instructor leads the group next on clarifying the behavioral anchors for the exemplary category. The group struggles with this for the subject of integrity. They tend to view integrity in terms of acceptable or unacceptable, with little ability for students to excel. After some discussion, they identify a few behaviors that illustrate exemplary conduct. As an example, the group identified courage to directly and appropriately challenge other students' poor behavior as a description of excellent conduct within the area of integrity.

The group then moves on to the next characteristic on the list and repeats the previous steps.

Portfolio projects can be used to evaluate different domains and appeal to different learning preferences. Portfolios take time for the student to complete, as components are usually developed over the duration of the course. This allows the project to serve both as a learning tool and as an evaluation tool. These projects can be a challenge for the instructor to grade, and rubrics may have to be created for each of the styles of presentation. Fortunately, generic rubrics are available. Typically, generic rubrics are designed for teachers in elementary and secondary schools; they may require some degree of modification by the EMS instructor.

Competency Portfolios

Beginning in 2009, paramedic education programs across the United States joined in a coordinated project to document psychomotor competency through a body of evidence. This body of evidence was known as a **competency portfolio**, rather than single skills attempts or a single summative exam. The group was convened by the National Registry of EMTs (NREMT), which was exploring a more effective method to demonstrate consistent skills proficiency than with a single skills exam. The concept in that initial group, and subsequently with additional programs, included (1) setting a minimum number of practice attempts for students in the laboratory setting; (2) having a **preceptor** evaluate those same skills in the hospital setting on real patients; and (3) field preceptor evaluation of the skills.

Documentation of the skills competency portfolio became a requirement for candidates to qualify for National Registry paramedic certification examination in 2017. The skills proficiency tools are provided to programs without cost and are available at www.NAEMSE.org on the *Trading Post* or on the National Registry website.

Components and Process

The laboratory component of the package includes 33 formative evaluation instruments that detail the skills to assist in learning. Peers are used to assist in the development of skills proficiency, allowing for more practice time in lab. Once proficient, as evaluated by an instructor in the discrete skills such as comprehensive adult physical assessment, intravenous (IV) therapy, or IV bolus medication administration, students move into a scenario phase where they begin to demonstrate competency in those same skills integrated within the context of a simulated patient situation. This is where the more complex responsibilities of patient assessment and management, along with the ability to correctly execute the individual skills, are learned. Scenario lab instruments include Team Leader and Team Member evaluation sheets, and students are evaluated by peers and instructors. The next progression of the portfolio package is demonstration of skills in the clinical setting on real patients and evaluated by a preceptor. The skills include clinical evaluation instruments for skills, such as medication administration, blood glucose measurement, and 12-lead ECG acquisition, and also include an "impression/differential diagnosis" section and a "treatment plan" section to facilitate discussion of these areas and development of clinical judgment. Students must interact with the patients and perform the skills.

The final component of the portfolio package is the field internship setting, with actual patients and with preceptor supervision and feedback. Preceptors who are trained in methods of evaluation and the specific internship tool are utilized to guide student practice and evaluate the student in all domains.

Advantages of Competency Portfolios

Documentation of competency through use of a competency portfolio presents significant advantages over a single summative examination. The portfolio can document proficiency through the combination of formative and summative assessments. Many skills are applied in scenarios that present differing complications and difficulties, such as successful IV cannulation in which difficulty varies widely between patients. A portfolio can document the body of evidence over many situations rather than a single examination of that skill.

Additionally, skills are learned and demonstrated over time. Often, student performance declines slightly at the beginning of each new phase of portfolio documentation. The goal of the portfolio package, however, is to document the development of proficiency over time, so variations in performance level are expected.

Documentation of skills acquisition can show the mastery of that skill. One tool used to assess skills proficiency is the "eureka point." While early attempts at a skill frequently show inconsistent success, a student who has mastered the skill shows consistent successful performance.

Portfolios are useful as a supplement to summative examinations, particularly for component skills used in patient management. Portfolios for component skills can replace skills stations and allow summative examinations to assess integrated scenario management and clinical judgment rather than rote skills performance. When programs can demonstrate a completed portfolio that documents multiple iterations of each skill and patient-management situation by multiple evaluators, including peer and faculty evaluators, over a sustained period of time, a final summative examination may not be necessary for program completion. The ability to do this may be limited by accreditation and state requirements.

Documentation of competency portfolios can be assisted by the use of databases of student skills performance in laboratory and clinical settings. Instructors can then monitor skills performance throughout the educational experience to ensure skills acquisition, retention, and competency.

As mentioned earlier, competency portfolios for EMS are now required for paramedic national certification examinations; they are also required for paramedic education program accreditation. As practice analyses and examination strategies evolve, the use of portfolios to document skills competency is likely to be a useful tool for assessment of student performance in the psychomotor domain.

Applied Care Evaluation

The primary goal of an EMS educational program is to prepare graduates to function competently as EMS providers. It is impossible for the instructor to fully simulate the environment and conditions of a medical emergency. Therefore, some degree of assessment in the actual setting in which care is being provided is necessary. Instructors must supervise the experience because the student's competency is not fully determined at this early stage. Assessing the student in the hospital and field environment is difficult. Among the challenges are maintaining appropriate patient care during the evaluation experience, ensuring reliability of the assessments, and working with a team of preceptors. Appropriately assessing student performance in the applied care environment requires well-constructed instruments that match the clinical experience to the objectives, a team of high-quality preceptors, and a systematic approach by the lead instructor.

Global Rating Scales

The most commonly used tool for assessing student performance in the clinical setting is a set of global ratings of performance. When this tool is used, a set of characteristics are listed, along with a Likert-type scale for each (**FIGURE 22.3**). In some cases, a short description is provided for each rating.

Global ratings are easy for the preceptor to complete. They can be constructed and completed quickly. The major difficulty with global rating scales is that without extensive training and continuous reminders, interrater reliability is impossible. Many instructors compensate for this lack of reliability by requiring that a large number of ratings be performed by multiple preceptors. Other instructors bolster reliability by providing detailed descriptions for each rating, effectively converting the global rating tool into a rubric.

Standardized global rating scales can be useful. Tavares et al discuss the development and evaluation of GRS, a global rating scale used in the assessment of Canadian paramedics.[22] Standardized tools with published performance criteria and wide applicability are a useful tool for educators, who would find it difficult or impossible to validate locally developed instruments.

Other Evaluation Tools

Neal Whitman, in *A Guide to Clinical Performance Testing*,[23] describes a model for using other tools to assess student performance in the clinical setting. Whitman draws distinctions between aspects of assessed performance that are related to a specific objective in the course and aspects that are not well described by course objectives. This is discussed in terms of whether predescribed specific steps are to be performed (as in patient assessment), or the specifics are not predescribed (as in scene management) as illustrated in the objectives matrix shown in **TABLE 22.2**.

TABLE 22.2 Objectives Matrix

	Specifics Preestablished	Specifics Not Preestablished
Objectives	Checklists	Observation logs
Other Aspects	Critical incident forms	Anecdotal records

Checklists as Whitman describes would be very similar to those checklists used in skills assessments and simulations. Observable aspects would be listed in well-constructed checklists, generally in the order in which they should be performed (**FIGURE 22.4**). The preceptor indicates whether the student performed the step or not. Preceptors should be discouraged from making qualitative ratings. In some variations, the checklist includes categories for whether the step was performed correctly, performed incorrectly, or not observed (**FIGURE 22.5**). Affective components can be assessed with rubrics that contain observable behaviors associated with levels of performance, instead of checklists.

Observation logs list the various objectives, and open space is provided beside each in which the preceptor can note how that objective was met during the encounter. For example, an objective might be: "The student keeps the patient's family informed." Preceptors would make notes next to this objective when they observe that objective being performed. Although checklists work well for those skills and qualities that can be standardized for nearly all patient encounters, observation logs can be used when the

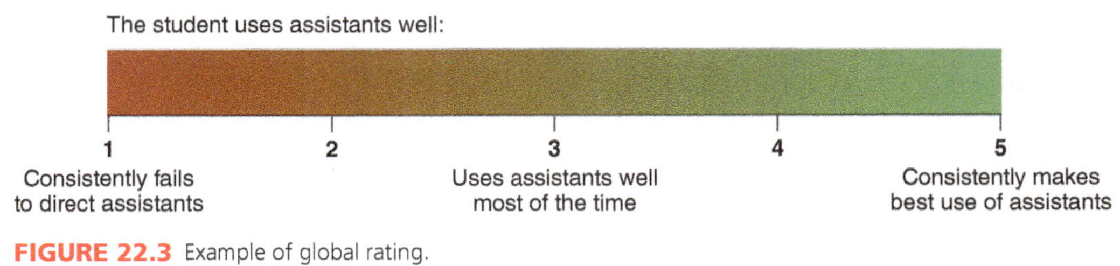

FIGURE 22.3 Example of global rating.

Directions

The contact should be rated by the student FIRST and the preceptor SECOND. Use the following standard for evaluation:
NA - Not Applicable ; Not needed or expected
0 - Unsuccessful; required excessive or critical prompting; not attempted when student was expected to try
1 - Marginal; Inconsistent; Not yet competent
2 - Successful; Competent; No Prompting

	Student				Preceptor			
Interview + HX Gathering	0	1	2	N/A	0	1	2	N/A
Physical Exam	0	1	2	N/A	0	1	2	N/A
Field Impression TX Plan	0	1	2	N/A	0	1	2	N/A
Skill Performance	0	1	2	N/A	0	1	2	N/A
Communication	0	1	2	N/A	0	1	2	N/A
Professional Behavior	0	1	2	N/A	0	1	2	N/A
Team Leadership	0	1	2	N/A	0	1	2	N/A

FIGURE 22.4 Sample call evaluation form.

Candidate: ______________________________ Date: ______________

ID#: ______________________________

Skill Drill 30-2: Applying a Commercial Tourniquet (Combat Application Tourniquet)

Task: Apply a commercial tourniquet.					
Performance Observations: The candidate shall be able to correctly apply a commercial tourniquet.					
Candidate Directive: "Properly apply a commercial tourniquet."					
No.	**Task Steps**	**First Test**		**Retest**	
		P	F	P	F
1.	Hold direct pressure over the bleeding site and place the tourniquet proximal to the injury, preferably at the groin or axilla. Wrap the band around the limb and fasten it to the buckle.				
2.	Pull the band tightly and secure the band back on itself. Ensure that the tips of three fingers cannot fit between the band and the limb.				
3.	Tighten the rod (windlass) until the bleeding stops.				
4.	Secure the rod inside the clip. Ensure bleeding is still controlled and assess for a distal pulse.				
5.	Wrap the rest of the band through the clips. Secure the rod with the strap labeled *TIME:* and document the time.				
Retest Approved By:		Retest Evaluation:			

Evaluator Comments:

Candidate Comments:

Evaluator	Date	Candidate	Date
Retest Evaluator	Date	Retest Candidate	Date

FIGURE 22.5 Sample skills evaluation form.

specifics of skills and qualities are heavily dependent on the situation.

Critical incident forms are used to identify a specific aspect of performance, and the preceptor describes the situation when a positive or negative example is observed. As an example, the characteristic might be: "Promotes interagency cooperation." When the preceptor observes the student bringing water to the incident commander on a fire scene, the preceptor would make notes on the critical incident form to describe the positive example.

Anecdotal records are simply a means of describing behavior that the preceptor deems relevant. Space for anecdotal comments is often provided on evaluation forms. Anecdotal records are valuable for capturing information that is not well described in advance by the other tools. Use of anecdotal records acknowledges that no assessment system is perfect and that all tools will invariably miss some important aspect of performance.

The effective instructor uses a combination of the previously described tools to form a system for observational reports of the experience to be completed by the preceptor. An effective strategy is to use a pyramid approach to the assessment system. This consists of a report for each clinical encounter; these reports form the base of the pyramid. These encounter reports could include components of checklists, observation logs, critical incident forms, and anecdotal records. The preceptor would then complete a report for the entire shift (the next tier on the pyramid) and combine information from encounter reports. This has the advantage of giving the student a degree of perspective on how the patient encounters combine to form a general impression for the shift. A number of shifts would be combined into a summative report for the entire rotation, forming the next higher tier on the pyramid. This builds from formative assessments into a summative tool. An overall summary would be included at the end of the clinical cycle. Each tier builds on information obtained from the tier below (**FIGURE 22.6**).

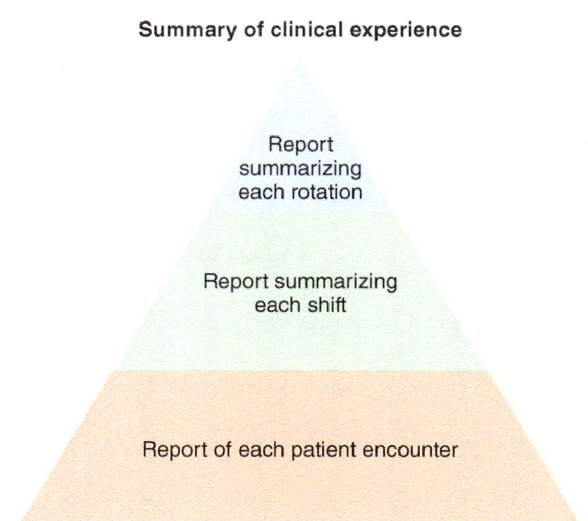

FIGURE 22.6 Pyramid approach to the evaluation system.

Selection of Experiences

The instructor should provide student experiences in relevant areas. For initial courses of instruction, guidelines for clinical experiences can be drawn from The National EMS Education Standards, accreditation standards, or state EMS regulatory agency documents. The instructor should review these guidelines before beginning to instruct a course. Working from these guidelines, the instructor can plan for relevant clinical experiences. Early clinical experiences are typically used to assess student performance of skills on actual patients.

The student is usually moved from specialized areas of the hospital (such as labor and delivery) to more relevant areas (such as the emergency department) and then to the field environment. This model illustrates the concept of scaffolding experiences. The instructor should assess each clinical area according to two dimensions. The first dimension is one of educational experiences. In other words, what can the student learn in this environment? Educational experiences in the applied care environment should be clearly linked to educational experiences in the classroom and lab to build relevance. The second dimension is one of assessment potential. In other words, what conclusions can the instructor draw from assessments of the student performance in the given environment? For example, say a paramedic instructor requires venipuncture experiences with the hospital laboratory team. The student will learn the variation of vein locations and will learn techniques for finding a vein. The student can be evaluated on finding veins, and successfully accessing the vein to draw blood. This may be a necessary precondition before IV infusions on patients are allowed. However, the instructor should not draw the conclusion that the paramedic student can initiate IV lines after observing performance only of venipuncture in lab settings. A variety of areas is useful, and the instructor should consider contextual differences in areas that are professionally distant from EMS.[24]

Preceptors

In most cases, the lead instructor is not able to directly observe the performance of all students in the hospital

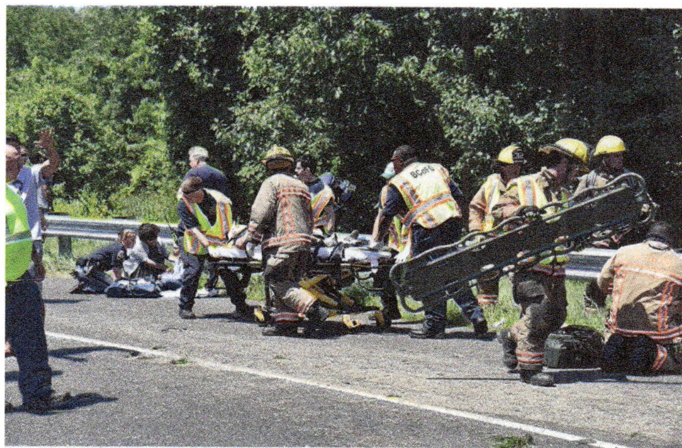

FIGURE 22.7 Feedback from preceptors is often instrumental in student learning. Feedback should be documented on the student evaluation tool.

or field setting, so preceptors must be used. A *preceptor* is defined as a teacher who is an identified, experienced practitioner who provides transitional role support and learning experiences during the hospital or field setting.

Preceptors should be proficient in the environment in which they perform. However, subject matter expertise is not enough. In fact, many students take lessons from preceptors to heart much more than they do lessons from the classroom instructor (**FIGURE 22.7**). This can be effective if the lessons from the preceptor are aligned with those given in the classroom. If the lessons conflict, significant problems can arise. Thus, preceptors must be aware of the basic principles of adult education. They must also be aware of their role, and they must know what is being taught in the classroom. Regular communication between preceptors and instructors is necessary. Preceptors should be trained in the use of the assessment tools they will be expected to use.

Some instructors experience difficulty in ensuring that negative impressions are appropriately documented in the hospital or internship phases of education. In some cases, the preceptor is willing to share the experiences informally with the instructor. There can be many reasons for this, ranging from difficulty in using the forms to fear of confrontation. Occasionally, meeting directly with preceptors informally can help the instructor identify mismatch between formal and informal communications. Training on assessment instruments and assuring preceptors that negative ratings are taken in context can also help. Ensuring that there are lines of reporting from the preceptor to the educational program that are independent of the student may be helpful in minimizing the fear of confrontation that some preceptors feel.

Integration of Evaluation with Patient Care

A unique challenge to assessing student performance in the applied care setting is the integration of educational goals, assessment goals, and provision of competent clinical care to the patient. It is essential that preceptors be prepared to meet this challenge. In terms of the educational goals of clinical experiences, the applied care setting is extremely effective in allowing students to experience the consequences of poor decisions. These lessons are extremely powerful and are likely to be retained by the student. However valuable these teachable moments may be, the educational value of having to deal with poor decisions must not be allowed to affect the patient. The preceptor must be prepared to intervene if it appears that the patient or family will suffer from a student's mistake. If the patient or family will not suffer, though, a valuable opportunity to drive a lesson home may be created.

CASE in Point

A clinical coordinator is revising the documentation tools used for students in a paramedic program during field internships. This program does not have access to a computerized system for documentation. The instructor decides that because different types of forms will be required for different elements, each student will be given a notebook with a set of forms to be completed by the preceptor. Each notebook contains the following, which are designed for up to 15 shifts with a preceptor:

- Forty call evaluations, each including an observation log that lists 10 objectives that can be demonstrated during any call
- Fifteen shift evaluations, each including an observation log that lists 10 objectives; these can act as a tool for the preceptor in summarizing the day's performance
- Twenty performance checklists for patient assessment, to be completed by the preceptor after observing the intern's performance of an assessment
- A knowledge checklist for each of several common protocols used by the service, to be completed by the preceptor after the student applies each protocol to an ambulance run
- Eight rubrics for affective objectives, to be completed by the preceptor on every other day of the internship
- One summary evaluation, along with a global rating for each objective, to be completed by the preceptor at the end of the internship

With regard to the goals of assessing student performance, preceptor intervention can present challenges. It is difficult for the preceptor to hold a student accountable for a mistake that was never allowed to occur. Intervention should occur just at the "point of no return," when it is apparent that the student will not realize and correct the mistake. If the preceptor repeatedly intervenes too early, the student may become hesitant and unwilling to commit to a decision. If the preceptor provides clues to the intervention, such as by asking, "Are you sure you want to do that?" on all critical steps, and not just when a poor decision is in progress, the assessment has greater validity. Mastering this fine balance is an important skill for preceptors.

Even with extensive clinical and internship opportunities, it is unlikely that the student will be assessed on all skills in the clinical environment. The instructor must be prepared to extrapolate from the results of assessments that have been conducted. This extrapolation should be reasonable, based on the types of situations in which the student has demonstrated acceptable performance. For example, it is unlikely that all students will have the opportunity to manage a cardiac arrest in the applied care environment.

The instructor may choose to extrapolate from the student's actual performance in caring for a critically ill patient and from simulations of cardiac arrest, to conclude that the student can adequately manage a cardiac arrest in the field. This is a matter of professional judgment for the instructor, who combines personal opinion with input from the program director and the medical director. It is helpful to have guidelines regarding minimum exposure to different types of patients experiencing different types of emergencies. However, it is not feasible to require every student to see all types of calls. Reasonable extrapolations must be made.

TEACHING TIP

State regulations and program accreditation requirements typically have rules regarding minimum exposure for patients chosen from various age groups (e.g., adult and various pediatric age groups), types of complaints and emergencies (e.g., cardiac and respiratory), and procedures (e.g., initiating IV access and medication administration).

Summary

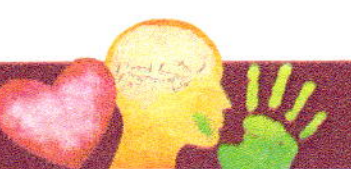

By combining written assessments with other tools, an integrated strategy can be developed for assessing each of the domains of learning. Creating an effective assessment strategy begins with careful consideration of the purpose of the assessment. This purpose may be tied to a curriculum, using established objectives to anchor the evaluation tools used; or, the purpose may be to verify competency using assessments that are based on a practice analysis. It is sometimes helpful for the instructor to divide course objectives among the domains of learning, as the domain will be a significant consideration in the selection of assessment tools. Cognitive objectives can be effectively assessed through the use of written examinations, oral examinations, and research projects. Psychomotor objectives can be assessed with performance examinations, simulations, and assessments of student care of patients in a supervised clinical experience. Affective objectives can be assessed through writing assignments, oral examinations, and surveys at lower levels. Higher levels can be assessed through behavioral observations (with rubrics) that occur during class and lab as well as during the clinical and field components of a course.

A number of tools are required for effective assessment of the student. No one single tool will be capable of assessing the depth and breadth of objectives for the typical EMS course. The use of multiple tools also helps to ensure reliability of the assessment process. The grade assigned to a course should include elements from each of the formal assessment tools. Each tool can be weighted according to the stated purpose of the assessment strategy and the course objectives.

Based on the strategy chosen, specific tools and items can be selected and edited, and testing instruments constructed. The resourceful instructor collects tools and items from commonly available sources, instead of constructing each from scratch. Effective instructors also carefully edit each item and tool to ensure that the item has content validity for their particular course. Items are then analyzed to confirm reliability and validity. Over time, instructors can collect a powerful toolbox of assessments.

Although security is an issue for written examinations, other types of evaluation instruments can be shared with students. For example, students can use performance checklists and rubrics for meaningful self-assessment.

Assessing student performance can be viewed as a set of progressive steps. Formative assessment and learning activities allow the student and the instructors to modify the learning strategy to ultimately master the course objectives. Mastery is then assessed through curriculum-based summative tools. The curriculum and the student together are tested through competency verification, which is a summative assessment based on a practice analysis.

Assessing student performance can be complex. Educators must remember that poor results may reveal that the student is performing poorly or that the instructor has not provided adequate learning opportunities for the student to master the material. Of course, this assumes that the assessment itself is giving accurate and meaningful results. To decipher these multiple messages requires an understanding of the fundamentals of student assessment.

Proper selection, construction, and analysis of assessment instruments help to ensure that assessment is providing meaningful results. Proper formative assessment provides feedback to the instructor about whether the learning activities have adequately prepared the student. With these fundamentals, the instructor can decode the results of tools that assess student performance.

Glossary

360-degree evaluation Feedback that utilizes many sources of evaluation, including peers.

competency portfolio Documented body of evidence that shows consistently acceptable performance of skills.

Cronbach's alpha Complex statistical method of assessing internal consistency.

dichotomous scoring Type of scoring in which the observable action is either performed or not, to the greatest extent possible.

equating Procedures used to control for examinations of varying difficulty.

polytomous scoring Type of scoring in which the examiner chooses a number of points indicating how well the step was performed; it is frequently less reliable and more difficult to standardize.

preceptor Teacher who is an identified, experienced practitioner who provides transitional role support and learning experiences during the hospital or field setting.

rubric Evaluation tool that defines criteria for each degree of expected performance when there are multiple facets to the evaluation.

task analysis Examination method that provides a comprehensive list of the steps to be performed for a skill or process.

References

[1] Gardner, Howard. 1993. *Multiple Intelligences: The Theory in Practice*. New York: Basic Books.

[2] Waterhouse, Lynn. 2006. "Multiple Intelligences, the Mozart Effect, and Emotional Intelligence: A Critical Review." *Educational Psychologist* 41, no. 4: 207–25. https://doi.org/10.1207/s15326985ep4104_1.

[3] Gardner, Howard. 2006. *Multiple Intelligences: New Horizons*. New York: Basic Books.

[4] Rogowksy, Beth A., Barbara M. Calhoun, and Paula Tallal. 2015. "Matching Learning Style to Instructional Method: Effects on Comprehension." *Journal of Educational Psychology* 107, no. 1: 64–78. http://dx.doi.org/10.1037/a0037478.

[5] Pashler, Harold, Mark McDaniel, Doug Rohrer, and Robert Bjork. 2009. "Learning Styles: Concepts and Evidence." *Psychological Science in the Public Interest* 9, no. 3: 105–19. https://doi.org/10.1111/j.1539-6053.2009.01038.x.

[6] Sparks-Langer, Georgea M., Alane J. Starko, Marvin Pasch, Wendy Burke, Christella D. Moody, and Trevor G. Gardner. 2003. *Teaching as Decision Making: Successful Practices for The Secondary Teacher,* 2nd ed. Philadelphia: Prentice Hall.

[7] Gaur, Lasya, and Susan Skochelak. 2004. "Evaluating Competence in Medical Students." *Journal of the American Medical Association* 291, no. 17: 21–43. http://dx.doi.org/10.1001/jama.291.17.2143.

[8] Seddon, G. M. 1978. "The Properties of Bloom's Taxonomy of Educational Objectives for the Cognitive Domain." *Review of Educational Research* 48, no. 2: 303–23. https://doi.org/10.3102/00346543048002303.

[9] Margolis, Gregg S., Gabriel A. Romero, Antonio R. Fernandez, and Jonathan R. Studnek. 2009. "Strategies of High-Performing Paramedic Educational Programs." *Prehospital Emergency Care* 13, no. 4: 505–11. https://doi.org/10.1080/10903120902993396.

[10] Jacobs, Lucy C., and Clinton I. Chase. 1992. *Developing and Using Tests Effectively: A Guide for Faculty*. San Francisco: Jossey-Bass.

[11] Harden, R. McG, Mary Stevenson, W. Wilson Downie, and G. M. Wilson. 1975. "Assessment of Clinical Competence Using Objective-Structured Examination." *British Medical Journal* 1: 447–51. https://doi.org/10.1136/bmj.1.5955.447.

[12] Tavares, Walter, and Kevin W. Eva. 2013. "Exploring the Impact of Mental Workload on Rater-based Assessments." *Advances in Health Sciences Education* 18, no. 2: 291–303. https://doi.org/10.1007/s10459-012-9370-3.

[13] Tavares, Walter, and Kevin W. Eva. 2014. "Impact of Rating Demands on Rater-based Assessments of Clinical Competence."

Education for Primary Care 25, no. 6: 308–18. https://doi.org/10.1080/14739879.2014.11730760.

[14] Tavares, Walter, Shiphra Ginsburg, and Kevin W. Eva. 2016. "Selecting and Simplifying: Rater Performance and Behavior when Considering Multiple Competencies." *Teaching and Learning in Medicine*, 28, no. 1: 41–51. https://doi.org/10.1080/10401334.2015.1107489.

[15] Davis, Barbara G. 2001. *Tools for Teaching*. San Francisco: Jossey-Bass.

[16] National Highway Traffic Safety Administration. 2009. "National Emergency Medical Services Education Standards." [DOT HS 811 077A]. Accessed January 15, 2019. https://www.ems.gov/pdf/National-EMS-Education-Standards-FINAL-Jan-2009.pdf.

[17] National Research Council. 1991. *Pay for Performance: Evaluating Performance Appraisal and Merit Pay*. Washington, DC: National Academy Press.

[18] National Highway Traffic Safety Administration. 2002. "National Guidelines for Educating EMS Instructors." Accessed March 2, 2019. http://www.nhtsa.dot.gov/people/injury/EMS/Instructor/Tableofcontents.htm.

[19] Papadakis, Maxine A., Carol S. Hodgson, Arianne Teherani, and Neal D. Kohatsu. 2004. "Unprofessional Behavior in Medical School Is Associated with Subsequent Disciplinary Action by a State Medical Board." *Academic Medicine* 79, no. 3: 244–9.

[20] Committee on Accreditation of Educational Programs for the Emergency Medical Services Professions (CoAEMSP). 2017, February 3. "CoAEMSP Interpretations of the CAAHEP 2015 Standards and Guidelines." Accessed February 10, 2019. https://coaemsp.org/Documents/Standards_Interpretations_CoAEMSP-2015%20approved%202017%2002%2004.pdf.

[21] RubiStar. 2003. *Create Rubrics for Your Project-Based Learning Activities*. Lawrence, KS: Advanced Learning Technologies Center for Research on Learning at the University of Kansas. Accessed March 5, 2019. http://rubistar.4teachers.org.

[22] Tavares, Walter, Sylvain Boet, Rob Theriault, Tony Mallette, and Kevin W. Eva. 2013. "Global Rating Scale for the Assessment of Paramedic Clinical Competence." *Prehospital Emergercy Care* 17, no. 1: 57–67. https://doi.org/10.3109/10903127.2012.702194.

[23] Whitman, Neal. 1982. "A Guide to Clinical Performance Testing." *IDEA Paper* no. 7. Manhattan, KS: Kansas State University Center for Faculty Evaluation and Development. Accessed March 5, 2019. http://web.archive.org/web/20130622102242/http://www.theideacenter.org/sites/default/files/Idea_Paper_07.pdf.

[24] Mausz, Justin, and Walter Tavares. 2017. "Learning in Professionally 'Distant' Contexts: Opportunities and Challenges." *Advances in Health Sciences Education: Theory and Practice*, 22, no. 3: 581–600. https://doi.org/10.1007/s10459-016-9693-6.

Additional Resources

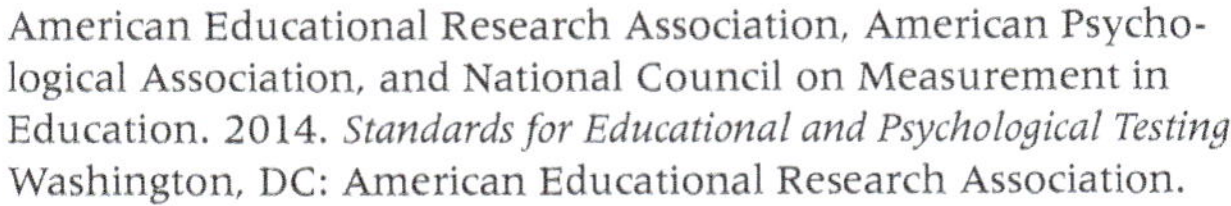

American Educational Research Association, American Psychological Association, and National Council on Measurement in Education. 2014. *Standards for Educational and Psychological Testing*. Washington, DC: American Educational Research Association.

Johnson, Robert L., James A. Penny, and Belita Gordon. 2009. *Assessing Performance: Designing, Scoring and Validating Performance Tasks*. New York: Guilford Press.

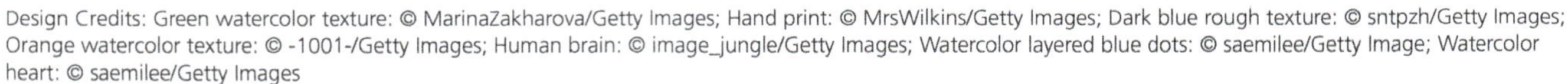

CHAPTER 23

Remediation

OBJECTIVES

At the conclusion of this chapter, the educator will be able to:

Cognitive Domain

1. Define *remediation*.
2. Describe situations that may merit remediation.
3. List strategies for remediation.
4. Outline the steps in the remediation process.
5. Discuss the role of attribution in the remediation process.
6. List the elements of a learning contract.
7. Given a student problem, develop a remediation plan based on the principles described in this chapter.

Psychomotor Domain

There are no psychomotor objectives for this chapter.

Affective Domain

1. Value the need for the remediation process to be proactive.
2. Justify the importance of remediation strategies to student success.

"Nobody cares how much you know until they know how much you care."

~ THEODORE ROOSEVELT

CHAPTER GOAL This chapter will define the purpose and process of student remediation.

Without question, as educators we realize in any educational endeavor we must ensure a process is in place to position faculty members to assist students, when needed, with appropriate **remediation**. Any quality educational program must proactively initiate steps before the need to remediate a student arises. This chapter will assist instructors in thinking about methods to design, develop, implement, and evaluate the process required to assist a student or students in remediation within emergency medical services (EMS) programs.

What should an educator do when a student does not meet the program's performance standards? Performance standards provide the foundation for all levels of the U.S. Department of Transportation National Highway and Traffic Safety Administration (DOT-NHTSA) *National Emergency Medical Services Education Standards* (the *Standards*) with terminology such as "competencies, clinical behaviors, and judgments."[1] However, education standards typically do not provide specific learning objectives or explicit guidance on how to measure goals or objectives, nor do they advise how to conduct an effective remediation (retraining and retesting) process. Although this allows for a great deal of flexibility, the novice instructor may need additional guidance.

In addition to the *Standards*, additional performance standards are often established in state, regional, and local regulations for EMS education. Because regional guidelines are typically written to allow for flexibility in programs, they also may not contain specific evaluation or remediation processes. An instructor should use these references to provide the foundation on which to build an evaluation system for an educational program.

When a student does not meet the established performance standard, two options are available to the instructor: (1) remediation or (2) removal of the student from the educational process. When an evaluation system is in place for an educational program, a remediation process should also be included as a component of that system.[2] To be most effective, the remediation process must be clearly articulated and understood by all members of the educational team and, perhaps more important, by the students.

TEACHING TIP

The instructor has the greatest control of the remediation process when policies and procedures are in place before remediation is needed.

Remediation Defined

The term *remediation* is derived from the root word *remedial*, which means to correct a deficiency.[3] The suffix to remediation is *-ation*, which refers to an act or process. Therefore, the definition of remediation is the process of analysis and identification of deficits (or problems) and a plan for retraining or improving performance before retesting is undertaken. The implication for assessment is that performance standards will be achieved by each student. One must realize, however, there is no guarantee that all students will achieve the performance standards following a remediation process.

Remediation is a critical component of any educational process because it provides solutions for situations in which students do not meet the performance standard. In these cases, the educational program must effectively respond with actions that go beyond the typical educational process (i.e., apply additional effort to help a student achieve competency). Research indicates that many, if not most, students require remediation at some point in their academic careers. It should be noted that up to 90% of community college students needed remediation in literacy and mathematical skills.[4] Based on this statistic, it is evident that any educational process must ensure remediation is included as an essential aspect of the program design and development of the instructional offering. If this vitally important aspect of instruction is not included in the process, one would surely expect to see a high failure rate.

Reasons other than the threat of low success rates must drive the need for remediation. The educational process is a partnership between the student and the educational team, and a successful student outcome is a reasonable expectation. In this partnership, it is also reasonable to assume the educational team will be an advocate for student success. In this environment, a remediation process is an appropriate tool designed to facilitate success.[5]

One aspect of the student–educator partnership that is difficult to design is a system that allows for remediation but does not compromise program integrity or fairness to the other students in the program. Based on student performance in a course, an instructor may feel one student deserves a second chance and another does not. Without a defined remediation system in place for guidance, the potential for bias is greater. Thus it is essential for any educational program to have a clearly established remediation process in place.

When to Remediate

Remediation should follow a student's inability to meet an expected standard during an assessment process. The remediation may be related to a deficiency in the cognitive, affective, or psychomotor domain. The remediation process should be initiated as soon as the breakdown is identified. Based on curricula design, students may or may not be permitted to continue in the program until the remediation is completed and successful reassessment is achieved. It is of utmost importance that programs, faculty members, students, and administration know the process of remediation prior to the first student being subject to it.

It is normal to have students with educational deficits in one or two areas. In other cases, students may have difficulties in several components of the educational offering. Unfortunately, an instructor may have many students who have difficulty throughout the entire program of instruction. These students will benefit from tutorial sessions to assist them in their learning. When offering tutorial sessions, they should be made open to the entire class. The instructor may find that the students in greatest need of the tutorial session do not attend, but others who attend gain even more knowledge and skills. Faculty members should consider assigning students to attend tutorial sessions, reducing the need for remediation. Tutorial sessions should be offered to all students seeking additional insight on any subjects or skills in an EMS program of instruction. Often, students who voluntarily attend additional learning programs have achieved mastery of the content or skills. Thus, faculty members may need to mandate that students who have not yet gained the expected knowledge or skills attend these sessions and continue to do so until mastery is obtained.

In some cases, in order to adhere to the program schedule, remediation must occur quickly. Frequently, educational systems allow students to proceed in their educational programs without establishing the foundation of instruction required to ensure success. Programs should create methods to provide counseling or tutorial programs for students who need additional information or clarification on a specific topic.

Any type of assessment, whether formal, informal, formative, or summative, can trigger the remediation process. (Chapter 20, *Assessing Learning,* describes different types of assessment in detail.) That remediation is an integral part of the evaluation process cannot be overemphasized. Student advocacy is a primary role for every EMS educator, just as patient advocacy is a primary role for every EMS provider.[1] In addition to discussing and describing student advocacy as a value, it is important for the instructor to provide the necessary tools to accomplish this task.

Although the range of students who may require remediation is not yet fully known, mounting evidence suggests there is a need for it in every educational program.[4] Given this need, educational programs must plan for remediation by establishing deliberate steps and processes. A defined procedure allows classroom educators to focus on *how* to provide remediation for specific students, rather than getting bogged down in determining whether they should or can provide remediation. The administrative team for the program should create the remediation policies and procedures. The student handbook, syllabus, policies and procedures manual, and other program documents should contain policies and procedures that clearly outline the process. The remediation policy should be provided to students during program orientation. Students should sign a copy of the program's policies and procedures, including those relating to remediation. Faculty and students should know where and how to access these.

A diligent educator reviews the steps of remediation and covers this information with the students at the beginning of the course, at a minimum. Once an

CASE in Point

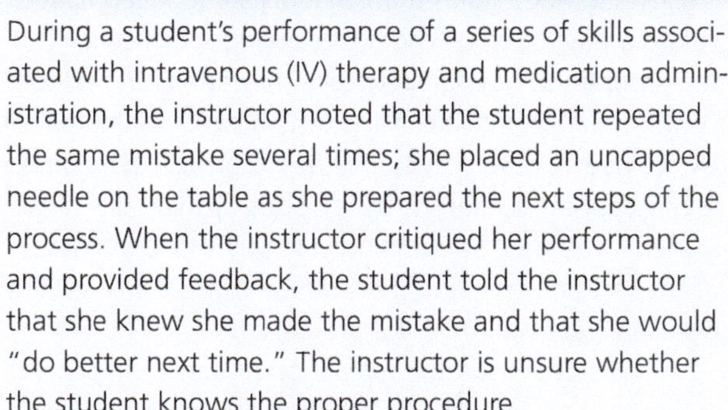

During a student's performance of a series of skills associated with intravenous (IV) therapy and medication administration, the instructor noted that the student repeated the same mistake several times; she placed an uncapped needle on the table as she prepared the next steps of the process. When the instructor critiqued her performance and provided feedback, the student told the instructor that she knew she made the mistake and that she would "do better next time." The instructor is unsure whether the student knows the proper procedure.

A formal remediation cycle followed by retesting may correct this mistake. In this case, the amount of time spent on the actual retraining may be minimal. In the remediation process, the student would be required to demonstrate proper skill performance and to provide evidence that she knows the procedure. The instructor may consider videotaping the student as she performs the skill(s) and allowing the student to watch and self-critique her progress.

inappropriate outcome occurs, the instructor should review the remediation policies and procedures early in the process to ensure compliance with established rules of the program.

Eligibility for Remediation

The following questions are useful in determining if a student is eligible for remediation, and in deciding whether remediation is possible and appropriate:

1. Is there a standard in place that indicates what level of student involvement is required for remediation to be provided?
   - Does the policy identify a score or range of scores required for remediation to occur?
   - Is there an attendance standard?
   - Are other criteria specified (e.g., limits on total number of attempts at remediation and retesting allowed in a program)?
2. Can remediation be accomplished in a timely manner to allow the student to continue in the program?
3. Are appropriate resources available for providing remediation?
4. How committed is the student to the remediation process and to improving their performance?

Time constraints are a critical factor to be analyzed. For example, if the course schedule does not permit enough time for remediation to take place, it may not be appropriate to proceed with retraining. This varies from student to student as well as from event to event. If the time frame for retraining is not adequate, a second inappropriate outcome may result during the retesting phase. As the course continues to move forward, the student will be faced with the additional burden of keeping up with new material while attempting to achieve success in the retraining required. Resource considerations are vitally important in the development and implementation of a remediation plan. Many programs have limitations on their equipment and supplies; some share resources among several simultaneous courses. Remediation requires careful scheduling and cooperation. The need to provide resources for remediation for one student can seriously disrupt programs that operate with tight resource constraints, emphasizing the importance of incorporating remediation considerations into the assessment process.

The costliest aspect of most remediation events is the cost for faculty and staff to plan and deliver retraining for a student. Some systems pay personnel for the additional time required for remediation. A program's design must accommodate costs for remediation. Programs with funding (or volunteers who are willing to assist) have the ability to offer remediation in a more structured manner. Programs in educational systems that lack funding or lack personnel to assist will need to find methods to assist students based on these constraints.

The final decision regarding eligibility for remediation usually requires an understanding of the reason for this outcome. If it is determined the decision rests solely with one instructor, bias can enter the decision-making process. Input from preceptors and other faculty members or a consistent committee of the educational team can help reduce this bias.

TEACHING TIP

Because of the commitment to student advocacy, when educators are unsure whether a remediation attempt should proceed or are unclear of the standard in place, it is best to allow the student to attempt the remediation process.

CASE in Point

(Part 1 of 2)

An educator is teaching an emergency medical responder (EMR) course. The course is 48 hours long and adheres to the *Standards* and to the state EMS agency regulations.

The syllabus states that students are required to successfully pass three testing cycles during specified parts of the program to be eligible to take the state EMR test for certification. Each test consists of two parts: 50 multiple choice questions and three psychomotor skills tests based on appropriate scenarios. The syllabus further states that students who fail the exam process can retake that part of the test one time and that a second failure will result in dismissal (removal) from the program.

One student failed the practical examination portion for the first testing cycle. What should happen next?

In this case, a process allowing for remediation is included in the evaluation system for this course, and it outlines three testing points that have relatively high stakes: (1) students must successfully complete each examination to be able to continue in the course; (2) in the event a student fails a test, one retest opportunity is provided before dismissal; and (3) remediation should occur after failure of the first attempt and before a retest is attempted.

When an assessment reveals the inability of a student to meet an expected standard, the educator should initiate the remediation process. In some cases, the student may independently recognize this inability to perform and will discuss concerns with the instructor; this discussion may result in initiation of the process.

Educators should refrain from using the word "failure" when communicating with a student. Instead, it is essential for educators to speak about outcomes and results in the educational process. In each of the three educational domains, the student must strive for and achieve success to the level defined by the program. In the educational process, scores are established that can determine whether students have met the expectations of the program or if remediation is required.

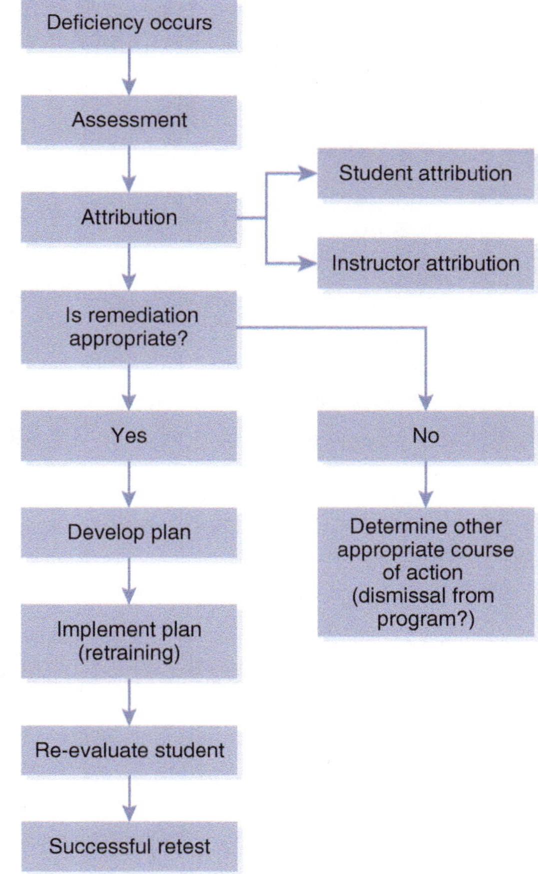

FIGURE 23.1 Remediation algorithm.

Steps in the Remediation Process

The remediation process includes the following five steps:

1. Assess possible reasons for the student's performance deficit.
2. Determine the cause of the performance deficit (attribution).
3. Develop a remediation plan.
4. Implement the plan.
5. Reevaluate.

Once the problem has been identified and retraining is determined to be possible and appropriate, a remediation plan is developed. For the plan to be finalized, the student must agree to the terms and conditions, including the consequences of repeated inappropriate outcome. Once the plan is in place, the retraining can begin. The progress of the student during the retraining process should be closely monitored. Once retraining has occurred, Step 5, reevaluation, can occur. **FIGURE 23.1** illustrates a remediation algorithm.

Step 1: Assess Possible Reasons for Failure

To ensure fairness in the remediation process and to maintain program integrity, a thorough assessment of the student's performance (be it cognitive, psychomotor, or affective) should take place prior to a remediation plan being developed and implemented (**FIGURE 23.2**).

Information gathered during this step assists the instructor in determining whether remediation is permissible, possible, and appropriate. Information from

Assessment Phase of Remediation

The assessment phase of the remediation process may reveal helpful information for the student on any of the following topics:

- Need for study skills enhancements
- Need for evaluation for learning disabilities
- Need for developmental or remedial classes
- Need to obtain additional clinical experience
- Need to work on affective skills such as communication
- Understanding of the sacrifices necessary for the course
- Contacts for helpful resources
- Schedule adjustments for work and family
- Access to financial or other support

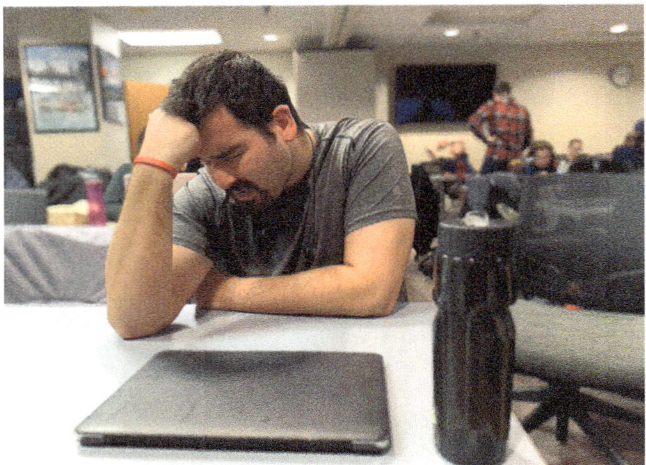

FIGURE 23.2 Whether the difficulty is in the cognitive, psychomotor, or affective domain, the student must be committed to improving performance in order to succeed.

Courtesy of Sydney Abbott.

TEACHING TIP

If the instructor does not conduct a thorough front-end analysis to identify the problem, the instructor may not identify the actual cause or causes of the student's inability to meet expectations, and the remediation plan may not be successful.

the student's perspective as well as from the instructor's regarding the cause of a student's inabilities (outcomes or results) is needed to make this decision.

Educational program strategies and educator knowledge and experience are important considerations in the assessment phase, but the student's role in the process is also critical. There is significant anecdotal evidence and action research (nonscientific or pseudoscientific evidence) on student attitudes and their impact on learning. Educational psychologists are placing greater emphasis on attitude. If the real cause of the inappropriate outcome or result is primarily attributed to the student and the student is unwilling to acknowledge that fact, then successful remediation may not be possible if the student is not willing to correct the behavior.

TEACHING TIP

The instructor must maintain the student's confidentiality during the assessment and attribution process. Discussion of the issue should be limited to appropriate members of the educational team.

The educator should demonstrate active listening and implement clear communication skills when interviewing the student. A seasoned educator realizes that most students are very emotional during this time, and it is important to maintain professionalism and perspective.

Step 2: Determine the Cause for Failure (Attribution)

The second step in the process, during which the root cause for the issues is identified, is known as **attribution**. Attribution helps to identify the level of responsibility shared by the instructional process, educators, and the student. Attribution has a significant impact on the remediation process.

Evidence suggests that attribution may be the single most vital component affecting the remediation process.[6] To develop a meaningful remediation process, the educator must identify the root cause of the student's inappropriate outcome.

Intuitively, we know that incorrect problem identification can lead to implementation of an incorrect or ineffective solution. Therefore, seeking multiple points of input can assist the instructor to identify the correct cause. In addition to reviewing the instructional process and assessment instruments, the educator should interview the student. As mentioned earlier, the instructor can consider seeking input from instructors in all settings in which the student has participated, including the classroom, lab, clinical, and field settings. It may also be appropriate to seek input from the medical and program director.

It is common for the educator's assignment of attribution to be different from what the student believes to be the cause. For example, a student believes the reason for inappropriate outcome was inadequate time to prepare for the examination, but the instructor believes the root cause is that the student missed a practical skills development section. The impact of conflicting attributions on the solution is significant.

TEACHING TIP

Often, failure of a student, regardless of the cause, affects the instructor as well as the student. Input from members of the educational team outside the situation should be considered to help limit bias and provide objectivity.

Student Attribution

One way that the educator can identify the student's attribution of the cause for inappropriate outcome is through an interview. The instructor should ask open-ended questions and should approach the interview in a nonjudgmental manner. It may be appropriate for the instructor to emphasize to the student that they are working on an educational solution to the problem. The instructor may find it helpful to tell the student that the goal of the remediation process is to determine strategies that will most likely result in the student's passing on the next attempt.

As the educator conducts the interview, it is important that the student's commitment to improving performance be assessed.[6] The instructor may find it necessary to make decisions regarding the student's abilities to succeed on future attempts. If the student does not possess the necessary tools (cognitive, affective, or psychomotor abilities), the resultant remediation plan may need to include strategies for developing these abilities. Inclusion of the program director, clinical coordinator, medical director, and others in the decision process may be required.

As the instructor works through the process of attribution, it is important to ascertain whether the student ever successfully demonstrated the standard. This may reveal whether the student can attain the standard. If success was demonstrated previously, then the instructor should determine what has changed. Perhaps the progress of the student was not monitored appropriately, which allowed for uncorrected deficient performance. If the instructor does not have evidence of successful attainment of the standards, corrective instruction should be provided to the student.

TEACHING TIP

Some students lack the maturity to accept responsibility for their action or inaction. The instructor should focus energies on developing a solid plan with the intent that the student will eventually accept responsibility in the failure. If the student's action or inaction cannot be rectified, additional steps will be required.

Program Attribution

It is important for the instructor to examine what possible role the educational process played in the inappropriate outcome or result. It must be ensured that the faculty understood and articulated the performance standard clearly to the student. Was the student informed of one standard, yet tested for another? The instructor must ensure that the goals and objectives of the course appropriately match the testing process.

The educator must analyze the assessment process. Were the correct instruments used to evaluate students? Have these instruments been validated? Are they reliable? Chapters 20 through 22 explain these processes in detail.

The educator must also analyze the learning plan. Was the plan appropriate and effective? Was adequate time allotted for students to learn the material? Were adequate teaching strategies used to appeal to the student's learning style or preference? Did the learning plan allow for reinforcement of concepts, and did it test for understanding? Were activities designed to facilitate the learning of critical-thinking processes?[7]

Findings from the program attribution may indicate the need for changes and improvements in the course.

CASE in Point

(Part 2 of 2)

The policies and procedures indicate that remediation is allowed and encouraged for the student who requires additional interactions. During the problem assessment interview, the student is unclear about why he believes he failed, but he says he wishes he had been allowed more time to practice the skill.

As the educator reviews the course syllabus and schedule, he notes that the practical skills development session has many skills listed on the sheet. Because of time constraints, although the instructor demonstrated all of the skills, the students did not get appropriate practice time. The instructor also determined that many of the students did not perform well on the practical exam, even though only one failed to demonstrate proficiency of the required skills. The educator contacts the program coordinator to discuss rearranging the schedule to allow for additional practical skills time and requests permission to retest the entire class. A private skills session is also arranged for the student who failed to complete the required tasks.

On retest, all students pass.

Multiple Attributions

Frequently, student inappropriate outcome is caused by multiple attributions. In many cases, the attributions identified by the student and the educational team do not match. The interrelationship between education, performance, environment, and student needs is complex. The instructor should consider the effect that each of these has on student performance.

The next *Case in Point* highlights two program problems: not enough manikins for students and not enough instructors. One-on-one instruction may result in successful retesting of the student in this case, but unless the program can allocate additional resources, the problem will most likely reoccur.

CASE in Point

A program has an inadequate number of manikins for all students to actively participate during class. A shy student feels that the instructor is paying more attention to the other students and does not actively participate. The instructor is dividing his attention between many students and does not notice that the student is withdrawing. When the student fails the examination, he blames the instructor for not providing appropriate instruction. The instructor counters that the student is not assertive and seems unwilling to practice skills. Every instructor must consider the impact these multiple attributions have on the development of a successful remediation plan.

People are often willing to listen to advice and direction provided by professionals during a teachable moment. However, the discussion of attribution with a student is not usually a teachable moment. Receiving a bad grade on an examination may be devastating to life plans and goals, and the student may be very emotional. It may not be helpful for the instructor to try to convince a student that their attribution is incorrect at this time.

Therefore, although students can benefit from understanding and accepting personal responsibility for an inappropriate outcome, the student attribution interview may not be the best time to approach the subject. Experience and strong interpersonal skills will assist an educator in deciding when it is appropriate to confront a student about their perception of attribution. It is critical for the instructor to determine whether the remediation plan can account for the student's attribution.

Step 3: Develop a Remediation Plan

Input from both the student and the educational team is used to develop the remediation plan (see sample remediation plan document in **FIGURE 23.3**). The remediation plan should clearly describe the process and the expected outcomes for the student and instructional team. It should define any work (e.g., reading assignments, homework, or self-study) that is to be completed independently by the student, and it should describe the type of assistance that is to be provided by the instructor. A timeline for the remediation should also be included, clearly identifying when the process will begin and end, including an estimated total number of hours the retraining process should require. The plan should describe the length of time the student and instructor may spend together and should suggest the amount of time the student will consider spending on independent work or study. If appropriate to the plan, the instructor can include the dates and times that progress reports will be issued.

TEACHING TIP

It is helpful for another member of the educational team to review the plan before it is finalized to ensure that it is reasonable and appropriate.

The plan should also identify the date and time of retesting, specify what type of retesting will occur, and list any observers (e.g., the medical director or other instructor) who will be present during retesting. The expected standard for successful completion should be reinforced, and the consequences of any inappropriate outcome to comply with the terms specified in the remediation plan should be described. The consequences of an inappropriate result of the retest should also be described.

The remediation plan should be presented in a positive light and set the student up for success. Remediation plans should engage the student in their need to gain the knowledge, skills, or attitude in the EMS domain. As field healthcare providers, students must know that developing mastery in these areas will benefit them and their patients. Remediation should not be viewed as a negative or punitive event. It should be viewed as part of the educational process that is known to be needed for those students who need a bit more time to achieve success.

The instructor should review the finished plan to ensure that it complies with the program remediation policy. The completed document, when signed by the student, instructor, program director, and medical director, is sometimes called a **learning contract**. Copies of the document should be provided to all parties involved, and a copy should be maintained in the student's permanent record.

If the educational methods are not identified as the cause for the inappropriate outcome, they may then become the basis for the retraining methods used in the remediation plan. For example, the teaching strategy can shift from a group approach to a targeted process for the student's individual learning style and preference. If, on the other hand, the educational method is attributed as the cause of the inappropriate result, adjustments to the educational methods should be made. An educator cannot continue to do the same thing and expect different results.

TEACHING TIP

Instructors should ensure that remediation plans are reasonable for both the students and the instructional staff. Plans should not be so complex that they set up either or both for failure.

A

<Employee Name> Education Plan
Date: *<date>*

Goals	**Behavioral Objectives** **(what they should know and able to do)** *Upon completion, the paramedic will:*	**Actions** (unbold) **Assessments (Bold)**	**Evaluated By & Date Completed**
Recognizes the need for a....	1. <list indications for> 2. <describe the benefit>	Complete: ***<assignment entered here>***	
Demonstrates an understanding of....	Outlines... Distinguish between...	Reads/prepares: ***<assignment entered here>***	
Understands....	1. <list>	Reads assigned articles: ***<assignment entered here>*** **Answers an open-book quiz xx with 100% accuracy.**	
Performs *xx* skill competently	1. Lists the steps to perform *xx* skill with 100% accuracy based on *xx* skill sheet. 2. On a manikin, with no critical errors, performs *xx*. 3. Given a scenario, performs *xx* skill, competently with no critical errors, in the correct sequence at the appropriate time. 4. In the prehospital setting, on a 9-1-1 call, performs *xx* skill successfully *xx*% of the time.	**1. Given a blank sheet of paper, lists the steps to perform *xx* skill.** **2. Using a task trainer, performs *xx* skill according to the steps of *xx* skill sheet with 90% accuracy and no critical errors.** **3. In a complex simulation with a paramedic partner, performs xx skill appropriately with no critical errors.** **4. Through direct observation on 10 emergency calls, the training officer verifies appropriate performance of *xx* skill.**	

I have read this educational plan, understand it and agree to complete it by ***<date>*** as specified in this document unless my Training Officer authorizes (in writing) a plan extension or alteration.

Employee Signature________________________ Training Officer ________________________

Witnessed________________________ Date ______________

Plan Completion Date: __________ Verified by: ________________________

Medical Officer

FIGURE 23.3 Examples of remediation plan templates. **A.** Education plan. **B.** Remediation plan.

A. Courtesy of St. Charles County Ambulance District.

(continues)

B

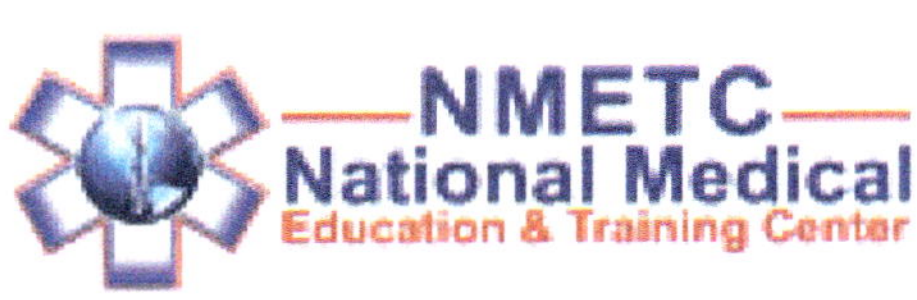

Remediation Plan

Student Name: ______________________________

Critical problem or area that needs remediation (academic or psychomotor skills)

____

____

____

____

Student to take ownership for actions: Please indicate what you feel is the cause of your current academic situation. (i.e., work, children, lack of study time, etc.) Also, please indicate what you plan on doing to improve your GPA or skill level, as well as what you expect from NMETC in an effort to bring you to a passing grade or skill sign off to competency.

Student Ownership of Problem: ______________________________

____

____

____

____

____

____

____

____

____

Educational Goals: ______________________________

____

____

Faculty Feedback: ______________________________

____

____

____

____

Faculty Action Plan for student: ______________________________

____

____

____

Re-evaluation Date:______________________________

Remediation Completed by: ______________________________

Student Signature: ______________________________

FIGURE 23.3 *(Continued)*

B. Courtesy of National Medical Education & Training Center.

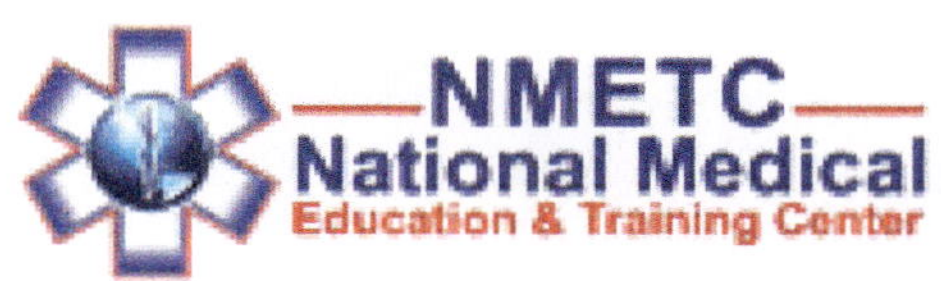

Follow-up review of remediation plan

Student: ______________________ **Date:** __________

Reviewed by: ______________________

Results of remediation: ______________________

____

____

____

____

____

____

Program Directors Final Review **Date:** __________

Recommendations: ______________________

____

____

____

____

Program Director Name: ______________________

Program Director Signature: ______________________

C.C. Student's File

FIGURE 23.3 *(Continued)*

Step 4: Implement the Plan

The instructor must monitor the student's progress closely during remediation, ensuring that all involved parties are performing as described in the plan. The instructor should maintain progress reports and regularly provide the student with corrective feedback. The student should be held accountable for their actions as outlined in the plan. Careful documentation is critical; in the event of legal challenge, the educational team will be called on to provide evidence to show how they advocated for the student.

TEACHING TIP

Instructors may need to address additional issues that arise while there is an active remediation plan in place. Strategies can include revising the current plan or creating an additional plan. The faculty or program has the right to determine how best to address additional issues.

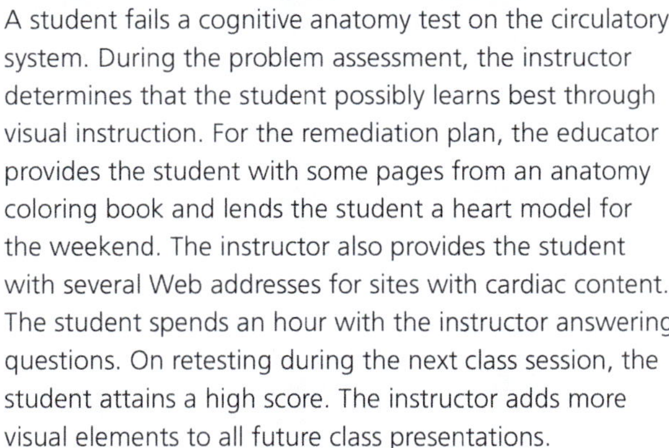

CASE in Point

A student fails a cognitive anatomy test on the circulatory system. During the problem assessment, the instructor determines that the student possibly learns best through visual instruction. For the remediation plan, the educator provides the student with some pages from an anatomy coloring book and lends the student a heart model for the weekend. The instructor also provides the student with several Web addresses for sites with cardiac content. The student spends an hour with the instructor answering questions. On retesting during the next class session, the student attains a high score. The instructor adds more visual elements to all future class presentations.

Step 5: Reevaluate

Remediation plans require sacrifices in time and resources from both the student and the educator, and the stakes are often high. The educator must carefully evaluate the tool that will be used to retest the student to ensure that it is fair and objective. All tools should undergo validity and reliability testing and should be approved by the program director as well as the medical director. The instructor must decide whether the same assessment tool will be used to retest the student. A psychomotor skills test will most likely use an identical tool, but the scenario used to prompt the student to perform the skill may be different.

Using the same tool for a written exam will likely increase the score without necessarily resulting in an increase in the student's knowledge level. Having seen the exam and identifying what was missed may lead the student to correct only those specific errors, with no increased knowledge or improved understanding. Consequently, retesting a written exam with a different tool provides a more accurate measure for determining that true remediation has occurred. If this approach is used, it is essential that the second assessment instrument be parallel to the first. In other words, it should assess the same learning objectives and have questions of similar difficulty levels as the first exam. Educators should seek advice from other members of the educational team if they are unsure about reevaluation decisions.

If retesting involves an instrument with an elevated level of subjectivity, such as a psychomotor skills test that uses an assessment instrument with a global rating scale, the instructor should consider using an independent evaluator who has limited knowledge of the student's previous results.

An educator must ensure that the grading of the reassessment tool complies with the policies for remediation. Depending on how the policy is written, it may be appropriate for the original grade to remain unchanged, with the grade book indicating that a "pass" occurred on retest, or it may be appropriate for the two grades to be averaged. Another process may be appropriate as well; this decision should be based on how the policy is written.

Performance Improvement Plans

A remediation plan for an EMS employee is often developed by the training officer or medical officer and contains the same elements described for a student in an education program; however, the resulting learning contract may be referred to as a performance improvement plan.

Remediation to Improve Outcomes on High-Stakes Certification Exams

Without question, EMS faculty members and the institution where students obtain their EMS instruction have a vested interest in the overall success of the candidate doing well on the final national or state certification or licensure examination. Thus, it is essential to have a process of final remediation in place. Students may have difficulty in the cognitive, psychomotor, or both exam portions of the final testing.

With regard to the psychomotor examinations, the institution should be positioned to assist the student with additional simulation practice scenarios. These should be offered in the same manner as the high-stakes testing format. Drill and practice should be conducted with the student until mastery is achieved. That said, often the problem is not with performing the individual skills, but with the sequencing of the skill or skills. This is a cognitive issue that requires the student and faculty members to ensure the sequencing of the steps in the skill stations is achieved. Again, this is a drill and practice exercise that is best accomplished by ensuring the right steps are done in the right order, simulating actual test conditions as closely as possible.

As for the cognitive examination, faculty should first explore and acknowledge the student's feelings after the failed attempt. In a study of nursing students who failed their licensure exam, researchers found these candidates lived the failure in a way that dominated their lives, experiencing feelings of isolation and self-doubt. They also reported feelings of emptiness and abandonment despite wanting support that they felt was lacking.[8] The instructor should reach out to the failed student early and establish a remediation plan.

The thought of re-studying an entire curriculum is often overwhelming. Faculty can help the student establish a plan with built-in checkpoints to assess progress. Students may need to return to the simulated testing programs. The student should complete any additional practice examinations until such time that they achieve the required scores (cut score as determined by the institution) to predict greater likelihood of success on the national or state examination.

Summary

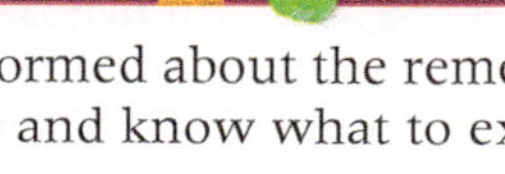

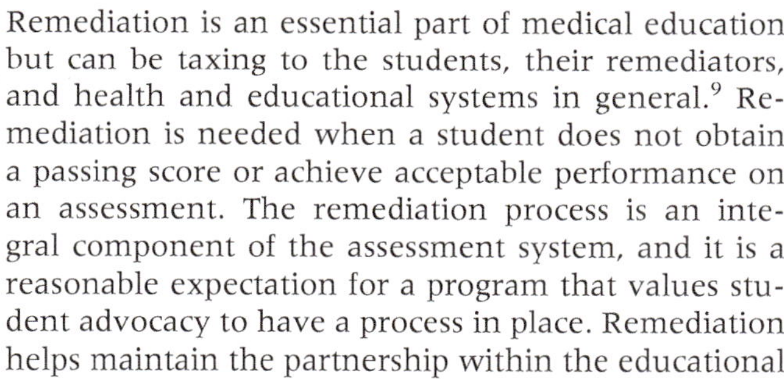

Remediation is an essential part of medical education but can be taxing to the students, their remediators, and health and educational systems in general.[9] Remediation is needed when a student does not obtain a passing score or achieve acceptable performance on an assessment. The remediation process is an integral component of the assessment system, and it is a reasonable expectation for a program that values student advocacy to have a process in place. Remediation helps maintain the partnership within the educational process. Students should be informed about the remediation process well in advance and know what to expect if they need it.

Remediation is necessary for many students. It will not be appropriate in all situations, but it is important that clear guidelines and policies be established before the need arises. With deliberate design, the process can maintain program integrity and provide fair criteria for all students.

Glossary

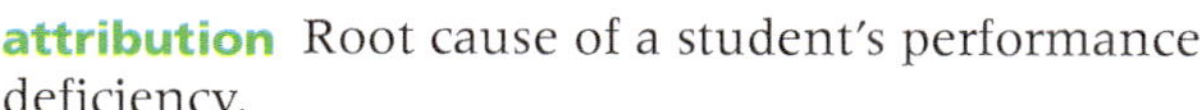

attribution Root cause of a student's performance deficiency.

learning contract Document mutually agreed to by the student and faculty that defines activities and behaviors that must be met in a specified time frame to achieve specific objectives.

remediation Process to analyze and identify performance deficiencies and develop a plan to improve performance.

References

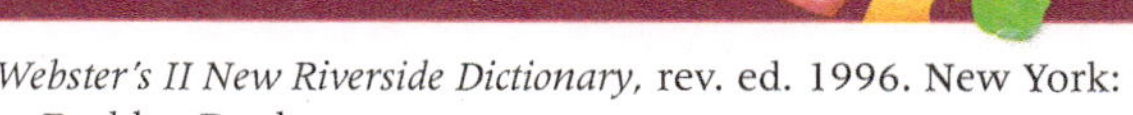

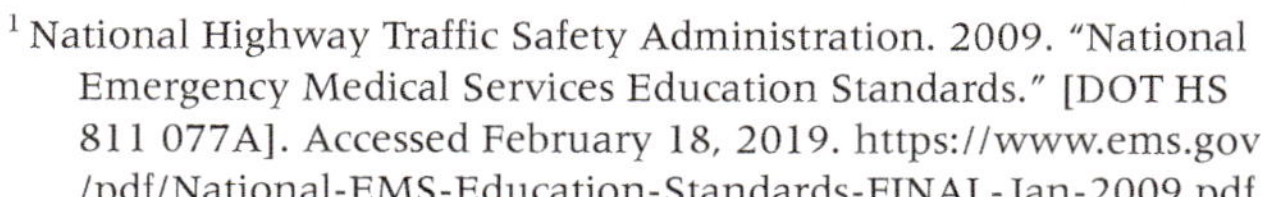

1 National Highway Traffic Safety Administration. 2009. "National Emergency Medical Services Education Standards." [DOT HS 811 077A]. Accessed February 18, 2019. https://www.ems.gov/pdf/National-EMS-Education-Standards-FINAL-Jan-2009.pdf.

2 Boylan, Hunter R., Barbara S. Bonham, and Lizette M. Rodriguez. 2000. "What Are Remedial Courses and Do They Work: Results of National and Local Studies." *Learning Assistance Review* 5: 5–14.

3 *Webster's II New Riverside Dictionary*, rev. ed. 1996. New York: Berkley Books.

4 Spann, Milton G., Jr. 2000. "Remediation: A Must for the 21st Century Learning Society." Policy Paper. Denver, CO: Center for Community College Policy, Education Commission of the States.

5 Colby, Anita, and Ron Opp. 1987. "Controversies Surrounding Developmental Education in the Community College."

Los Angeles: ERIC Clearinghouse for Junior Colleges. Accessed June 5, 2019. https://files.eric.ed.gov/fulltext/ED286557.pdf.

[6] Benner, Patricia. 1982. "From Novice to Expert." *American Journal of Nursing* 82: 402–7.

[7] Adult Education Resource Information Service. 1999, September. "Adult Learning. ARIS Information Sheet." Melbourne, Australia: National Languages and Literacy Institute of Australia. Accessed April 14, 2019. https://files.eric.ed.gov/fulltext/ED434223.pdf.

[8] Poorman, Susan G., and Cheryl A. Webb. 2000. "Preparing to Retake the NCLEX-RN: The Experience of Graduates Who Fail." *Nurse Educator* 25, no. 4: 175–80. http://dx.doi.org/10.1097/00006223-200007000-00013.

[9] Kalet, Adina, Calvin L. Chou, and Rachel H. Ellaway. 2017. "To Fail Is Human: Remediating Remediation in Medical Education." *Prospective on Medical Education* 6, no. 6: 418–24. https://doi.org/10.1007/s40037-017-0385-6.

Additional Resources

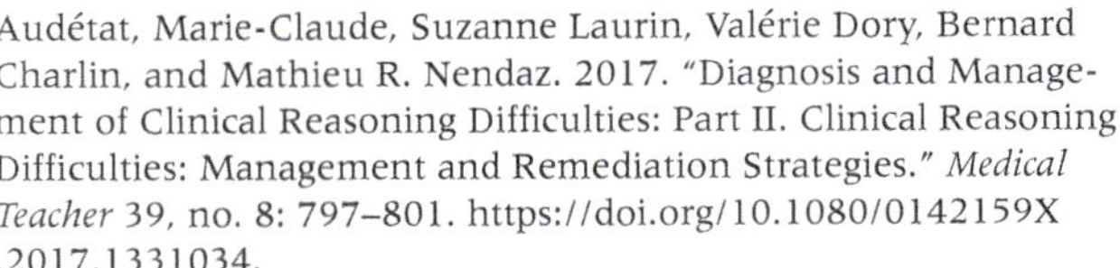

Audétat, Marie-Claude, Suzanne Laurin, Valérie Dory, Bernard Charlin, and Mathieu R. Nendaz. 2017. "Diagnosis and Management of Clinical Reasoning Difficulties: Part II. Clinical Reasoning Difficulties: Management and Remediation Strategies." *Medical Teacher* 39, no. 8: 797–801. https://doi.org/10.1080/0142159X.2017.1331034.

Corrigan-Magaldi, Maryann, Georgina Colalillo, and Janice Molloy. 2014. "Faculty-Facilitated Remediation: A Model to Transform At-Risk Students." *Nurse Educator* 39, no. 4: 155–57. http://dx.doi.org/10.1097/NNE.0000000000000043.

Ellaway, Rachel H., Calvin L. Chou, and Adina L. Kalet. 2018. "Situating Remediation: Accommodating Success and Failure in Medical Education Systems." *Academic Medicine* 93, no. 3: 391–8. http://dx.doi.org/10.1097/ACM.0000000000001855.

Gaither, Gerald H. (Ed.). 1999. *Promising Practices in Recruitment, Remediation and Retention. New Directions for Higher Education*, No. 108. San Francisco: Jossey-Bass.

Hayden, Jennifer. 2010. "Use of Simulation in Nursing Education: National Survey Results." *Journal of Nursing Regulation* 1, no. 3: 52–7. https://doi.org/10.1016/S2155-8256(15)30335-5.

Humphrey, Charlotte. 2010. "Assessment and Remediation for Physicians with Suspected Performance Problems: An International Survey." *Journal of Continuing Education in the Health Professions* 30, no. 1: 26–36. https://doi.org/10.1002/chp.20053.

Kaslow, Nadine J., Muriel J. Bebeau, James W. Lichtenberg, Sanford M. Portnoy, Nancy J. Rubin, Irene W. Leigh, Paul D. Nelson, and I. Leon Smith. 2007. "Guiding Principles and Recommendations for the Assessment of Competence." *Professional Psychology* 38, no. 5: 441–51. http://dx.doi.org/10.1037/0735-7028.38.5.441.

McLaughlin, Michael P. 2010. "Medical Simulation in the Community College Health Science Curriculum: A Matrix for Future Implementation." *Community College Journal of Research and Practice* 34: 462–76. https://doi.org/10.1080/10668920903235811.

Pennington, Tracy D., and Darrell Spurlock. 2010. "A Systematic Review of the Effectiveness of Remediation Interventions to Improve NCLEX-RN Pass Rates." *Journal of Nursing Education* 49, no. 9: 485–92. https://doi.org/10.3928/01484834-20100630-05.

Yeom, Yei-Jin. 2013. "An Investigation of Predictors of NCLEX-RN Outcomes among Nursing Content Standardized Tests." *Nurse Education Today* 33, no. 12: 1523–8. https://doi.org/10.1016/j.nedt.2013.04.004.

PART VI

Administration

In education, administrative responsibilities have long been an integral component of the job. Many educators come from a diverse clinical background and may not have a strong foundation in administrative, legal, and accreditation-related issues. This section has been expanded to include chapters on legal issues and accreditation processes and was designed to assist all levels of emergency medical services (EMS) educators as they evolve into more defined administrative roles. It can be daunting for both novice and experienced educators to ensure that all stakeholders work collaboratively on the development and implementation of policies, procedures, budgets, assessment tools, and safe environments for learning. The administrative chapter provides guidance on best practices for the development of a business plan by utilizing local, state, and federal recommendations to assist educators who assume administrative leadership roles and responsibilities in sustaining positive student and program outcomes.

Major administrative challenges can take the form of liability issues related to the students enrolled in EMS programs. The legal chapter addresses basic areas of liability, whether it be technology, policies, students, classes, or clinical areas. This chapter includes a discussion of legal terminology, concerns related to program and curriculum development, nondiscrimination, and preceptor issues; these discussions are designed to inform the educator regarding the implications of legal and ethical responsibilities as they relate to EMS education. The information provided is not intended to replace accessing legal counsel who specialize in local and state education and health laws.

The addition of the *new* accreditation chapter provides instructors who teach any level of EMS education with information about how the accreditation of a program, hospital, community college, or university provides consumers with the assurance there are standards, reviewed by an external entity, that support successful student, program, and institutional outcomes.

The information in the administrative, legal, and accreditation chapters encourages the professional growth of EMS educators into successful leaders within their institutions and in their communities.

CHAPTER 24

Administrative Issues

OBJECTIVES

At the conclusion of this chapter, the educator will be able to:

Cognitive Domain

1. Outline national, state, and local documents that influence emergency medical services (EMS) program design and operation.
2. Outline the institutional infrastructure needed to operate an EMS program effectively.
3. Recognize key elements of formative and summative program evaluations.
4. Describe how to use program evaluation findings to shape program changes.
5. Detail the steps to develop an operational budget.
6. Discuss the role of the medical director.
7. Describe considerations in program director administrative issues such as instructor contracts, course syllabi, affective assessment, and academic dishonesty.
8. Describe elements for effective general classroom management.
9. Outline steps needed when planning a new educational program.

Psychomotor Domain

There are no psychomotor objectives for this chapter.

Affective Domain

1. Value the need to manage program resources effectively.
2. Promote the need for frequent program evaluation as an improvement tool.

"It is a mark of an educated mind to be able to entertain a thought without accepting it."

~ Aristotle

CHAPTER GOAL This chapter discusses general administrative matters common to programs and instructors as well as issues with which the program director or primary instructor should be familiar.

Whether a seasoned veteran or a new education program administrator, conducting a successful class is much like running the hurdles at a track meet. Good preparation and a solid administrative infrastructure help the program director or primary instructor scale the "hurdles" with deftness and finesse. EMS educators live in a VUCA world—that is, characterized by volatility, uncertainty, complexity, and ambiguity. A masterful academic leader thrives in this environment by setting the vision, assessing the environment, building consensus, and encouraging and mentoring the team to create Relevant Authentic Engaging Learning (REAL) opportunities so that students acquire contemporary knowledge and skills—communicating effectively with stakeholders, abating risk, ensuring quality, creating the budget, monitoring financial performance, and planning and evaluating the work. Lack of effective planning can leave the track littered with frazzled and discouraged educators, grievances, budget variances that threaten program viability, and students who fail to meet academic goals, or worse, experience harm due to program liability. As the saying goes, every system is perfectly designed to achieve the results that it gets.

Although tending to administrative issues may be the responsibility of a program director or lead instructor, every educator has a role in administration of the course, from documenting attendance and enforcing conduct rules, to completing student evaluations. Additionally, every educator should have a basic understanding of, and appreciation for, administrative tasks to maintain order; to protect the institution, program, and faculty from liability; and to ensure fairness and consistency with students. Paying close attention to administrative policies and procedures can also promote the best possible educational experience for students and everyone else involved in the program.

Chapter Format

Administrative issues are not just the purview of the program director. Every member of the educational program team—from director, to instructor, to medical director, to administrative and support staff—needs to appreciate the importance and necessity for administrative issues and proper administrative follow-through. This is especially challenging in EMS education because educational programs are defined and regulated by a number of external forces. The first part of this chapter presents an overview of administrative issues germane to all EMS educational programs, regardless of venue or offering institution. The second part of the chapter addresses those issues of importance to the program director, and the final section describes issues and information important to the individual course instructor.

The reader is encouraged to review Chapter 25, *Legal Issues for EMS Educators*, as a number of issues discussed in this chapter have a basis in laws and regulations presented in the chapter.

It may seem that running an EMS educational program is a confusing and monumental undertaking, especially if the program is a "one-person shop" or "one full-time person shop" supplemented by part-time instructors. The difficulty lies in determining how to juggle national, state, local, and institutional issues and still teach. This can indeed be a challenge, and one way to transition into this role is to find a strong and effective mentor.

Conducting a program with excellent results takes more than transitioning good street providers into the classroom to impart their knowledge to the next generation of EMS personnel. It is a good place to start, but most quickly discover that they do not even know what they do not know and need to come up to speed as fast as possible. *Details make a difference; foundational competency in the principles of teaching and learning is essential, and egos need to be left at the door!*

The best place to begin is to find a program demonstrating best-practice models and superior outcomes, and seek a mentoring relationship with that instructor or program director. This program need not be in EMS; it could be another health-related field or one suggested by a dean or other academic leader. This can assist in creating an administrative infrastructure that provides a sound foundation upon which an excellent program can be built, sustained, and ever improved.

Administrative Foundation

This section provides an overview and introduction to national, state, and local issues; consensus documents; and regulations that affect EMS education. As with any broad overview, the reader is cautioned that state and local authority has final jurisdiction; thus, not all of the material presented may be applicable to each specific program.

National Curricular and Administrative Issues

The National Highway Traffic Safety Administration (NHTSA), a division of the U.S. Department of Transportation (DOT), is currently recognized as the lead federal agency for the development of national EMS consensus documents. The Emergency Medical Services for Children (EMSC), a division of the Maternal and Child Health Bureau (MCHB) within the Health Resources and Services Administration (HRSA), partners with NHTSA to support and promote many EMS activities.

The original *EMS Agenda for the Future* (Agenda) was a federally funded position paper completed by the National Association of EMS Physicians (NAEMSP) in conjunction with the National Association of State EMS Directors (NASEMSD) and published in 1996. The purpose of the document was to "predict the future by creating it."[1] It served as the guiding force to drive change across the country and to impact EMS providers, healthcare organizations and institutions, governmental agencies, and policy makers for 20 years. Notable among its many recommendations was that EMS educational programs should seek affiliations with academic institutions to enhance their professional standing.

The Agenda sunsetted in 2016. During that time, health care experienced a revolution of reform to a person-centered model characterized by value-based, coordinated, humanistic, and population-based care with risk capitation and new payment models that required sophisticated data and care environment interoperability. Using EMS personnel as navigators in the new care integration model required enhanced planning for EMS education programs as well.

To meet these challenges, the 1996 Agenda has been updated to the *EMS Agenda 2050* (**FIGURE 24.1**).[2] NHTSA hosted a national implementation forum in September of 2018. Speakers challenged EMS leaders to begin making changes necessary to achieve a people-centered EMS system. "Doing things that are truly people-centered will take hard work and create bruised egos," said Andy Gienapp, director of the Wyoming Office of EMS. "But that's our challenge. Stop doing things because they are convenient"[3] (EMS.gov). The EMS Agenda 2050 sets the course for the next 30 years.

The following relevant background information is important: After the Agenda was published, NHTSA and EMSC convened a task force in January of 1998 to discuss the EMS educational system and the high variability of EMS scopes of practice around the country.

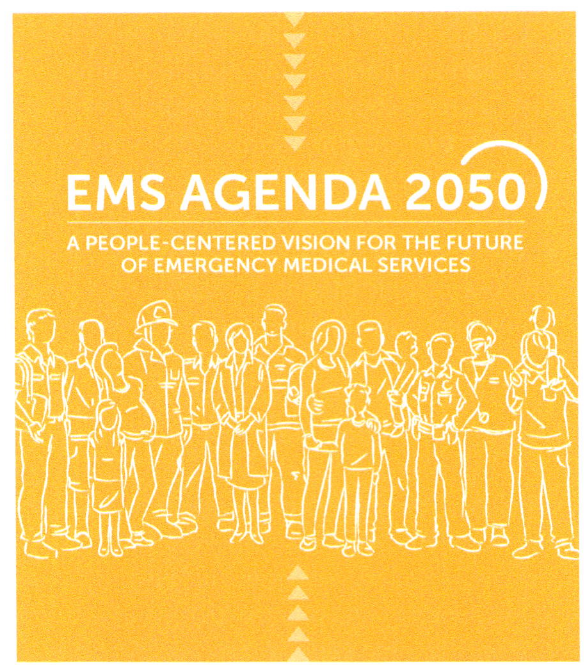

FIGURE 24.1 *EMS Agenda 2050.*

Reproduced from EMS Agenda 2050 Technical Expert Panel. 2019, January. *EMS Agenda 2050: A People-Centered Vision for the Future of Emergency Medical Services* [DOT HS 812 664]. Washington, DC: National Highway Traffic Safety Administration. Accessed February 12, 2019. https://www.ems.gov/pdf/EMS-Agenda-2050.pdf.

Out of that task force, the *EMS Education Agenda for the Future: A Systems Approach* (EMS Education Agenda) was developed and published in 2000 using the same extensive, peer-reviewed process that was so successful for the Agenda (**FIGURE 24.2**).[4]

The Education Agenda set the vision for increasing the quality, structure, professionalism, and accountability for EMS education, thus advancing EMS education standards in alignment with medical, nursing, and other allied health programs. It declared that EMS education programs should support, not define, the scopes of practice by teaching to national standards. It built upon the Agenda to outline steps to enhance the consistency, quality, and efficacy of EMS education with the goal of increased competency among program graduates. The Education Agenda set forth a model with five integrated components:

- National EMS Core Content
- National EMS Scope of Practice Model
- National EMS Education Standards
- National EMS Testing and Certification
- National EMS Education Program Accreditation[4]

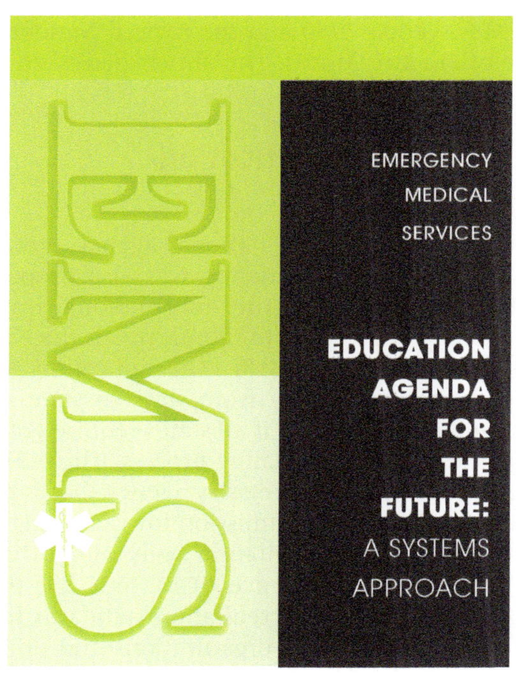

FIGURE 24.2 *EMS Education Agenda for the Future.*

Reproduced from National Highway Traffic Safety Administration. 2000. *Emergency Medical Services Education Agenda for the Future: A Systems Approach*. [DOT HS 809 042]. Washington, DC: U.S. Department of Health and Human Services. Accessed May 10, 2019. https://www.ems.gov/pdf/education/EMS-Education-for-the-Future-A-Systems-Approach/EMS_Education_Agenda.pdf.

The Education Agenda prescribed a high degree of structure, coordination, and interdependence among the five components. Both the Agenda and EMS Agenda 2050 are important reading for anyone who is or wishes to become an EMS administrator or educator. These documents may be obtained from several websites: www.naemse.org and www.ems.gov are good resources.

National EMS Core Content

The National EMS Core Content document was published in 2005 by NHTSA. Led by the NAEMSP and the American College of Emergency Physicians (ACEP), the document defines the entire domain of EMS knowledge and skills without assigning the skills into any specific provider level.[5] This document falls primarily within the medical domain and is led by the medical community with input from multiple stakeholders.

National EMS Scope of Practice Model

Practice as an EMS provider is dependent on education, certification of competency, state licensure, and medical director credentialing of practice privileges.

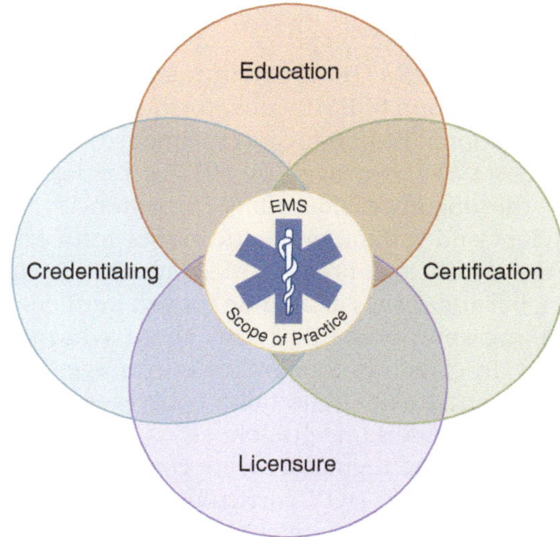

FIGURE 24.3 The National EMS Scope of Practice Model is the intersection of education, certification, licensure, and credentialing of EMS professionals.

Reproduced from Friese, Greg. 2018, December 19. Quick Take: Introducing the 2018 National EMS Scope of Practice Model. Accessed March 28, 2019. https://www.ems1.com/ems-education/articles/393090048-Quick-Take-Introducing-the-2018-National-EMS-Scope-of-Practice-model/.

The National EMS Scope of Practice Model (2007 Model) is at the intersection of each of those elements (**FIGURE 24.3**). The 2007 Model project was led by the National Association of State EMS Officials (NASEMSO) and the former National Council of State EMS Training Coordinators with multiple other EMS community and stakeholder participants.

The document was published by NHTSA and identified four levels of EMS providers: emergency medical responder (EMR), emergency medical technician (EMT), advanced EMT (AEMT), and paramedic.[6] It was updated in November 2017 to add narcotic antagonists, tourniquets, and wound packing to the EMR and EMT licensure levels.

In 2016, NASEMSO, under contract with NHTSA and HRSA, launched an initiative to revise the 2007 Model. It used an extensive representative process to provide an evidence-based approach to identify practice gaps between the old model and emerging science, current EMS practice, and community needs. When scientific literature was inconclusive, expert opinion was used to inform the document. The work of the expert panel concluded in June of 2018, and their findings were presented in a webinar format in the fall of 2018.[7]

Each provider level is assigned specific skills that are intended to be a floor for that level nationally. The NASEMSO update is recommended to states for adoption to ensure consistency and promote reciprocity and serves as the basis for updating the National EMS Education Standards.

National EMS Education Standards

NHTSA and HRSA (EMSC) contracted with the National Association of EMS Educators (NAEMSE) to create the National EMS Education Standards (Standards) (**FIGURE 24.4**).[8] Approved by NHTSA on January 30, 2009, the document identifies competencies, clinical behaviors and judgments, educational infrastructure, and the depth and breadth of content to include at each level and serves as a guide for program personnel in making appropriate decisions about what material to cover in class. The document encourages educator creativity and flexibility to tailor courses to local needs while meeting national guidelines.

Educators and regulators were concerned that transitioning from the DOT curriculum to the Standards would be a difficult paradigm shift. In response, companion documents, called *Instructional Guidelines* (Guidelines), were simultaneously published for each level of practice. The Guidelines provided elaboration of the content included in the Standards, but quickly became outdated as the body of EMS knowledge evolved. They were intended to provide short-term guidance to help programs adapt to the new model and were specifically *not* intended to be part of the Standards.

In 2018, NAEMSE and the RedFlash Group were awarded the contract to update the National EMS Education Standards based on the new vision set forth in the EMS Agenda 2050 and the revised National EMS Scope of Practice Model. The anticipated issue date is 2021.

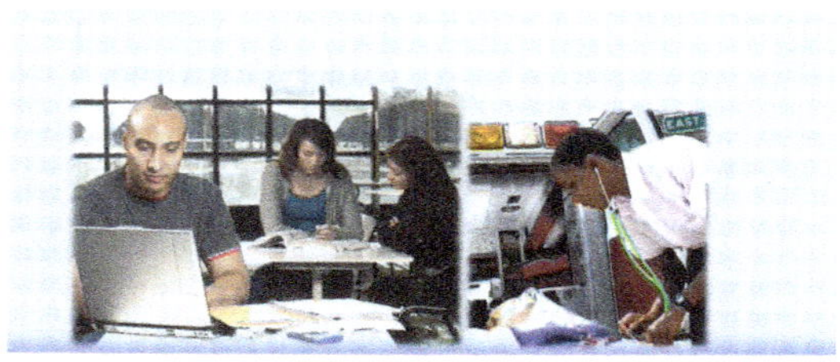

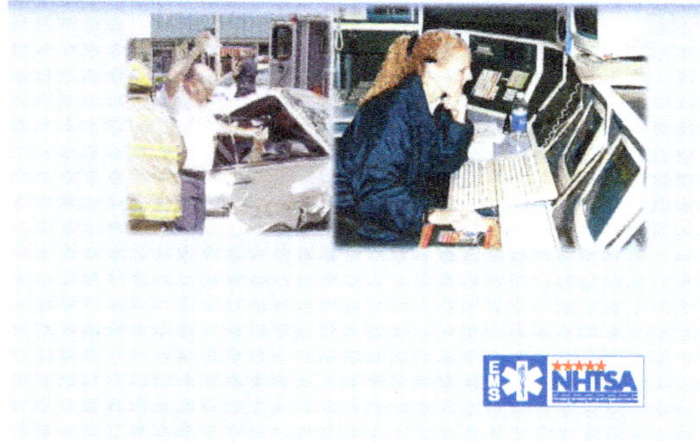

FIGURE 24.4 The National EMS Education Standards.

Reproduced from National Highway Traffic Safety Administration. 2009. "National Emergency Medical Services Education Standards." [DOT HS 811 077A]. Accessed January 15, 2019. https://www.ems.gov/pdf/National-EMS-Education-Standards-FINAL-Jan-2009.pdf.

National EMS Certification/Credentialing

The creation of a single national agency process for EMS testing and credentialing was also proposed in the Education Agenda. The only national organization that currently exists to fill this role is the National Registry of EMTs (NREMT). The Education Agenda proposes that reciprocity from state to state will be easier and more efficient if all states require graduates to use the same credentialing process. The NREMT is currently the only EMS registry agency that is accredited by the National Commission for Certifying Agencies (NCCA), the accreditation body of the Institute for Credentialing Excellence (ICE). NCCA is the recognized authority on accreditation standards for professional certification of organizations and programs. The NREMT also identifies requirements for renewal of registration. In many states, continuing education (CE) and recertification or relicensure requirements are also managed through the biennial NREMT reregistration process.

The NREMT has candidate handbooks for those pursuing their initial certification that provide a step-by-step process for submitting applications and taking the certification exams. They are available on the NREMT website (www.nremt.org) in a downloadable digital format. Handbooks are available for EMR, EMT, AEMT, and paramedic certifications.

More information on the psychomotor exam can also be found at the NREMT website (www.nremt.org/rwd/public/document/psychomotor-exam).

National EMS Education Program Accreditation

The last pillar of the Education Agenda is National EMS Education Program Accreditation. In the Agenda, the accreditation described is programmatic and is intended to be tied to national certification. Currently, only paramedic candidates who have graduated from a **Commission on Accreditation of Allied Health Education Programs (CAAHEP)**–accredited program are eligible to take the NREMT paramedic cognitive and psychomotor exams.

Although the concept of national certification married to national accreditation proposed in the Agenda includes all levels of EMS practitioners, only the paramedic level has currently operationalized this requirement with variable state adoption. CAAHEP does not accredit programs that are shorter than one academic year (two semesters).[9] Standards have been developed for accreditation of AEMT programs.

Chapter 26, *Fundamentals of Accreditation and Program Evaluation*, provides a foundation in accreditation and related topics. For more information on credible education through accreditation, go to www.coaemsp.org.

Although not mentioned in the Education Agenda, accreditation also exists for CE programs in EMS. The Commission on Accreditation for Prehospital Continuing Education (CAPCE) reviews and accredits EMS-related CE including live, online, and virtual instructor-led training refresher classes. Applicants must demonstrate sound educational design, physician oversight, relevant references that are current and appropriate in breadth of coverage, and appropriate educational infrastructure.[10] CAPCE accreditation is particularly useful as it is possible for participants to earn CE credit at national or regional EMS conferences and workshops conducted outside the person's home state or for students to obtain CE through distance-learning options.

State-Level Administrative Issues

The governance of EMS is the responsibility of each state and territory. Each jurisdiction's laws or statutes and their attendant regulations or administrative rules contain specific directives regarding the education, scope of practice, certification, licensure, credentialing, and renewal of EMS licenses/certificates.

The location of each state's lead EMS agency varies, but it is typically found inside the Department of Public Health, the Department of Public Safety, or the Office of Emergency Management, or it is established as a separate state agency or division. The state EMS agency is often organized into sections that may include (but not be limited to) testing and licensure or certification; education; trauma systems; special populations (e.g., EMSC, ST-elevation myocardial infarction [STEMI], elderly, stroke); data management, emergency preparedness, and response; vehicle licensing and operation; other strategic trends; communications; information technology; resource funding, allocation, and utilization; and medical oversight. Each state should have an EMS Act or other enabling legislation outlining its scope, function, and authority.

The state EMS agency is usually given the authority to develop, adopt, and periodically update rules and regulations that implement the relevant laws or statutes. Time is generally allowed for input and comment from stakeholders who have an interest in or are impacted by proposed changes in laws, rules, and/or regulations. The state legislature, via bodies such as the joint committee on administrative rules, is responsible for ensuring that the intent of the statute is preserved and rules are fully consistent with law.

Each state has statutes unique to its jurisdiction. Some are more prescriptive than others, and some delegate more responsibility to the state EMS agency or a local governmental office. In addition to the state EMS agency, the Department of Education of each state frequently has additional or similar laws that regulate the establishment of educational institutions and the qualifications of instructors, including those who offer EMS education.

Each EMS educator must be familiar with the state's laws, rules, and regulations regarding education where they teach. States may require that EMS program directors, primary (lead) instructors, or classroom educators have particular education and/or credentials in order to teach, as well as appropriate CE to continue their eligibility to teach.

To fill the need for initial education and certification, NAEMSE created the instructor courses and the national EMS educator certification (NEMSEC) exam. For more information, see www.naemse.org/page/aboutnemsec. States may also require that educational programs meet specific minimum regulations before beginning operations. The states, in most cases, do not accredit educational programs, although they may use the terms "accredit" or "accreditation." The states typically provide authorization to the program based on content, organization with time specifications, objectives, operation, educators, and/or outcome criteria. Accreditation is, by nature, based on a structured self-appraisal that is overseen by professional peers, not by state regulators or any governmental entity.

Instructors must be able to access the statutes and/or rules if students request the information or ask questions that must be answered within the context of the law of regulations. It is a good idea for instructors to include information regarding how students can access these documents within the student handbook or orientation materials.

Local Issues

Most local jurisdictions do not have specific regulations related to EMS or emergency services education. However, general local ordinances and regulations such as zoning laws, noise regulations, taxes, and so on, may apply to an educational institution providing EMS education. The other possible source of local administrative issues may relate to EMS educational programs that are designed to serve the needs of a specific response agency such as a local ambulance district or city fire department. Admissions, class schedule, length of program, location of classes, and so forth may be specified in the training-program contract. It is important that any such contractual relationships clearly define the role of the instructor, the educational institution, and the response agency, as related to student performance, discipline, and dismissal. These issues may have special implications for personnel employed by unionized agencies. However, the educational institution should not compromise its educational standards or quality to meet such requirements.

Institutional Issues

Each educational institution has its own set of rules, regulations, and procedures for delivery of an educational program. It is imperative that the program director, instructors, medical director, and administrative staff know and follow them. Failure to do so may result in, at the least, confusion and inconvenience, and more seriously, harm to students academically and financially. Program and institutional accreditation is predicated on adherence to such regulations.

Program Director-Related Administrative Issues

Each program must have a program director and primary (lead) instructor; in some cases, this may be the same person. The program director is responsible for all aspects of the program, including, but not limited to, the following:

- Administration, organization, and supervision of the educational program
- Continuous quality review and improvement of the educational program
- Long-range planning and ongoing development of the program
- Effectiveness of the program, including instruction and faculty, with systems in place to demonstrate the effectiveness of the program
- Cooperative involvement with the medical director
- Orientation/training and supervision of clinical and field internship preceptors
- Effectiveness and quality of fulfillment of responsibilities delegated to another qualified individual[11]

Admission Policies

Admission to an EMS program may be open to anyone, with or without meeting minimum eligibility criteria (open vs. limited enrollment). Some programs require minimum English, reading, writing, and math placement criteria that should be specified in the admission requirements. These prerequisites are designed to ensure that students have the necessary reading comprehension, computational, and written communications skills to be successful in the program prior to enrolling in the course.

The admissions process may require a prospective applicant to attend an informational meeting and submit the following: an application, verification of meeting the minimum age requirement by the time of credentialing, official documentation of high school enrollment in good academic standing, transcripts, or general education development (GED) results, college transcripts, proof of a current driver's license, current EMT license (if applying to AEMT or paramedic classes), and a current cardiopulmonary resuscitation (CPR) for healthcare provider card. It is important to note that it is not appropriate to ask a potential student's age; only whether or not the individual will meet the minimum age requirement by the time of credentialing testing.

Some programs have a competitive admission process that gives higher standing for admission to those with general or science-specific academic course credits, EMS or other patient care affiliations and/or experience, military service, or higher assessment scores. Regardless of the setting or type of admission process, it should be fair, be nondiscriminatory, with objective and defendable criteria, and meet the needs of the local EMS community and education program.

Criteria should be clear and published so they are easily accessed by all applicants. Prospective students should be given information on the content and nature of preadmission tests to help optimize their performance on those assessments. Admissions policies should be carefully crafted with the assistance of subject matter experts (admissions personnel at a college or university) and receive the approval of deans or comparable administrators who oversee the EMS educational program. Policies must be closely aligned and consistent with state and federal laws and regulations. (See Chapter 25, *Legal Issues for EMS Educators*, for additional information on legal requirements related to program admission.)

Course Policies/Handbook

There are many layers of rights, obligations, deliverables, expectations, consents, and agreements inherent in a student–program relationship. The names of these documents may vary from institution to institution, but the contents should always include the key issues identified in this section. The more common names for these collections of policies and documents are "student policies" or "student handbook."

Elements for inclusion in course policies or a student handbook may include, but not be limited to, the following, in no specific order:

- Program core values
- Student accountability statement
- Program accreditation or approvals
- Safe, inclusive campus environment/equal opportunity statement
- Program description; core courses, methods of instruction
- Student outcomes/competencies; general goals, objectives, and expected learning outcomes
- Academic calendar and/or schedule of topics with corresponding readings, possible references, useful websites; general activities by course or dates
- Explanation of major classroom assignments or required projects and due dates
- Explanation of hospital and field clinical rotations, including scheduling required hours, unit assignments, minimum patient contacts and number of skill revolutions, documentation requirements, and criteria for successful outcomes
- Required textbooks (print or digital options)
- Explanation of portfolio creation, if required
- Requirement to purchase and/or use specific learning management system software to log and track patient care contacts and skill completion
- Equipment or supplies needed for class, labs, and/or clinical experiences to be provided by the student (e.g., pencils, whiteboard markers, erasers, stethoscope, penlight)
- Health, criminal background check, and immunization requirements
- Insurance requirements: health, liability
- Attendance and class participation policies; how each affects students' grades, if applicable
- Special instructions for items that are not self-explanatory (e.g., parameters for an oral report, lab etiquette, or logistics for student participation)
- Code of student and faculty conduct: Statements of expected behaviors at all times during any component of the program. These may include provisions such as uncompromising academic and research ethical behavior based on the standards and codes of professional conduct established by statute, rules, EMS organizations, and program policy; adherence to all statutes, rules, protocols, and procedures that govern the program and EMS care, which includes compliance with the federal Health Insurance Portability and Accountability Act (HIPAA) Privacy Rule requirements; and policies regarding academic dishonesty and compliance with the Family Educational Rights and Privacy Act (FERPA)
- Required professional interpersonal skills
- Consequences for violations of professional conduct rules based on verification of prohibited behaviors
- Just culture and corrective actions: Disciplinary policies, including student and faculty grievance policies, due process rights, filing an appeal, and recovery of damages/restitution
- Evaluation and measurement of student, program, faculty and preceptor performance; how objective achievement is measured in all three domains of learning; also includes scheduled examination dates, policy on missed exams and late assignment submissions, grading and retest policies, and explanation of final computation of grade point averages
- Course completion criteria
- Options for credentialing exams
- General course policies: classroom civility and language; counseling opportunities; dress and decorum guideline that include the wearing of ID badges, approved jewelry, body art, and piercings; hygiene; food in the classroom; harassment; discrimination; diversity, inclusion, and cultural awareness; inclement weather; parking; drug, smoking, and tobacco product use; social media and technology use; tuition and fees; course drop dates and payment refund policy; veterans' benefits; and withdrawing from class
- Safety policies: Classroom, lab, clinical, and field policies and procedures, including emergent reporting and evaluation of substance exposures or injuries
- Standard precautions and body substance isolation methods and the proper use of personal protective equipment (PPE)
- Students with disabilities and academic accommodation policies
- Student resources: May include, but not be limited to, student development, access and disability services (ADS), health and psychological services and wellness programs, student activities, fitness center, academic support services (reading and writing resource for learning division, support for English language learners, math credit recovery), college and career counseling to help students make informed career decisions; library and computer lab

- Essential job functions and functional job description of an EMS professional, which may include, but not be limited to, the following: Requirements for language and mathematical competency; intellectual and reasoning ability; ability to cope with stress and emotional intelligence; the ability to safely operate equipment generally found on an ambulance for the level of practitioner being taught; the ability to operate communications equipment and enter and retrieve data from a computer; use of program-approved software to specified standards of competency; and physical demands for vision, hearing, strength, endurance, conditioning, motor control, and manual dexterity
- Work environment elements that can place an EMS professional at risk despite appropriate mitigation
- Roles and responsibilities of the program medical director in student evaluation, terminal competency verification, and sign-off for NREMT or state testing
- Any program disclaimers, faculty contact information, and hours of availability
- Terms and reach of policy application. For example:

  The student, by virtue of applying for or accepting a position in the class, assumes the responsibility to conform to all applicable governmental laws, regulations, ordinances, policies, procedures, and protocols governing citizen conduct as well as those addressing students and licensed emergency medical services (EMS) personnel, including all federal, state, local, and program requirements.

  These standards of conduct apply to:

  - *Applicants who become students, for offenses committed as part of the application process.*
  - *Applicants who become students and program faculty, for offenses committed on the program's campus and/or while engaging in program-related events or activities that take place following a student's submittal of the application or an instructor's submission of the independent contractor agreement and throughout his or her tenure with the program. They also apply to former students and faculty for offenses committed while a student or faculty member.*

Agreements/Learning Contracts

It is imperative that each student and faculty member sign a statement that provides written proof that they have been given access to the policies/handbook, understand their meaning, and agree to follow them. Without this written verification, students and faculty could challenge sanctions for noncompliance, claiming that they were never informed, and be successful in their appeals. The signed acknowledgment page from each agreement, with a copy of the specific handbook/policies, should be kept on file for each one. Students may also be asked to sign forms for release of academic information, consent for invasive procedures, photo consent, and agreement to participate in emergency preparedness exercises, based on program policy.

Instructors should also read every word of the student handbook/policies and follow the policies to the letter. The documents(s) should be reviewed before the beginning of each new program and edits made as needed. Every class seems to have someone who artfully uncovers an unsuspected loophole and challenges program conventions, governance, or operations because the policies were unclear, ambiguous, or silent on a particular topic. Thus, experience becomes a painful catalyst for closing those gaps.

If the program is conducted in collaboration with or under the jurisdiction of a college or university, they will already have general policies in place that have been vetted by the institution's attorneys. Instructors must align any program-specific policies with the college's documents. If a student handbook must be created for the first time, a good strategy is to find examples from respected high-performing programs or templates published in peer-reviewed literature. Veteran instructors are usually more than willing to share resources if asked. Obtain permission prior to using or adapting their verbiage and cite sources in your document. The handbook/policy manual forms the basis of an enforceable covenant between the program and students. Thus, it must be thoughtfully prepared in full compliance with laws, rules, and guidelines and have requirements that are specific, measurable, attainable, realistic, and defendable, and that change as little as possible during each course.

Disability Accommodations

EMS educational programs should not discriminate against otherwise qualified individuals who have a disability. However, students must be able to demonstrate the physical, intellectual, and emotional capacity to perform all of the essential functions of the profession during the course, with or without reasonable accommodation. Information on access and disability services may be included in the syllabus, student policies/handbook, or both. It is important that the program specify the essential functions of the profession so that prospective students can self-identify their ability to successfully complete the class. Several examples of a functional job analysis for EMS personnel are available online. See the NHTSA or International Association of Fire Fighters (IAFF) websites for excellent templates.

After admission to the program, students should be instructed, if applicable, to make written requests for accommodations for documented disabilities to the program director or lead instructor. Programs may not discriminate based on a disability covered by Americans with Disability Act of 1973 if the student can (with reasonable accommodations) otherwise perform all of the essential elements in the functional job description and meet program objectives in all three domains of learning. (See Chapter 25, *Legal Issues for EMS Educators*, and Appendix B, *Disabilities in EMS Education*.) Processing such requests may take a few weeks, so the request should be submitted before the course begins or as early in the course as possible, and must be accompanied by documentation from a medical professional confirming and describing the disability with recommended accommodations. An individual representing the teaching institution with expertise in disability issues may be needed to ascertain whether the individual making the disability diagnosis and recommending the accommodation is qualified to do so. The program will need to review whether the accommodations requested are reasonable for the program to make based on resources. Applicants should be counseled that, although all students with a disability may not be able to successfully complete the course, the law was enacted to provide access to job training for those who are otherwise qualified. Reasonable accommodations made during the course by a particular program do not guarantee a similar accommodation for the NREMT or state exams. Students should address specific accommodation requests to the NREMT and/or the state EMS office according to their criteria.

Religious and Cultural Accommodations

With the ever-increasing diversity of the population, it is common to have class participants from different cultural backgrounds, with different gender identities, and a wide variety of world views and sincerely held beliefs. Students may request accommodations due to their religious practices and cultural norms. How the instructor responds to these requests is often guided by institutional policy. Program policies may not impose restrictions on outside-of-class activities unless the individual is representing themselves to be an agent of the program and policies specifically reference the scope of the policy's reach.

One of the more common issues encountered involves student participation in class and/or clinical rotations on days with a religious observance or prohibition to work. Observance of a Sabbath may prevent a student from scheduling a clinical or field internship shift from Friday at sundown through Saturday or on a Sunday. Traditionally, academic calendars observed major federal as well as Christian holidays such as Christmas and Easter. However, more and more institutions, school systems, and governments are recognizing the Jewish high holy days and other ethnic or religious holidays as being acceptable for an excused absence for a student's personal observance. Most policies encourage instructors to allow makeup of assignments or testing missed during one of these absences. The student remains accountable for knowing content covered and completing work that was missed during their absence. Whenever possible, instructors should avoid scheduling major class activities such as tests or mandatory labs on these days.

Muslim students are required to pray several times per day. There are restrictions on where these prayers can occur, such as in an area where blood is present. Thus a student in a clinical setting may not be able to meet this obligation or will need assistance to find a suitable area. Students may also bring their prayer rug or mat with them to class, clinical, and/or field sites.[12]

A concern that may arise with some students is a religious requirement to maintain a beard. Agencies used for field internships may have requirements related to using self-contained breathing apparatus (SCBA) that preclude the wearer from having facial hair that would prevent a tight mask seal. This issue has been addressed in a number of legal challenges, and the outcomes most often come down on the side of provider and patient safety. EMS services should have a policy to address or accommodate this religious practice.

Dress codes also need to take into consideration religious and cultural norms with respect to head covering and clothing requirements that may pose a concern for freedom of movement, work safety, infection control issues, and professional identity. Be sensitive to the needs for student modesty in lab sessions where areas of the body are exposed to practice assessment or skills. The instructor should provide reasonable accommodation if safely possible and within program guidelines.

Equal Opportunity Statement

Programs that receive federal dollars are required to have an Equal Opportunity Statement that declares the program's commitment to nondiscriminatory practices. Statutory references that support the statement may also be listed. For example:

> To the extent provided by applicable law, no person shall be excluded from participation in, denied the benefits of, or be subject to discrimination under any program or activity sponsored or conducted by The Program or any of its component institutions, on the basis of race, color, national origin, ancestry, religion, gender, sexual orientation, age, marital status, physical or mental disability, or veteran's status as long as

> the individual is otherwise qualified to perform all the essential elements of a [practitioner's] scope of practice and meets eligibility requirements for [practitioner's] licensure. It is the policy of The Program to strive to maintain an educational and work environment free from impermissible discrimination.

Discipline Policies, Grievances, Appeals Process; Restitution

All programs should encourage accountability and behaviors that reflect program values and policies within a **culture of safety**.

Any student or faculty member suspected of, or alleged to have demonstrated, behavior that is unprofessional, unethical, inappropriate, inconsistent with program values or policies, or illegal must be awarded due process during the discovery of facts, determination of findings, and resolution processes.

As a first step, the alleged wrongdoer and instructor should discuss the situation and their points of view face-to-face with a witness present. The alleged wrongdoer should be able to present a defense or rebuttal to the allegations against them, explaining their reasons for unacceptable performance. Programs should have form templates for conducting an investigation so no process steps or due process rights are omitted or violated.

Students and faculty also have the right to file complaints and to receive due process for the resolution of grievances that may be lodged against the program, instructors, or other students. Programs should follow policies that address the process steps and protections inherent in a grievance process. A grievance should be resolved at the lowest level possible.

Ensure that all investigative materials, findings, and meeting proceedings are maintained in strictest confidence and are disseminated only to the parties permitted access due to their direct involvement in the situation. The person bringing the grievance or allegation must be afforded full immunity from reprisals or retaliatory actions stemming from the act of bringing a grievance (whistleblower protections).

If the allegations are sustained, the alleged wrongdoer should receive corrective coaching, penalties, or disciplinary action. Corrective coaching is generally progressive and shall be communicated privately and delivered in a timely manner. Corrective action is generally intended to be a positive, nonpunitive intervention that allows an individual time to correct an identified deviation from expected behavior. Personal coaching, a verbal warning, a written warning, a written reprimand, or a last chance agreement may precede suspension or dismissal. However, for more severe offenses, the disciplinary process may begin with suspension or expulsion. In each instance, consequences are to be fair, just, and proportionate to the seriousness of the offense.

The program should include an appeal process for sanctions that prevent a student's academic progression and/or result in suspension or dismissal prior to the terms of the discipline being imposed, unless the nature of the allegation is so egregious that an immediate suspension or dismissal is deemed necessary by the program and medical directors.[1]

Some programs have a standing student affairs committee composed of class peers who are empowered to hear an appeal on matters related to discipline in an informal process and to render an opinion. This opinion may or may not be binding on the student or the faculty member depending on program policy.

If a student remains dissatisfied with the outcome, the student should have the option of appealing to a program administrator or a hearing board that is empowered to review the facts and affirm, modify, or reverse the disciplinary recommendation(s). The student and the faculty member recommending disciplinary action should have the right to be heard by a neutral fact-finder in a fair and unbiased hearing.[13]

Recovery of Damages/Restitution

If a student or faculty member is found to have defaced or damaged program or another person's property, policies should stipulate that they will be assessed the cost for expenses incurred by the program or other parties resulting from the student's or instructor's infraction. Such reimbursement may take the form of monetary payment or appropriate service to repair or otherwise compensate for damages to program property or equipment. Restitution may be imposed on any student who alone, or through group activities, participates in causing the damages or costs to the program. Policy may stipulate that the student will not graduate or a faculty member will not receive full remuneration until full restitution has been made.

Inclement Weather Policy

It is a matter of policy whether an educational program stays open or adjusts its academic schedule during inclement weather (**FIGURE 24.5**). This may be determined at the program level or it may be imposed by the academic institution with which the EMS program is affiliated. The policy should affirm that the foundational concern is always student and faculty safety. Possible language is as follows:

> The Program will make their best assessment of the safety and practicality of travel due to adverse weather. No pressure is extended from the Program on any

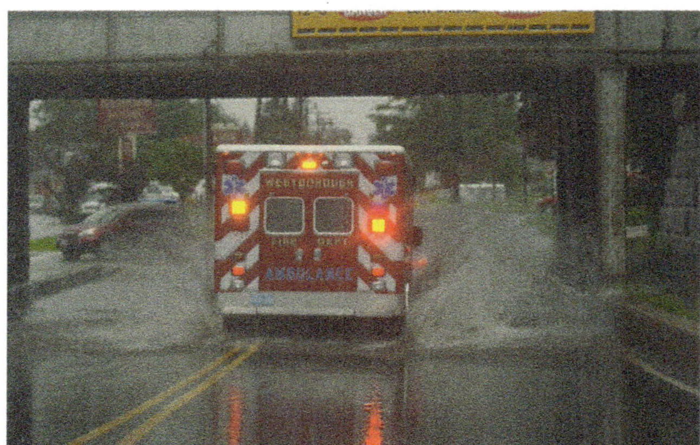

FIGURE 24.5 It is a matter of policy whether an educational program stays open or adjusts its academic schedule during inclement weather.

educator or student to take unsafe chances to attend a class. The safety and well-being of our educators and students is of paramount importance in all situations.

The policy should specify conditions under which class schedules may need to be altered or modified and to allow flexibility to usual and customary attendance policies. The policy should stipulate who is authorized to make the decision to invoke the policy, cancel class, or resume normal class schedules. The following questions should be considered as the policy is developed or reviewed.

- What are the implications if a class is canceled in terms of student objective achievement (is it the day of a major exam?), financial considerations, and work hours of EMS agency employees who are detailed to class as their duty assignment, and how should these be addressed?
- What elements need to be included in the policy, such as a flexible approach authorizing a late start or an abbreviated class schedule for the session, authorizing students to arrive late without penalty, up to canceling the class?
- What is to be included in the notice, and how long in advance of the cancellation must it be issued?
- How will the program communicate to students and faculty that the schedule is altered or a class has been canceled? One of the greatest challenges is the method by which these changes are effectively conveyed to all students and faculty with enough advance notice for them to take appropriate action. Variations in commute times, distances, and methods of transportation pose different challenges to each student. Communication options may include local radio or television community-service announcements; phone tree activation; auto-calls with a recorded message; website notice, group email, text message, or use of other social media platforms; and/or a voicemail message on the program's main phone line. Also specify how long the policy will remain activated or classes will remain canceled, depending on the significance of the weather disruption.

Program Evaluation

A major administrative responsibility is program evaluation, oversight, and management of necessary changes. Periodic evaluation of achievement of program goals is essential to maintain and continuously improve program quality. The Educational Infrastructure section of the National EMS Education Standards describes needed evaluation of program instructional effectiveness and evaluation of program organizational and administrative effectiveness.[8] Additionally, the Committee on Accreditation of Educational Programs for the Emergency Medical Services Professions (CoAEMSP) requires that accredited paramedic programs annually assess their resources and program outcomes.

As deBoer states, "Effective assessment of student learning in any context represents a significant challenge, and controversies persist at all levels of education about which methods of data collection and analysis are most effective and appropriate."[14] EMS program evaluation can be extensive, involving a number of different evaluative dimensions and perspectives with sophisticated metric reporting. However, for the purposes of this text, a simple approach designed to help an EMS instructor evaluate their education program will be presented. It is important to stress that program evaluation is just one part of a larger scheme of assessment and measurement that includes faculty, preceptor, clinical unit, and student evaluation and outcome reporting.

Evaluations include a variety of tools that are administered at specific points throughout the program. They are divided into two major types (just like the student evaluation process): *formative* and *summative*.

A **formative course evaluation** is designed to measure program effectiveness while the class is still in progress, allowing changes and improvements to be implemented right away. It could include trending student cognitive or psychomotor examination results, student achievement of objectives, compliance with program policies, as well as having students and faculty evaluate the program's instructional design, organization, methods of instruction, clarity and completeness of information delivered, student engagement, and the degree to which the program is meeting their expectations.

Gagné and Briggs, in their book, *Principles of Instructional Design*, list the following as examples of data that can be collected during a formative evaluation.[15]

From the observer:

- In what respects are (are not) the materials and media employed in the manner intended by the designer?
- In what respects does (does not) the instructor carry out the procedures and make the decisions intended?
- In what respect do (do not) the students follow the general procedures specified?

From the instructor:

- What practical difficulties are encountered in conducting the lessons?
- How would you estimate the degree of interest or absorption of students in the lesson?
- What difficulties were encountered in carrying out the intended teaching procedures?

From the student:

- How likely are you to choose to do the things you learned in this lesson?
- How likely are you to recommend this lesson to a friend?
- What are the results of a test of performance based on the lesson's objectives?

How the instructor goes about obtaining these data will depend on a number of factors, including course length, course type, number of students, and available time. Some possible approaches to evaluation include the following:

- Giving a course evaluation questionnaire to students periodically
- Taking time out from class to discuss with students how the course is going
- Using standardized measures such as giving the same test to all sections of a course, or comparing results of previous course measures with those of the current course. The assumption behind standardized assessments is that they reflect particular abilities and skills of the students being tested, and that these abilities and skills extend beyond the particular test questions and instruments.[14]
- Using an outside observer of a course lesson as a resource
- Having a "neutral third party" visit with students alone and discuss the course(s)
- Asking students to list the pros and cons of the course anonymously

A practical example of a formative evaluation would be an informal discussion with students following the first lab session on the design and timeliness of station set-ups, available equipment and resources, completeness and accuracy of skills sheets, attentiveness and effectiveness of preceptors, adequacy of time for instruction and skills revolutions so students begin to gain competency in the presented skills, and timely orchestration of station assignments and rotations.

Formative program evaluation can prompt "in-flight corrections" to adjust materials and/or delivery to better meet student needs. Ideally, formative evaluations provide ongoing feedback to the teaching staff and the program administrative team on all aspects of the course, including instructional effectiveness, the classroom/lab environment, hospital and field experiences, and student performance. Formative evaluations can identify whether stated goals and objectives are being achieved or not achieved, the degree of opportunity, and root causes of nonachievement, so corrections can be made as quickly as possible.

A **summative course evaluation** is a retrospective review of the entire program after the class has been completed. This would potentially include graduate, employer, faculty, preceptor, and clinical unit surveys that evaluate course organization; how well the course met the educational needs of the students; the appropriateness of presented material to the learner's scope of practice; effectiveness of the lead instructor; knowledge and effectiveness of instructors/lab/field preceptors; effectiveness of labs skill stations; alignment of lab instruction with classroom content; effectiveness of the course in preparing the practitioner to function as an EMS provider in all three domains of learning; and evaluation of the hospital clinical experience and field internship experience. Obtaining information from others who participated in or were impacted by the program is also helpful.

For example, hospital personnel can identify whether clinical instruction plans were communicated adequately to define student and preceptor objectives and expectations; if preceptor orientation was adequate to prepare them to serve in that role; and if students were appropriately prepared for the clinical rotations and remained adequately engaged while there. Field experiences should be evaluated from the student and field preceptor perspective, so that any problems or suggestions can be identified and corrected or improved for the following class. Obtaining a summative program evaluation from advisory committee members is also beneficial for informing program strengths and opportunities.

Ideally, formative and summative evaluations should complement each other and provide a total evaluative picture of the program. The collective evaluation results should be reviewed by the program director and shared with the medical director, faculty, management team, and advisory committee. The major positive points should be compiled into a course summary format. Opportunities should be similarly identified and discussed at staff meetings and documented in minutes. Action plans should be created to address priorities for change with strategies, milestone dates, and accountability assigned.

Terms often associated with course and program evaluations are "outputs" and "outcomes." While there is a technical difference between the two, practically speaking, they are generally collectively referred to as outcomes. For example, CoAEMSP requires the following outcome thresholds to be measured and included in the annual reports and posted to the websites of accredited paramedic programs: number of students enrolled versus the number completing the course (retention and attrition rates), job placement rates, and pass rates on credentialing exams. The minimum threshold for each is specified as 70%.[16] Colleges or universities will similarly require an annual assessment plan and results with actions report that includes the outcome to be measured, assessment year, method of measurement, criteria for success, program results, whether thresholds were met (Y/N), and use of results (action plan). CE programs can also measure outcomes in the form of quality improvement metrics before and after class instruction.

The key to performing any type of evaluation is determining the elements to be measured, how they are to be measured, and the threshold or benchmarks to be met. Benchmarks may be set internally by the program based on historical trending and desired outcomes, or they can be matched against national standards where they exist. Possible measures or sources of measurement include the following:

- **Course objective achievement in all three domains of learning**. This is the gold standard for evaluation because it measures whether or not the participants met each of the objective requirements for the course. This information can be obtained through graduate and employer surveys distributed between 6 and 12 months following class completion.
- **Student retention/attrition rates**. The number of students successfully completing the course provides some indication as to the effectiveness of the course, provided a uniform standard for determining successful completion is applied.
- **Certification/licensure rates**. If a course prepares the student for some level of certification or licensure, attainment of that certification level is one measure of course success.
- **Exam analysis**. These include measures of central tendency, item analysis and performance, and actions taken.
- **Job placement and continued employment**. Are students who have completed a course able to obtain jobs in that field and function effectively in those jobs? Graduate and employer surveys sent between 6 and 12 months after completing the program give feedback about employment and how prepared graduates were to function in an EMS role.
- **Standardized testing results.** Passing rates on standardized tests taken by students or graduates can be compared year-over-year to previous students or to state or national average pass rates for that exam. These standardized tests need to be validated examinations that are appropriate for the level of students in the educational program. Examples of summative standardized testing would be state or NREMT testing results.
- **Graduate, faculty, and employer satisfaction**. Feedback helps to fully evaluate whether the program is meeting the needs of its communities of interest. These surveys are designed to help the program determine areas of strength and those that need improvement. They can be given at the conclusion of the course and followed up some time later, perhaps after the provider has been employed in the field for a specified time. The survey could include an evaluation of administrative support, program resources, faculty teaching effectiveness, curriculum effectiveness in meeting program goals, clinical and field coordination, identification of program strengths, and opportunity to improve.
- **Faculty evaluations**. Evaluations of faculty by students, peers, or the program director, and after a course is completed.
- **Financial evaluation**. This may include positive or negative variances from the budgetary plan.

Just as programs are evaluated, individual courses should be evaluated as well. A competent instructor will ensure that the course they are teaching is accomplishing its objectives and outcome measures. If a problem is noted, it can be corrected to ensure a positive learning experience.

The bottom line is this: Instructors must be prepared to render some judgment regarding a course or program's quality, suitability, effectiveness, efficiency, and importance based on qualitative and quantitative data.[17] By using a combination of formative and summative evaluations, they will be better able to evaluate a program in the many dimensions required to provide an effective learning experience.

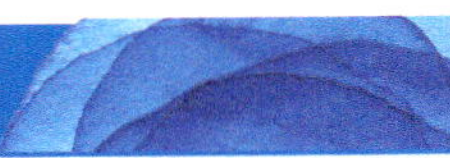

CASE in Point

Battalion Chief Monroe supervises the training division in his mid-sized EMS agency. The department leadership have determined that a pediatric emergency course will be mandatory beginning in the next fiscal year and he must develop a budget to support it.

BC Monroe first runs a report to determine how many of his 200 paramedics currently have the certification or an approved equivalent credential, and how many will need renewal. Based on these numbers, he determines how many courses and how many instructors will be needed and in which months they will need to be held. Knowing this, BC Monroe realizes at least 8 additional instructors will need to be educated or hired from outside the department to meet the needs. He is fairly sure some of the costs of the new program can be offset by also offering the course to outside candidates. Costs for the program will be significant. He calculates the fixed and variable direct and indirect costs that may include salary plus overtime for employees to attend; call-back pay for those who will work for a person who is at class if the staffing plan requires set coverage; instructor costs (time, travel, per diem); initial book, handout, and/or printing costs; refreshments; course completion cards; and teaching supplies.

In an attempt to keep the costs affordable and to increase the expertise of faculty, BC Monroe reaches out to the tertiary pediatric center in his city for support and is thankful when they agree to provide one instructor per course at no charge to his department. After calculating all costs to conduct the classes, he does a comparative analysis of the market for local tuition costs and sets his price for outside candidates based on a reasonable income-to-cost ratio. Although the final costs submitted in his budget still reflect a deficit (negative variance), the department agrees to proceed with the program because of its value to their employees and the community they serve.

Budgeting and Financial Planning

A suggested core value for all educational programs is as follows: *Fiscal responsibility and careful stewardship of all resources are the cornerstone of business planning.* A key part of the planning process is creating a balanced budget. A **budget** is a financial plan for coordinating revenues (inflows) and expenditures (outflows) over a selected period of time in a manner that hopefully provides a net positive margin. Hospitals, EMS agencies, and educational institutions prepare many types of budgets, such as capital, cash flow, and operating budgets. The capital budget plans for the acquisition of major assets with a dollar value over a predetermined threshold and with an anticipated life cycle of 3 to 5 years or more. The cash flow budget is typically a month-by-month plan for revenues received and expenses paid. A program director is most directly concerned with the operating budget.

An **operating budget** identifies the expected resources and expenditures of an entity for a given future period, usually spread by month over 1 year. It provides a basis for evaluating the financial performance of the program while helping to control costs and communicating financial requirements within the program and externally to the communities of interest.

Prerequisites for the development of an operating budget are as follows:

- Include a statement of the purpose or mission of the program.
- List the specific objectives that the program is expected to accomplish during the budget year.
- Identify who is responsible for submitting specific sections of the budget.
- Describe the current operations in terms of revenues, expenses, and services accomplished.

This requires an intact reporting system that highlights program activities and the attendant financial information.

Steps in Developing an Operating Budget

An orderly, systematic approach to developing a budget will assist in ensuring that resources are available to meet program needs. The budget must account for all foreseeable income and expenditures and ideally accounts for unforeseen costs in the form of contingency plans.

1. Justify Work Units Consumed, Programs Conducted, Outputs and Outcomes Produced. Does the program need to continue what it does in the way that it is currently being accomplished? Is there any opportunity for economies of scale or increased efficiency? Because salaries typically consume over 60% of an educational program's operating budget, *efficiency is important and is often gauged in terms of staff productivity.*

Productivity is defined as the amount of output (service) per unit of input (hours of work), student-contact hours, or semester hours. Consider how many educator hours are budgeted per class hour or per number of students. Is valuable educator time consumed in clerical tasks? Consider whether an investment in technology or the addition of support staff would actually pay for itself in improved efficiency.

Additionally, the institutional and program mission for research and professional service may be components of academic institutions, and time should be included for those activities when possible.

Programs use different metrics to measure productivity. Each program should create measures that work for them based on institutional guidelines. If the program runs low on educator-to-student productivity ratios and outcomes are poor, additional faculty may be needed. If the program runs high on educator-to-student ratios and outcomes are poor, processes and/or instruction/learning is inefficient or ineffective and money is likely being wasted. An evaluation of the current plan is called for and action plans are needed.

Examine the **effectiveness** of the program. The metrics used may vary; some will use pass/fail rates on credentialing exams; student retention/attrition rates; job placement rates; or satisfaction rates on performance assessments from students, faculty, stakeholders, and employers. Perhaps the best measure would be the quality of patient care performed by graduates after they transition from class to the workforce. Adding dollars to a program's budget is not a guarantee of improved effectiveness. It is necessary to conduct a complete root-cause analysis of any performance gaps before determining whether a budget adjustment is the answer to the problem.

2. Prioritize Program Outputs and Outcomes. What would be the impact to the program, organization, EMS service providers, community, or patients if any item in the education budget were denied or cut? What are the core services or line items that must be preserved and protected at all cost? Can the program manage without that extra box of 4 × 4s, but not without a working bag-valve-mask? Although this is a somewhat simplistic analogy, program managers must often operate in an environment of limited resources, and educators must find creative cost savings whenever possible. Reasoned justifications should be included in the plan for each line on the chart of accounts so that higher-level administrators understand the need if they are to sign off on the final figures.

3. Forecast Service Demand. In the case of an educational program, the budget must consider student enrollment projections and whether they are increasing or decreasing. If possible, analyze trends in admissions and completions for the past 3 to 5 years. Service providers can predict their needs for more, less, or the same number of EMTs and/or paramedics in the next year based on their resources and volumes. Consider whether members of the current workforce are expected to retire and whether or not they will be replaced. Also consider whether other environmental factors may impact enrollment, such as an economic downturn or recovery, availability of EMS jobs, or increases in college tuition and fees. Consider whether a competing program has closed or expanded, or whether a fire-science program at your college made EMS education a mandatory part of their curriculum. Consider also how National EMS Education Standards and/or Scope of Practice changes may impact class length and resource needs.

4. Project Revenues. Consider all possible revenue streams. These may include tuition, student fees, grants, donations, or subsidies (depending on your affiliation). As tempting as it sounds, the program cannot just raise tuition or student fees to meet inflated cost projections. Anyone affiliated with a college is locked into a tuition cost per credit hour cap that cannot be changed mid-year just because program faculty have overspent and more money is needed. Thus, if a program is to operate within allowable profit or loss margins, it must maximize revenue and minimize costs or it will not be sustainable over time.

5. Estimate Personnel and Other Expenses. An essential component of zero-based budgeting is to project all costs to the program as accurately as possible and align expenses with projected revenues so there is a balanced budget. It is not wise financial stewardship to simply rely on historical trends and add 5% to each line item per year.

A *general ledger chart of accounts* is used as a framework to project costs. These are program and institution specific, and may include, but are not limited to, the following, in any particular order:

- Human resources costs (employees): Regular and overtime wages; other pay: paid time plan (vacation, sick, personal time), meetings, orientation, education, military deployment, bereavement, jury duty, disability; FICA; pension, 401(k) contributions, retirement plans
- Professional fees (nonemployees/independent contractors): Medical director, guest faculty, preceptors, consultants, patient models, legal consultation
- Physical plant/facilities: Rent, lease, mortgage; utilities; cleaning, repair, and maintenance; furnishings; taxes, landscaping, snow removal; garbage and waste removal
- Automotive (vehicle owned by program): License plates, inspection sticker, insurance, car loan payments, repairs, tires, maintenance, fuel
- Phones: Data plans; air cards
- Computer hardware and software: Learning management system, test item banks, exam analysis; simulation; ePCR and general operating system software products

- Supplies: Instructional (pharmaceutical, medical-surgical)
- Supplies: Noninstructional (office supplies)
- Minor equipment: Durable and consumable that fall under threshold of capital expenses
- Educational equipment: Repairs, maintenance, service contracts
- Educational equipment: Rental
- Books and publications: Print and electronic (digital)
- Printing, copying, scanning
- Postage, delivery service
- Business travel (local and out of town): Ground mileage, fuel, tolls, parking; auto rental; ground transport; airfare; lodging
- Food and beverage; meals and entertainment
- Marketing and communications: May include cost of maintaining a website; mass communication software
- Professional dues, subscriptions, licenses; permits; accreditation fees
- Uniforms; clothing allowance
- Testing and credentialing fees
- Insurance: Medical, dental, vision, life, disability, worker's comp; retirement, liability; vehicle
- Staff education and development: Initial, continuing (conferences, seminars, professional development)
- Charitable donations or contributions
- Business gift expense or recognition awards
- Bank charges; debt repayment and opportunity costs (interest)
- Costs for criminal background checks, drug screening, physical examinations, and immunizations/titers may be paid for by the program and passed through to the students so they become budget neutral to the program as long as revenues can be shown to offset the expenses.

Accounts may be added or adjusted based on specific program configuration, needs, inflows, and outflows.

At the outset, program managers must consider whether a cost is responsive or driven by changes in service volume or the number of students. Those that fluctuate by volume are considered a **variable cost**. One that remains constant, uninfluenced by volume, is called a **fixed cost**. For example, the program director and lead instructor's salary costs are typically fixed if they are salaried and hired at a specific full-time equivalent (FTE) allowance. The time spent in the administrative work of curricular design, development, and classroom instruction should vary little whether there are 5 or 60 students, but the time spent in grading, evaluating, processing files, examination authorizations, student communication, and counseling etc., may vary significantly based on class size. Thus, it is preferable to fill all class openings to maximize revenues for programs that have heavy fixed costs.

Other costs, such as those incurred related to preceptors, or printing and consumable supplies, are strongly driven by volumes (number of students and nature of class activity). If one assumes a consistent ratio of five or six students per lab preceptor, far more instructors would be needed for a class of 40 than for a class of 5. Staffing for a class of 30 and then only enrolling 20 students will result in the law of diminishing returns. Staffing plans must be optimized to the actual number of students present.

Creating a **staffing plan** for the budget is an art. The need for human capital and productivity measures can be heavily influenced by staff maturity in terms of experience and ability. Time needed to mentor and orient new faculty must be factored into the budget. It is expected that novice educators will take longer to prepare and process class materials than those who have greater proficiency and can operate more independently. Mentoring takes time, but it is well worth the investment. Consider the costs if new educators are left on their own to conduct a program by trial and error, fail, become discouraged, and resign, requiring that new staff be onboarded on a frequent basis.

Asking seasoned educators to do things in a new way, such as using online teaching or new technology, may also result in a temporary erosion in productivity that requires additional staff hours during the transition and skill acquisition phase. One must also consider the educator administrative time and resources needed for program updates and revisions as standards and/or new medical advances are published.

A place to start in building the staffing budget is to measure work inputs and outputs in relative value units (RVUs). For example, if an RVU is defined as 60 minutes of an employee's time, all work taking 60 minutes (or a proportion of an hour) would be one RVU (or a corresponding fraction of one). Consider all the tasks that must be completed by staff members based on current and projected student and class volumes and work flow. Determine a target RVU by conducting time and motion studies where staff are actually observed and timed while doing these tasks. Plot the findings and distill them into a reasonable and expected norm and assign a time value to them. Compare the anticipated work units against the number of hours staff are authorized to work to see if the staffing plan is aligned with needs. The process is laborious when done the first time, but it is necessary for informed planning.

One full-time equivalent (employee) (1.0 FTE) is usually budgeted for approximately 2,080 work hours per year (40 hours per week). Both productive and nonproductive hours, such as those consumed when using vacation, sick, bereavement, jury duty, education, leave of absence, military deployment, meetings, CE, orientation, or holiday time, should be included within this total. Those items may be factored in as a general productive to nonproductive time ratio, depending on the nature of the benefit package and budgeting model. For employees, it is also necessary to factor in FICA expenses and other benefit costs, such as insurance coverage and matching funds for pension plans.

FTE allowances may need to be adjusted from full-time to part-time if it is shown that work units do not support a full-time employee. Some programs also consider the flexibility and advantages that two part-time employees may provide over one full-time employee in meeting simultaneous competing priorities. Lean, nimble, and adaptable are watchwords for the current economic environment.

The program director must evaluate assets in terms of capital and noncapital supplies and equipment, compare current inventories against par levels, and determine needed purchases to conduct a quality class based on student and program projections and stakeholder feedback.

Look at all class activities and program needs. What disposable or consumable supplies, equipment, or resources are needed for each class or lab based on the number of students? What is the cost of each item? How many will each student use or need? This provides the **per capita cost per student**. Multiply these variables by the number of students to obtain projected cost figures. EMS programs are often lab intensive. Instructors need to create authentic simulations and scenarios that require the use of real equipment in good working order. These instructional costs can be large and must be well-planned to conduct a quality program. Positive **variances** are welcome, negative are not; and all must be explained.

When budgeting, consider the following points:

- **Try to never pay full or list price**. Make it a practice to work closely with vendor representatives to negotiate discounted or preferred pricing and locked-in pricing for several years in return for a commitment to use their product for a specified period of time or to guarantee a minimum order number during that time. Also work with vendors to borrow rather than purchase equipment needed for limited times in class.
- **Be a wise consumer**. Compare cost, quality, features, and vendor support for all goods and services.

  The competitive market economy can help reduce costs when vendors know that they do not have a lock on a company's business. Programs have the option of selecting from a large variety of texts, tools, supplies, software, and equipment. Price points, warrantees, and customer service can vary widely for products of reasonably equal quality. Continuing to buy from the same vendor year-over-year may not be cost effective. Although it may take some time to investigate various options for purchases, it will pay off in the long run. One limitation to changing vendors is whether an institution has a purchasing agreement with a particular company; contracts may need to be established before a purchase order can be submitted. Some institutions are reluctant or resistant to process special orders outside of their standard practices and purchasing agreements as they may compromise economies in place. If a better price from another vendor is found when there is a strong loyalty to a great product representative, then the vendor should be asked if they can provide rebates or adjusted pricing. Most will try to do so rather than lose existing business.
- **Seek out economies of scale**. Program personnel should attempt to negotiate a better cost per item by purchasing products in bulk that will be used during the fiscal year. This can also be achieved by creating or joining a buying group to become more attractive for preferred pricing.
- **Institute tight inventory controls**. The cost of waste and creative procurement (theft) from supplies can be significant, and measures to minimize or eliminate these problems are worthwhile.

Lastly, consider indirect costs related to overhead if a prorated fee for classroom/office space, housekeeping, maintenance, utilities, insurance, and so on is paid.

6. Adjust the Figures to Reach a Balanced Budget. If there is a disparity between resources available and resources needed, cut costs or increase revenues if possible to reach a balanced budget (revenues should equal or exceed expenses) unless an unfavorable variance (negative profitability margin) is acceptable. This process may involve difficult decisions, belt tightening, or dreams deferred. Adding FTEs is challenging for most programs in an economic climate of scarcity, but reducing FTEs should not be a knee-jerk response when asked to cut the budget. Educators are the program's most valuable asset. Be certain that *all* other options have been robustly explored before cutting needed staff. Skillful budget preparation requires accurate data, accurate information, and careful planning. Managers should not submit a pie-in-the-sky budget that cannot be justified. It will immediately tarnish credibility with higher-level administrators who may then mistrust other initiatives brought to them for consideration.

Medical Director's Role in an EMS Program

The medical director is an essential component of an EMS educational program and can be a potent force for positive change in the classroom or in the clinical and field settings (FIGURE 24.6). Physician oversight is commonly required by the state EMS agency and is identified in the EMS Education Standards as a necessary component at all levels of EMS education. Additionally, active participation of the medical director is required for the national accreditation of paramedic programs (CoAEMSP) standards.

As a practicing physician, the medical director can be a powerful advocate and therefore instrumental in moving a program toward its organizational development goals. The medical director interaction should occur in a variety of settings, such as lecture, laboratory, clinical, and field internship. Interaction may be by synchronous electronic methods. The medical director can also be responsible for securing the financial and community support necessary to be successful. Too often, the medical director is not used to their full advantage and programs struggle to meet student needs without the assistance of this important ally.

The general program duties of a medical director are as follows:

- Be responsible for medical oversight of the program.
- Serve as an active advisory committee member.
- Review and approve the educational content of the program curriculum for appropriateness, medical accuracy, and reflection of current evidence-informed prehospital or emergency care practice.
- Review and approve the required minimum numbers for each of the required patient contacts and procedures.
- Review and approve the instruments and processes used to evaluate students in didactic, laboratory, clinical, and field internship.
- Review the progress of each student throughout the program, and assist in the determination of appropriate corrective measures, when necessary. Corrective measures should occur in the cases of adverse outcomes, failing academic performance, and disciplinary action.
- Ensure and attest to the competence of each graduate of the program in the cognitive, psychomotor, and affective domains.
- Engage in cooperative involvement with the program director.
- Ensure the effectiveness and quality of any medical director responsibilities delegated to another qualified physician.
- Ensure educational interaction of physicians with students.[18]

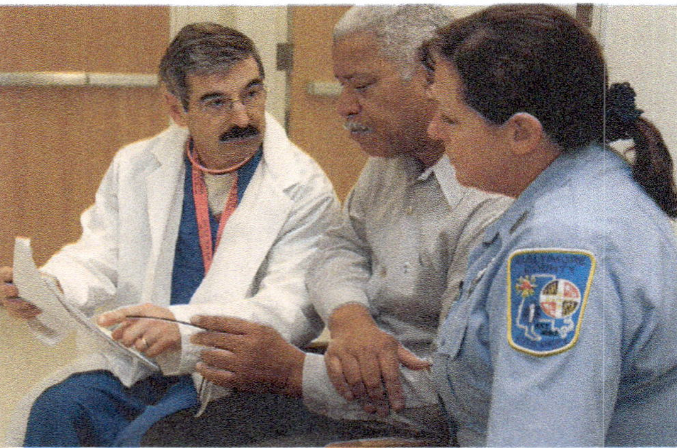

FIGURE 24.6 The medical director is an essential component of the EMS educational program and should approve the medical accuracy of the course content and all examinations.

For all of these duties and others that may arise during the medical director's tenure, the medical director should likely be provided some amount of monetary compensation. Payment for serving as an EMS education program medical director should be commensurate with the time and complexity committed toward meeting the program's goals and objectives.

Instructor-Related Administrative Issues

The role of primary (lead) and secondary instructors goes beyond that of being a well-prepared, knowledgeable, and effective classroom or lab instructor. All instructors have a duty and responsibility to know, understand, follow, and enforce rules, regulations, and program policies. Often the classroom or lab instructor is on the front line for questions, maladaptive behavior, or challenge to or noncompliance with program policy. This section presents some common administrative issues relative to EMS instructors.

Instructor Contract or Agreement

All instructors and preceptors who are not sponsoring institution/agency employees must be vetted for their qualifications and eligibility to teach, and they all should have a written independent contractor or work-for-hire contract or agreement. This protects not only the individual instructor, but the organization and EMS program as well. The program director and even a part-time course instructor generally find it necessary to ask colleagues to help teach or precept specific parts of a course. It is important from a legal vantage point that all such arrangements be formalized in compliance with organizational standards and guidelines, especially if compensation is involved.

An independent contractor agreement may include, but not be limited to, the following:

- Names of the parties involved in the contract
- Recitals: Mutual promises and covenants contained in the agreement
- Terms of engagement: Qualifications, compliance with law, relationship between parties
- Responsibilities of both parties: The agency agrees to provide workspace, equipment, supplies, and information generally required to do the work; the contractor is responsible for devoting time, attention, and energy to faithfully and diligently perform the services in a professional, competent, and satisfactory manner in adherence with all statutes, rules, regulations, bylaws, policies, procedures, and requirements of the government, program, or other entities having jurisdiction over or providing reimbursement to the program.
- Qualifications of the contractor: Generally stated to be commensurate with the knowledge and skills set forth in the National EMS Education Standards and Scope of Practice Model for the level of practitioner being taught; and qualifications of EMS educators specified in national and state statutes, rules, guidelines, and local policy, which may include academic preparation, licensure/certifications; teaching experience, and demonstrated expertise.
- Confidentiality and conflict of interest statements, if required by the organization
- Requirement to immediately notify the program if any action is being taken on their professional license or if they have been convicted of a felony
- Insurance and indemnification: Defines who is responsible for providing professional liability and healthcare coverage during contractor service delivery
- Compensation: Lump-sum agreement or rate per hour; any caps on hours or amounts to be paid
- Time records: How evidence of work and/or expenses are to be documented for compensation
- Tax withholdings: Statement as to whether taxes will be withheld by the agency or are the responsibility of the contractor
- Term of contract and termination clauses; auto-renewal provisions if applicable
- Assignment clause: Limits the contractor from delegating the duties or responsibilities in the contract to another without prior written consent
- Nondiscrimination clause
- Names and contact information for persons responsible for the contract
- Signatures of parties to the contract
- Appendix documents: May include a full description of duties and services; information on how the instructor will be evaluated; time sheet examples

It is important that contracts be in full force and effect and on file for all instructors for each semester or program period. Ensure that the contract-signing process is begun with sufficient advance time to ensure execution prior to any services being provided.

Course Syllabus

A syllabus usually describes the body of instruction to be conducted within a specific class. This document is a supplement to school or program policies and procedures or handbooks. The form and title of this document may vary based on local requirements. The format may be set as a standard by the educational institution with which the EMS program is affiliated or it may be created at the instructor's discretion based on the nature and complexity of the class. It may be as short as a couple of pages, or it may be much longer, depending on the level of detail presented. Many elements noted as general statements in the syllabus may be provided in greater detail in the student handbook or course policies if not included fully in the syllabus.

Whatever the form, the syllabus is an important resource for students and faculty. Educators should design a clear, concise, complete, and current document that specifies important points of information about the class in an effort to prevent misunderstanding and ambiguity about requirements. A well-written syllabus can determine the outcome of a dispute between the instructor and a student. Careful writing is essential to develop a document that stands the test of an institutional or legal challenge. Each student should receive their own copy of the syllabus and/or student handbook or be directed to where they may find these documents online on or before the first class meeting. Any questions they may have should be clarified during orientation. Instructors should review key points in the syllabus and student handbook and make sure all students are informed about and agree to follow each section. Copies of these documents should be available through electronic media and/or posted to the program's website.

A syllabus may contain, but not be limited to, the following:

- Course title and description, course number; semester or credit hours awarded
- Instructor's name, contact information (email and/or telephone number), office location, and hours of availability
- Course dates, times, location(s)
- Course general description
- Any pre- or corequisites
- Program goal
- Topical outline
- Methods of presentation
- Student outcomes
- Methods of evaluation
- Course grading policies
- Assignments
- Attendance policies
- Makeup test/assignment policies
- Student behavior expectations
- Required textbooks and/or educational resources plus details on where these can be purchased or consulted
- Equal opportunity statement
- Students with disabilities; how to request accommodation
- Method(s) of student notification

Academic Dishonesty

Academic integrity and honesty are essential values for all health professionals. EMS personnel must often care for patients who require the most urgent and possibly invasive interventions without benefit of immediate medical consultation or assistance. Their ability to perform swiftly and competently may impact patient outcomes. Educators must ensure that all participants in their programs (entry level or CE) possess and demonstrate the knowledge, skills, and behaviors required to perform the job well. Academic dishonesty transcends more than social mores or professional ethics. It can negatively impact the quality of care rendered to a patient. A dishonest or incompetent student who becomes a dishonest or incompetent EMS practitioner produces unconscionable consequences.

Academic dishonesty is defined as a breach of the standards of academic integrity and typically includes engaging in, assisting in, or condoning lying; cheating (looking at someone else's exam during a test or allowing other students to look at your exam; giving or receiving information that is on a test by any electronic or other communication; talking to another student during an assessment without permission; using notes, resources, or devices not authorized for use on an assessment; consulting websites or other resources without being granted permission to do so by the instructor); plagiarism; furnishing unauthorized information; unauthorized collaboration on graded work; collusion; falsifying academic records; and any act designed to give unfair advantage to a particular student. A founded allegation of academic dishonesty may result in suspension or separation from the program on the first offense. Consequences could also include a failing grade along with a disciplinary record that may affect the student's future employment or educational opportunities.

Similarly, faculty members can be guilty of academic dishonesty by awarding credits or certifications where they have not been earned, falsely attesting to time in class or content covered, or grading unfairly or capriciously to give a higher score than earned to a participant.

In today's culture, many believe that cheating is appropriate to help them get results at all costs and is not morally wrong.[19] Multiple high-profile stories have chronicled the pervasive culture of academic dishonesty in EMS programs around the country, giving rise to public uncertainty regarding those they traditionally regarded as heroes and an emergency healthcare safety net.

It is critical that educators understand why cheating or educational fraud occurs, do everything possible to correct the root cause, and engineer process controls to abate the risk. A survey conducted by NAEMSE to educators in 2008 indicated that the leading causes of cheating in EMS were failure to study, laziness, a "desire to just get their ticket punched," time pressure, and poor supervision. There was a prevailing attitude that accomplishing CE hours was not as important as personnel and vehicles remaining in service; staying compliant with requirements and regulators by the most expeditious means possible was considered more important than honesty.

Researchers at the University of British Columbia (2010) examined the behavior of university students over 10 years and found that many who cheated were not afraid of punishment, were amoral, and had a strong sense of entitlement. They reported that students who cheat ranked high for three personality disorders: psychopathy, Machiavellianism (manipulativeness), and narcissism. Others were simply unprepared.[20]

An evolving area of concern is online education, where the opportunities for academic dishonesty abound, including "short cutting" or "beating the system"— for example, spending little or no time with the educational content, going straight to the test and completing it in a matter of minutes (using the questions and/or key already in their possession), or learning how to change an answer after it had been marked incorrect. CAPCE has created rigorous standards for content and testing standards for CE vendors and educators who seek approval for online courses.[21]

Institutional policies vary regarding what an instructor should do when they suspect that academic dishonesty is occurring or has occurred. All instructors should be familiar with institutional policies on confronting a student, taking up an exam, documenting the allegation, and recommending consequences and/or disciplinary action. Academic dishonesty is typically considered by institutions as a disciplinary issue rather than an academic issue, and students are entitled to full due process. It is paramount that nothing be done to prejudice the student's rights. (See Chapter 25, *Legal Issues for EMS Educators*, for more information.)

The following box entitled "Sample Code of Student Conduct" shows a general code of conduct, including issues of academic dishonesty.

Sample Code of Student Conduct

Paramedic students have the opportunity to participate in a worthy, honorable, and progressive profession. This opportunity is not without obligation. The profession's viability rests on the integrity and capability of its members. See the Program's Core Values.

Students will have exposure to diverse learning environments, including, but not limited to classroom, hospital, and out of hospital settings and must behave professionally in each.

Students must take responsibility for their own learning and conduct themselves at all times as practitioners who already have a paramedic license.

We believe in uncompromising ethical behavior based on the standards and codes of professional conduct established by statute, rules, EMS organizations and Program policy. See the Program's Code of Ethics.

We are dedicated to excellence as our performance standard. All services provided in the context of EMS care shall be delivered in a consistently superior manner. Working together, we will approach everything as an opportunity for continuous improvement.

Expected Behaviors

Students shall:

- Comply with all statutes, rules, protocols, and procedures that govern the program and EMS care.
- Comply with Federal Health Insurance Portability and Accountability Act (HIPAA) Privacy Rule requirements, and respect patients' autonomy, confidentiality, and right to privacy.

Professional Interpersonal Skills

- Treat others with respect, civility, courtesy, and dignity, and conduct self in a professional and cooperative manner at all times.
- Work cooperatively and harmoniously with peers, preceptors, and educators.
- Respect cultural differences and protect the rights, privileges, and beliefs of others.
- Avoid threatening, profane, and/or abusive language or actions and refrain from verbal or written communication that defames any person or organization or would be considered harassment.
- Address concerns or conflicts with associates in a direct, prompt, yet sensitive manner in an appropriate setting. If this fails, go through proper channels to appropriately resolve the conflict.

Strive toward Academic and Clinical Excellence

- Encourage and assist colleagues in the pursuit of excellence through approved team activities.
- Practice ONLY within the scope of approved clinical privileges.
- Adhere to the guidelines prescribed by the Program in completing all assignments and exams.
- Report to class/clinical rotations on time and complete objectives by stated deadlines.
- Mitigate safety risks by protecting self and others from exposure to foreseeable and preventable risks.

Violation of Code of Conduct

Whenever a student is alleged to have committed a violation of the student Code of Conduct while on hospital premises or at an activity, function, or event sponsored or supervised by the program, an investigation will be conducted. If the allegation is sustained, disciplinary action and/or a corrective action plan will be imposed per Program and College policy. The conduct will be documented in the student's file. Discipline may also be imposed if student conduct off campus or on social media adversely affects the hospital, Program, or the College.

(continues)

Sample Code of Student Conduct *(Continued)*

Examples include, but may not be limited to, proof that the person:

- is guilty of fraud or deceit in procuring or attempting to procure admittance into the Paramedic program;
- has demonstrated a gross lack of integrity;
- has engaged in dishonorable, unethical, or unprofessional conduct of a character likely to deceive, defraud or harm the public.

  This may include actions that create the potential for harm through negligence or willfulness; providing patient care without proper preparation or authorization; lying, covering up or failing to report an error in the clinical setting; and falsification of any documents;
- has violated the handbooks, contracts, or behavioral agreements specific to the paramedic program;
- has violated any law, ordinance, College or Program rule or regulation while enrolled as a student;
- is unfit for duty or nondecisional by reason of illness, drug/chemical use, or gross negligence;
- is found in possession of, or has used or distributed a controlled substance or look-alike drug in an illegal manner;
- is guilty of unauthorized and/or illegal possession, use or distribution of any alcoholic beverage or product;
- has presented to class impaired, intoxicated, under the influence and/or with the odor of drugs or alcohol on their person;
- has brought a weapon or explosive device of any kind to class or to a clinical area;
- is guilty of theft of property or services;
- is guilty of intentional or willful destruction of property;
- has abused College or hospital technology resources, or medical equipment;
- is guilty of assault and/or battery;
- is guilty of academic dishonesty: engaging in, assisting in, or condoning lying, cheating, plagiarism, furnishing unauthorized information, unauthorized collaboration, or other similar activities. A founded allegation of academic dishonesty may result in separation from the program on the first offense. Cheating on exams transcends more than social mores or professional ethics. It can negatively impact the quality of care rendered to a patient.

  Examples of prohibited behaviors:
  - Blatant copying of content sources for student assignments or failure to cite references
  - Written information found on a student's person, clothing, skin, personal effects or property, book edges, notebook covers, etc. that could provide information about exam content
  - Use of any outside source in violation of policy to obtain an answer on an exam
  - Removal of an exam booklet from the testing site unless authorized by the instructor
  - Audible noises, gestures, or body language used to alert others to exam answers
  - Use of digital pens during exams
- is guilty of disruptive behavior and/or conduct, bullying, harassment, discrimination, or abuse that threatens the physical or mental well-being, health or safety of any individual.

  Disruptive behavior is defined as student-initiated acts that range from tardiness to violence. It may consist of behavior that is argumentative, disrespectful, offensive, or threatening and may present itself physically, verbally, or psychologically. It has a negative impact in the learning environment and interferes with the learning activities of the perpetrator and other students. Examples include, but are not limited to the following:
  - has demonstrated insubordinate or inappropriate behavior towards any instructor or preceptor;
  - is guilty of disrupting the peace, the education process or related activity;
- has violated the terms of any corrective action plan imposed in accordance with program procedures.

Just Culture/Corrective Action

The program encourages accountability and behaviors that reflect program values within a *culture of safety*.

Communication Openness

Students are expected to report any misconduct, errors, or violation of policy to an Instructor or Program Director without fear of retribution. Students should speak up if they observe anything that may negatively impact themselves, peers, or patient care. They should feel free to respectfully question the decisions or actions of those with more authority.

Any student suspected of academic dishonesty or is alleged to have demonstrated behavior that is unprofessional, unethical, inappropriate, or illegal may be academically suspended pending an investigation.

Reporting Alleged Academic Dishonesty

Faculty are asked to fill out an Academic Dishonesty Reporting form located on the System website under the Education tab/Paramedic Class and forward to the EMS Program Director to trigger an evaluation and response.

- **Reporting behaviors inconsistent with program values and/or policy.** Any student, faculty, or system member may fill out a *Behavioral Incident Reporting form* to inform the program of behaviors and/or practices inconsistent with program values or policies to trigger an evaluation and response. The form is also found on the System website in the same location as mentioned above.

- **Faculty members** may file a Grievance using the G1 policy and Request for Clarification form.

If the allegations are sustained, the student or alleged wrong doer will receive corrective coaching, penalties or disciplinary action.

Corrective coaching is generally progressive and shall be communicated privately and delivered in a timely manner. Corrective action is generally intended to be a positive, non-punitive intervention that allows an individual time to correct an identified deviation from expected behavior. Personal coaching, a verbal warning, a written warning, a written reprimand, or a last chance agreement may precede suspension or dismissal. However, for more severe offenses, the disciplinary process may begin with suspension or expulsion. In each instance, it is to be fair, just, and proportionate to the seriousness of the offense.

Due process rights are specified in System Policy G1 Grievance Recourse Step 1: Request for Clarification; reporting complaints and D1 Due Process: Disciplinary Action and the College Catalog/Student handbook.

Appeal Policy

Students and faculty members have 24 hours from the time of an invoked *disciplinary* action to appeal the action taken against them. All appeals must be in writing (e-mail is acceptable) and addressed to the Program Director.

General Classroom Management

Managing students in any classroom can be a challenge. Decisions about classroom management require knowledge of students' rights.

Right to Fail

It is important for instructors to recognize that students have a right to fail. This means that if a student elects to not meet course requirements as clearly delineated in the syllabus, the student will receive the appropriate grade. An instructor may establish expected classroom behaviors such as no talking, no use of earbuds, directed use of electronic devices, and so forth in the best interest of the class as a whole. However, if a student's behavior is not illegal, immoral, disruptive, or distracting, they have the right to engage in such actions and accept the consequences. Of course this does not abdicate the instructor's responsibility to coach and counsel students to desired behaviors and levels of achievement.

Right to Access

Students pay tuition to attend an entry-level educational program and thus have access rights to unrestricted program resources. This may seem straightforward, but it is not uncommon for instructors to inadvertently violate this right. A common example is the "locked-door policy" in which an instructor locks the classroom door at the beginning of class, preventing late-arriving students from entering. In denying access in this manner, they attempt to reinforce the need for on-time arrival. However, the student has paid for the right to attend that class, and as long as coming late is not disruptive to the class, the student has the right to do so. This does not, however, prevent an instructor from specifying when late arrivals may take their seat and/or connecting tardiness to disciplinary consequences and/or the course grade.

Instructors should also be aware of institutional policies that define a class distraction and/or disruption and their responsibility to deal with students who cause them. In an EMS academy setting, the instructor can set more stringent classroom behavior requirements due to the formal relationship with the students.

Arbitrary and Capricious Grading

Even with the best-written syllabus and clearly defined criteria, a student may challenge a grade, accusing the instructor of unfair scoring practices. Ideally, a face-to-face meeting between the parties can redress any misunderstandings and settle the dispute. In some instances, an impasse arises where the student believes they are not receiving fair due process from the instructor and they escalate their concerns to the program director or department chair. Students often erroneously believe that a director or chair can overturn or change a grade assigned by the instructor, which may not be the case. In principle, an instructor is the sole master of the classroom in academic matters stemming from the tenets of academic freedom. A program director can serve as a mediator between the student and instructor. If mediation fails, institutions usually have a policy in place for addressing adjudication of such disputes, especially in cases of alleged arbitrary or capricious grading on the part of an instructor.

To prevent such disputes, it is important for the instructor to grade all assignments fairly and accurately, without partiality or bias and to carefully follow all grading criteria listed in the syllabus or student handbook. The use of a scoring rubric that clearly shows the criteria, weight, and value of each component of an assignment or the critical facts or concepts that must be included in written assignments helps an instructor award an appropriate grade. These keys also provide an objective reference if a student questions their score. A rubric is also useful for maintaining grading consistency when sections of a course are taught by multiple instructors.

Electronic Devices

Limiting student use of electronic devices in the classroom remains controversial. Prohibitions against ringing cell phones are well established, but limiting the use of electronic devices and social media present a number of legal and logistical challenges. If the program or agency has policies regarding electronic device and social media use, an individual instructor must follow them. However, if instructors must create their own policy, it is imperative to research legally defensible language. While the motivation for prohibiting use may be to motivate student engagement in classroom activities rather than having them distracted by playing games, watching movies, or streaming on social media during class, policy language may be too restrictive and violate a student's civil liberties. Conversely, unregulated use of social media makes possible unintended self-disclosure by students, which may result in violations of confidentiality policies and federal laws.[22]

Today's students live in a world dominated by electronic devices. Social communication is more likely to be electronic than verbal. Information is immediately available via the Internet and Web-enabled smartphones. Many entering college freshmen cannot write in cursive and have not read a print textbook in high school. Given this demographic, is it a good educational strategy to deny students the tools that have become an integral part of their daily lives? A better strategy would be to educate them in the proper etiquette of using such devices in class. Even better would be designing educational activities to integrate the devices into the learning schema.

The following sample language is from Yale University Publications:[23]

> In many circumstances, the use of computers and similar devices in the classroom may enhance teaching and learning. However there are other circumstances, such as small interactive seminars, in which individual use of, for example, laptop computers may interfere with the pedagogical model of the course.
>
> Except in cases in which a student has a registered and documented disability that requires the use of assistive devices, instructors may, at their discretion, restrict the use of computers and other electronic devices in their classroom. Such electronic devices include, but are not limited to, laptop computers, cell phones, and tablets. Again with the exception of students with registered disabilities, students who have been permitted the use of laptops or other devices in most sessions of a course may still be barred from using them in sessions in which quizzes or tests are administered. Instructors who wish to restrict the use of such devices from any or all sessions of their courses should consider stating their policy on the syllabus from the outset of the course.

Instructor Evaluations

The instructor plays a central role in the teaching and learning dynamic (**FIGURE 24.7**). In the case of EMS education, an **instructor evaluation** is required by accrediting bodies and often by state regulatory agencies. This is especially true for educational programs that result in professional certification or licensure. In institutions of higher education, these evaluations serve a number of purposes, such as forming the basis for contract renewal, pay increase, tenure review, accountability, or union contract requirements.

Most evaluations follow an approved and standardized format and are conducted by a program director, chair, or dean based on personal observation, student evaluations, peer evaluations, and outcome criteria. They should also include a self-evaluation completed by the instructor.

For a proper instructor evaluation to occur, it is imperative that the purpose and nature of the evaluation be clearly defined and not be a vehicle for retaliation. Instructor evaluations fall into two broad but overlapping categories: evaluations done to evaluate the

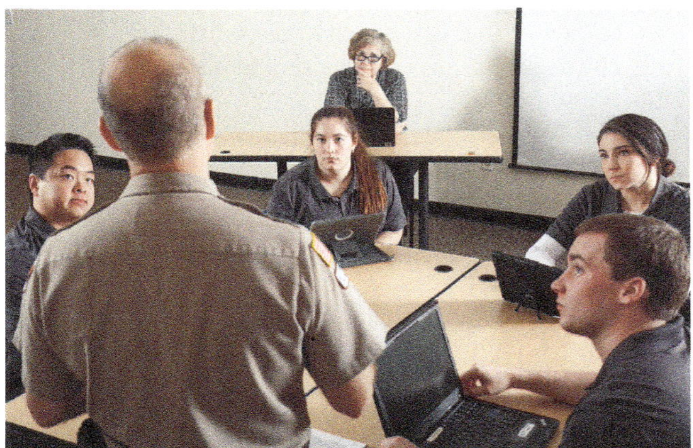

FIGURE 24.7 Most instructor evaluations follow an approved, standardized format and are conducted by a program director, chair, or dean.

CASE in Point

Lilia, a new adjunct instructor, was hired this semester after completing the required education, credentialing, and mentoring by a full-time faculty member. She was assigned to independently teach selected sections of the EMT program.

Her mid-semester evaluations were below the expected performance level. Students complained that Lilia's approach suggested that some of the material in some of the introductory chapters wasn't important and that she tended to just "read the slides." When the program director conducted her scheduled on-site observation, she noted that while Lilia's appearance was professional and she began class on time, she launched into the lecture without an instructional set or creating a "need to know." The content did not vary from that provided by the publisher slides and she did not incorporate active learning or student-centered methods or activities. As a result, all learning was passive, and both Lilia and her students appeared disengaged.

Later, when the program director sat down with Lilia, they reviewed her performance based on a pre-established evaluation tool rubric that identified areas of strengths as well as specific opportunities for her to improve. Then, using the next lesson plan as an example, they explored ways to inspire interest in the subject matter by leading with a compelling real-life case study or dispatch recording. The program director emphasized that the publisher materials were just a starting point, and discussed how to highlight key content in a way that encouraged participants to apply the concepts presented in the reading assignments. She also encouraged Lilia to delete slides that only cover foundational content so there is time for a simulation, scenario, role-play, creation of a mind map, or debate that engage all students in active learning strategies.

The day after her next class, the program director bumped into Lilia, who was bubbling with excitement. She admitted that she had been afraid to try something new because she had always been taught by lecture, but that the new strategy worked. Lilia said that both she and the class had fun, and that the students asked great questions and gave positive feedback. As they headed down the hallway, Lilia explained how she was going to approach the next lesson and the program director smiled, knowing this instructor was now on the road to success!

performance of the instructor and those obtained for the purpose of improving the instructional experience. It may seem that both ultimately accomplish the same objective—to improve the learning experience. They ultimately do, but for different reasons.

Faculty evaluation may include, but not be limited to, the following:

- **Preparation and professional knowledge**. Demonstrated an understanding of the curriculum, subject content, and the needs of students by providing relevant learning experiences; provided thorough, clear, and organized presentation and explanation of content with no content errors and delivered in a manner that was understandable to learners
- **Instructional strategies**. Promoted student learning by using research-based instructional strategies relevant to the content area to engage students in active learning and to facilitate their acquisition of key knowledge and skills, diversifying methods to a variety of preferred learning styles, and meeting all class objectives; remained on-task
- **Communication**. Clearly communicated instructional purpose of the lesson and need to know; connected learning outcomes to previous and future learning, including how this presentation fits into context of whole course
- **Explained content clearly and imaginatively**. Used appropriate examples and experiences to bring content to life; explained procedures and directions clearly
- **Language/speech/verbal skills**. Used expressive, well-modulated voice; varied tone and tempo to maintain interest; volume of voice could be heard throughout room; language professional and appropriate; found opportunities to extend students' vocabularies (understanding of medical terminology); displayed a good sense of humor
- **Body language**. Conveyed openness and invited participation; gestures and gait natural, appropriate, and not distracting
- **Positive learning environment**. Provided a well-managed, safe, and orderly environment that was conducive to learning; class interactions highly respectful, reflecting genuine warmth, caring, and sensitivity to students as individuals and involved everyone
- **Invited intellectual engagement**. Posed questions with high cognitive challenge to encourage participants to think critically, advance high-level thinking, problem-solve effectively, and check for understanding; used active listening skills; encouraged high-quality responses; inspired students to learn
- **Students-initiated higher-order questions**. Led students to correct answers and provided feedback that furthered learning

- **Adjusted pace of presentation appropriately**. Immediately identified student misconceptions and addressed them before proceeding; allowed sufficient time for questions, used time well
- **Visual aids**. Audiovisual aids were well-developed and enhanced learning; used AV equipment effectively
- **Classroom management**. Managed classroom procedures involving noninstructional duties such as transitions, materials and supplies, and supervision of guest faculty/preceptors
- **Mentoring.** Served as a role model; fostered personal relationships; gave of self; willing to help on a personal level; expressed believed in students; challenged students; suggested specific ways to improve; encouraged independence
- **Helpfulness**. Made self available for consultation; provided positive feedback and corrective coaching effectively; made self available outside of class time; returned graded assignments promptly; provided meaningful feedback on written work
- **Measurement of learning**. Quizzes and exams measure achievement of key objectives based on a blueprint and table of specifications tied to a practice analysis; items well constructed in compliance with standards of testing and measurement; scoring accurate, fair, and nondiscriminatory; results communicated in a timely manner; formative and summative assessments well written and communicated to students with fair and substantiated documentation of ratings and delivered in a timely manner
- **Discipline**. Provided verbal and written feedback as needed in implementing progressive discipline

Using student evaluations of the instructor as part of an annual performance review is a reasonable approach given that the instructor's role is to assist students in meeting course objectives. However, such evaluations must be considered within the full context of the instructor's **key performance indicators (KPIs)** and the standards established by the program.[24] Consider whether the student's evaluations reflect a true measure of the instructor's performance or their personal feelings and biases. An instructor with rigorous standards and professional values and ethics may receive low ratings because students perceive their expectations as unreasonable or unattainable, even though the instructor is meeting or exceeding national teaching standards. Instructors may teach entry-level EMS courses to personnel who have other interests but are required to complete EMS training as a condition of continued employment. Such students may express their frustration or anger through critical and unfair evaluations. Conversely, students may rate an instructor as exceptional when they have low standards, release them early, socialize with them as "one of their own," and give consistently high marks for easy exams. These programs likely have poor performance on national high-stakes exams if they are taken, but students may be very happy with the instructor. The honest appraisal from others should reflect a consistent trend when determining the validity of feedback for inclusion in a composite performance evaluation.

All instructors should have professional development support regardless of the ratings received in their performance reviews. In academic institutions, a faculty development center or teaching laboratory can provide help in evaluating classroom performance and providing strategies for improvement. In smaller programs, money should be budgeted for faculty development.

A performance evaluation for one class or based on one observation is merely a snapshot in time of the instructor's performance. Everyone has good and bad days, and some topics and subjects are taught better than others. To provide a more complete picture of an instructor's performance, a more comprehensive tool, such as a **teaching portfolio**, is needed. The teaching portfolio provides an opportunity for the instructor to present their "teaching life" in a complete and organized manner. A teaching portfolio could contain the following items:

- List of all courses taught over a particular time
- Syllabi of past and present courses
- Past evaluations—both performance and student-based
- Examples of innovative or creative teaching approaches or student-centered strategies developed by the instructor
- Statement of the instructor's teaching philosophy and what the instructor expects to accomplish through the teaching
- Instructor's future plans related to instruction and teaching

More information on teaching portfolios can be obtained through the Vanderbilt University Center for Teaching (see https://cft.vanderbilt.edu/guides-sub-pages/teaching-portfolios/).

When conducting a performance evaluation or classroom observation, the evaluator should do the following:

- Use a standardized form that has been institutionally or agency approved.

- Provide a means for the instructor to acknowledge that the evaluation has occurred, most often by signing the form. This acknowledges that the evaluation has taken place, but not that the instructor necessarily agrees with or accepts the findings of the evaluation.
- Provide a time for consultation with the instructor after the evaluation has been completed to discuss the findings and to identify strengths and weaknesses.
- Provide the instructor with a copy of the evaluation.
- Provide a means by which the instructor can refute evaluation findings in a formal manner. This is especially important when the evaluation has a direct effect on continued employment and promotion.
- Consider videotaping the instructor during the class in which the evaluation is done as a means of recording instructor performance and minimizing subjectivity.

Formative Instructor Evaluations

If an instructor evaluation is to be a truly useful tool to drive improvement, consideration should be given to conducting formative evaluations during the course. This allows the instructor to receive feedback while there is still time to make changes to improve performance, and thus better assist students in meeting their objectives. A good time to give such evaluations is at midterm or after major module completion during the course. Conducting such evaluations lets students know that the instructor values their input and is willing to make changes in their best interest. It also signals that the instructor is seeking meaningful feedback. Depending on the course length, students may be given multiple opportunities to evaluate the instructor. Because such formative assessments are often not "official," the instructor can tailor the evaluation instrument to provide the opportunity to receive the broadest and most honest and transparent feedback from students.

Summative Instructor Evaluations

This evaluation usually occurs at the end of the course and is often completed by course participants. End-of-course instructor evaluations are often mandated by institutions and accreditation bodies. Feedback to the instructor is provided so that the instructor may recognize strengths and areas for improvement or change. Some institutions use a two-part evaluation consisting of a standardized form that may be machine-readable and a second form that contains open-ended questions. The open-ended form is designed exclusively for feedback given directly to the instructor; the machine-readable form may be used to rank instructors on an institution-wide basis, for accreditation reports, and may be used as a portion of the instructor's performance evaluation.

The common practice of gathering course evaluations from participants at the end of the course has positive and negative aspects. Positive aspects include the following:

- Convenience—participants are in class and have scheduled time to complete the evaluation.
- Response rates are high because the participants are in class.
- Students have the entire course perspective on which to base their evaluation.
- Evaluations given after final participant course evaluation and results are anonymous, so students have no fear of retaliation by the instructor.

However, some disadvantages to this approach should be considered, including the following:

- Participants may feel "forced" to complete an evaluation.
- If the evaluation is the last thing to be completed before the student leaves, especially with 1-day seminars, the participant may rush through the evaluation and not give it much thought.
- Any corrective feedback given to the instructor is not actionable for this offering because the course has already been completed.
- The participant may be "motivated" or "pumped up" about the course, especially if it will result in a new certification with the expectation of being able to perform at a new level. This may cause the participant to have a positive bias toward the instructor and the course.
- The participant may focus unduly on a recent negative or positive event with the instructor instead of on the whole course experience.

Given the limitations of the traditional end-of-course evaluations, some instructors and institutions wait for a time after the course has been completed to send participants the final instructor evaluation. The main advantage to this approach is that students have had time to reflect on their educational experience as a whole and the instructor's ability to facilitate their learning. The downside is that return rates may be poor in that participants can self-select to respond. In addition, responses may be slanted toward those participants with strong opinions, either positive or negative, about the instructor.

Starting a New Program

Creating a new educational program is a major undertaking, and the amount and degree of planning depend on the type, nature, location, and resources of the program to be conducted. An essential first step is to engage in an environmental needs assessment followed by a planning process with the goal of writing a clear and compelling business plan that identifies tactics and strategies to implement over the short-, intermediate-, and long-range planning horizons. If done well, this document serves as a blueprint for success, gives the program clear direction, helps it adapt to environmental threats and challenges, and secures needed resources.

Components of a Business Plan

The six major sections of a business plan are as follows:

- An executive summary: Create a one- to two-page abbreviated summary of the plan.
- A business problem to be addressed: Conduct an environmental assessment (assess the considerations driving the requested change).
- The available options to address a problem or an opportunity: Use the SWOT (strengths, weaknesses, opportunities, and threats) analysis technique. Then define the best options and provide an analysis of the benefits and risks, feasibility, direct and indirect costs, and issues and assumptions for each option. Options may be rated based on criteria such as efficiency, enhanced quality, staff needs, productivity, capital and operational costs, feasibility, and marketing requirements.
- Select the preferred options: Summarize rationales for preferred options.
- Implementation and evaluation: State the required activities, timelines, responsible individuals, milestones of progress, and measures of success.
- Appendix: Provide feasibility studies, research or surveys, quotes from vendors, worksheets with cost detail, and other supporting documentation.[25]

Planning

Practical steps in planning new start-up programs include the following:

- Identify all stakeholders and solicit their input and support for the program.
- Conduct an environmental assessment that may take the form of a community needs assessment/market analysis:
    - Identify potential student volume by forecasting market size and projected demand for the program. Complete a quantitative assessment (demographics, utilization rates) and qualitative assessment (other education options, practice, or technological advances that may affect demand).
    - Demonstrate that the program characteristics and operational strengths will be positively received by the market to forecast its potential for success.
    - Look at existing programs to review drivers and barriers for program success.
- Identify target student populations and educational needs, as well as relevant consumer preferences.
- Map out the program description and design. Questions to ask and answer:
    - What needs support the development of the program? Why should the program exist?
    - What should be the core values of the program?
    - What ethical or philosophical constructs will be embraced?
    - What growth, direction, milestones, and outcomes are desirable in the next year, 3 years, and 5 years?
- Create a clear, concise, and easily articulated statement of the program's "mission" or "purpose." In one or two sentences, distill the essence of why the program exists. Most organizations write very comprehensive, sometimes flowery, and wordy mission statements that almost no one can recall or recite. In stark contrast, one of the most profound healthcare organization mission statements is simply phrased "Patients first." Everyone, at every level, can remember that, and it leaves no doubt in anyone's mind as to what the organization stands for.
- Create a vision of where the program should be in the next 3 to 5 years. Consider how the program should be viewed in the broader educational arena, what linkages or accreditations will be accomplished, what services will be provided, and the desired levels of excellence or outcomes to be achieved.
- Identify core values that should drive all educational planning and decisions. Consider the beliefs and world views that are embraced by the organization and program.
- View the impact to the program from a perspective that considers internal and external factors such as a change in national education standards and/or scopes of practice or a tight economy. Consciously position the program to drive innovation, rather than being reactionary and a victim of change.

- Conduct a "SWOT analysis" to identify the following components (FIGURE 24.8):
  - **S** Strengths: Analyze program strengths.
  - **W** Weaknesses: Identify program weaknesses.
  - **O** Opportunities: Determine areas for growth or improvement.
  - **T** Threats: Consider potential present or future threats to the program.

Internal strengths and weaknesses should be evaluated based on potential for financial return on investment and budget; quantity and quality of education based on defined outcome measures; and anticipated performance based on assessment of leaders, educators, preceptors, and providers; physical facilities; and technological resources. It may be helpful to group external considerations into categories such as professional or practice; economic and financial; legal or regulatory; political; competitive or collaborative.

Armed with this information, develop practical goals, objectives, and tactics to address the key issues. Segregate the tasks into functional units. These units are sometimes called key result areas (KRAs) or KPIs that may include, but not be limited to, the following:

- **Program leadership/management**. Structure and reporting relationships; staffing plan (instructors and clerical support)
- **Medical oversight**. The physician(s) who will oversee the program.
- **Collaboration and communication**. Relationships with local EMS educational programs, hospitals, EMS agencies, and other stakeholders
- **Partnership agreements**. Agreements between institutions, for example, between an EMS program and a hospital where field internships occur

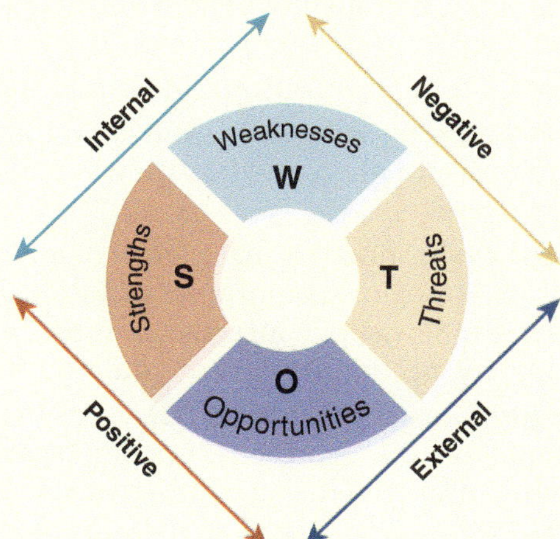

FIGURE 24.8 SWOT analysis.

- **Program accreditation**. Approvals needed; plan to achieve those requirements
- **Curriculum design and development**. Research best-practice models and/or use institutional or accreditor templates and guidelines to develop admissions policies, leadership, faculty, and preceptor job descriptions and contracts, syllabi, student policies/handbook, learning contracts and student agreements, academic calendar, instructor lesson plans, goals and objectives, content outlines, measurement and evaluation instruments, clinical unit instruction plans, agreements, and forms; field internship policies, procedures, forms
- **Asset management**. Determine needs for initial and ongoing space, supplies, equipment, and technology resources
- **Quality outcomes**. What is the expected level of detail, content, and construct excellence? Who has the final say over the quality of the outputs? (Peer review; quantitative and qualitative assessments)
- **Project deliverables/outputs**. What must the project deliver to meet the goals? How will the final deliverables be provided to the stakeholders? What will success look like?
- **Communications and marketing**. Who needs to be kept informed? How will they receive the information? When or how frequently will progress reports be issued? What will be communicated with respect to milestone achievement?
- **Feasibility and risk assessment**.
  - Potential business feasibility is assessed, as are degrees of risk and possible barriers to implementation.
  - Probability of achieving overall performance targets is "pressure tested."
- **Contingency plans**. These are in place if:
  - Time estimates are too optimistic.
  - Stakeholder review and feedback/approval cycle is too slow.
  - Unexpected resource constraints exist.
  - Technical limitations prevent implementation as proposed.
  - Roles and expectations are unclear.
  - Stakeholder needs are not properly understood.
  - Stakeholders have changing requirements after program is launched.
  - Stakeholders add new requirements after program is launched.
  - Poor communications result in quality problems and rework.

(continues)

Starting a New Program (*Continued*)

- **Financial analysis/plan**.
  - Pro forma results yield an assessment of the true economic value of the program and likely financial worthiness (sustainability).
  - Revenue streams and adequate resources are available to meet program objectives.
  - Opportunities for grant funding.
  - Review of the innovation landscape, forecasting how processes will need to change, and possible opportunities for cost savings.
  - Balanced zero-based budget creation and approval
  - Anticipated measurable return on investment (ROI).
- **Dependencies**. Board, agency, and regulatory approval.

While it is important to be visionary, as champions see and often achieve the impossible, the plan must also be practical. It is frustrating and counterproductive to create a program that has no chance of being successfully implemented. If a large gulf exists between the present and desired states, identify and prioritize steps to bridge the gap to achieve a successful program inauguration based on available resources. This permits reasoned decisions in an economically challenging environment. Create an implementation plan that details and sequences the steps, assign the persons accountable for completing each task, and specify due dates, keeping in mind that these are dynamic, rather than static documents.

Summary

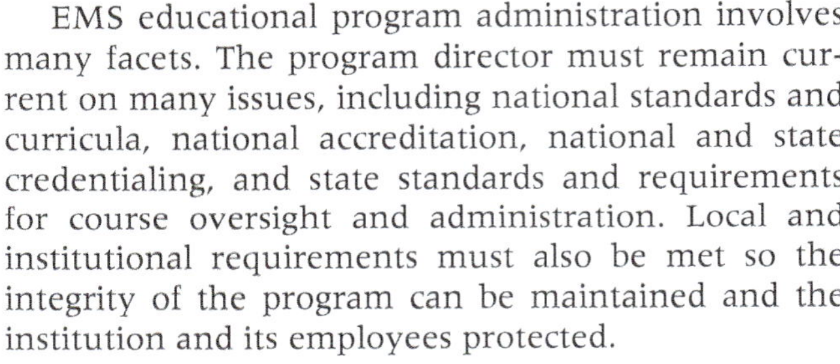

EMS educational program administration involves many facets. The program director must remain current on many issues, including national standards and curricula, national accreditation, national and state credentialing, and state standards and requirements for course oversight and administration. Local and institutional requirements must also be met so the integrity of the program can be maintained and the institution and its employees protected.

Administrators should work toward the goals of increased innovation, decreased duplication, enhanced quality, and better use of resources.[26] Attention to administrative matters is essential for safeguarding the reputation of the program and its faculty and for raising the professional standards of EMS. Beyond the legal and ethical considerations, doing so will enhance the quality of the program, abate risk, and protect the public.

Glossary

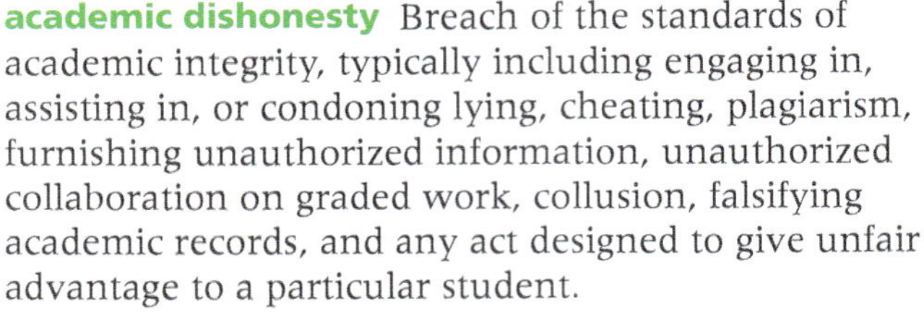

academic dishonesty Breach of the standards of academic integrity, typically including engaging in, assisting in, or condoning lying, cheating, plagiarism, furnishing unauthorized information, unauthorized collaboration on graded work, collusion, falsifying academic records, and any act designed to give unfair advantage to a particular student.

budget Financial plan for coordinating revenues (inflows) and expenditures (outflows) over a selected period of time in order to provide a net positive margin.

Commission on Accreditation of Allied Health Education Programs (CAAHEP) Approving entity for accreditation of EMS education programs.

culture of safety Values and behaviors that prioritize the safety of EMS providers and their patients.

effectiveness In terms of program evaluation, a measure of the outcome of the program. May be measured by pass/fail rates on credentialing exams, student retention/attrition rates, job placement, satisfaction rates, or quality of patient care by graduates after they transition to the workforce.

fixed cost Cost that is constant (does not fluctuate).

formative course evaluation Course evaluation designed to measure program effectiveness while class is still in progress.

instructor evaluation Formal review of an instructor by their employer for the purposes of forming a basis for contract renewal, pay increase, tenure review, accountability, or union contract requirements.

key performance indicators (KPIs) Attributes or functional units that represent core, important aspects that can be measured to gauge program success.

operating budget Budget that identifies the expected resources and expenditures of an entity for a given future period, usually spread by month over 1 year.

per capita cost per student Total cost of supplies, equipment, and resources needed for each student.

productivity Amount of output (service) per unit of input (hours of work), student-contact hours, or semester hours.

staffing plan Documented analysis of the number of educators needed to achieve program goals, and the expertise required for each educator role.

summative course evaluation Retrospective review of the entire program after the class has been completed.

teaching portfolio A collection of documents or other evidence that shows an educator's work over the course of their career, and that can be used for an educator's development and reflection.

variable cost Cost that fluctuates by volume.

variances Differences from the budgeted projections.

References

[1] National Highway Traffic Safety Administration. 1996. *Emergency Medical Services Agenda for the Future*. Washington, DC: U.S. Department of Transportation.

[2] EMS Agenda 2050 Technical Expert Panel. 2019, January. *EMS Agenda 2050: A People-Centered Vision for the Future of Emergency Medical Services* [DOT HS 812 664]. Washington, DC: National Highway Traffic Safety Administration. Accessed February 12, 2019. https://www.ems.gov/pdf/EMS-Agenda-2050.pdf.

[3] EMS.gov. "NHTSA Hosts EMS Agenda 2050 National Implementation Forum." Accessed February 12, 2019. https://www.ems.gov/newsletter/january2019/ems-agenda-2050-forum.html.

[4] National Highway Traffic Safety Administration. 2000. *Emergency Medical Services Education Agenda for the Future: A Systems Approach*. [DOT HS 809 042]. Washington, DC: U.S. Department of Health and Human Services. Accessed May 10, 2019. https://www.ems.gov/pdf/education/EMS-Education-for-the-Future-A-Systems-Approach/EMS_Education_Agenda.pdf.

[5] National Highway Traffic Safety Administration. 2005. *National EMS Core Content*. [DOT HS 809 898]. Washington, DC: U.S. Department of Transportation.

[6] National Highway Traffic Safety Administration. 2007. *National EMS Scope of Practice Model*. Washington, DC: U.S. Department of Transportation.

[7] National Association of State EMS Officials. 2018. "National Model EMS Clinical Guidelines, June 2018, Version 2.1." Accessed February 12, 2018. https://nasemso.org/wp-content/uploads/National-Model-EMS-Clinical-Guidelines-2017-Version2.1-29June2018-1.pdf.

[8] National Highway Traffic Safety Administration. 2009. "National Emergency Medical Services Education Standards." [DOT HS 811 077A]. Accessed January 15, 2019. https://www.ems.gov/pdf/National-EMS-Education-Standards-FINAL-Jan-2009.pdf.

[9] Commission on Accreditation on Allied Health Educational Programs. 2016, October. "Policies and Procedures." Accessed March 2, 2019. http://www.caahep.org/documents/file/PolicyManual.pdf.

[10] Commission on Accreditation for Pre-hospital Continuing Education (CAPCE). 2019. *Accreditation Guidebook*. Accessed March 2, 2019. http://capce.org/docs/Accred%20Guidebook.pdf.

[11] Committee on Accreditation of Educational Programs for the Emergency Medical Services Professions (CoAEMSP). 2015. "Standards and Guidelines for the Accreditation of Educational Programs in the EMS Professions." Accessed November 2, 2018. https://www.caahep.org/CAAHEP/media/CAAHEP-Documents/EMSPStandards2015.pdf

[12] Anwar, Lubna Shah. 2007, March-April. "Muslim Student Needs on U.S. Campuses." *Foreign Student Affairs. International Educator*. Accessed February 13, 2019. https://www.nafsa.org/_/File/_/ie_marapr07_fsa.pdf.

[13] Haidinyak, Gina, and Glenda C. Walker. 2005. "Don't Let the Grievance Process Cause Grief." *Nurse Educator* 30, no. 2: 73–5.

[14] deBoer, Frederick. 2016, March 22. "Standardized Assessments of College Learning Past and Future." Accessed March 28, 2019. https://www.newamerica.org/education-policy/edcentral/standardized-assessments/.

[15] Gagné, Robert M., and Leslie L. Briggs. 1979. *Principles of Instructional Design*, 2nd ed. Fort Worth, TX: Harcourt, Brace, Jovanovich.

[16] Committee on Accreditation of Educational Programs for the Emergency Medical Services Professions. 2015, August 1. "CoAEMSP Outcomes Assessment Thresholds." Accessed March 1, 2019. https://coaemsp.org/Documents/Thresholds-2015.pdf.

[17] Boyle, Patrick G. 1981. *Planning Better Programs: The Adult Education Association Professional Development Series*. New York: McGraw-Hill.

[18] Committee on Accreditation of Educational Programs for the Emergency Medical Services Professions. 2015. "Standards & Guidelines: 2015 CAAHEP Standards and Guidelines." Accessed February 14, 2019. Retrieved https://coaemsp.org/Standards.htm.

[19] Callahan, David. 2004. *The Cheating Culture: Why More Americans Are Doing Wrong to Get Ahead*. Orlando, FL: Harcourt.

[20] Williams, Kenneth M., Craig Nathanson, Delroy L. Paulhus. 2010. "Identifying and Profiling Scholastic Cheaters: Their Personality, Cognitive Ability, and Motivation." *Journal of Experimental Psychology: Applied* 16, no. 3: 293–307. http://dx.doi.org/10.1037/a0020773.

[21] Eastham, J. N., and Zietlow, V. 2004, September 1. "Will Cheating Kill EMS Online Education?" *EMSWORLD* 89–93. Accessed March 1, 2019. https://www.emsworld.com/article/10324488/will-cheating-kill-ems-online-education.

[22] Emergency Nurses Association, and Joop Breuer. 2018. "Position Statement. Social Networking by Emergency Nurses." Accessed March 27, 2019. https://www.ena.org/docs/default-source/resource-library/practice-resources/position-statements/socialnetworkingbyernurses.pdf?sfvrsn=5e069b1a_8.

[23] Yale University Publications. 2018–2019. "The Use of Computers in the Classroom." Accessed March 1, 2019. http://catalog.yale.edu/handbook-instructors-undergraduates-yale-college/teaching/use-computers-classroom/.

[24] Himelein, Melissa J. 2018, December 17. "Pitfalls of Using Student Comments in the Evaluation of Faculty." *Academic Briefing*. Accessed March 1, 2019. https://www.academicbriefing.com/human-resources/faculty-evaluation/pitfalls-of-using-student-comments-evaluation-of-faculty/.

[25] Berg, Judith G. 2010, November 8. "Getting Down to Business with a Business Plan." *Nursing Spectrum (Illinois)* 26–31.

[26] Youngberg, Barbara J., and Diane R. Weber. 1998. "Integrating Risk Management, Utilization Management, and Quality Management: Maximizing Benefit through Integration." In *The Risk Manager's Desk Reference*, edited by Barbara J. Youngberg, 27–42. Gaithersburg, MD: Aspen Publishers.

Additional Resources

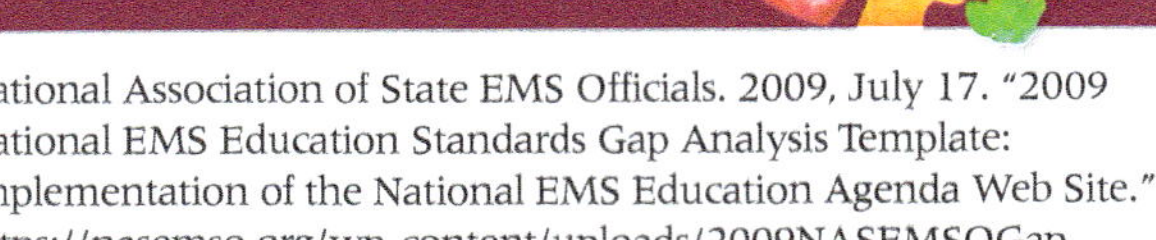

Alexander, Melissa. 2006. "Packaging the Program." In *Foundations for the Practice of EMS Education*, 168–71. Upper Saddle River, NJ: Pearson Prentice Hall.

Association for Supervision and Curriculum Development (ASCD). *Educational Leadership*. www.ascd.org/el.

Bastable, Susan B., Margaret M. Braungart, Pamela R. Gramet, Karen Jacobs, and Deborah L. Sopczyk. 2020. *Health Professional as Educator: Principles of Teaching and Learning*, 2nd ed. Burlington, MA: Jones & Bartlett Learning.

Beloit College. 2014. "The Beloit College Mindset List for the Class of 2014." *The Mindset List*. http://themindsetlist.com/.

Bloom, Benjamin S., George F. Madaus, and J. Thomas Hastings. 1981. *Evaluation to Improve Learning*. New York: McGraw-Hill.

Board of Regents of State Colleges v. Roth, 408 U.S. 564. 1972. [Student discipline policies].

Cannon, Sharon, and Carol Boswell. 2016. *Evidence-Based Teaching in Nursing: A Foundation for Educators*, 2nd ed. Burlington, MA: Jones & Bartlett Learning.

Cooper, James M. (Ed.). 2005. *Classroom Teaching Skills*. Lexington: Wadsworth Publishing.

Covey, Stephen R. 2004. *The 8th Habit: From Effectiveness to Greatness*. New York: Simon & Schuster.

Crowe, Remle C. 2015. "Are Paramedic Instructors Overworked and Under-Resourced?" *EMSWORLD* 44, no. 1: 56–60.

Danielson, Charlotte. 2013. *Framework for Teaching Evaluation Instrument*. Princeton, NJ: The Danielson Group.

Finn, Amber N., and Paul Schrodt. 2016. "Teacher Discussion Facilitation: A New Measure and Its Associations with Students' Perceived Understanding, Interest and Engagement." *Communication Education* 65, no. 4: 445–62. https://doi.org/10.1080/03634523.2016.1202997.

Gushee, Matt. 1984. "Student Discipline Policies." Eugene, OR: ERIC Clearinghouse on Educational Management. http://www.ericdigests.org/pre-922/policies.htm.

Institute of Medicine (IOM). 2014. "Assessing Health Professional Education: Workshop Summary." Washington, DC: The National Academies Press.

JEMS.com. 2011, June 10. "Former Massachusetts Firefighter Guilty in EMT Fraud." Accessed March 2, 2019. https://www.jems.com/articles/2011/06/former-massachusetts-firefighter-guilty.html.

Leger, Michael J., and Janne Dunham-Taylor. 2018. *Financial Management for Nurse Managers: Merging the Heart with the Dollar*, 4th ed. Burlington, MA: Jones & Bartlett Learning.

Magna Publications. 2018. *Fundamentals of Faculty Development: An Academic Briefing Special Report*. Madison, WI: Magna Publications.

National Association of State EMS Officials. 2009, July 17. "2009 National EMS Education Standards Gap Analysis Template: Implementation of the National EMS Education Agenda Web Site." https://nasemso.org/wp-content/uploads/2009NASEMSOGapAnalysisTemplate.pdf.

Nichols, James O., and Karen W. Nichols. 2000. *The Departmental Guide and Record Book for Student Outcomes Assessment and Institutional Effectiveness*, 3rd ed. New York: Agathon Press.

Page, James O. 2004. "Discipline with Due Process." In *Prehospital Care Administration*, 2nd ed., edited by Joseph J. Fitch, 73–82. San Diego: JEMS Communications/Elsevier.

Pozgar, George D. 2014. *Legal and Ethical Essentials of Health Care Administration*, 2nd ed. Burlington, MA: Jones & Bartlett Learning.

Steinhauer, R. 2016. "Transformational Leaders: Change Agents for Good." https://www.reflectionsonnursingleadership.org/features/more-features/Vol42_4_transformational-leaders-change-agents-for-good.

Stepien, William, and Shelagh A. Gallagher. 1997. *Problem-Based Learning across the Curriculum: An ASCD Professional Inquiry Kit*. Alexandria, VA: Association for Supervision and Curriculum Development.

Suver, James D., Bruce R. Neumann, and Keith E. Boles. 1995. *Management Accounting for Health Care Organizations*, 4th ed. Santa Monica: Bonus Books.

University of California, Office of the President. 2019, March 1. "100.00 Policy on Student Conduct and Discipline." https://policy.ucop.edu/doc/2710530/PACAOS-100.

Vaughan v. State, 456 S.W.2d 879, 833. 1970.

Weimer, Maryellen. 2015. *What Ethical Issues Lurk in My Grading Policy? Magna 20-Minute Mentor*. Madison: Magna Publications.

Weimer, Maryellen. 2016, May 11. "How Teaching Is Like Composting." https://www.teachingprofessor.com/topics/for-those-who-teach/teaching-like-composting/.

Wiggins, Grant, and Jay McTighe. 2012. *Understanding by Design Framework*. Alexandria, VA: Association for Supervision and Curriculum Development (ASCD). www.ascd.org.

Yee, Kevin, and Diane E. Boyd. 2018. "How Can We Amplify Student Learning? The ANSWER from Cognitive Psychology." *Faculty Focus*. https://www.facultyfocus.com/articles/teaching-and-learning/how-can-we-amplify-student-learning-the-answer-from-cognitive-psychology/.

Zoll Data Systems. 2006. "Defining KPIs to Maximize Business Performance." KPI White Paper. http://docplayer.net/19853119-Defining-kpis-to-maximize-business-performance.html.

CHAPTER 25

Legal Issues for EMS Educators

OBJECTIVES

At the conclusion of this chapter, the educator will be able to:

Cognitive Domain

1. Outline aspects of tort law that impact emergency medical services (EMS) educators.
2. Describe measures to manage risk within EMS programs.
3. Describe nondiscriminatory laws that can impact the EMS classroom.
4. Identify the potential liability concerns of poorly written policies, procedures, and affiliation agreements.
5. Discuss how EMS program policies and design can reduce legal risk.
6. Outline the requirements of Family Educational Rights and Privacy Act (FERPA) as it relates to EMS education.

Psychomotor Domain

There are no psychomotor objectives for this chapter.

Affective Domain

1. Value the need to maintain legally defensible practices within the EMS classroom.
2. Defend how progressive discipline and grievance policies can impact litigation in EMS education.

"No man is above the law and no man is below it; nor do we ask any man's permission when we require him to obey it."

~ Theodore Roosevelt

CHAPTER GOAL The primary goal of this chapter is to help EMS educators and others involved in EMS education understand the basic legal issues associated with educating students and preceptors of hospital and field clinicals. A second goal is to avoid the circumstances that give rise to lawsuits. The last goal is to limit the potential for liability and damages should a lawsuit be brought.

Since enactment of the federal Highway Safety Act and the formal beginning of EMS,[1] the goal of EMS has been to reduce avoidable death and disability.[2] While this goal has remained constant, EMS may not always meet the public's expectations for successful prehospital intervention.[3] Both the expectations for emergency care and the likelihood of lawsuits have increased, as have the number of claims filed by the public, as well as by EMS students (hereinafter simply referred to as students in this chapter).

This chapter focuses on legal issues related to educating students in EMS programs. Clearly, those who deliver prehospital interventions must first be properly trained. Furthermore, those who teach emergency response must be knowledgeable of both the legal issues related to the delivery of emergency medical care and the legal issues associated with teaching. This chapter is not provided as a substitute for legal advice or training. When legal questions arise, EMS programs and educators should seek the service of competent attorneys with expertise in health law and education law.

While many people consider the United States to be a litigious society, all U.S. citizens have a fundamental right to file meritorious lawsuits and seek the redress of their legitimate grievances. However, no one has the right to abuse the process by filing frivolous lawsuits, and attorneys are legally and ethically responsible for screening suits to make sure they have merit. Still, baseless claims are not always preventable. The best way for EMS educators to avoid being sued is to have a sound understanding of basic legal concepts and terminology and an appreciation for the facts and circumstances that have caused others to be sued. Such an understanding begins with a brief overview of the U.S. legal system.

Areas of Law

The American legal system can be divided into two broad categories: criminal law and civil law. **Criminal law** refers to public wrongs or crimes that violate laws at the state or federal level. Criminal cases are prosecuted by an attorney for the government, such as a district attorney, state's attorney, or attorney general. Violation of criminal laws can result in fines and imprisonment, among other sanctions.

Civil law involves private matters such as contracts, business transactions, and domestic relations. In civil cases, the injured party, known as the plaintiff, seeks recovery of money or other forms of relief for a claimed act or omission. This claim is made against another person or entity, called a defendant. A defendant who claims to have been injured by a plaintiff may also file counterclaims against the plaintiff as part of the same lawsuit.

Tort Law

A **tort** is a private or civil wrong or injury, other than a breach of contract, for which the law allows a remedy. A tort is an act that causes personal injury or property damage. It is committed by one party against another party, in either an intentional or negligent manner. A claim of medical negligence or professional malpractice is a tort action, as are assault, battery, defamation, misrepresentation, and fraud.

TEACHING TIP

EMS educators should be alert to high-risk activities in the classroom, lab, clinical setting, or field that could result in a tort claim. For instance, special precautions or safeguards should be in place when students are lifting and moving live persons on any device. Spotters, lab instructors, or safety officers should be in place to observe for proper techniques and focus on safety issues. In addition, EMS programs and educators should ensure that appropriate preventive maintenance is performed on stretchers used to move participants.

Assault and Battery

Although assault and battery are frequently discussed in combination as a single phenomenon, they are actually separate torts. An **assault** occurs when one person places another person in reasonable fear of immediate harm or physical contact. For instance, if a student raises their fist in a menacing manner toward someone as if about to strike them, causing the person to fear being struck, the student has assaulted that person. Verbal assault occurs when a person states the intent to harm another person. Nonverbal assault occurs when a person creates an atmosphere of intimidation, such as when brandishing a weapon or advancing toward another person.

Battery is the physical, unlawful touching of another person without consent. It is important to ensure students understand that even well-intentioned treatment can later be the subject of a battery claim. Some religions forbid the use of blood transfusions, and doing so on a prehospital patient of that persuasion may constitute battery if no defenses are available. EMS educators must also be aware that whenever an EMS program is dependent on the completion of clinical training, students might feel pressure to tolerate instances of harassment to obtain a good recommendation from a preceptor and to be offered a permanent position. This abuse of power could give rise to a claim for battery.

Consent is a defense to any claim for assault or battery. It is always advisable to obtain a person's consent prior to making physical contact with them. This includes making physical contact with a student for demonstration purposes in a classroom setting.

Defamation

Defamation can be the intentional or reckless making of a false statement, or the sharing of true, but private information that injures the reputation of another. Libel is the written or printed form of defamation. Slander is the spoken or oral form of defamation. Truth is one potential defense to a claim of defamation; it is, however, not a defense when private, sensitive information is willingly shared without permission.

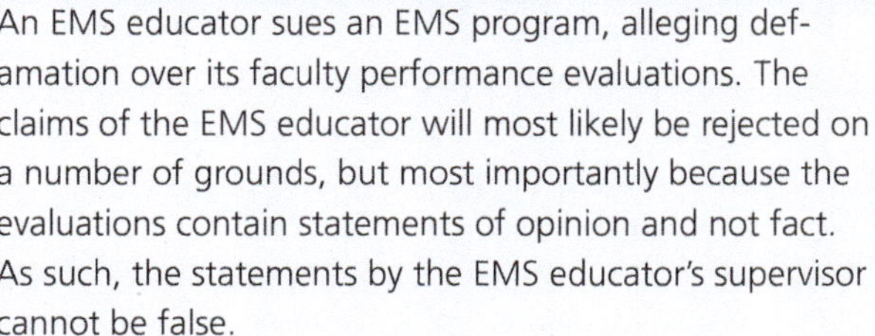

CASE in Point

An EMS educator sues an EMS program, alleging defamation over its faculty performance evaluations. The claims of the EMS educator will most likely be rejected on a number of grounds, but most importantly because the evaluations contain statements of opinion and not fact. As such, the statements by the EMS educator's supervisor cannot be false.

CASE in Point

A student sues an allied health program alleging, among other claims, that statements by an allied health educator to the certification agency about the eccentricity of the student constituted defamation. The claims of the student will probably fail because the educator is not liable when their opinion is based on truth, namely that (1) the student discussed termination of another healthcare provider in a public setting during the student's hospital and field clinicals; (2) educators and preceptors of the student were contacted and the student was found to be difficult to work with; (3) the student told patients that their medical insurance would not fully cover their hospice stay; and (4) the student was not able to accept feedback or constructive criticism from educators and preceptors, all of whom suggested that the student displayed eccentric behavior. This eccentric behavior, in conjunction with other academic shortfalls, will most likely result in dismissal of the student from the program; the defamation claim by the student will probably fail.

Misrepresentation

Misrepresentation is the making of a false statement with intent to deceive, that causes actual harm to someone who reasonably relies on the falsity of the statement. It is a polite way of saying **fraud**. In EMS programs, misrepresentation or fraud could occur when marketing material for an EMS program indicates that it is something other than what it is. For instance, if a marketing brochure indicates that a program is accredited by certain organizations, when it is not, someone who attends EMS classes may have a cause of action for misrepresentation or fraud. The U.S. Department of Education is focusing on misrepresentation or fraud regarding the number of students who are employed upon graduation, whether graduates are employed within their fields of study, and the salaries of graduates.[4]

Training Fraud

Over the past several years, reports of training fraud in EMS programs have increased. This practice jeopardizes EMS programs, and everyone involved in EMS, and in some cases, anyone receiving prehospital interventions. The following hypotheticals will most likely result in termination of EMS educators and students, licensure actions, and in some cases criminal charges:

- Numerous states investigated claims that paramedics falsely reported attending advanced cardiac life support, basic life support, and pediatric life support training classes.
- Paramedics involved in training fraud voluntarily surrendered their licenses and certification from the NREMT, and numerous paramedics had their license revoked.[5]
- Fire fighters and EMTs faked both fire and medical training records.
- EMS educators who submitted false training records were sentenced to 2 or more years in prison and fined, with fines averaging $5,000.[6,7]

When accrediting or regulatory agencies find that an EMS agency, program, or educator has misrepresented or fraudulently documented training information, the EMS program is subject to loss of accreditation. Commonly, everyone involved in the training fraud is terminated, along with supervisors who knew or should have known of the fraud and yet condoned it. If anyone receiving prehospital interventions was harmed, the top managers of the EMS program will often face termination. When anyone is actually harmed, criminal charges are usually brought against the EMS program, as well as against everyone who knew or should have known about the misrepresentations and overlooked them. Substantial fines are commonly assessed against the EMS program and often against everyone who knew about the training fraud. It is the EMS educator's duty to ensure that honest documentation of training occurs. Accurate records must be maintained in all cases.

Negligence

Negligence is the failure to exercise the care that a reasonably prudent person would have exercised in a similar situation that causes damages to another. In everyday life, everyone is held responsible to act as the fictional reasonably prudent person would act under similar circumstances. This applies when driving, cooking, or engaging in other normal activities.

However, people who have specialized skills and training, such as physicians, nurses, paramedics, and EMTs, are held to a higher standard of care when acting in their respective professional capacities. A professional is held to the standard of care that the reasonably prudent professional of like skill and training would exercise under like circumstances. As such, a paramedic is held to the standard of the reasonably prudent paramedic, and an EMT is held to the standard of the reasonably prudent EMT. EMS educators are responsible to make sure that appropriate, safe educational practices are being provided to students and ensure that their students deliver competent emergency care.

Negligence claims must establish four elements:

1. A legal duty
2. Breach of the requisite standard of care
3. Injury or damages
4. The resulting injury or damage was caused by the breach of the standard of care

A claim of medical negligence brought against an EMS facility or program would likely be brought in conjunction with a claim for professional malpractice; the elements are the same, with the caveat that the EMS defendant is a professional held to the higher standard of care exercised by other similar professionals under

CASE in Point

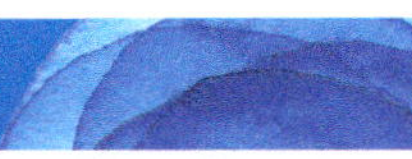

An EMS educator is teaching a class on patient lifts and carries. A student is asked to serve as a patient and is seated on a stair chair as two other students attempt to carry their classmate down a flight of stairs. The EMS educator does not instruct the students to secure the student seated on the stair chair using the attached straps, and in fact observes the students lift their classmate and start to carry the student on the stair chair with the straps dangling. One student steps on a strap, causing the student on the stair chair to fall and injure their back and neck.

An analysis of these hypothetical facts follows in light of the elements of negligence:

1. The EMS educator has a legal duty to students to exercise reasonable care.
2. The EMS educator very likely breached the standard of care by (a) failing to properly train students before allowing them to engage in a dangerous activity and (b) failing to stop the students from engaging in a dangerous activity even though the EMS educator observed an obvious safety risk. What needs to be determined is what a reasonably prudent EMS educator would have done, and if the EMS educator's conduct in this instance met or failed to meet that standard. The EMS educator's actions will then be compared to that of other EMS educators in like circumstances.
3. A student was injured.
4. The EMS educator's breach of the standard of care caused the injuries to the student who fell off the stair chair.

like circumstances. In many states, **expert** testimony is required in order to establish that all elements of professional malpractice have been met. In such states, a suit based on the negligence of a professional cannot legally be successful without the testimony of an expert. In some states, lawsuits may not even be filed without an expert's certification that the suit has merit. This is because a baseless accusation of professional negligence has serious repercussions against the professional's career and reputation; in some instances, the professional may countersue the plaintiff for defamation.

Duty

The first element of any negligence claim, *legal duty*, is usually undisputed in actions against EMS providers because the duty exists by virtue of providers being on the job and responding to a call for emergency assistance. However, duty to act is actually a challenging area of the law. Duty to act often becomes an issue for off-duty personnel who come upon an injured person.

As a general rule, no one has a legal duty to come to the aid of another person, absent some special relationship. Relationships that create a duty to act include parent to child, spouse to spouse, and teacher to student. Thus, an EMS educator would have a legal duty to come to the aid of a student who is stricken or injured during a class. An EMS educator would also have a legal duty to take reasonable precaution to protect students from foreseeable, preventable harm.

Breach

The second element of a negligence claim, breach of the standard of care, asks what a reasonably prudent person, or a professional would have done in the same or similar situation.

Evidence of the applicable standard of care may come from many sources, including the following:

- Expert witnesses
- Authoritative, peer-reviewed textbooks and training materials
- Industry-wide standards
- EMS program operating procedures, policies, and rules
- Federal and state laws
- State and local protocols for emergencies
- Federal education standards from the U.S. Department of Health and Human Services, U.S. Department of Labor, and the U.S. Department of Transportation
- Accreditation agency standards

The term **standard of care** is commonly used in two different senses. In one sense, a standard of reasonable care refers to prevailing or routine practice that a provider of equal training or certification would administer; in another sense, the duty of care refers to the legal obligation to conform to a minimum level of safe care.[8] In any event, the totality of the circumstances is always taken into consideration. EMS programs must ensure that their education is offered according to current training standards and that their EMS practices protect student rights. Furthermore, the EMS educator must follow safety standards during training activities to ensure the safety and well-being of students.

TEACHING TIP

EMS educators have an affirmative legal duty to take reasonable precautions to protect students from foreseeable, preventable harm.

Injury

The third element of negligence, injury or damages, is required in order to pursue a claim of negligence. That injury may be academic, including dismissal from an EMS program or delay in graduation, or physical, in cases where a student is harmed during a training exercise. A breach of the standard of care that does not produce appreciable injury or damages will not give rise to a negligence claim. Some states do not allow recovery for injuries that are purely psychological, such as emotional distress, in the absence of some physical symptom. In some states, damages may not be allowed for a purely economic loss.

Causation

The final element of negligence is causation. Causation requires that the negligent act or omission be the legal cause of the damages or injuries to the person harmed or injured. A lack of causation is often raised as a defense in negligence cases. For instance, just because someone is injured does not mean that the EMS program, or an EMS educator or student, committed negligence, or that the injury was the result of a careless act or failure to act. A common defense is to assert that the injured party contributed to the negative outcome, such as by ignoring advice.

Defenses to Negligence

There are three common defenses to negligence claims:

1. Assumption of risk
2. Release of risk
3. Contributory or comparative negligence

Assumption of Risk

The assumption-of-risk doctrine generally indicates that anyone who willingly participates in an activity known to involve risk (including hospital or field clinicals) cannot recover damages resulting from an injury due to the materialization of risks generally associated with that activity. Upon assumption of the risk, there is no longer a duty of care running from anyone who assumed the risk; without a duty owed, there can be no negligence. It cannot, however, always be assumed that someone has accepted the inherent risks involved in a particular activity.

Release of Risk

EMS programs frequently require students (or parents/guardians) to sign release or waiver-of risk forms. This is done to establish the assumption of-risk doctrine. The signed release form is evidence that the student was aware of, and assumed, the risk involved with the activity.

EMS educators should be cautious when creating release-of-risk and waiver-of-risk forms. These forms should be clearly written and in compliance with federal and state laws. Minors may be owed a greater duty of care than adult students, and in addition, minors may not be legally able to sign a waiver for themselves. It is vital that legal counsel review any proposed release and waiver forms before they are used by an EMS program. An EMS educator must never take another organization's release or waiver and adapt it for their own needs.

Contributory or Comparative Negligence

Up to this point, the focus of this chapter has been on liability concerns when one person was totally at fault for another person's injuries. What happens if the injured person bore some responsibility for their own injuries? This is known as *contributory negligence*. Until recently, no one could obtain compensation for an injury if they, themselves, were negligent. If there was contributory negligence, the injured person was completely barred from any compensation if the injury suffered was only partly their fault.

Today, nearly all states have abandoned contributory negligence in favor of a doctrine known as *comparative negligence*. Under comparative negligence, the injured party's damages are reduced in proportion to their degree of fault in causing their own injury. For instance, if someone is found to be 30% at fault for an injury, their award of damages would be reduced by 30%.

CASE in Point

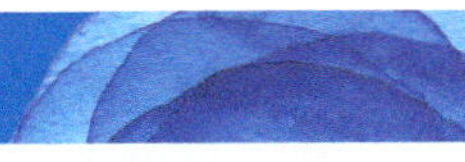

Students engaged in horseplay that resulted in severe injuries to one of the students. If it is determined that each student was 50% responsible for the injuries, then the injured student could only recover 50% of the damages.

CASE in Point

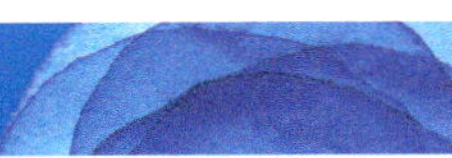

A student who was injured as a result of horseplay in the classroom sues another student and the EMS program. The injured student claimed that the negligent supervision by an EMS educator played a role in their injuries. If the other noninjured students, as well as the EMS educator, are found to be liable, then fault would be apportioned, accordingly. The injured student could conceivably receive 100% of the damages from the other student and the EMS educator.

Risk Management

Risk management is the process of preventing, or at least minimizing, harm or loss. The discussion of risk management fits the topic of tort law by showing that sound risk management principles may reduce liability exposure. While reducing liability is an important consideration in risk management, there is a more important factor: *safety*. Risk management steps taken to prevent lawsuits and liability have the advantage of enhancing safety.

Consider the risk management value of a driver training program. By training EMS drivers with a standardized curriculum, liability exposure to the EMS program is reduced. In the event of a lawsuit stemming from a vehicle collision, showing that all EMS drivers have met a minimum level of training and competence may prove valuable in limiting liability and monetary damages. Just as important, the workplace is made safer by ensuring EMS drivers are better trained and less likely to get into a preventable collision.

Whenever an injury occurs, the injured party may likely attempt to place blame and seek compensation. Risk management helps to focus EMS educators on preventing such injuries from occurring. In addition, risk management can help mitigate the liability costs associated with injuries when they do occur.

Methods of Risk Management

EMS educators should consider two principal methods of risk management. The first method, risk control, is the process of reducing the rate and intensity of potential harm. This is a preventive process where safety methods are employed to modify potential activities or equipment that could lead to EMS program or personal liability to EMS educators. The second method of risk management is risk transfer. Waivers, releases, and insurance policies are all forms of risk transfer.

EMS educators should be actively involved in risk management in their classrooms and clinical education settings. Based on the nature of the EMS profession, safety is of critical importance. Safety education should be an initial component of any EMS curriculum. Safety tests should be given to students, and a high level of success should be required for continued participation in the program.

The results of safety exams should remain on file with the EMS program. Clear record keeping is critical for establishing a strong defense against litigation when the EMS facility, program, or educators are facing litigation. Two examples of high-risk, high-frequency activities that warrant risk management attention by EMS programs and educators are stretcher handling and sharps handling.

Student Supervision

No laws directly govern the supervision of students while engaged in classroom, laboratory, hospital, or fieldwork. EMS educators must therefore be guided by considerations of what the reasonably prudent educator of like skill and training would be expected to do under similar circumstances. EMS educators should adhere to all applicable program policies, as well as all relevant federal and state laws and policy statements.

EMS educators should consider the maturity level of their students, their level of safety education, and the type of emergency services activity being engaged in before leaving students unsupervised. EMS educators should be alert for any student who may have mental health or behavioral problems that are not properly controlled. Clearly, these may affect the student's ability to competently and effectively perform EMS tasks. In such a situation, the EMS educator should follow the protocol of the EMS program when documenting their observations and referring the student to mental health assistance, keeping in mind the student's right to privacy.

Emergency Protocol Procedures

It is doubtful that anyone is more familiar with the value of emergency protocol procedures than EMS educators. EMS educators must be familiar with emergency response procedures at each teaching venue and be able to implement the procedures quickly and properly in emergency situations. Educators should also inform students of emergency procedures at the outset of the course, which may simply include references to emergency procedures in the course syllabus. This includes how to summon help, the address of the venue, and the location of available equipment such as defibrillators.

Hazardous Events in Clinical Education. Whenever students are placed at risk in an educational situation, special care should be taken by EMS educators. Students are owed a duty of protection from reasonably foreseeable dangers that are known to exist in their assignments. EMS programs that require students to drive emergency vehicles should be particularly cautious given the high-risk nature of operating emergency vehicles. Other areas of concern include exposure to infectious diseases and helicopter transport.

Bloodborne Pathogens and Infectious Diseases. EMS educators and students are at occupational risk of exposure to blood and other bodily fluids that might contain the hepatitis B virus (HBV), hepatitis C virus (HCV), or human immunodeficiency virus (HIV), among other infectious diseases.[9] EMS educators should ensure that students are provided with and are required to use appropriate protective barriers (such as gloves, gowns, aprons, masks, or protective eyewear) during time spent in labs, hospitals, or ambulances (**FIGURE 25.1**). Training records should document that students have been trained in proper bloodborne pathogen and infectious disease procedures, and counseling should be documented when deviations occur.

All occupational exposures to pathogens should be considered urgent medical concerns to ensure timely management and administration of postexposure prophylaxis. Students should be given a written, easily accessible policy concerning what to do once they have an exposure and to whom they should report. Hospital and field personnel should also be clear about the process to follow for their students. In addition, consultation with local experts and the **National Clinicians' Post-Exposure Prophylaxis Hotline** (1-888-HIV-4911) is advised.

TEACHING TIP

EMS educators should require students to employ standard precautions when exposed to blood, as well as when exposed to other bodily fluids containing visible blood, semen, or vaginal secretions. This includes exposure to tissues and cerebrospinal, synovial, pleural, peritoneal, pericardial, and amniotic fluids, as advised by the Centers for Disease Control and Prevention. This also includes exposures during lab work in addition to fieldwork.

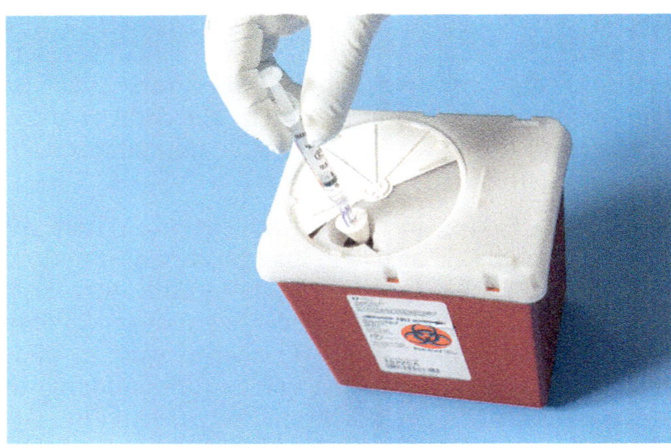

FIGURE 25.1 Students should be fully trained in infection control as required by OSHA regulations before being potentially exposed to bloodborne pathogens and infectious agents, especially when using sharps.

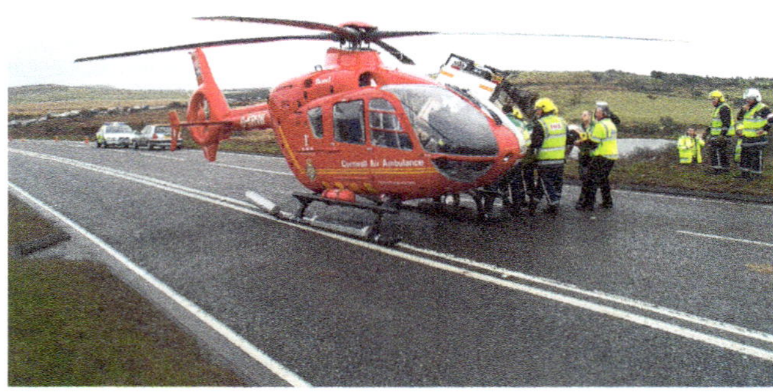

FIGURE 25.2 Helicopter EMS flights are inherently dangerous, and educators should carefully consider alternatives prior to assigning students to this type of prehospital intervention.

Courtesy of Mark Woolcock.

Helicopter Emergency Medical Service Flights. Helicopter emergency medical service (HEMS) flights carry certain inescapable risks, causing many EMS educators to question the advisability of unnecessarily exposing students to this activity during their clinical education (**FIGURE 25.2**). Undoubtedly, the risks and benefits of such training must be evaluated by each EMS program.[10] Because HEMS flights are inherently dangerous,[11] EMS educators might consider restricting students to accompanying persons receiving emergency care on HEMS flights to hospitals only in situations where other methods of EMS transportation are impractical or impossible.[12]

Site Selection

EMS educators should be cognizant of inherent dangers when selecting educational sites for clinical affiliations. Although no guarantee may be made to ensure the safety of students as they complete clinical rotations, EMS educators should be aware of potential risks based on site selection, including where reductions in EMS services leave insufficiently trained or supervised staff to provide proper student supervision.

Clinical Instruction

Clinical and field experiences are essential elements of entry-level EMS education. Aside from safety considerations, key aspects ensure an effective, legally defensible clinical experience that is safe for anyone receiving prehospital interventions. EMS educators must follow state laws in their clinical instruction. In many cases, this means that students must maintain basic life support certifications, or when attending a paramedic program, an EMT license. Other state policies often include the requirement that students work under the direct supervision of a clinician licensed at or above the level the student for which is being trained. In all cases, students should perform invasive skills or administer medication only with direct observation and supervision of their clinical preceptor. To ensure the appropriate supervision of students, EMS programs must make sure their clinical preceptors have the appropriate training regarding student policies and their level of preparation. Students must have adequate knowledge and skills practice in a lab or simulated setting prior to performing skills and care on real persons receiving emergency services. Failure to do so can subject the EMS program and clinical preceptors to litigation.

Clinical objectives should clearly define expectations and should be written to progressively higher levels as the student moves through the EMS program. A student who can master entry-level clinical objectives and perform isolated skills may struggle when asked to synthesize information and apply it within the context of a fast-paced EMS call. The student's performance must be assessed at each experience and the student made

TEACHING TIP

Anyone who receives emergency medical services may sue if they are injured by an EMS student. Thus, EMS programs and their clinical preceptors have an obligation to provide adequate supervision and should not allow students to make independent medical decisions in emergency situations.

TEACHING TIP

Sometimes students pass all of their didactic classes but fail their clinical courses. Most of these students repeat their clinical courses with a different EMS preceptor and pass; however, some will continue to fail. EMS programs will generally prevail in clinical instruction claims if they have detailed anecdotal notes that document instances of unsafe or incompetent student behavior.

aware of their progress no less often than at the midterm. If a student fails during the latter part of a course, it is essential to identify the objectives that they were unable to meet. Specific examples of situations where the student failed to meet objectives should be provided, with additional details regarding how the student was notified of the deficiencies before the end of the program and any remediation measures attempted.

Civil Rights and Nondiscrimination Laws

The U.S. Constitution and numerous federal and state civil rights and nondiscrimination laws prohibit **discrimination** in a variety of settings, including in the workplace, public spaces, and EMS facilities and programs. EMS educators should be familiar with the ethical, legal, and practical considerations of discrimination and civil rights laws, and in particular, with the specific applications of these laws to their classroom and clinical programs.

TEACHING TIP

EMS educators must ensure that students understand their obligation to promote universal respect for, and observance of, all human rights and freedoms. This respect must be without distinction as to color, disability, gender, language, national origin, race, religion, or any other type of distinction that is based on group characteristics. During their clinical experiences, the best way for EMS students to understand and learn to respect other people is for EMS educators to consistently model empathy and appropriate nondiscriminatory behavior. EMS educators must also be mindful that as role models they cannot condone others who demonstrate a lack of empathy and respect for the rights of others. An EMS educator who observes discriminating behavior and does not stop it, condones it.

Federal Constitutional Protections

The U.S. Constitution prohibits any level of government from violating the constitutional rights of its citizens—a concept called **constitutional protections**. Federal and state civil rights law allow U.S. citizens, and anyone else who is lawfully in the United States, to sue any **governmental actor** who violates their constitutional rights. EMS facilities and programs may be considered governmental actors if they receive any type of public funding.

Other factors are considered in determining whether EMS educators or students are acting under **color of law**. To the extent that EMS educators are governmental actors, they can be sued in their individual capacities for violating the constitutional rights of others. While aggrieved persons face significant obstacles to successful litigation, constitutional mandates serve as an important guide for EMS educators, and discrimination lawsuit victories do occur.

Search and Seizure Clause of the Fourth Amendment

The Fourth Amendment provides that U.S. citizens have the right to be free against unreasonable searches and seizures by the government. This Fourth Amendment right extends to anyone who is lawfully in the United States, but does not apply to anyone who is in the United States illegally. Generally, the right to privacy is protected during the treatment and transportation of persons receiving emergency services. While people who are not in the United States legally may receive the benefit of the Fourth Amendment in emergency circumstances, they usually are not considered to be in custody when receiving emergency services for purposes of the Fourth Amendment. At the same time, in some jurisdictions, whenever a person cannot walk away, they may be considered to be in custody and subject to arrest or deportation.

Search and seizure laws commonly come up in an educational context with regard to locker searches. The protections of the Fourth Amendment against unreasonable searches and seizures applies to any location wherein someone has a "reasonable expectation of privacy." Courts have found that EMS educators, as well as students, may enjoy a reasonable expectation of privacy in locations such as lockers, desks, backpacks, and briefcases.

What can an EMS educator do if informed by a student that another student has illegal drugs in their locker? Would it matter if it was a handgun? EMS programs are well advised to address these concerns proactively by adopting policies that inform everyone that EMS facilities or locations such as a locker are not

CASE in Point

A student sues the EMS program in which they are enrolled for violations of their Fourth and Fourteenth Amendment rights when the EMS program ordered the student to either undergo a urinalysis for drugs or face expulsion upon refusal. The urinalysis was requested after determination by EMS educators that drug use may have been the cause of some of the inappropriate behavior that had warranted past discipline of this student. In this instance, the intrusiveness of the search was minimal, and the student was not singled out arbitrarily or capriciously. The needs of the EMS program entitled the EMS educators to immunity. Thus, the constitutional rights of this student were not violated.

private. Such a policy should clearly indicate that the EMS program reserves the right to search areas such as lockers at any time.

Due Process and Equal Protection Clauses of the Fourteenth Amendment

The Equal Protection Clause of the Fourteenth Amendment provides that people have the right to equal protection of the laws, while the Due Process Clause provides that no person can be deprived of their "life, liberty, or property, without due process of law." In general, students cannot be arbitrarily dismissed from an EMS program. Accordingly, EMS educators must demonstrate fair and impartial treatment of students. Discipline or program dismissal must be carefully documented and grounded in an unbiased assessment of performance. Published **grievance** policies must be followed.[8] The reason for dismissal must be readily evident and should be supported by progressive documentation of performance that deviates from expectations described in EMS program policies and syllabi.

Federal Nondiscrimination Laws

The U.S. Constitution prohibits governments from violating the civil rights of U.S. citizens. Congress has gone a step further by enacting federal laws that prohibit various types of discrimination. Although this list is not all-encompassing, these five federal nondiscrimination laws impact EMS facilities, programs, EMS educators, and students:

TEACHING TIP

To protect against lawsuits, EMS educators should do the following:

- Have a clear syllabus and handbook outlining EMS program policies related to attendance, grading, classroom and clinical behaviors, and appropriate interpersonal interactions.
- Review policies with the students at the beginning of each class and have them acknowledge receipt.
- Ensure that students understand how they will be graded and what criteria may constitute failure (including any required assessments).
- Inform students of their progress, especially if they are at risk of failing.
- Consistently follow course policies and apply them equally to all students.
- Avoid labeling students.
- Document problems and disciplinary actions as they arise.
- Approach each potential disciplinary action objectively and document facts, not opinions.
- Follow established protocols for grievance and appeals.

- Americans with Disabilities Act (ADA)[13]
- Title VI of the Civil Rights Act[14]
- **Equal Employment Opportunity Act (EEOA)**[15]
- **Pregnancy Discrimination Act (PDA)**[16]
- **Title IX of the Education Amendments Act**[17]

The Americans with Disabilities Act and the Rehabilitation Act

The federal ADA was enacted in 1990. Before that time, the key piece of legislation addressing persons with disabilities was the Rehabilitation Act.[18] Both the Rehabilitation Act and the ADA prohibit disability-based discrimination. The ADA states, "No covered entity shall discriminate against a qualified individual on the basis of disability in regard to job application procedures, the hiring, advancement, or discharge of employees, employee compensation, job training and other terms, conditions, and privileges of employment."[19] Several terms with which students should be familiar are defined in **TABLE 25.1**.

This dual commitment is particularly important in the context of situations wherein students with special needs may require certain accommodations in order to fulfill their requirements for professional EMS certifications or licensure. Mentally and physically

TABLE 25.1 ADA Terminology

Term	Definition	Comments
Qualified individual with a disability	Any individual with a disability who, with or without reasonable accommodation, can perform the essential functions of the employment position that they hold or desire.	The term "handicapped" has been replaced by "disability." The term "alcohol and illegal drug abuse" has been replaced by "substance use disorder."
Reasonable accommodation	Making existing facilities used by EMS educators and students readily accessible to and usable by persons with disabilities, examples include job restructuring; part-time and modified work schedules; acquisition or modification of equipment or devices; appropriate adjustment or modifications of examinations, training materials, or policies; provision of qualified readers or interpreters; and other similar accommodations.	An interactive process involving representatives from the existing EMS facility and the disabled student determines student accommodations to be provided.
Undue hardship	Nature and cost of accommodations, including the overall financial resources of the existing EMS facility.	Financial burden may be respected in light of establishing undue hardship for the existing EMS facility.
Major life activities	Functions such as caring for oneself, performing manual tasks, walking, seeing, hearing, speaking, breathing, learning, and working.	To qualify for disabilities, persons must have substantially limited activity or activities.
Substantially limited	Unable to perform a major life activity that the average person in the general population can perform.	Factors to consider in determining whether someone is substantially limited include the nature and severity of the impairment, duration of impairment, and permanent or long-term impact of the impairment.

Data from Federal law codified in the U.S. Code at 42 U.S.C. §§ 12101-12213, with implementing regulations in the U.S. Code of Federal Regulations at 42 C.F.R. §§ 12101-12213.

TEACHING TIP

It is important for EMS educators to understand that the ADA and the Rehabilitation Act establish a dual mandate of nondiscrimination and accommodation. These laws not only prohibit discrimination, but also mandate that affirmative steps be taken to accommodate the needs of students with disabilities.

challenged students face many hurdles when seeking to establish a *prima facie* ADA case in which their evidence is strong enough to create a presumption that a disability exists. To prevail in any discrimination litigation, students must be able to demonstrate the following:[20]

- They are disabled within the meaning of the ADA.
- They are otherwise qualified to perform the essential functions of EMS activities with or without reasonable accommodations.
- They suffered an adverse decision with regard to their professional EMS certifications and licensure due to their disability.

Disabilities are interpreted in a broad and inclusive manner. The exception to this statement of defining what is interpreted as a disability is students with substance use disorder. Students with substance use disorder are not considered disabled under the ADA.[21] Otherwise, the definition of disability under the ADA is construed in favor of the broadest coverage.[22]

Civil Rights Laws

Whereas the federal ADA and Rehabilitation Act protect persons with disabilities from discrimination,

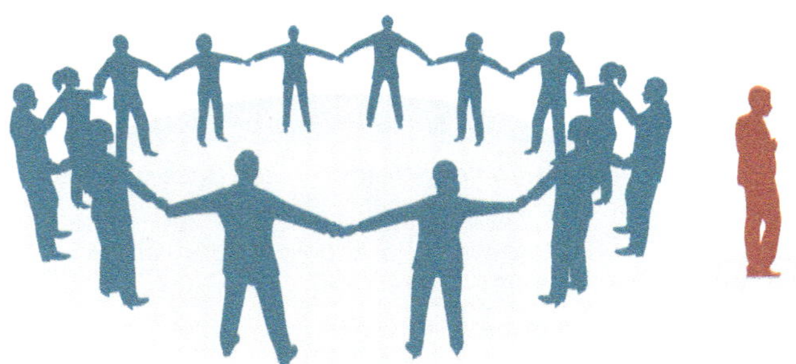

FIGURE 25.3 This classic illustration of discrimination demonstrates exclusion of a person on the basis that they are not part of a group, or are different.

interpretations of the U.S. federal and state civil rights laws have been significantly expanded to prohibit discrimination by any EMS facility or program receiving federal funding or any EMS educator benefiting from federal funding. The law prohibits EMS facilities and programs, as well as EMS educators, that receive or are benefited by public funds, from engaging in discrimination. Discrimination is prohibited on the basis of color, disability, gender, language, national origin, race, religion, or any other type of expansive distinction that is based on group characteristics, economic class, or category to which someone may perceive themselves to belong (**FIGURE 25.3**).

Equal Employment Opportunity Act

Under Title VII of the federal Civil Rights Act, it is illegal to discriminate in the hiring or terminating of employees, or in any other act of employment training, such as in EMS certification or licensure programs, based on age, race, color, religion, sex, or national origin.[23] Students, as well as applicants to an EMS program, are afforded the same rights as EMS educators within the EMS facility and program.

Pregnancy Discrimination Act

Pregnancy discrimination has been a longstanding problem. What makes it particularly challenging is that some well-intentioned efforts to "protect" pregnant women, have the "effect" of discriminating against women. Pregnant women cannot be categorically excluded or restricted from EMS programs based on their pregnancy. The federal Pregnancy Discrimination Act requires EMS facilities and programs to provide pregnant women the same accommodations they provide to other temporarily disabled workers with similar levels of incapacity.[24]

TEACHING TIP

EMS educators should be aware that female students who become pregnant during their EMS certification and licensure training may need to delay some clinical experiences (in hospitals or the field) if recommended by the pregnant student's physician. The ultimate decision rests with the student and her physician, not the EMS program or its preceptors. EMS programs may wish to include special provisions addressing pregnancy in release and waiver forms.

Title IX of the Education Amendments Act

Title IX of the Education Amendments Act provides that students may not be excluded from participation in, be denied the benefits of, or be subjected to discrimination by any EMS program or clinical or fieldwork in the EMS program receiving federal funding on the basis of their gender or category to which someone may perceive themselves to belong, such as transgender students.[25] Discrimination cases are frequently filed under Title IX, Title VII (federal Equal Employment Opportunity Act), or a combination of these two federal laws. EMS programs that receive public funds may not discriminate in admission, dismissal, or any other way based on any type of gender characteristics or gender category to which someone may perceive themselves to belong. Even though not required by law, EMS programs that are not federally funded would be wise to follow the same nondiscriminatory practices.

Public Health and Safety Laws

Various federal, state, and environmental workplace regulations require EMS programs and educators to assess and improve the quality of equipment and clinical education provided to students who work with organic hazardous waste materials, such as bodily fluids and tissues. These regulations also assess and improve training for situations involving chemical hazardous waste. Workplace safety cases are being prosecuted with increasing frequency and success, so it is critical that federal, state, and local regulations be clearly understood. As with any type of EMS activity, response is much more effective if potential problems are examined beforehand and procedures are developed, such as by having an emergency protocol in place for chemical or bodily fluid exposure.

Federal Health and Safety Laws and Affirmative Duties

On both the federal and state levels, environmental laws are increasingly being used in combination with workplace safety regulations whenever death or serious injury occurs due to inadequate safety equipment or protocols. Environmental regulations, unlike the relatively modest penalties of traditional workplace regulation, carry the possibility of substantial financial penalties, as well as felony convictions and lengthy incarceration. This regulatory interplay is of particular consequence to EMS educators dealing with hazardous substances, because even routine safety incidents may subject EMS facilities, programs, and educators to increased scrutiny in both the workplace safety and the environmental spheres. Fit testing for high efficiency particulate air (HEPA) masks and ensuring latex-allergic students can obtain nonlatex gloves are some examples of how EMS educators can make sure the environment is safe for EMS educators and students.

Occupational Safety and Health Act

The **Occupational Safety and Health Act (OSH Act)** ensures safe and healthy working conditions in EMS facilities and clinical sites. The federal law is overseen by the Occupational Safety and Health Administration (OSHA).[26] Congress enacted federal OSHA legislation upon a finding that workplace injuries and illnesses impose a substantial burden on the economy in terms of the following:

- Disability compensation payments
- Lost production
- Medical expenses
- Wage loss

For decades, EMS workplace injuries and illnesses have been addressed by the following:

- Encouraging EMS programs and educators, as well as students, to reduce the number of safety and health hazards at the workplace when providing prehospital interventions
- Ensuring that EMS programs and educators, as well as students, share in this responsibility
- Establishing and enforcing occupational health and safety standards
- Encouraging EMS educators and students to jointly reduce workplace injuries and disease in their clinical training

EMS educators should be familiar with all OSHA guidelines that impact prehospital interventions. While the safety of students must always be considered, EMS programs must also do the following:

- Acquire and inspect relevant safety gear to be used by students.
- Conduct applicable safety education.
- Routinely inspect potential sources of health hazards.

While OSHA regulations are not legally binding on students *per se*, they do apply to anyone who is an employee at an EMS facility, which may include students. In any event, EMS programs are wise to implement OSHA policies, whether mandatory or not.

OSHA is authorized to investigate, with no advance warning, suspected safety hazards and violations of its regulations. Harsh penalties and restrictions may be imposed for safety violations. Workplaces cited for safety violations may be fined. Those found guilty of second offenses may face more substantial fines, and a third offense could put programs under OSHA oversight with the federal government determining what safety steps must be taken.

Emergency Planning and Community Right-to-Know Act

The federal **Emergency Planning and Community Right-to-Know Act (EPCRA)** gives EMS educators and students the right to better understand the risks posed by chemicals and toxins present in EMS facilities and hospitals. EMS educators are required to obtain material safety data sheet (MSDS) information on all applicable toxins or chemical hazards present in the EMS facility and provide training to students so they understand the need for gloves, face shields, masks, or respirators to protect themselves when exposed to potentially harmful substances. EMS educators should also include this chemical and toxin information on waivers and releases signed by students.

State Public Health, Safety, and Education Codes

Each state has a lead agency that has overall responsibility for occupational safety and health. Although OSHA is a federal law, states have been offered the

Occupational Safety and Health Administration

One of OSHA's missions is to keep EMS educators and students healthy and safe.[27] Personal injuries and illnesses arising out of EMS activities impose a substantial burden upon and are a hindrance to the success of EMS programs in terms of lost production, wage loss, medical expenses, and disability compensation payments. Occupational health and safety are improved in the following ways:

- Encouraging EMS programs and educators, as well as students, to reduce the number of occupational safety and health hazards at their EMS facility and clinical field sites
- Ensuring that EMS educators and students share in this responsibility
- Advancing EMS program initiatives to provide safe and healthy conditions in EMS facilities and clinical sites
- Providing occupational safety and health research
- Exploring the relationship between diseases and environmental conditions
- Providing medical criteria for safe and healthy EMS facility conditions
- Providing training for EMS programs
- Establishing occupational health and safety standards
- Enforcing standards
- Encouraging states to assume full responsibility for administration and enforcement of federal OSHA policies
- Creating appropriate reporting procedures
- Encouraging EMS educators and students to jointly reduce injuries and disease in their EMS facility and clinical sites

opportunity to accept responsibility for administration and enforcement of OSHA policies. Nearly half of the states assume this responsibility. EMS educators should be familiar with their own state's OSHA requirements for compliance.

State EMS Standards of Education

Besides the state lead agency responsible for managing federal occupational safety and health policies, states have generally assigned responsibility for management and administration of EMS-related oversight to a state regulatory agency. Some states assign responsibility for EMS to the state health department, while others assign it to the state fire marshal. EMS educators should be familiar with the licensure, certification, and instructional regulations that the applicable state agency has issued. In this regard, state EMS offices are an important source of regulatory and administrative rules for EMS educators.

For instance, some states require students to have a current state EMT license to participate in hospital clinicals as paramedic students. States may also regulate what students can or cannot do when working as a student versus what that student can do when employed. Typically, paramedic students can perform advanced skills under specific circumstances during their hospital or field clinicals but cannot perform any advanced skills when functioning in an employment situation.

Accreditation by the Commission on Accreditation of Allied Health Education Programs (CAAHEP) and the Committee on Accreditation of Educational Programs for the Emergency Medical Services Professions (CoAEMSP) indicates the meeting of a minimum national level of educational standards. In following federal guidelines, states may establish standards of instruction required of all EMS educators. Frequently, EMS educators must hold teaching certifications or credentials. Clearly, it is critical that EMS educators meet or exceed the minimum standards for both the EMS and teaching professions established by accrediting bodies and states.

State Immunity Laws

In order to encourage EMS educators and students to participate in hospital or field clinical programs, most states have enacted broad general immunity laws for EMS educators. EMS educators cannot be made a party in legal actions. Nevertheless, immunity generally is not granted for gross negligence or willful misconduct.

Program Clinical Affiliation Agreements

EMS is a highly complex system and **affiliation agreements** to educate students account for most of this complexity. EMS programs should have affiliation agreements with all clinical sites involved in EMS activities. A standard affiliation agreement should be clearly written and approved by legal counsel. Clinical sites generally require that affiliation agreements be reviewed by legal counsel.

CASE in Point

A student at a field clinical site filed a lawsuit after suffering injuries during a rope-training exercise. The student claimed that the negligence in supervision of the preceptor caused the student's injury. State immunity laws, however, grant immunity to EMS educators based on the express intent of promoting the development, accessibility, and provision of emergency medical care. The student claimed that the rope training was beyond the scope of training for prehospital interventions, even though rope training is appropriate training for situations requiring extrication and mountain rescues. EMS educators may, however, develop training programs based on the geographic challenges students might encounter in their respective environments. The student further claimed that the preceptor was not properly qualified in rope techniques, but finding liability on this basis would defeat the intent of state laws to provide immunity for EMS educators. EMS programs are immune from liability for personal injury; such laws do not violate due process because state immunity laws apply to all students, not just students in EMS programs.

Emergency Protocols and Procedures

Affiliation agreements establish guidelines that are mutually acceptable to both the EMS program and clinical sites. Well-written agreements identify obligations required by EMS programs, by students, and by the clinical sites. Emergency protocols and procedures should be clearly defined. In the event that policies conflict, the affiliation agreements should indicate which should be followed. Addressing this information in the affiliation agreements before students are assigned to clinical sites is useful in addressing potential conflicts before they arise.

Framework for Clinical Education Agreements

To minimize litigation potential, affiliation agreements should contain basic components. The following basic components are particularly important in affiliation agreements.

Introductory Clause

Affiliation agreements should clearly identify the parties involved. At a minimum, the parties include identification of the EMS program and the clinical site. The introductory clause also often includes the date of the contract.

Dates

Affiliation agreements should identify the starting and terminating dates of the contract. Multiple-year affiliation agreements are generally advantageous in that they eliminate the need for annual renegotiations. In consultation with legal counsel, the EMS program and clinical sites must determine if affiliation agreements should be developed on a year-by-year basis or as a multiple-year contract.

Performance Objectives

Affiliation agreements should provide measurable achievement-based objectives for students, including knowledge and skills to be achieved, and identification of the abilities required to make judgments. In this way, everyone will be aware of their duties in the clinical sites. Where student achievement falls short of the learning and performance objectives, the affiliation agreement should define who evaluates students and how students may be remediated.

Student–Employee Relationships

Affiliation agreements should also define the relationship between students and the clinical sites. In most cases, students do not receive remuneration for their clinical experiences. In addition, EMS educators should be aware of federal, state, and accreditation policies and should clearly identify these in the affiliation agreements. Some states and CAAHEP require that EMS programs not substitute students for paid hospital or field personnel.[28]

Liability Expectations

This section of the affiliation agreements is designed to define the liability responsibilities and expectations of both the EMS program and the clinical sites. Indemnification information should identify who has a duty to remediate any loss, damage, or liability incurred. Inherently dangerous activities should be addressed, such as the protocols that students should follow when dealing with bloodborne pathogens or infectious disease exposures.

Mutual Obligations

This part of affiliation agreements should be specific as to the exact steps necessary to ensure compliance with the agreements themselves. Generally, this part addresses obligations of the EMS program to students and to cooperating clinical sites, as well as obligations of the clinical sites to students and to the EMS program.

Key Contacts

Names, titles, mailing addresses for formal notifications, and contact numbers for both the EMS program and the clinical sites should be included. All parties to the affiliation agreements should have immediate access to their counterparts.

Signatures

Signatures are required on affiliation agreements. These agreements are considered legal documents, meaning only authorized persons should affix their signatures. EMS programs should determine who this is and should notify EMS educators. State law varies as to whether signatures need to be witnessed and notarized in order to make the contract valid. State law also varies as to how the signature block is to be formatted such that the entities that are party to the contract are held liable for any breach and that whoever signed on behalf of the entities is not held personally liable.

Curriculum Issues

EMS educators should establish curricula that are in compliance with the U.S. Department of Transportation's educational standards. Clearly, curricula must be compliant with federal and state laws and adhere to accreditation standards. Beyond that, EMS educators have the right to adapt curricula within their EMS programs to meet local needs.

Student Issues

Student issues in EMS programs are similar to those of most education programs. Common student issues include, among others, the following:

- Institutional relationships
- Enrollment and dismissal
- Background checks and drug screening
- Discipline in the classroom
- Professional appearance
- Academic dishonesty
- Bullying (including cyberbullying)

The issues identified in this chapter merely provide a brief overview. EMS educators should become familiar with all local, state, and federal regulations under which their program operates. It is vital that educators have access to appropriate support by legal counsel to avoid being placed in positions of potential liability.

Student/EMS Program Interactions

Interactions with students are among the most critical and most challenging components of any EMS program. Establishing positive student interactions is critical to the success of EMS programs and their graduates. EMS documents, including but not restricted to catalogs, handbooks, course syllabi, and advertising materials, play an important role in promoting positive interaction with students. All information should be correct, current, detailed, and readily available to students.

Catalogs

Catalogs, electronic or otherwise, are perhaps the most enduring document of the EMS program/student relationship. Information generally provided in catalogs includes the following:

- Institutional data
- Academic requirements
- Enrollment and dismissal rules and regulations
- Student support services

Student Handbooks

Depending on the size and type of the EMS educational program, students may receive a variety of handbooks that provide rules, regulations, and information pertinent to their education. Some programs combine general student handbooks with the educational institution's handbooks. Traditionally, student handbooks are broad in scope and include information pertinent to the entire EMS program.

EMS educators may develop handbooks specifically for students in their educational program. This handbook may provide specific information on the following:

- Attendance guidelines
- Curricula
- Uniform or dress code
- Code of conduct

EMS educators may also create handbooks that provide rules, expectations, and guidelines relevant to activities in the hospital and field clinicals. (See Chapter 24, *Administrative Issues*, for more information on syllabi, student handbooks, and student/institutional relationships.)

When developing program policies, EMS educators may establish standards that are stricter than those of the federal and state government and accrediting agencies. No policies should be established that are less stringent or that conflict with governmental or accreditation policy. EMS educators should use the policies approved by their program and legal counsel before the time of publication. EMS educators should avoid changing program policies after a term or semester begins. If this is necessary, the EMS program should make clear that there are valid, carefully considered reasons to do so and make adequate notification to students.[8]

Related EMS Program Documents

EMS educators may use documents for recruitment or enrollment activities. All published documents may provide information that may lead to litigation and should first be approved by the EMS program and legal counsel. All EMS programs that participate in federal financial aid programs must provide key information to all prospective and current students. Materials must include information on the following:[29]

- ADA support
- Confidentiality of records
- Descriptions of in-class or online programs, as well as hospital and field clinical activities
- Financial assistance opportunities
- Nondiscrimination policies
- Refund policies
- Program costs
- Veterans' benefits

Student Challenges to EMS Program Documents

Today, catalogs and handbooks are perceived by students as legal documents that create a binding, inflexible obligation on the part of the EMS program. Many EMS programs include disclaimer statements to protect themselves from potential litigation. Most misrepresentation or fraud claims originate from EMS program documents. Many students view these EMS program documents as containing promises made to students. Understandably, students expect these promises to be fulfilled, particularly when they have taken out substantial student loans in order to undertake an EMS certificate or licensure program.

Students have rights and do not lose their basic constitutional freedoms when they enter an EMS program. Thus, EMS educators should be careful not to violate the constitutional rights of students when making programmatic changes. Students' constitutional rights include:

- Freedom from discrimination (including the right to due process and equal protection of the laws)
- Freedom of assembly
- Freedom of speech

Enrollment and Dismissal

The enrollment process in EMS programs begins with recruitment. All applicants and students should be treated equitably and according to published guidelines. The ultimate goal is to see students successfully complete the EMS certificate and licensure programs and become gainfully employed. On some occasions, however, students must be dismissed from EMS programs. When this occurs, students should be treated in a fair and equitable manner so potential litigation can be avoided.

Recruitment

When recruiting students, EMS educators should be certain that unlawful discrimination does not occur. Printing a nondiscrimination statement on all recruiting documents is a good starting point. Policies, however, should go beyond official policy statements; all EMS program policies should be implemented and strictly enforced. The two most common areas of recruitment-related litigation are breach of contract and misrepresentation or fraud.

Breach of Contract Claims. The relationship between an EMS program and its students is based on a contract. The EMS program agrees to provide an educational opportunity, and the student agrees to pay a fee and attend classes and clinicals. However, numerous subtle details between the parties also exist and become part of the agreement, including the following:

- Student will obey the rules.
- EMS program will hold classes and provide clinicals that the student needs.
- Student will attend classes and participate in clinicals.
- Classes and clinicals will be held at the place and time scheduled.

When EMS programs do not meet a written or implied expectation of students, it may be considered to be a breach of contract.

Claims of Malpresentations or Fraud. Misrepresentation or fraud claims may occur when an EMS program intentionally provides false or misleading information to students to induce their attendance. In cases claiming misrepresentation or fraud, students must show reasonable evidence of the following:

- A false statement of material fact
- A statement that was known to be false or uttered with reckless disregard for the truth or falsity of the statement upon which the students reasonably relied
- A claim that resulted in damages to the students

EMS programs should be extremely careful in determining the factual accuracy of all program material used for recruitment and enrollment of students, particularly regarding employment and compensation rates of graduates. Nonaccredited and provisionally accredited programs should clearly acknowledge this fact. For instance, students should be advised that they will *not* be eligible for any NREMT examination if they attend an EMS program that is either not fully accredited or is seeking accreditation by CoAEMSP and CAAHEP.[30]

Acceptance

Once accepted, students have a right to know what is expected of them, not only in the general EMS program, but also in specific clinicals. Also, once accepted, students should be asked if accommodations are necessary to meet essential functions. Student handbooks may provide most of this information. During the first session of each class, EMS educators should provide students with course syllabi. Each syllabus should be clearly written and adhere to EMS program guidelines. All program expectations and grading criteria should be set forth unambiguously. Well-written syllabi limit the ability of students to threaten or pursue successful litigation.

Dismissal

EMS educators like to see their students succeed. Occasionally, however, students fail to meet the standards and for that or other reasons, must be dismissed from the EMS program. This difficult situation should be handled carefully. Attention should be paid to fully documenting the entire situation. Just as with other aspects of interaction with students, fair treatment is critical. If EMS educators follow their own program rules, their academic judgments will be upheld. In terms of student issues, litigation may result if EMS educators fail to do the following:

- Regularly and objectively document student behavior
- Provide EMS experiences, both academic and clinical, directed toward student success
- Keep evidence of both positive and negative completed student work
- Maintain fair and objective student assessments
- Communicate as though every word, written or spoken, would be broadcast in public
- Treat all students the same and objectively
- Maintain the confidentiality of students

Most EMS educators recognize the importance of careful documentation. Accordingly, EMS educators should adapt the ability to document their EMS activities. Again, it is critical that all students be treated equitably, and it is vital that this equitable treatment be documented.

Background Checks

EMS programs typically require students to pass criminal background checks, including fingerprinting that screens for violent criminals and registered sex offenders. In addition, EMS programs generally require review of tracking systems for incidents of child abuse and neglect. Almost all clinical sites require this in their contracts.

Without screening and background checks, clinical sites might be exposed to claims that they did not sufficiently screen students. Such claims could be brought under the existing tort liability doctrine of negligent hiring and retention. This could subject EMS programs to liability if they fail to gather or act on relevant background information indicating someone was a dangerous fit for EMS.

Criminal Convictions

The Joint Commission, an entity that accredits hospitals, verifies state and/or organizational requirements regarding background checks for staff, volunteers, and students to ensure compliance with those requirements.[31] These criminal background checks are also generally required by state law, regulation, or clinical site policy. Student failure to disclose a felony conviction often results in dismissal from an EMS program, suspension from a current job, and forfeiture of their license or certification. Felony convictions must generally be disclosed to state EMS agencies within days of entry of final judgment; a failure to disclose results in a temporary suspension of a license or certification. Some felony convictions may prohibit student participation in clinical experience and prevent NREMT certification and EMS state licensure.

Screenings for Illegal Drug Use

EMS programs may require drug tests for illegal drug use. Test results may be validated by asking about lawful medication use or possible explanations for the positive results other than illegal use of drugs. However, disability-related questions are prohibited and students who take medications under medical supervision should not be compelled to disclose their medical condition unless it affects their ability to safely participate in the program or serve in the EMS profession.

Therefore, while follow-up questions in response to a positive drug test are permitted, there are specific limitations on the types of information that can be elicited by someone other than a medical review officer (MRO). For instance, a student who is taking antiseizure or antiretroviral medications should not be compelled to disclose that they are epileptic or HIV-positive unless such disclosure is made to an MRO. The MRO then must make a determination if the medical condition is one that might be dangerous in an EMS setting. No one other than a MRO should ever be present during this follow-up questioning of students.

Social Networking and Credit Record Screening

Neither social network screening nor credit record screening is recommended; it risks claims of unfair discrimination based on embarrassing but otherwise legal behavior. Other pitfalls include violating equal opportunity employment laws like the ADA or Title VII, and could implicate fair credit-reporting standards that require an opportunity to respond to any damaging information a background search could produce.

Discipline in the Classroom

One of the most common problems faced by EMS educators is addressing student misconduct in the classroom or clinicals. There are two primary pathways for dealing with problems related to student conduct. One pathway is academic, and the other is disciplinary. EMS educators are traditionally supported when dealing with professional conduct issues as academic issues rather than disciplinary issues, provided that student rights are not violated.

Academic requirements should include specific professional behavioral expectations and assessment, which in EMS are identified by the National EMS Education Standards. These include the following behaviors:[32]

- Appearance and personal hygiene
- Careful delivery of emergency medical care
- Communications
- Empathy
- Integrity
- Patient advocacy
- Respect
- Self-confidence
- Self-motivation
- Teamwork and diplomacy
- Time management

These characteristics should be evaluated during each course, and it should be verified that they are adequate or the student will not pass. A specific problem with any one of these items should indicate a need for an additional evaluation to point out and direct the student to appropriate behavior. Failure of that evaluation at whatever point is identified would result in failure of the course. Students who fail their affective or professional behavior requirements are entitled to the same grievance for that failure as they would be for a failure of any examination or course. Academic decisions by EMS educators are generally supported, as long as they are not arbitrary or capricious.

The disciplinary process is the other pathway to deal with behavioral issues. It is up to each EMS program to develop its own disciplinary process, which may vary according to the offense. For instance, dismissing a student for cheating may take time for verification of the cheating. Thus, the EMS program might not be able to immediately dismiss the student unless there is a specific threat for the student to be in the classroom or clinical. Dismissal depends on the specific disciplinary policy and procedure of the EMS program.

Prior to a student being dismissed, due process must be provided in disciplinary dismissals at EMS programs. Undoubtedly, due process can be rigorous in terms of disciplinary hearings and the various levels of appeals that must be followed. Consequently, it is generally to the advantage of an EMS program to use the academic pathway rather than go down the disciplinary path. The disciplinary pathway should be determined by the written grievance policies provided to students, and each progressive step along this path should be fully documented and supported should the student turn to litigation after dismissal.

CASE in Point

A student sued a program after he was dismissed for failing to attend orientation or giving a reason for his absence. The student filed suit to be let back into the program. Programs will generally prevail in such claims because educators are better suited to evaluate the suitability of students than are courts of law.

Professional Appearance

EMS educators and students are traditionally held to a higher standard of professional appearance than the general public. The appearance of EMS educators and students not only establishes a level of professionalism, it also is a matter of hygiene and safety. Educators should expect students to adhere to dress codes as approved and provided by the EMS program. Dress code policies may address the following:

- Body piercings
- Fingernails
- Hairstyles, including facial hair
- Jewelry
- Tattoos
- Uniforms
- Other related personal hygiene issues

Policies regarding student uniforms and personal hygiene should be established in accordance with input from advisory committees, and they should be written in compliance with clinical expectations. If clinical sites have dress codes or personal hygiene policies that are stricter than those of the EMS program, EMS educators may enforce such guidelines, provided that such requirements are reasonable.

Policies should be clearly presented to students in their handbooks and syllabi. EMS educators should not assume that students know what acceptable appearance is. If students are required to wear identification badges or name tags, it is the responsibility of EMS educators to notify students of this requirement. If stethoscopes and bandage scissors are part of the uniform, students should know this in advance.

Depending on the EMS program, students may be required to be in uniform at all times. It is also possible that they may be required to wear uniforms only during time spent in their hospital or field clinicals. Again, it is important that students are provided this information as early in their educational process as possible. By informing students, the EMS educator has clearly identified the standards and has established a basis for expectations.

Although student appearances may be perceived as problematic, EMS educators should use caution in dealing with issues such as clothing and hairstyles. EMS programs may establish dress codes to restrict clothing or other appearances deemed to be unsafe, offensive, or unsanitary. Students with offensive tattoos can be required to cover them before being allowed in a hospital or field clinical. While observing health and safety practices regarding hairstyles, EMS educators should be cognizant of prohibitions that may be deemed unconstitutional. Ethnic hairstyles are generally protected, even when they violate professional dress codes.

Academic Dishonesty

Academic dishonesty is not a new concept. It is, however, on the rise with an increase in the uses and capabilities of technology. Printed information in catalogs, handbooks, and syllabi should contain clearly established policies on academic dishonesty. Such policies should be made available to students upon enrollment and should be reinforced at the beginning of each course. In the event that academic dishonesty does occur, students will have already received the EMS program policy and will know the related penalty. The most common current form of academic dishonesty is plagiarism.

Bullying

EMS programs should have a strict policy that prohibits hazing and bullying of anyone. This policy should be broad enough to include hazing and bullying in all of its various forms, including cyberbullying. Thus, it is important for EMS programs to adopt a formal policy on hazing and bullying. In the absence of such a policy, it is likely that an offender may successfully claim a First Amendment right to use the Internet. It is also important to recognize that such a policy may not extend to all online hazing and bullying activities, only those that impact the EMS program.

Grievance Policies

Every EMS program should have a published formal grievance policy. Although policies may differ according to the nature of the relationship (students aggrieved by an EMS educator or vice versa), the concepts are the same. EMS programs accredited by CAAHEP are required to have a defined and published policy and procedure for processing grievances.

Students

Grievance policies should be made readily available to all students upon enrollment in an EMS program. Many EMS programs elect to publish the grievance procedure in their catalogs or handbooks. When disciplining students, EMS educators should attempt to resolve issues at the lowest possible level. If unable to resolve student issues, educators should be certain that the steps in the student grievance policy are carefully followed and documented. Failure to adhere to published policies may enhance student opportunities for successful litigation.

EMS Educators

EMS educators should also have published grievance policies relative to their employment. Just as students do not sacrifice their constitutional rights when they enroll in an EMS program, EMS educators should be afforded the opportunity to respond when their rights appear to have been violated. These rights, however, have limitations.

Whereas EMS educators might have a constitutional claim under the First Amendment for adverse job actions based on their freedom of speech, this right is restricted if their words are uttered or their deeds done in the course of their employment duties. In particular, when a public employee is acting as a spokesperson for an employer, the employee does not enjoy complete First Amendment protections. Employers may lawfully discipline educators who publicly voice concerns about issues such as fraud, mismanagement, misuse of funds, student discipline, and discrimination practices in instances wherein the educator fails to clearly establish that they are speaking as a private citizen.

Safe Environment Laws

While safe environments are established on the basis of laws and consistent enforcement of safety programs, the recent frequency of mass shootings has highlighted school violence. EMS facilities were once considered secure. However, today, no space is exempt from violence.

Federal Safety Laws and Directives

EMS educators should strive to provide safe, disciplined, and drug-free learning environments for their students. Among the federal laws requiring safe environments with which EMS educators should be familiar are the following:

- **Safe and Drug-Free Schools and Communities Act (SDFSCA)**[33]
- **Gun-Free Schools Act (GFSA)**[34]
- **Jeanne Clery Disclosure of Campus Security Policy and Campus Crime Statistics Act (Clery Act)**[35]

Safe and Drug-Free Schools and Communities Act

The SDFSCA introduced zero-tolerance policies with regard to any type of disruption in educational environments, such as EMS facilities and clinical sites. Hate speech, harassment, fighting, and inappropriate attire are now prohibited at EMS facilities and clinical sites. Consequently, strictly speaking, EMS educators are responsible for safeguarding students from activities occurring outside their gates that ultimately have an impact inside their gates, such as cyberbullying.

Whether EMS educators choose to severely punish students who disrupt academic achievement is a question that must be answered by individual EMS programs.

It is uncontroverted that educators have the legal authority to do so. Through SDFSCA, EMS facilities, programs, and EMS educators have been mandated to establish clear and consistent programs of drug and violence prevention, education, and rehabilitation referral for students. This law also encourages the sharing of disciplinary records of students who transfer between EMS programs.

Inappropriate Social Media Posts

The issue of inappropriate student posts on social media sites is complicated, and the position of the courts varies depending on each specific case. Violations of the **Health Insurance Portability and Accountability Act (HIPAA)** and social media posts that fall in the category of "true threats" are clearly violations of the law. Issues related to student rights to free speech when posting inappropriate comments, even when they relate to the EMS program or clinical experiences, are sometimes less clear. Program policies related to social media posts must by clearly drafted and approved by legal counsel. Likewise, when electing to dismiss a student based on a social media post, it is often advisable to consult legal counsel.

CASE in Point

A student was dismissed from an allied health program for posting graphic and violent content related to animal cruelty, sexual violence, torture, and murder. In this instance, the student's First Amendment rights will likely be upheld despite the fact that the social posts were racist, sexist, homophobic, insensitive, degrading, and contained graphic descriptions of violent behavior, as the posts were not aimed at anyone specifically. If there is no evidence that the student intended to cause harm, the social postings do not meet the characteristics of a true threat.

CASE in Point

A student was dismissed from a program based on violation of the honor code and the professional code of ethics. The student posted graphic and disparaging information related to women in labor encountered during a school-related clinical experience. The court did not agree with the school's argument because it said the concept of professionalism was not adequately explained in the school's policies.

Crime Categories to be Reported Under the Clery Act

- Aggravated assault
- Arson
- Burglary
- Manslaughter (negligent)
- Murder and nonnegligent manslaughter
- Motor vehicle theft
- Robbery
- Sex offenses (forcible)
- Sex offenses (nonforcible, incest, and statutory rape)
- Other hate crimes involving bodily injury

Gun-Free Schools Act

Despite the prevalence of zero-tolerance policies for disruptive behavior by students, it is deadly legal fiction to assume EMS facilities are free of guns. While some states apply the federal GFSA to EMS facilities, most state laws allow gun possession if allowed by the EMS program. While some state laws restrict guns in EMS facilities, almost all states explicitly permit adult students to have firearms in locked cars; other states allow licensed guns to be stored in student dormitory rooms.

Clery Act

The federal Clery Act[36] was named in memory of a Lehigh University freshman in Pennsylvania, who was sexually assaulted and murdered in her residence hall. Her murderer was another student whom she did not know. After investigation, the parents of Jeanne Clery learned that 38 undisclosed crimes had occurred on the Lehigh University campus during the 3 years before their daughter's death.

Today, all higher education institutions (including EMS facilities) receiving public funds are required to publish annual reports on crime statistics. Within this document, 3 years of statistics must be reported. The report must be provided to all current students and employees. Additionally, this information may be provided to prospective students and employees, as well as the public upon request. Crime statistics must include data from all campus and local law enforcement agencies, and must also include incidents that occurred on the campus and in public areas surrounding the campus.

Higher educational institutions (including all EMS facilities) are also required to issue annual statements of current policies regarding immediate emergency response and evacuation procedures. The policy statement must articulate procedures that will be used to notify the campus community upon confirmation of a significant emergency or dangerous situation involving an immediate threat to the health or safety of students occurring on the campus. EMS educators may want to review or even reconsider whether their campus emergency response efforts are sufficiently coordinated for maximum effect.

Negligent Referrals

EMS programs and educators should be aware of potential litigation that may result from a **negligent referral** or inaccurate referral. Anyone who writes letters of recommendation owes a duty to not misrepresent the qualifications or character of another educator or students. This is especially the case if such action could result in harm to prospective third parties; for instance, when EMS educators or students have a known history of actions that may put others at risk.[37] Reference information can no longer be intentionally withheld if that causes injury to prospective third parties. This essentially renders "no comment" policies of the past useless.

Workers' Compensation and Other Public Benefits Laws

Workers' compensation and other public benefits laws usually supplant tort litigation as a method of resolving disputes over workplace injuries. Workers' compensation laws have been established to determine who will be eligible for benefits such as the following:

- Family support
- Medical expenses
- Wage loss

Workers' compensation is a type of strict liability, no-fault insurance in the event of injuries or illnesses related to EMS activities, whether in the classroom or at clinical sites. In such cases, the EMS program does not admit fault for the injury and the injured third party agrees to receive benefits without litigation. Workers' compensation benefits are not generally provided for injuries resulting from intentionally harmful conduct, horseplay, alcohol, or illegal use of drugs. Students would not typically be covered by workers' compensation unless on-duty and being paid by an employer at the time of the injury during training.

Coverage

Each state determines workers' compensation coverage. As penalties against employers who fail to provide workers' compensation insurance can be severe, EMS educators should check and monitor the coverage of clinical sites. Because EMS programs have the potential for injury, educators should be aware of program policies and should follow procedures exactly.

In many cases, injury or incident reports must be completed within a specified time frame. Injured students or EMS educators may be required to visit a physician who has contracted with the EMS facility or clinical site or state workers' compensation insurance. EMS educators also should be familiar with the status of students in their programs regarding workers' compensation coverage. Some states may cover students in clinical education; other states may provide no workers' compensation coverage for students under any circumstances.

Fraud

Misrepresentation of injuries might result in charges of fraud. As workers' compensation benefits are determined by physicians' reports, injured students and EMS educators should be sure to provide accurate and detailed information. Most states have laws that require everyone—including students, EMS educators, insurance carriers, and the public—to report suspected cases of workers' compensation fraud. States frequently allow the informer to remain anonymous. Fraudulent workers' compensation claims may be subject to criminal proceedings.

Health and Malpractice Insurance

Traditionally, students who are enrolled in an EMS program must show proof that they have health insurance coverage. If unable to provide such proof, students may be required to purchase health insurance through the EMS program. Some students may be employed by an EMS provider and covered under their plan as an employee. In addition to health insurance coverage, some EMS programs, clinical affiliations, and certification boards require that students carry malpractice insurance in the event that students cause injury to third parties. EMS educators should comply with EMS program expectations in advising students regarding health and malpractice insurance.

EMS Educator Malpractice

Malpractice insurance is generally not a covered benefit, so EMS educators should determine the necessity of carrying such insurance themselves. In some institutions, EMS educators are required to carry malpractice insurance. The value of carrying malpractice insurance is that the attorney for the malpractice carrier will always seek to protect the certification, registration, or licensure of EMS educators in the event of injury to a third party.

Confidentiality and Data Privacy Laws

Based on their medical experiences, EMS educators are already familiar with privacy rules and patient confidentiality. As educators, the rules of data privacy and confidentiality extend to students.

Federal Privacy Laws and Directives

The three most important federal laws regarding data privacy are the following:

- The **Family Educational Rights and Privacy Act (FERPA)**[38]
- The **HIPAA Privacy Rule**[39]
- The **Freedom of Information Act (FOIA)**[40]

Family Educational Rights and Privacy Act

FERPA, also known as the Buckley Amendment, was enacted in response to concerns that personal information was being maintained and disseminated by the government and other public entities. The Buckley Amendment prohibits the release of any type of personally identifiable information to anyone without a legitimate educational interest in the information. All EMS facilities, programs, EMS educators, and students who receive or benefit from public funds are required to comply with the Buckley Amendment.

FERPA Guidelines

The Family Policy Compliance Office in the U.S. Department of Education interprets and enforces FERPA and publishes advice letters to clarify the law. FERPA guidelines, established to protect the confidentiality and handling of student records, clarify the following:

- Student records must be kept confidential, with access provided to outside third parties only with parental consent or with the consent of adult-aged students.
- Student records must be accessed on request by the student's parents/guardians (for minors) or adult-aged students.
- Student records may be challenged by parents or adult-aged students who think that the records are misleading, inaccurate, or a violation of their privacy rights.

Under federal law, EMS programs and educators must inform students or their parents or guardians of FERPA guidelines. Students under age 18 years, the legal age of full responsibility, are generally considered minors, and their parents or guardians have legal access to their educational records. Once students turn 18, they are considered adults under FERPA; at this point, parents and guardians have no legal right to access student information.

Educational Records

Documents maintained at an educational institution that specifically relate to students are considered educational records. These records may take the form of written documents, video or audiotapes, films, photographs, or computer files. Five types of documents are excluded from FERPA regulations:[41]

- Sole possession notes (notes by the EMS educator) that are not accessible or revealed to any other person (such as grade books)
- Medical records of adult students (such as letters from physicians, psychiatrists, or psychologists for the purpose of treating adult students)
- Law enforcement records
- Student employee records
- Alumni records unrelated to their attendance as students[41]

While the definition of educational records has been the subject of significant litigation, the term has been broadly defined to cover disciplinary records.

Disclosure Policies and Practices

Single acts do not violate FERPA; instead, EMS programs must have a policy or practice governing conditions under which unauthorized release of student records may be permitted.[42] Thus, FERPA does not govern every single disclosure that might constitute an unauthorized release of educational records. Instead, FERPA forbids only policies or practices that condone such releases.

According to FERPA regulations, student records may be disclosed in only three ways:

- To students directly
- To third parties with written permission of students (or parents/guardians)
- To third parties without written consent

EMS educators should understand the circumstances under which educational records have been requested and should be certain to comply with federal regulations. For instance, law enforcement may obtain student health data only with a court order.[43]

Legitimate Educational Interests

Student records may be obtained by EMS educators who have legitimate educational interests. While student records may be accessed for information pertinent to employment, each situation should be handled individually and on a need-to-know basis.

HIV/Acquired Immune Deficiency (AIDS) Status. FERPA does not allow EMS programs to disclose the HIV status of anyone solely for the promotion of general health and safety.[44] EMS educators have to decide whether HIV status poses a special health risk in EMS clinical education. Today, only a narrow set of deserving persons with HIV-positive status qualify for confidentiality protection under state confidentiality laws. Two facts point to this lack of general protection: there is no cure for HIV/AIDS at this time, and widely disseminated preventive vaccines or curative medicines are likely years away.

Student Health Emergencies. FERPA allows for parental notification, without student consent, in cases of health emergencies where knowledge of the information is necessary to protect a student.[45] While such emergencies often involve potential suicides, it is not clear what constitutes a health emergency and whether hospitalization is required before parents/guardians may be notified. A second exception is rare infectious outbreaks such as methicillin-resistant *Staphylococcus aureus* (MRSA). Such outbreaks are clearly covered by the health emergency exception to FERPA.[46]

Employee Reimbursement Disclosures. It is common in the EMS profession for employers to pay for the education of its employees. In return, employers expect to remain informed about student academic standing. This is a contractual issue between the employer and the student employee. It is the student employee's responsibility to provide this release. EMS educators should not release information to employers without written permission from the student or parent/guardian.

Circumstances Under Which Educational Records May Be Released

Under the following circumstances, educational records may be released without previous written consent:

- Directory information (unless a written request denying the publication of this information is provided by the student or parent)
- Information required by a school official who has a legitimate educational interest (Educators should be careful to demonstrate the legitimate educational interest, or they could be in violation of FERPA.)
- Information requested from an educational institution into which the student plans to enroll
- Financial aid documentation
- Documents necessary for accrediting bodies (It is best to remove student identification whenever possible.)
- Information necessary for studies on behalf of the institution regarding financial aid, testing, and other related research (Again, if possible, it is best to remove any personal identification.)
- Health and safety information necessary to protect other persons in the event of an emergency
- Documents or data required under lawfully issued subpoenas or orders

Moreover, reimbursement contracts should be established with employers before students enroll in EMS programs. These contracts should clearly identify the expectations of both parties and should be signed and dated. For instance, employers might agree to pay for tuition, books, supplies, and all related educational expenses. In return, students may be expected to provide records of attendance and transcripts at the completion of each grading session.

Challenges to Educational Records

Students have no enforceable right to sue to enforce provisions of FERPA, which prohibits the federal funding of EMS education facilities that have a policy or practice of releasing educational records to unauthorized persons. Under FERPA, only parents/guardians and adult students have the right to review and challenge educational records. Such a request must be made in writing and provided to the EMS education program or educator. Financial records and confidential letters of recommendation are not subject to this review.

HIPAA Privacy Rule

The HIPAA Privacy Rule requires EMS educators and students to safeguard the privacy of persons receiving prehospital interventions in a variety of ways.[47] For instance, with some exceptions, EMS educators and students must do the following:

- Obtain the permission of anyone receiving emergency care before speaking to third parties about the person's medical condition.[48]
- Distribute privacy notices containing information concerning the use and disclosure of health records of anyone receiving emergency care.[49]
- Allow people who received prehospital interventions the opportunity to inspect their health records and request that they be modified or used restrictively.[50]

Oversight

The Office for Civil Rights within the U.S. Department of Health and Human Services is responsible for enforcement of HIPAA. As the first federal legislation to protect medical privacy, HIPAA established the norm to be used throughout the nation. No state may be less restrictive than the national law; however, states may be more restrictive. Thus, EMS programs should establish written policies and procedures to adequately segregate and protect patient health information that may be received inadvertently as a result of student assignments. Collecting any personally identifiable information should be avoided in student assignments as much as possible, and any sensitive personal information collected with other information should be destroyed.

TEACHING TIP

EMS educators should ensure that students diligently strive to protect the privacy of everyone receiving prehospital interventions.

Federal and State Freedom of Information Acts

Federal and most state FOIAs require EMS records and reports to be available upon request to law enforcement officers investigating criminal conduct.[51] Such requests may be made under federal or state public records law, and may also be made for civil litigation purposes. What information requests will be honored is not clear.

Security Camera Surveillance Systems

EMS educators should be knowledgeable of any closed-circuit television (CCTV) program policies in the municipalities where their students have clinical education. CCTV programs increasingly place government-owned cameras in public areas of cities and stream video feeds from the cameras to an observation room, where employees view multiple screens and see multiple areas of a city at the same time. By monitoring video feeds, EMS educators could use CCTV information to review student clinical activities and assist students in making the best decisions.

Practical issues as well as constitutional issues arise when balancing security, privacy rights, and EMS program transparency. For an effective, efficient CCTV program, EMS educators should clearly articulate their end goal in education as well as the means for which they plan to use CCTV technology for their students. Citizens may request recorded CCTV footage, and attorneys may subpoena either recordings or governmental employees who watched an incident unfold on a CCTV monitor.[51] Students should be made aware of the possibility that the emergency medical care they are delivering in a public place is being recorded and could possibly be used in any subsequent litigation.

Legal Research

Because this chapter provides limited information on legal issues for EMS educators, additional research may be of value. When completing legal research, EMS educators should be cognizant of copyright laws and intellectual property. It is highly recommended that EMS programs and educators work with qualified legal counsel to review their legal research.

Federal Copyright Laws and Protection

Copyright protection is afforded to original works of authorship fixed in any tangible medium of expression.[52] Many think of January 1, 2019, and the so-called "Public Domain Day" when hundreds of thousands of copyrighted works entered the public domain for the first time in more than 20 years, when they hear the term copyright (think *Mary Poppins*). Today, works published on the Internet are also fully protected and subject to the same qualifications and limitations as nondigital works. Copyright protection extends to any original work of authorship in physical or electronic format. This includes written and recorded classroom or clinical site lectures, including PowerPoints, as well as videos of classroom or clinical sites. Copyright protection, while undergoing a fundamental rethinking, endures for the following terms:[53]

- General works (single author): The life of the author plus 70 years after the author's death
- Joint works: The life of the last surviving author plus 70 years after the last surviving author's death
- Anonymous works, pseudonymous works, and works made for hire: For 95 years from the year of the work's first publication, or a term of 120 years from the year of its first creation, whichever expires first

Fair Use Doctrine in Education

While many exceptions exist, U.S. copyright law provides no definitive legal standard for the acceptable scope of copyright exceptions and limitations. "Fair use doctrine" is the first listed and best known of the exceptions listed in the Copyright Act; surrounding case law provides some guidance on how exceptions can be crafted to permit beneficial and reasonable uses without causing undue harm to rights holders. Nonetheless, fair use is a difficult concept to master. Fair use is fact-specific and unique to any given situation, with four factors determining if the exception will apply (**TABLE 25.2**).

With the increased number of distance-education degrees now available, EMS educators should be cognizant of copyright issues. It may be tempting to copy sections of text into Web-based courses or distribute text via interactive video. However, educators should be aware that the same potential copyright violations

TABLE 25.2 Fair Use Factors

Fair Use Factor	Generally Accepted
Purpose and character of use	Nonprofit, educational, and/or personal use
Nature of work to be used	Fact-based research and publication
Amount and substantiality of material	Small amounts of copyrighted information
Effect on the potential marketplace	No concrete response as it stands alone; depends on the nature of the previous three factors

Data from 17 U.S.C. §§ 101–102.

apply to distance education as they do in the traditional classroom. When determining whether permission is needed for making copies of copyrighted material, it is best to err on the side of caution.

Digital Millennium Copyright Act

The **Digital Millennium Copyright Act (DMCA)** addresses the Internet and digital communications technology.[54] Among other things, the DMCA helps protect the integrity of copyright-protected content while creating processes to permit Web-based service providers some modicum of assurance that good-faith posting of content will not be held against them. Note, however, that the "safe harbor" provisions of the DMCA that limit service provider liability do not extend to the original poster of infringing content; EMS educators still must ensure that their use of others' materials complies with copyright law.

Legal Resources

The primary legal resource for any EMS educator should be the legal counsel for the EMS program or the risk management office. EMS educators who work for public or private EMS providers should have access to their city or county attorney, or corporate attorney for private entities. The greatest single access to printed legal resources is found in public law libraries, but not every educator has such a library near where they live or work. Electronic legal research is also valuable. Remembering that EMS educators are not always experts in the field of law, EMS educators should rely upon formal legal counsel for advice and direction.

Summary

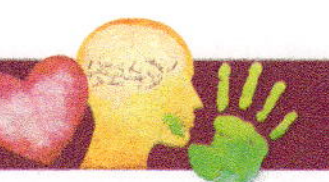

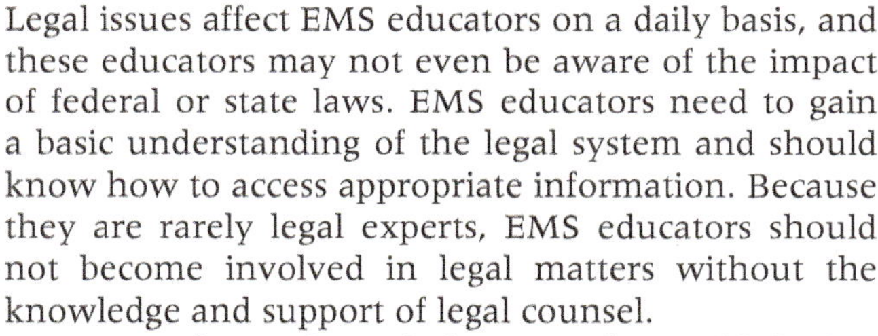

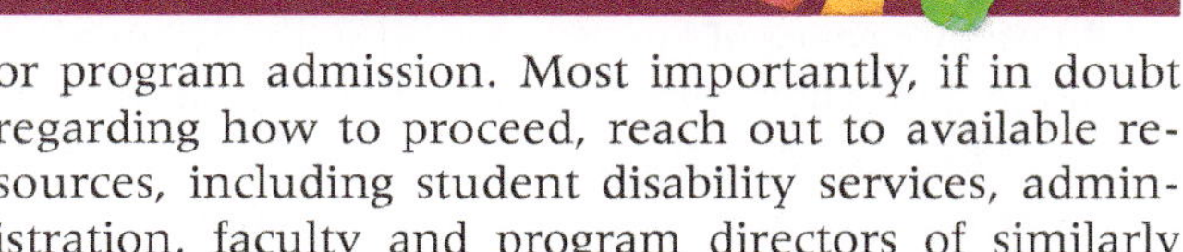

Legal issues affect EMS educators on a daily basis, and these educators may not even be aware of the impact of federal or state laws. EMS educators need to gain a basic understanding of the legal system and should know how to access appropriate information. Because they are rarely legal experts, EMS educators should not become involved in legal matters without the knowledge and support of legal counsel.

Laws, rules, and regulations may be established at the federal, state, or local level. The U.S. Constitution is the supreme law of the land, and no laws may be in conflict with it. Although federal laws establish a basis for national EMS standards, state laws may be more restrictive. At no time are state or local laws allowed to be in conflict with or allow for lower expectations than federal laws.

Standards for EMS facilities, programs, or activities should uphold the integrity of the profession. EMS educators should be familiar with nondiscrimination laws. Students should be treated fairly and in a nondiscriminatory manner from the time of initial recruitment through graduation. All EMS program information should be accurate and reflect what actually exists.

Learning to assess and accommodate students with disabilities in the environment of EMS education is complicated and understandably intimidating. The primary factors to remember are that the characteristics and *abilities* of students with disabilities are individual and neither can nor should be assumed or generalized. Accommodations should be student-specific, as well as with any decision to deny an accommodation request or program admission. Most importantly, if in doubt regarding how to proceed, reach out to available resources, including student disability services, administration, faculty and program directors of similarly situated programs, or legal counsel.

Students have the right to access and challenge their educational records in compliance with FERPA guidelines. Every EMS program is required to have formal, published grievance policies in place for EMS educators and students.

Tort law is especially important to EMS educators. Care should be taken to avoid assault and battery, defamation, misrepresentation or fraud, and negligence. The best protection against tort liability is to implement effective risk management practices. Some of these practices include waivers and releases, safety instruction, student supervision, and careful selection of clinical sites. Affiliation agreements should be developed and should include all necessary components.

Educational programs should be as safe as possible. Federal laws, such as the Safe and Drug-Free Schools and Communities Act, the Gun-Free Schools Act, the Clery Act, and OSH Act provide direction in establishing and maintaining a safe and secure environment.

EMS educators should become familiar with the rules on workers' compensation insurance in their own states. Printed information should be available regarding who and what is covered under workers' compensation. False claims of workers' compensation are considered fraud and punishable by law.

It is important for EMS educators to know which health and malpractice insurance is provided for them, or whether they are expected to provide their own insurance coverage. The same is true with regard to students.

Confidentiality is critical for EMS programs, educators, and students. FERPA and HIPAA clearly define federal guidelines and standards regarding confidentiality. HIPAA, however, does not apply to records covered by FERPA.

Copyright issues should always be reviewed with students. EMS educators involved in research and publications should comply with all copyright laws. EMS educators should not reproduce material from other sources without appropriate citation and permission when required.

EMS educators should be familiar with legal issues that affect their programs. Although EMS educators are not expected to be legal experts, a basic knowledge of legal concepts and an ability to apply them are critical in alleviating potential litigation, as is the ability to identify situations in which legal counsel should be consulted.

Glossary

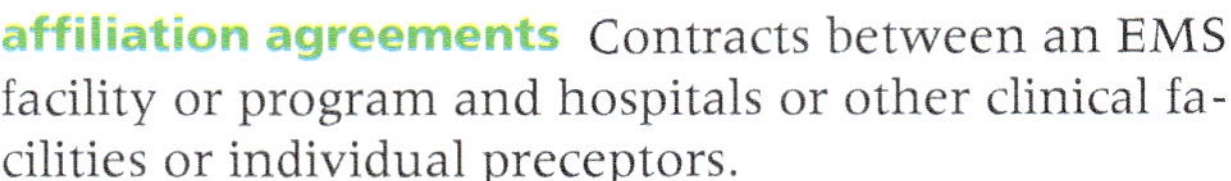

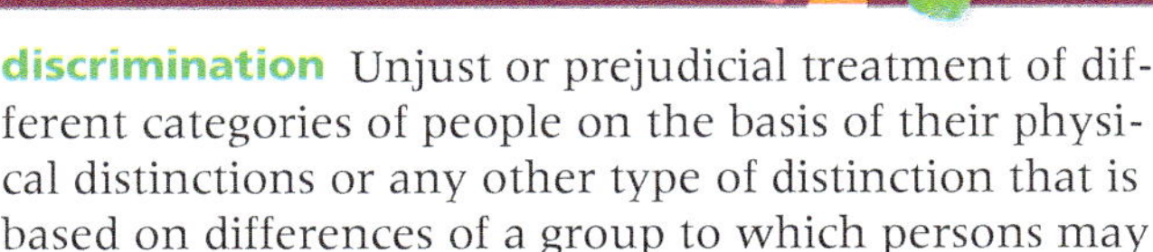

affiliation agreements Contracts between an EMS facility or program and hospitals or other clinical facilities or individual preceptors.

assault Occurs when one person places another person in reasonable fear of immediate harm or physical contact.

battery Physical, unlawful touching of another person without consent.

civil law A system of law concerned with ordinary private matters between members of a community.

color of law Implies the mere semblance of legal rights or the appearance of rights; recognition of novel rights that resemble legal rights and adjusts the law to the circumstance.

constitutional protections The U.S. Constitution prohibits the government from violating the constitutional rights of its citizens; U.S. federal civil rights laws allows U.S. citizens to sue governmental actors who violate their constitutional rights; EMS facilities and programs, as well as individual EMS educators themselves, may be considered governmental actors if they receive or benefit (directly or indirectly) from any type of public funding.

copyright protection Safeguards the original works of authorship fixed in any type of communication material or statements of expression.

criminal law System of laws concerned with the punishment and rehabilitation of those who commit crimes that are prohibited by law because their conduct is deemed harmful to society.

defamation Sharing of true but private information that injures the reputation of another, or the intentional or reckless making of a false statement; two types are libel and slander.

Digital Millennium Copyright Act (DMCA) Implements treaty obligations of the World Intellectual Property Organization and helps move the U.S. copyright law into the digital age.

discrimination Unjust or prejudicial treatment of different categories of people on the basis of their physical distinctions or any other type of distinction that is based on differences of a group to which persons may perceive themselves to belong.

Emergency Planning and Community Right-to-Know Act (EPCRA) Helps communities, including facilities or programs, and educators plan for chemical emergencies; requires facilities, programs, and educators to report on the storage, use, and releases of hazardous substances to federal, state, and local governments.

Equal Employment Opportunity Act (EEOA) Gives the Equal Employment Commission (EEOC) authority to sue in federal courts, when it finds reasonable cause to believe that there has been employment discrimination, including discrimination in or by EMS programs or by EMS educators and students (including any program that leads to or results in employment requiring a certification or licensure).

expert Anyone who, through their education and experience, has developed special skills or knowledge of a particular subject, so that they may develop an informed opinion.

Family Educational Rights and Privacy Act (FERPA) Governs the access of confidential information and the data privacy of records to any publicly funded EMS facilities or programs and EMS educator or activity that receives or benefits from government funds; prohibits the release of any type of personally identifiable information about a student or EMS educator except under certain, limited circumstances; this confidentiality and data privacy law is commonly referred to as the Buckley Amendment and named after its principal legislative sponsor, Senator James Buckley of New York.

fraud Misrepresentation, or the making of a false statement with intent to deceive that causes actual harm to someone who reasonably relies upon the falsification.

Freedom of Information Act (FOIA) Provides that everyone, including EMS educators and students, has the right to request access to government records or information except to the extent the government records or information is protected from disclosure.

governmental actor Any person who acts on behalf of the government and is subject to the U.S. Constitution's Bill of Rights, which prohibits the government from violating certain civil rights and freedoms.

grievance Wrong considered as grounds for a claim and potential lawsuit.

Gun-Free Schools Act (GFSA) Directs education programs, including EMS programs in some states, to develop policies requiring referral to the criminal justice or juvenile delinquency system for anyone who brings a firearm or weapon in or around a school campus; mandates expulsion of students for at least 1 year.

Health Insurance Portability and Accountability Act (HIPAA) Establishes national standards for the confidentiality and data privacy and security of healthcare information.

HIPAA Privacy Rule Protects the medical privacy of everyone receiving prehospital intervention services.

Jeanne Clery Disclosure of Campus Security Policy and Campus Crime Statistics Act (Clery Act) Aims to provide transparency around campus crime policy and statistics; EMS programs, educators, and students must understand what this federal safety and security law entails and where their responsibilities lie.

National Clinicians' Post-Exposure Prophylaxis Hotline Phone line on which consultation is available, or questions are answered about occupational exposures to HIV and other bloodborne pathogens from needlesticks and splashes.

negligent referral Latest *new* civil wrong that represents an entire *new* line of litigation that strongly suggests that programs and educators have a duty to be honest in comments made about another educator or student; includes inappropriate recommendations by a program or educator that misrepresents someone's qualifications or character.

Occupational Safety and Health Act (OSH Act) Federal labor law governing employment-related health and safety.

Pregnancy Discrimination Act (PDA) A federal labor law that amended Title VII of the Civil Rights Act that prohibits gender discrimination on the basis of pregnancy; covers discrimination on the basis of pregnancy, childbirth, or related medical conditions.

risk management Process of preventing, or at least minimizing, harm or loss to an EMS facility, program, EMS educator or student, or anyone receiving emergency care.

Safe and Drug-Free Schools and Communities Act (SDFSCA) Encourages the creation of safe, disciplined, and drug-free environments, including support for EMS programs to be free of drugs and violence.

standard of care Prevailing or routine practice patterns; the legal obligation to conform to a minimum level of safe care to protect others from reasonable and foreseeable harm.

Title IX of the Education Amendments Act A comprehensive labor law that prohibits discrimination on the basis of gender in any place or by anyone, including any federally funded EMS facility or program and EMS educator.

tort Private or civil wrong, injury, or legal action that is not necessarily the result of criminal action but for which the law allows a remedy; other than for a breach of contract, the harm in civil torts may be due to negligence, which does not amount to criminal negligence for which the law allows a remedy.

References

[1] Federal law codified in the U.S. Code at 23 U.S.C § 401 *et seq.* with implementing regulations in the U.S. Code of Federal Regulations at 23 C.F.R. § 401 *et seq.*

[2] National Highway Traffic Safety Administration (NHTSA) and NHTSA Interagency Committee on EMS (FICEMS). 2013. *Advisory Recommendations from the National EMS Advisory Council.* Washington, DC: U.S. Department of Transportation (DOT), NHTSA and FICEMS; NHTSA and Health Resources and Services Administration (HRSA). n.d. *A Leadership Guide to Quality Improvement for Emergency Medical Services Systems.* Washington, DC: Rockville, MD: U.S. Department of Health and Human Services, HRSA.

[3] National Highway Traffic Safety Administration (NHTSA). 2019. *National EMS Information System (NEMSIS).* Washington, DC: U.S. Department of Transportation (DOT), NHTSA; *see also* Bureau of Labor Statistics (BLS). 2018. *Occupational Outlook Handbook.* Washington, DC: U.S. Department of Labor, BLS; NHTSA. 2014. *EMS System Demographics.* Washington, DC: DOT, NHTSA; MacKenzie, Ellen J., and Anthony R. Carlini. 2013. *Characterizing Local EMS Systems.* Washington, DC: DOT, NHTSA.

[4] U.S. Department of Education. 2016, October 28. "U.S. Department of Education Announces Final Regulations to Protect Students and Taxpayers from Predatory Institutions." [Press release]. Washington, DC: U.S. Department of Education.

[5] Matheson, Abbi. 2018, November 7. "Officials: Mass. Paramedics Falsified Training Records." *EMS1.com*. Accessed November 25, 2018. https://www.ems1.com/education-and-training/articles/392837048-Officials-Mass-paramedics-falsified-training-records/.

[6] States News Service. 2012, April 24. "Former Mass. EMT Sentenced to Jail for Falsifying Training Records." *EMS1.com*. Accessed November 25, 2018. https://www.ems1.com/ems-training/articles/1276302-Former-Mass-EMT-sentenced-to-jail-for-falsifying-training-records/.

[7] Moran, Robert. 2018, October 24. "Former NJ EMT Chief Charged with Insurance Fraud." Accessed May 13, 2019. https://www.ems1.com/certification/articles/392746048-Former-NJ-EMT-chief-charged-with-insurance-fraud/.

[8] Smith, Mable H. 2012. *The Legal, Professional, and Ethical Dimensions of Education in Nursing*, 2nd ed. New York: Springer Publishing Company.

[9] National Institute for Occupational Safety and Health. 2016. *Bloodborne Infectious Diseases: HIV/AIDS, Hepatitis B, Hepatitis C.* Atlanta, GA: Centers for Disease Control and Prevention.

[10] National Transportation Safety Board (NTSB). 2017. *Special Investigation Report: Improving Pilot Weather Report Submission and Dissemination to Benefit Safety in the National Airspace System.* Washington, DC: NTSB.

[11] Rasmussen, Kristen, Jo Røislien, and Stephen J. M. Sollid. 2018. "Does Medical Staffing Influence Perceived Safety? An International Survey on Medical Crew Models in Helicopter Emergency Medical Services." *Air Medical Journal* 37, no. 1: 29–36. https://doi.org/10.1016/j.amj.2017.09.008.

[12] American College of Emergency Physicians (ACEP). 2018. *Policy statement: Appropriate and Safe Utilization of Helicopter Emergency Medical Services.* Dallas: ACEP.

[13] Americans with Disabilities Act of 1990, As Amended. Accessed March 22, 2019. https://www.ada.gov/pubs/adastatute08.pdf.

[14] Federal civil rights law codified in the U.S. Code at 42 U.S.C. § 2000d0200d-7, with implementing regulations in the U.S. Code of Federal Regulations at 42 C.F.R. § 2000d0200d-7.

[15] Federal labor law codified in the U.S. Code at 42 U.S.C. §§ 2000e *et seq.* with implementing regulations in the U.S. Code of Federal Regulations at 42 C.F.R. §§ 2000e *et seq.*

[16] Federal labor law further codified in the U.S. Code at 42 U.S.C. § 2000e(k), with implementing regulations in the U.S. Code of Federal Regulations at 42 C.F.R. § 2000e(k).

[17] Federal education law codified in the U.S. Code at 20 U.S.C. § 1681 *et seq.* with implementing regulations in the U.S. Code of Federal Regulations at 20 C.F.R. § 1681 *et seq.*

[18] Federal law codified in the U.S. Code at 29 U.S.C. § 794 with implementing regulations in the U.S. Code of Federal Regulations at 29 C.F.R. § 794.

[19] Federal law codified in the U.S. Code at 42 U.S.C. § 12112, with implementing regulations in the U.S. Code of Federal Regulations at 42 C.F.R. § 12112.

[20] 42 U.S.C. § 12112.

[21] Federal law codified in the U.S. Code at 42 U.S.C. § 12114, with implementing regulations in the U.S. Code of Federal Regulations at 42 C.F.R. § 12114.

[22] Federal law codified in the U.S. Code at 42 U.S.C. § 12102(4)(A), with implementing regulations in the U.S. Code of Federal Regulations at 42 C.F.R. § 12102(4)(A).

[23] 42 U.S.C. § 2000e.

[24] 42 U.S.C. § 2000e(k).

[25] 20 U.S.C. § 1681.

[26] 29 U.S.C. § 651 *et seq.*

[27] Federal gun-free environmental law codified in the U.S. Code at 29 U.S.C. § 651 *et seq.*, with implementing regulations in the U.S. Code of Federal Regulations at 29 C.F.R. § 651 *et seq.*

[28] Commission on Accreditation of Allied Health Education Programs, Committee on Accreditation of Educational Programs for the Emergency Medical Services Professions (CoAEMSP). 2015. *Standards and Guidelines for the Accreditation of Educational Programs in the Emergency Medical Services Professions.* Rowlett, TX: CoAEMSP.

[29] 20 U.S.C. § 1001 *et. seq.* and 42 U.S.C. § 2751.

[30] National Registry of Emergency Medical Technicians. n.d. "Paramedic Program Accreditation Policy." Accessed November 25, 2018. https://www.nremt.org/rwd/public/document/policy-paramedic.

[31] The Joint Commission. 2019. "Criminal Background Checks—Requirements." Accessed March 5, 2019. https://www.jointcommission.org/standards_information/jcfaqdetails.aspx?StandardsFaqId=1592&ProgramId=46.

[32] National Highway Traffic Safety Administration. 2009. "National Emergency Medical Services Education Standards." [DOT HS 811 077A]. Accessed January 15, 2019. https://www.ems.gov/pdf/National-EMS-Education-Standards-FINAL-Jan-2009.pdf; *see also* MacKenzie, E. J., and Carlini, A. R. 2013. *Characterizing Local EMS Systems.* Washington, DC: U.S. Department of Transportation, NHTSA.

[33] Environmental safety law codified in the U.S. Code at 20 U.S.C. § 7101 *et seq.*, with implementing regulations in the U.S. Code of Federal Regulations at 20 C.F.R. § 7101 *et seq.*

[34] Gun-free safety law codified in the U.S. Code at 20 U.S.C.A. § 7151, with implementing regulations in the U.S. Code of Federal Regulations at 20 C.F.R. § 7151.

[35] Campus safety law codified in the U.S. Code at 20 U.S.C. § 1092 *et seq.*, with implementing regulations in the U.S. Code of Federal Regulations at 20 C.F.R. §1092 *et seq.*

[36] 20 U.S.C. § 1092(f).

[37] Hammaker, Donna K., and Thomas M. Knadig. 2018. *Health Care Management and the Law,* 2nd ed. Burlington, MA: Jones & Bartlett Learning; *see also Lentz v. Perskie & Fendt* (Superior Court of NJ, Appellate Division 2018) (holding negligent referral is not a recognized cause of action in New Jersey).

[38] Federal privacy law that protects personally identifiable information; codified in the U.S. Code at 20 U.S.C. § 1232g, with implementing regulations in the U.S. Code of Federal Regulations at 20 C.F.R. § 1232g; *see also* Hammaker, Donna K. 2020. *Health Records and the Law,* 5th ed. Burlington, MA: Jones & Bartlett Learning.

[39] Federal privacy law that enforces HIPAA; codified in the U.S. Code at 42 U.S.C. § 1320d-6, with implementing regulations in the U.S. Code of Federal Regulations at 42 C.F.R. § 1302d-6; *see also* Hammaker, Donna K. 2020. *Health Records and the Law,* 5th ed. Burlington, MA: Jones & Bartlett Learning.

[40] Federal privacy law codified in the U.S. Code at 5 U.S.C. § 552, with implementing regulations in the U.S. Code of Federal Regulations at 5 C.F.R. §552.

[41] 34 C.F.R. pt. 99 regulates the personal records to which FERPA applies.

[42] Clery Center. 2019. *Summary of the Jeanne Clery Act.* Strafford, PA: Clery Center; *see also Bragdon v. Abbott,* 524 U.S. 624 (U.S. Supreme Court 1998).

[43] 34 C.F.R. § 300.535b(1).

[44] 20 U.S.C. § 1232g(b)(1)(A).

[45] 20 U.S.C. § 1232g(1)(I).

[46] 20 U.S.C. 1232g.

[47] 42 U.S.C. § 1320d-6.

[48] 45 C.F.R. § 164.510.

[49] 45 C.F.R. § 164.520a.
[50] 45 C.F.R. §§164.520 to 164.522.
[51] 5 U.S.C. § 552.
[52] 17 U.S.C. § 102.
[53] 17 U.S.C. § 302.
[54] Federal copyright law codified in the U.S. Code at 17 U.S.C. §§ 512, 1201 *et seq.*, 1301 *et seq.*, 4001; amending the Copyright Act codified in the U.S. Code at 17 U.S.C. §§ 101, 104 *et seq.*, 108, 112, 114, 117, 701, with implementing regulations in the U.S. Code of Federal Regulations at 17 C.F.R. §§ 101, 104 *et seq.*, 108, 112, 114, 117, 512, 701, 1201 *et seq.*, 1301 *et seq.*, and 4001.

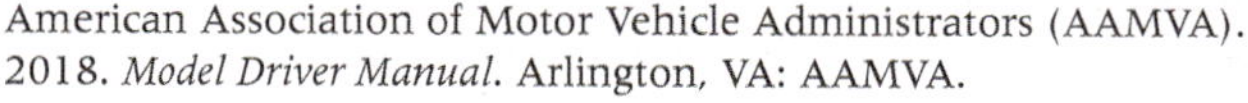
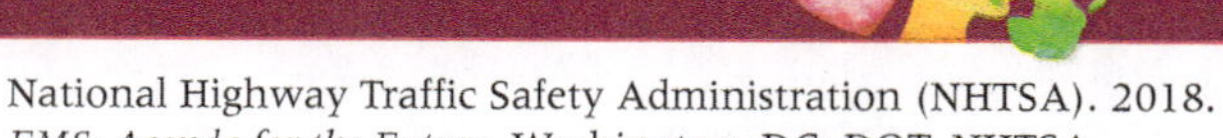

Additional Resources

American Association of Motor Vehicle Administrators (AAMVA). 2018. *Model Driver Manual*. Arlington, VA: AAMVA.

Dotson, Marc P., Mark L. Gustafson, Alfred Tager, and Leslie M. Peterson. 2018. "Air Medical Simulation Training: A Retrospective Review of Cost and Effectiveness." *Air Medical Journal* 37, no. 2: 131–7. https://doi.org/10.1016/j.amj.2017.11.012.

Health Resources and Services Administration (HRSA). 1997. *A Leadership Guide to Quality Improvement for Emergency Medical Services Systems*. Washington, DC: DOT, NHTSA and Rockville, MD: U.S. Department of Health and Human Services, HRSA.

MGA Research Corporation and National Highway Traffic Safety Administration (NHTSA). 2013. *Heat Stroke Evaluation: The First Years True Fit iAlert*. Manassas, VA: MGA and Washington, DC: U.S. Department of Transportation, NHTSA.

National Highway Traffic Safety Administration (NHTSA). 2018. *Additional Analysis of National Child Restraint Use Special Study: Characteristics of Those Not Restrained*. Washington, DC: U.S. Department of Transportation (DOT), NHTSA.

National Highway Traffic Safety Administration (NHTSA). 2018. *EMS: Agenda for the Future*. Washington, DC: DOT, NHTSA.

National Highway Traffic Safety Administration (NHTSA). 2018. *The Emergency Medical Services Workforce Agenda for the Future*. Washington, DC: DOT, NHTSA.

Occupational Safety and Health Administration (OSHA). 2017. *Training Requirements for Emergency Response Medical Service*. Washington, DC: U.S. Department of Labor (DOL), OSHA.

Occupational Safety and Health Administration (OSHA). n.d. *Checklist of Healthcare Wide Hazards*. Washington, DC: DOL, OSHA.

Occupational Safety and Health Administration (OSHA). n.d. *Checklist of Highlighted Hazards in Emergency Department*. Washington, DC: DOL, OSHA.

Occupational Safety and Health Administration (OSHA). n.d. *Checklist of Highlighted Hazards in Heliport*. Washington, DC: DOL, OSHA.

Waltz, Bruce J., and Jason J. Zigmont. 2017. *Foundations of EMS Systems*, 3rd ed. Burlington, MA: Jones & Bartlett Learning.

CHAPTER 26

Fundamentals of Accreditation and Program Evaluation

OBJECTIVES

At the conclusion of this chapter, the educator will be able to:

Cognitive Domain

1. List the principles of accreditation.
2. List the benefits of accreditation.
3. Describe the difference between institutional and programmatic accreditation.
4. Discuss the pillars of accreditation.
5. Describe the steps in the Commission on Accreditation of Allied Health Education Programs (CAAHEP) accreditation process.
6. Describe the relationship between CAAHEP and the Committee on Accreditation of Educational Programs for the Emergency Medical Services Professions (CoAEMSP).
7. Identify common citations in the accreditation process.
8. Identify multiple methods of program evaluation.
9. Locate tools to assist in developing and maintaining a quality program.
10. Describe the importance of outcome thresholds in higher education.

Psychomotor Domain

1. Develop an action plan to prepare a self-study for accreditation.

Affective Domain

1. Value the benefits of programmatic accreditation.

"The biggest room in the world is the room for improvement."

~ Helmut Schmidt

CHAPTER GOAL This chapter on accreditation is new to this text edition. The goal is to provide an overview of the types of accreditation and the processes specific to paramedic education at this time in the United States.

Accreditation of educational institutions has a long history in the United States and dates back over 100 years. The development of accreditation was rooted in concerns to protect public health and safety, to serve the public interest, and to provide a mechanism for quality assurance of educational institutions and programs. In the United States, accreditation of educational institutions and programs of study is organized under a decentralized, voluntary system of private, nonprofit organizations. There is no centralized federal authority with control over the quality of postsecondary education. This approach is in contrast to most other countries where a governmental ministry is responsible for reviewing and approving higher education.

Both degree-granting and non–degree-granting organizations participate in accreditation processes. Numerous organizations are involved at various levels, and funding is primarily through dues from institutions and programs and fees for the review process. There are more than 80 recognized accrediting organizations charged with oversight of more than 50,000 institutions and programs.[1] To the uninitiated, the various components that work together to oversee higher learning in the United States can appear complex and confusing.

Accreditation is an external quality review process. Both federal and state governments rely on accreditation to evaluate academic quality. In addition, federal funds and federal student aid rely on accreditation status. Eligibility for professional credentialing exams in various states can depend on the accreditation status of the institution or program.

Ensuring quality is a primary consideration in the accreditation process. When an institution is accredited, prospective students can feel confident that acceptable standards regarding curricula, faculty, and student services are met. Accreditation does not rank or grade institutions or programs, but it does provide periodic review to determine whether standards and outcomes are consistently met. Core tenets of accreditation are quality assurance and quality improvement. *Quality assurance* entails ensuring threshold quality; *quality improvement* requires institutions and programs to continue to evolve and improve processes. Accreditation is awarded when an institution or program is in substantial compliance with relevant standards and involves both qualitative and quantitative assessments. An important aspect of the process is creating a culture of continuous improvement of academic quality and increasing educational standards and methodologies.

The Accreditation Process

The accreditation process includes several common elements or components. Standards are developed by the accreditor in collaboration with subject matter experts from the communities of interest. These standards include content areas such as the following:

1. Mission
2. Integrity and ethical, responsible conduct
3. Sponsorship
4. Goals and objectives
5. Resources
6. Quality and institutional effectiveness
7. Evaluation
8. Assessment and improvement
9. Fair practices

Institutions and programs entering the accreditation process must first prepare a **self-study report**. While formats vary, the self-study document typically includes an analysis of the performance of the institution or program based on the relevant standards. The self-study report is then reviewed by the accrediting agency to determine if a site visit is appropriate or if additional information is required. Once the self-study is accepted, trained and approved peer faculty and administrative personnel conduct an onsite review or site visit to evaluate compliance with the standards. Finally, all documents and information are reviewed and evaluated by the decision-making body of the accrediting agency, and a judgment is made regarding compliance and the award of accreditation. The final step is periodic review, which may or may not include interim site visits and reporting.

The decision-making body consists of faculty, administrators, and public members and is typically referred to as a *commission*. Reevaluation is required, and the process continues.

Accreditation is a cyclical process, and the length of the award varies by accreditation agency and program. Some approvals are granted for a few years and others for as many as 10 years. Various factors are involved in determining the length of the cycle for re-review, including the type of accreditation (institutional or programmatic), type of program, complexities of the profession, rate of change within the profession, and other internal and external factors. According to the Council for Higher Education Accreditation (CHEA), "Accreditation is a standards-based, evidence-based, judgment-based, peer-based process."[2]

Several principles underlie accreditation of educational institutions and programs and have been identified by Michael Hamm in *The Fundamentals of Accreditation*. These include protection of the public, improving the quality of the accredited entity, providing education and training for the accredited entity, conducting and promoting research for the advancement of the accredited entity, increasing public awareness of the meaning of accredited entities, serving as a clearinghouse of information source on accredited entities, assuming a voluntary self-regulation role as an alternative to some form of government intervention, and achieving customer satisfaction.[3]

Types of Accreditation

Accreditation is either institutional or programmatic. As the name implies, **institutional accreditation** refers to the college, university, or institution and not a specific program of study. Institutional accreditation reviews the academic and organizational structure as a whole for compliance with established standards.

There are four types of accrediting organizations (accreditors); three are institutional and a fourth is programmatic.

A **programmatic accreditor** serves specific programs, professions, or schools and includes law, medicine, engineering, and health, conducting in-depth review and assessment of the program. The programs include public, private nonprofit, and private for-profit models and may or may not award a degree. Currently there are more than 60 programmatic accreditors recognized by either CHEA, the U.S. Department of Education (USDE), or both. In all instances, institutions and programs, *not* courses or individuals, are accredited.

In the United States, seven regional accreditors serve public and private, mainly nonprofit and degree-granting institutions, awarding 2- and 4-year degrees. **Regional accreditation** is viewed by some as a more rigorous process than career-related (programmatic) accreditation. Regional accreditors include the following:

1. Accrediting Commission for Community and Junior Colleges, part of the Western Association of Schools and Colleges (WASC)
2. Higher Learning Commission
3. Middle States Commission on Higher Education
4. New England Association of Schools and Colleges, part of the Commission on Institutions of Higher Education
5. Northwest Commission on Colleges and Universities
6. Southern Association of Colleges and Schools Commission on Colleges
7. WASC Senior College and University Commission

Seven national career-related accreditors serve mainly for-profit, career-based, single-purpose institutions, including distance-learning colleges and universities. These include the following:

1. Accrediting Bureau of Health Education Schools
2. Accrediting Commission of Career Schools and Colleges
3. Accrediting Council for Continuing Education and Training
4. Council on Occupational Education
5. Distance Education Accrediting Commission
6. National Accrediting Commission of Career Arts and Sciences, Inc.
7. Accrediting Council for Independent Colleges and Schools

There are five national faith-related organizations that accredit primarily religiously affiliated or doctrinally based, mainly nonprofit, degree-granting institutions. These organizations are as follows:

1. Association of Biblical Higher Education Commission on Accreditation
2. Association of Advanced Rabbinical and Talmudic Schools Accreditation Commission
3. Association of Institutions of Jewish Studies
4. Commission on Accrediting of Association of Theological Schools
5. Transnational Association of Christian Colleges and Schools Accreditation Commission

An important step in ensuring the quality of accrediting organizations is the process of recognition. **Recognition**, or the review of the quality and effectiveness of accrediting organizations, is based on a set of standards. The two organizations responsible for providing recognition of accreditors are CHEA and USDE. CHEA is a private organization that reviews the ability of accrediting bodies to meet established standards regarding attaining and maintaining academic quality of institutions and programs.[4] The USDE focus is on institutions and programs eligible for federal student aid and other funds and ensuring that federal funds are used for tuition for quality courses and programs.[5] Institutions must comply with all responsibilities under Title IV of the Higher Education Amendments of 1992.[6] Standards also include recruitment and admissions practices and fiscal and administrative capability. The review and approval process through CHEA and USDE is similar to institutional or programmatic review: Standards have been developed, a self-evaluation is required, a site visit and staff report may be required, and recognition is awarded. Periodic review is required to maintain the recognition status. CHEA and USDE do *not* accredit individual institutions.

Benefits of Accreditation

An institution must be accredited for students to be eligible for federal student financial aid. In addition, states require accreditation of institutions in order for students to receive available funding. In some occupations and industries, graduating from an accredited program is an important consideration in hiring decisions and increases the confidence of the employer in the competency of the individual. In higher education, increasing the option for mobility between institutions by transfer of credits is also an important benefit to the student.

Several studies have demonstrated a positive correlation between attending an accredited paramedic program and success on the National Registry of Emergency Medical Technicians (NREMT) paramedic credentialing exam. Dickison and colleagues reviewed the results of 12,773 students completing the NREMT exam and concluded that attendance at an accredited program was independently associated with passing the exam.[7] Studnek, Fernandez, and Margolis surveyed 5,509 students on six parameters and found that accreditation was the most significant in achieving success on the NREMT exam.[8] In 2017, Rodriguez and colleagues reported on 8,404 graduates attempting the NREMT cognitive exam and found that cognitive mean ability estimates were significantly higher for paramedic students graduating from an accredited program.[9] While success on the credentialing examination is only one outcome measure, it is an essential requirement for employment as a paramedic in the field of emergency medical services (EMS).

Accreditation: A National Conversation

Recent events in higher education have raised concerns regarding accreditation oversight and protection of the public. Some institutions have closed precipitously, leaving students without a path to complete their education. Responsibility and accountability of accreditors have been questioned. As a result, institutions, programs, and accreditors are increasingly challenged to develop and monitor student outcomes, provide external information about institutional and program performance and outcomes, provide greater transparency, and improve the ability to transfer credits. Institutions are expected to provide information on outcomes, including student retention (graduation rates), federal loan repayment defaults, success on credentialing examinations (where applicable), employment placement or the ability to obtain employment in the profession or field of study, and job earnings of the graduates. The amount of student debt incurred is also a major concern.

The growth in distance education has also created challenges in the accreditation environment. Increasingly, approval may be required in the state where the student resides and not just the where the program is located. Furthermore, the offering institution or program may be required to meet all requirements of educational institutions in the student's state of residence, including approval as an institution of higher learning in that state. Institutions and programs must be cognizant of applicable state regulations regarding the ability to offer distance-education options in locations other than their declared home state. As additional concerns develop, especially abuse and fraud related to federal student financial aid and distance education, other regulations may be enacted at the federal and/or state level.[10]

The national conversation continues regarding the future and the role of accreditation. Topics include competency-based education, assessment of prior learning, experiential learning, establishing minimum requirements for student achievement, expectations of student learning, and improving completion rates. Accrediting organizations must be transparent in all aspects of operation to protect the student and provide accurate information to the public. Finally, accrediting organizations must be aware of the outcomes and practices of the institutions and programs they accredit.

Accreditation and Emergency Medical Services

History

For many in the field of EMS education, accreditation is a relatively new concept. However, in 2018, paramedic program accreditation celebrated its 40th anniversary. In 1978, the Joint Review Committee on Educational Programs for the EMT-Paramedic (JRCEMT-P) was formed under the auspices of the Committee on Allied Health Education and Accreditation (CAHEA) of the American Medical Association.[11] The *Essentials and Guidelines* was established as a minimum requirement for programmatic accreditation; this document eventually became the *Standards and Guidelines* (*Standards*) in effect today.[12]

Although the accreditation review process was voluntary, a few states enacted legislation that required all currently existing paramedic programs to become accredited within a specified period of time. New programs were given a maximum amount of time to complete the process. Even in states where accreditation was not required, high-achieving programs voluntarily undertook the rigorous process of self-reflection, analysis, and action planning to meet the *Essentials and Guidelines*. The number of accredited programs grew gradually and reached approximately 220 programs by 2007.

Nationally, neither paramedic program accreditation nor national certification/licensure was required. State certification and/or licensure testing at the paramedic level was still prevalent in many states; this could result in challenges when moving between states. The *EMS Agenda for the Future*, published in 1996, called for national certification/licensure of paramedics and national accreditation of paramedic education programs under the **Commission on Accreditation of Allied Health Education Programs (CAAHEP)**; however, adoption of the process remained low.

The Roles of CoAEMSP and CAAHEP

In 1994 the JRCEMT-P became the **Committee on Accreditation of Educational Programs for the Emergency Medical Services Professions (CoAEMSP)** under CAAHEP. That same year, the role of programmatic accreditor moved from CAHEA to CAAHEP. As a programmatic accreditor, CAAHEP works with 26 committees on accreditation, representing 33 diverse health-related professional groups, such as surgical assisting, anesthesia technology, cardiovascular technology, and clinical research. As more health-related professions seek accreditation for their education programs and develop committees on accreditation, the number of programs under the CAAHEP umbrella may increase.

The committees on accreditation do the day-to-day work of accreditation, reviewing program self-studies, coordinating site visits, serving as each program's main contact throughout the review process, and formulating accreditation recommendations that are then considered by the CAAHEP board of directors. CAAHEP is approved as an accreditor by CHEA.

A common misconception is that paramedic programs are accredited by CoAEMSP; however, the approving entity is CAAHEP. This is an important distinction, and programs must correctly represent the accreditor in all program materials.

The nomenclature of CoAEMSP (Emergency Medical Services Professions) intentionally provides for the possibility of accreditation review of other levels of EMS providers, and interest has been expressed from various stakeholders regarding the potential to accredit advanced emergency medical technician (AEMT) programs. The volume of paramedic programs in the system has precluded movement in that direction, but future opportunities exist. The CAAHEP *Standards* are written in language that provides a path for that provider level. The potential for accreditation of emergency medical technician (EMT) programs has also been discussed; however, CAAHEP accredits only programs that are a minimum of 1 academic year in length, and therefore a different review and approval path may be considered in the future. Requests have also been received for accreditation of paramedic programs in foreign countries. Future plans include a path to review and accredit foreign programs if they meet the requirements of the *Standards*.

Who Are CoAEMSP and CAAHEP?

The member sponsor organizations of CoAEMSP include:

1. American Academy of Pediatrics
2. American Ambulance Association
3. American College of Cardiology
4. American College of Emergency Physicians
5. American College of Osteopathic Emergency Physicians
6. American College of Surgeons
7. American Society of Anesthesiologists

8. International Association of Fire Chiefs
9. International Association of Fire Fighters
10. National Association of Emergency Medical Services Physicians
11. National Association of Emergency Medical Services Educators
12. National Association of Emergency Medical Technicians
13. National Association of State Emergency Medical Services Officials
14. National Registry of Emergency Medical Technicians

Each organization sponsors two professional peers to serve on the board of directors. In addition, two public members are seated as board members.

CoAEMSP is governed by bylaws and operating policies. Core principles include confidentiality of program information, fiduciary responsibility to the board, and strict adherence to a conflict-of-interest policy. Board members may not participate in or attend a discussion related to any program that could potentially be considered a conflict of interest, including programs in their home state or an area that could be considered a competitor, programs where the member participated in a prior site visit, or any other situation where the member could be judged as potentially not able to be objective.

CAAHEP is governed by a commission that elects a board of directors. Over 100 commissioners represent committees on accreditation, professional associations, credentialing agencies, health care, educational institutions, Department of Veterans Affairs, Department of Defense, recent graduates, and the public. The commission is responsible for approving the bylaws, mission, and vision statements of CAAHEP and also for determining which healthcare professions are eligible for participation in the organization. The board of directors is a smaller group and is responsible for establishing board policies and objectives and making decisions on accreditation status based on recommendations from the committees on accreditation. Remaining abreast of trends and issues in the various professions represented and the accreditation process is an important function of CAAHEP members.

NREMT Initiative and the Growth of Accreditation

The 2000 National Highway Transportation and Safety Administration (NHTSA) document *EMS Education Agenda for the Future* tied programmatic accreditation to national certification.[13] In 2007, the NREMT took the bold step of requiring that all candidates for NREMT testing at the paramedic level must have completed an accredited program as of January 1, 2013. This timeline provided adequate notice for paramedic programs to come into compliance. At the time this initiative was announced, there was no reliable data available on how many paramedic programs existed across the country. Therefore, it was difficult for the CoAEMSP to determine what the impact would be as programs entered into the accreditation process. The best estimate developed by the CoAEMSP staff and board was that there could potentially be 700 existing programs.

The response to the new NREMT initiative was fairly swift and by January 1, 2016, 260 new programs had entered the system. It was also necessary to develop a "letter of review" path that made it possible for a graduate of a paramedic program that was in the accreditation process, but had not yet been awarded accreditation by CAAHEP, to sit for the NREMT exam. This was an important initiative that provided a pathway for these graduates to achieve national certification or licensure.

In 2018, there were nearly 700 programs either accredited or in the letter of review process. While there have been some program closures, CoAEMSP continues to receive new requests for accreditation services. As of October 2018, only four states did not require NREMT certification for licensure/certification at the paramedic level.[14] However, many programs within those states have voluntarily entered the accreditation process.

With the relatively slow growth of accredited programs over the first 3 decades, one frequent question from programs was: Why should we go through the accreditation process? Many of the early adopters viewed the process as an opportunity for external review and consultation, obtaining input on ways to continue to improve their programs and processes, identifying any gaps in those processes, standardizing paramedic education, providing more mobility for graduates, and meeting a national benchmark. An additional rationale for programs in some states that were not affiliated with a college was the potential to receive approval from the Veterans Administration that would allow qualifying students to access their veteran's benefits for funding.

Today, those same motivations continue to exist. Students can feel confident that an accredited program has met minimum standards and is reviewed periodically by a group of peers to verify continued compliance. Students from accredited programs also have mobility when relocating to a new state, because most have an NREMT credential that facilitates reciprocity in other states and a path to obtain certification or licensure. This is an important factor in a society that tends to be mobile and in an industry where job opportunities, sign-on bonuses, and other local attributes in a new location can be attractive. Perhaps the most important reason, however, for paramedic program accreditation is the potential to improve patient care through verifying competency of paramedic graduates. Patients are the reason why programs exist, and preparing competent entry-level paramedics is the driving goal. Requiring minimum standards of competency is an important step in quality patient care.

The EMS industry is diverse and exists in multiple types of models, including public and private ambulance services, fire service, hospital-based providers, governmental organizations, the military, and other variations. Likewise, paramedic programs vary by participating sponsor type. Approximately 52% are offered by a community or junior college, 15% by a vocational school or technical college, 11% are university based, 10% are hospital sponsored, 7% have a consortium sponsor, 3% are sponsored by fire services, 1% are county/municipality based, 0.2% are ambulance-service sponsored, and 0.1% are military.[15] Of course, programs of all types must meet the eligible sponsor requirement in the CAAHEP *Standards*.

Other EMS Professional Accreditations

Accreditation in the EMS industry is not limited to paramedic education programs. The avenue to accredit continuing education (CE) offerings is available through the **Commission on Accreditation for Prehospital Continuing Education (CAPCE)**, formerly the Continuing Education Coordinating Board for Emergency Medical Services (CECBEMS). CAPCE maintains the standards for the delivery of CE for EMS. Standards include requirements for active medical direction, valid post-tests, quality infrastructure, and sound educational design, including delivery methodology, marketing, fees, evaluation, student record keeping, and data reporting.

CAPCE accreditation provides EMS personnel access to high-quality, relevant, standard-driven CE activities that award appropriate credit. This mechanism allows providers to apply credits from any CAPCE-approved program to local or national recertification requirements. EMS personnel who participate in accredited CE activities are also less likely to be subject to audit by NREMT or by individual state EMS offices. EMTs and paramedics depend on CAPCE to provide accredited programs that are as follows:

- Relevant for EMS CE
- Medically accurate
- Properly referenced
- Original work that is correctly cited
- Grammatically correct and spelled accurately
- Not misleading

CAPCE also requires the following:

- CE providers cite and reference recent peer-reviewed journals as much as possible.
- Content areas cannot be skipped, and post-tests cannot be completed until the content has been viewed.
- CE hours are correctly applied; for example, a provider cannot award 2 CE hours for a 20-minute activity.
- Student activities and interactions are recorded, tracked, analyzed, and reported to the CAPCE data management system.
- Students are required to evaluate the program on completion of the lesson.
- The program committee analyzes the evaluations to make decisions on how they need to improve their activities.
- Needs assessments are performed and the results are applied to future educational content.

EMS educators can achieve a credential through the **National Emergency Medical Services Educator Certification (NEMSEC)**. The goal is to promote excellence in EMS education. In addition to an examination process, additional eligibility requirements must be met.

Accreditation in the ambulance industry is available through the Commission on Accreditation of Ambulance Services (CAAS). In the aeromedical industry, the Commission on Accreditation of Medical Transport Systems (CAMTS) provides this service. Fire service accreditation is offered by the Commission on Fire Accreditation International (CFAI). These recognitions are voluntary, and participating agencies and organizations elect to enter the process to evaluate performance based on a set of standards and to establish a method for achieving continuous organizational improvement.

Accreditation of EMS programs is not unique to the United States. Accrediting authorities exist in other countries; examples include the Health and Care Professions Council in the United Kingdom, Council of Ambulance Authorities Inc. in Australia, and Accreditation Canada in Canada.

Other Regulators

Programmatic accreditation is only one of the oversight mechanisms in EMS education. Depending on

CASE in Point

A new program director was hired by an established, accredited paramedic program that had completed two accreditation reviews. The next review was on the horizon and a self-study was due in 6 months. As a candidate for the position, the program director was assured that the program was operating smoothly and that there had been no issues from the previous site visits.

As the new program director began preparing for the self-study, he reviewed the last communication from CoAEMSP and CAAHEP and found that while the program was indeed accredited, there had been several citations that were not resolved until the third progress report. One of the citations related to lack of preceptor training and another to failure to complete a terminal competency attestation by the medical director for each student prior to graduation. A third citation revealed that not all graduates had met the stated minimum competency requirements. The program had eventually submitted satisfactory evidence that each of these issues had been satisfactorily addressed. However, since that time, the new program director found that new preceptors were not being trained, completion of terminal competency forms was inconsistent, and no one was monitoring minimum competency requirements.

The program director clarified the requirements by reviewing the CAAHEP *Standards and Guidelines* document from the CoAEMSP website and also reviewed the *Interpretations* document to gain a better understanding of the processes that needed to be in place. He also established collegial relationships with other paramedic programs in the area to solicit their best practices and discussed how they could potentially share preceptor training. They also discussed tracking and available tools. The program director met with the other staff and the medical director and clearly established the expectations and processes required, and assigned responsibilities, milestones, and timelines to evaluate progress.

After reviewing available tools on the CoAEMSP website for self-study completion and site visit planning, he developed a schedule for completion of all requirements to meet the self-study submission date and included the staff and medical director in the preparation of the documentation. In the process of a thorough evaluation of the current status of the program, he also discovered that not all of the required representation was present on the advisory committee and that a resource assessment matrix had not been completed annually, and he was able to address both issues prior to the site visit.

location, various regulatory agencies require program submission and approval. These regulatory agencies include state and/or regional approving agencies. However, state/regional approval and accreditation are not the same. Each state has promulgated statutes and/or rules that govern not only individual credentialing, but also requirements and approval processes for programs offering all levels of EMS education, including initial education programs such as emergency medical responder, EMT, AEMT, and paramedic. Regulations may also include authorization to provide CE programs.

Some states, regions, or districts have also defined requirements for education and approval, or credentialing, of instructors. In some cases, this may be an initial education requirement only, while in others the approval or credential must be renewed at specified intervals, and documentation of CE is required.

For programs outside of a college-based system, approval through a private postsecondary approver may also be required, for example the Bureau for Private Postsecondary Education in California, the Higher Education Coordinating Commission Office of Degree Authorization in Oregon, or the Nevada Commission

CASE in Point

A program struggled with graduate performance on the NREMT written exam. Students were passing course exams with mostly A and B grades. Certification results however, averaged around 64% on the cognitive exam. The accreditation body was recommending probationary status due to poor certification exam performance.

The program director and dean decided to explore the situation further. Students said the certification test "wasn't fair," and the course instructors agreed. Analysis of the program's exams revealed that most of the exam questions were low-level, basic knowledge questions. Conversely, the questions on the certification exam were more difficult, requiring candidates to diagnose conditions from scenarios and indicate appropriate treatments.

The program director arranged for the instructors to attend an item-writing workshop. After attending, the instructors had a much better grasp of the process and were able to offer the students exams that better prepared them for practice as well as certification.

on Postsecondary Education. The approval does not typically take the place of accreditation; it is a separate process to protect the public.

Paramedic Education Accreditation

The accreditation process is not a one-time activity, and it should be viewed as an important part of the quality assessment and improvement cycle. Initial accreditation is an opportunity for self-reflection and assessment of processes and policies and to adopt changes and establish best practices. However, the process should not end with the award of accreditation, but should continue to build on progress and successes. Programs are always in an accreditation cycle and must submit an annual report of performance on student achievement outcome thresholds.

The road to initial CAAHEP accreditation begins with a request for accreditation. An accreditation review cannot occur until a cohort has completed the program. Therefore, a mechanism is needed to allow the program to enter into the process. For CoAEMSP, this is the letter of review route. The program completes a letter of review self-study report (LSSR) for evaluation. Once approved, the program is granted the letter of review by CoAEMSP, and the program is considered to be making satisfactory progress in the accreditation process. The program then has 6 months to submit a completed initial self-study report (ISSR) following graduation of the cohort that was first enrolled after submission of the CoAEMSP letter of review.

FIGURE 26.1 illustrates the entire CoAEMSP letter of review and CAAHEP accreditation process for paramedic educational programs. While time frames are not included, it is clear that the process is detailed and transparent. It is significant to note that numerous procedures, professional peers, and CoAEMSP executive office staff are involved in review and evaluation of the program. No single individual determines the outcome of the accreditation decision for any program.

Standards

Standards are qualitative and quantitative measures used to assess compliance with established national norms and identify essential elements for educational quality. Guidelines are included in the CAAHEP *Standards* document in italics; they are descriptors that provide additional guidance and clarification. The CAAHEP *Standards* are typically revised every 5 years to remain current with the profession. CAAHEP *Standards* is based on a template organized under five categories: sponsorship, program goals, resources, student and graduate evaluation and assessment, and fair practices. Some language in the *Standards* is required by CAAHEP and cannot be changed. Other profession-specific language and specifications are formulated by the CoAEMSP board of directors. Once consensus is reached and a final draft is generated, input is sought from the various professional groups that comprise the CoAEMSP board, and each sponsor organization is requested to endorse the revisions. Comment is also sought from other interested professional and industry stakeholders. The draft is posted and opened for public comment. Following draft completion, the entire process of obtaining comment and ratification typically takes a year.

Process

As described earlier, the first major step in the accreditation process is to complete a written self-study report. The document required by CoAEMSP is detailed, and specific instructions are provided. The purpose is to provide all parties in the review and decision process with accurate and succinct information regarding the program. The ISSR and the continuing self-study report (CSSR) are Excel-based forms. Various other required documents must be submitted in a specific folder structure dictated by CoAEMSP, and all documents are uploaded electronically to CoAEMSP. The self-study is data-driven, and most information should be readily available. The program director should include all faculty in self-study report development, including the medical director.

The best means of reducing stress when preparing a self-study report is to allow adequate time to complete the process: begin early, review all of the requirements, make assignments to staff, and continue to evaluate adequate evidence of compliance. Tackling the document one section at a time, scheduling time to work on the document, and pacing help ensure on-time completion. Once received in the CoAEMSP executive office, an executive analysis is prepared by an expert reviewer that provides an overview of areas that appear to meet the *Standards* or are a potential *Standards* violation.

Once the self-study report has been evaluated by the CoAEMSP executive office, the next phase for the program is the site visit. Adequate notice is provided, and the date is mutually agreed upon. A regular site visit is a 2-day event with a minimum of two site visitors. Additional day(s) and/or site visitor(s) may be required if there are special circumstances that require more than a regular site visit. These include, but are not limited to, programs with one or more satellite campuses or online/distance learning. The team visiting the site includes one paramedic educator and

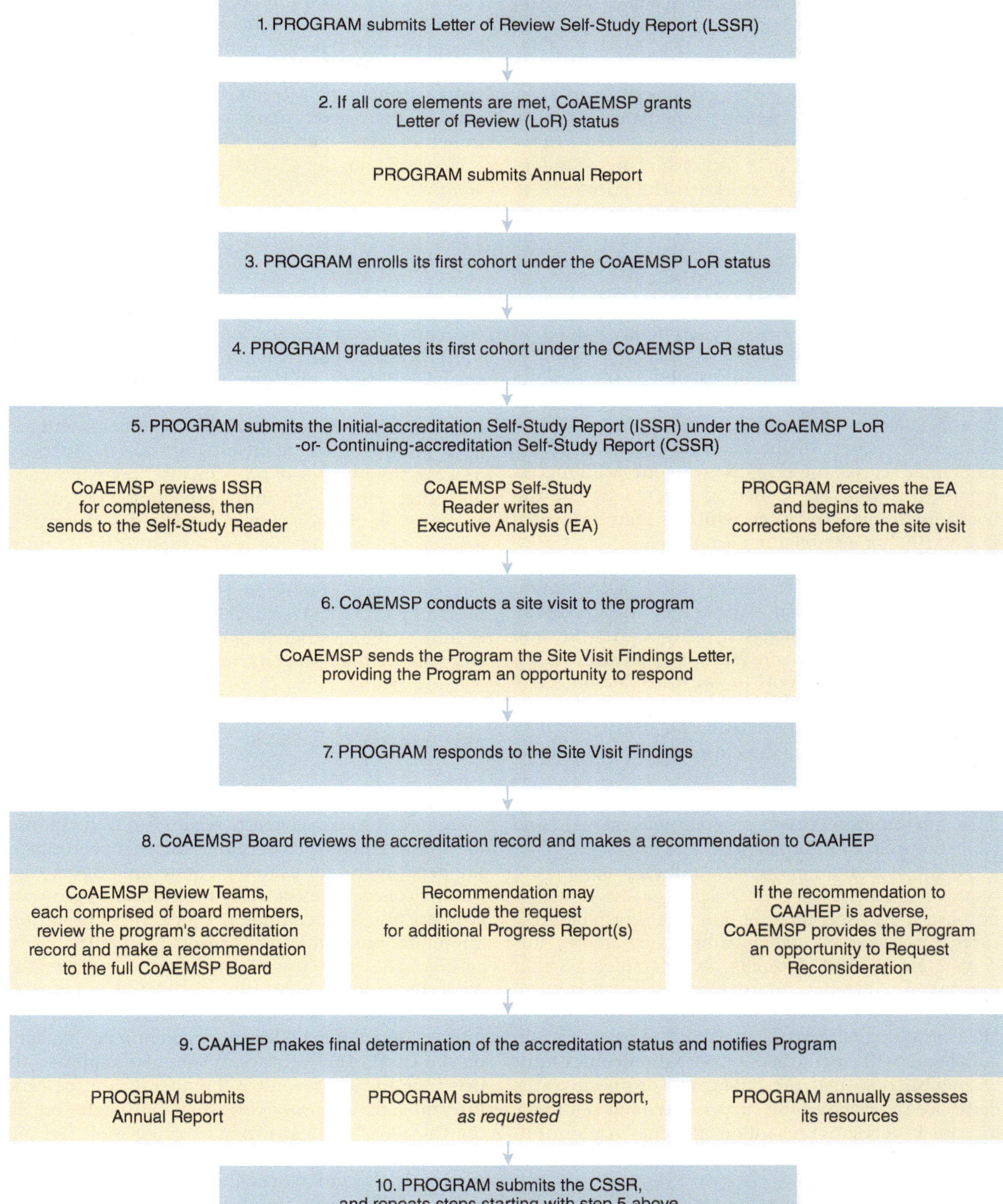

FIGURE 26.1 The CAAHEP accreditation process for paramedic educational programs.

Reproduced from The Commission on Accreditation of Allied Health Educational Programs. 2018, March." The CAAHEP Accreditation Process for Paramedic Educational Programs – from Start to Finish." Accessed April 16, 2019. https://coaemsp.org/seeking-ems-accreditation.

a physician or two paramedic educators. The team captain communicates with the program director regarding details of the visit, the process, and the schedule. Once onsite, the team meets with the program director, administrative personnel, the program medical director, faculty, students, graduates, advisory committee members, and employers, as well as preceptors at clinical and field internship sites. Student and program records are reviewed. The purpose is to verify information, learn additional details about the program, and identify evidence of compliance. The team prepares a report based on compliance with the CAAHEP *Standards* and reviews the findings at an exit summation.

The program then receives a findings letter that identifies any potential *Standards* violations. The program then has the chance to respond to the findings letter and submit any requested documentation. A CoAEMSP board of directors' review team, comprised of a subset of board members, evaluates the response, and either accepts the response or requests a progress report. The program is then considered by the full board for recommendation, which is then forwarded to CAAHEP for accreditation action.

Various tools and resources exist to assist throughout the process. Such resources include accreditation workshops and conferences hosted by the CoAEMSP and the executive office staff. The CoAEMSP and CAAHEP websites contain numerous forms, articles, webinars, and other tools to assist in obtaining and maintaining accreditation and continuing program improvement. Electronic newsletters are distributed on a regular basis to program directors and any other interested individuals and provide news on changes, new interpretations, articles, reminders regarding deadlines, and other important program management and education-related information.

As the accreditation cycle continues, programs are required to submit an annual report each spring. The purpose is the assessment of outcome threshold measures for success on credentialing examinations, student retention, and placement as a paramedic. Other information includes information on graduate and employee assessments. Programs that continue to fall below the established threshold must enter into a dialogue with the accreditor. Those outcomes must be published so that the public and prospective students are informed of the success rates and can make informed decisions regarding their education options. **FIGURE 26.2** demonstrates the cyclic nature of accreditation.

CAAHEP initial accreditation for paramedic programs is awarded for a period of 5 years and automatically expires if the renewal process is not completed. Continuing accreditation is the designation following the first successful renewal. Other potential designations include inactive, probation, administrative probation, withhold of accreditation, and withdrawal of accreditation (involuntary, voluntary, and voluntary in lieu of adverse action). Each potential designation is described in the CoAEMSP *Policies and Procedures Manual*.[16]

Length of Time to Complete the Process

CAAHEP surveys programs following award of accreditation regarding the length of time to complete the process. Reported times from program directors vary significantly and can be impacted by a variety of factors, including the dates a program selects for the site visit based on availability of students and program personnel, where the program falls in the review process, the number of programs in the review cycle, and other reasons. The initial preparation process also tends to take longer than reaccreditation cycles. The general period from first notification of the required submission date until receipt of the CAAHEP award letter is typically between 14 and 18 months as reported by CoAEMSP staff. It is important to note that as long as the program is in the accreditation process, students in that program are eligible to sit for the NREMT exam.

Associated Costs

Paramedic programs are resource- and equipment-intensive and often operate on a narrow financial margin. Costs are a concern, regardless of the sponsor (a sponsor could be a college, hospital, consortium, or fire department, for example). State funding for community colleges is more likely to shrink than grow and costs are also a concern for all other types of sponsors. Therefore, programs and sponsors are naturally concerned about the costs of accreditation. Committees on accreditation are basically self-funded and must be able to balance expenses and revenue. Fees are formulated based on services provided and are available on the CoAEMSP webpage.[17] Some fees apply to the first-time application only; subsequently, the fee structure remains relatively consistent. First-time fees in the CoAEMSP process include a submission fee, self-study report evaluation fee, and technology fee. Continuing accreditation fees include annual CoAEMSP and CAAHEP fees, and a fee for self-study report evaluation due with the submission of the self-study

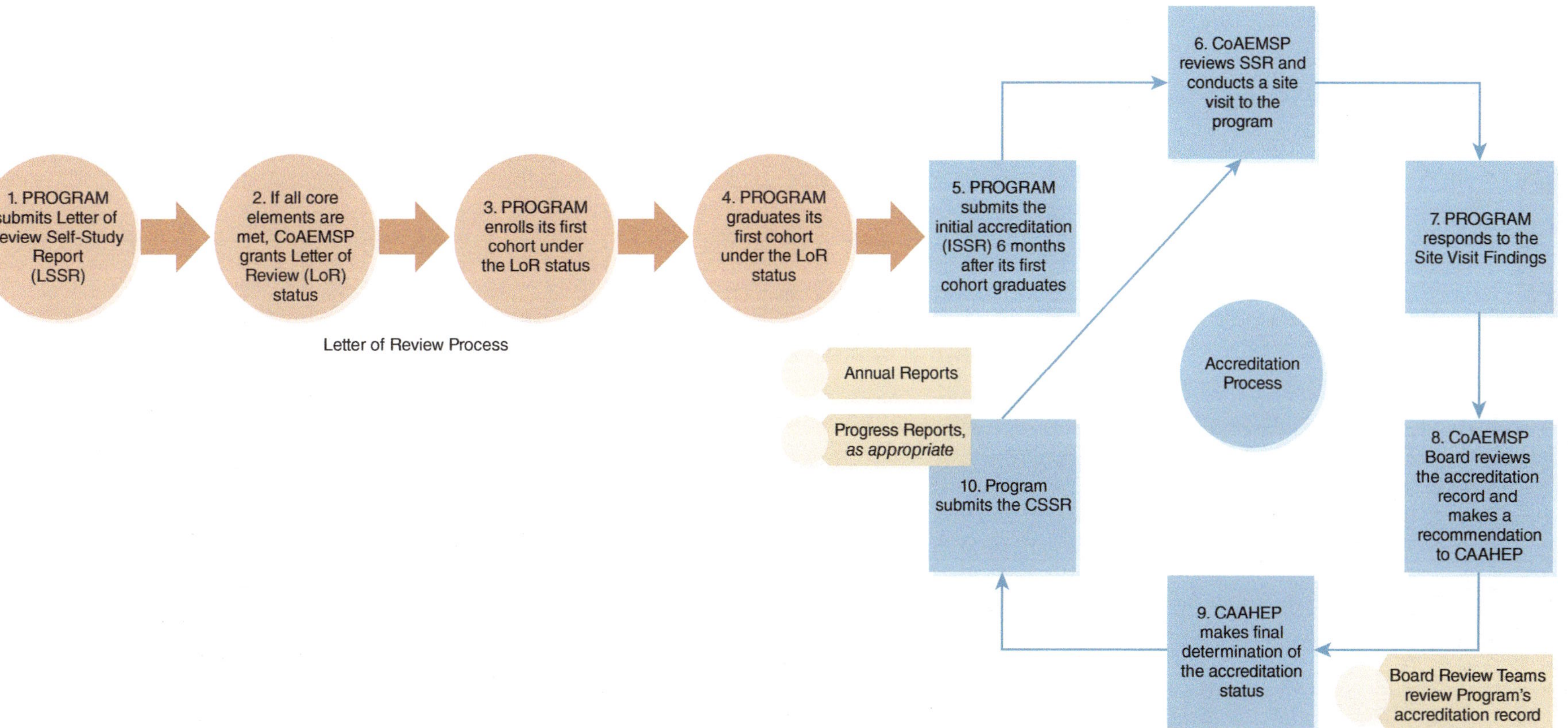

FIGURE 26.2 The CoAEMSP letter of review process and the CAAHEP accreditation process for paramedic educational programs.

Reproduced from The Commission on Accreditation of Allied Health Educational Programs. 2019, May. "The CoAEMSP Letter of Review Process and the CAAHEP Accreditation Process for Paramedic Educational Programs, CoAEMSP." Accessed June 4, 2019. https://coaemsp.org/seeking-ems-accreditation.

report. A flat fee for all site visits is assessed and is based on historical site visit cost data. Other additional costs can include visits to satellite locations, late fees, transfer of sponsorship, and an annual satellite fee. Site visitors are volunteers and receive no compensation. Likewise, members of the board of directors are not compensated. These volunteers are committed to improving education and outcomes.

TEACHING TIP

The goal of EMS education is to be outcomes oriented. Two survey processes are required by CAAHEP to assess specific outcomes. Outcomes include graduate success on credentialing exams and graduate and employer surveys. CoAEMSP provides required survey tools for graduates and employers. The questions are focused on the program goal—to prepare competent entry-level paramedics. Programs may add additional survey items, but must include CoAEMSP-required elements.

Other Delivery Options and Considerations

To meet the need for paramedic education in less populated locations, some programs have developed satellite locations. A **satellite** is an off-campus location where a student can complete a portion or all of a course of study without ever attending the main campus. The satellite location is under the administrative control of the sponsor. The satellite location must provide the necessary equipment, personnel, and other resources to meet the objectives of the course content offered at that location. Satellite locations must be approved by the CoAEMSP and are reviewed at the time of the site visit. Developing a satellite can be resource intensive. Students must receive the same level of instruction and clinical and field internship experiences as at the main campus.

Distance education is an increasingly popular method of delivering educational content. The definition and description of distance learning varies by authority. (See Chapter 17, *Tools for Distance Learning*.) In the simplest form, distance education is program delivery that allows completion of an entire curriculum without the need to attend any instruction on a campus location. EMS education is heavily oriented toward hands-on skills practice and highly developed scenarios and simulations that require in-person student and instructor interaction, so pure distance learning is rare. High-performing programs in today's environment use a variety of technological modalities to enhance the learning environment, including learning management platforms, online assignments, videos, video (and other Web-based) conferencing, and other technology. Hybrid programs help blend the nontraditional classroom delivery and the need for practical application. As technology continues to advance, new opportunities for meeting the needs of students in more remote areas may evolve.

Faculty Considerations

Institutions of higher education typically require that instructors possess an academic credential at least one level higher than the educational level offered in the course of instruction. CoAEMSP moved in that direction as well and, effective with the 2005 revision of CAAHEP *Standards*, program directors were required to have completed a bachelor's degree from an accredited institution of higher education with an implementation date of 2013 to allow time for programs to comply. Existing program directors of accredited programs were provided grandfather status; however, when a new individual is appointed to the position, the degree requirement is in effect. To assist in the transition, for new programs seeking accreditation prior to 2011, the program director was required to provide a transcript of 15 semester hours of credit per year toward the degree until completion. Beginning in 2011, all programs applying for accreditation were required to appoint a program director that met the degree requirement. The 2015 CoAEMSP *Standards* recommend a master's level degree.

Of note, education credentials for directors of accredited programs in 2018 were as follows: 54% of program directors held a bachelor's degree, 41% a master's degree, and 5% a doctorate.[18] The same desire to improve the educational preparation of individuals identified as lead instructors led to a similar requirement in the 2015 revision of the CAAHEP *Standards*. A minimum of an associate's degree was specified for individuals in this role. Existing lead instructors were provided grandfather status. CoAEMSP recommends a bachelor's level degree for lead instructors.

Common Challenges, Frequent Citations

Failure to meet a *Standard* results in a citation. Citations may be classified in three broad categories. These include foundational issues, process issues, and administrative issues. The most challenging are foundational issues, such as lack of an acceptable sponsor as defined in the *Standards* or a medical director who does not meet the required involvement in the program. Process issues are typically relatively easy to address but may take time for full implementation. This type of challenge often involves issues such as identifying required minimum competency numbers and implementing a tracking mechanism to verify that all graduates have met these minimums. The third type of citation is often easily correctable and may only require clarification, for example, not including all required policy statements, such as advanced placement or credit for prior learning, in program materials.

Typically, citations can be avoided through careful review of the CAAHEP *Standards* and the CoAEMSP *Interpretations* documents and addressing each content area. The CoAEMSP *Interpretations* of the CAAHEP *Standards* is reviewed by a board committee at least twice annually and provides additional information on what is meant by a specific CAAHEP *Standard* statement or provides suggestions on evidence that could meet the requirement.

In the CoAEMSP/CAAHEP process, programs have access to a sample site visit report on the CoAEMSP website. This document identifies all of the required standards and the potential evidence the reviewers use to evaluate the program, so the program can rate itself using the same tool. Even with these available tools, CoAEMSP staff report that programs average two to three citations on either the initial or continuing review.

The following is a list of the most frequent citations resulting from the CoAEMSP/CAAHEP accreditation review process, shown in descending order of frequency, as reported by CoAEMSP staff:

1. Failure to provide evidence of orientation of preceptors
2. Lack of medical director review of student progress throughout the program
3. Frequency of student assessment is inadequate, including assessing the validity of high-stakes examinations
4. Hospital and field internship sites that provide inadequate exposure to required patient types
5. Inappropriate sequencing of curriculum to provide adequate opportunity to attain competencies
6. Advisory committee membership not specified
7. Lack of a summary tracking mechanism that demonstrates that all graduates met minimum competencies
8. Lack of engagement of the medical director with the program director
9. Lack of medical director review of instruments to assess students
10. Lack of team lead experience
11. Lack of long-range planning
12. The required competencies for competent entry-level practice are not established or have not been reviewed and endorsed by the medical director and advisory committee

This list is not exhaustive but does include the most common occurrences. Familiarity with the CAAHEP *Standards* and understanding the application of the *Standards* are essential in operating a well-developed program that serves students, the EMS community, and patients.

Program Review, Evaluation, and the Quality Review Process

Continuous review of all components of a program is essential to ensure that quality is maintained. This type of review is also key to long-range planning and continued success of the program. The goal of paramedic education is to prepare competent entry-level graduates; three key metrics are success on the NREMT exam and the evaluation of that competence by both graduates and their employers.

The tools for evaluation by graduates and their employers are the graduate and employer surveys, administered 6 to 12 months following program completion. Three questions relate to competence in the cognitive, psychomotor, and affective domains. Programs can include additional questions to whatever depth desired, but CoAEMSP requires the three cited. While return rates can be challenging, the information received is critical for a program to determine whether it is meeting the needs of the profession. A similar tool can be used to assess graduate and employer satisfaction for other levels of EMS provider.

The resource assessment is another important tool and is used for students, program personnel, the medical director, and the advisory committee to evaluate the adequacy of resources within the program. Once again, a specific CoAEMSP set of survey questions to

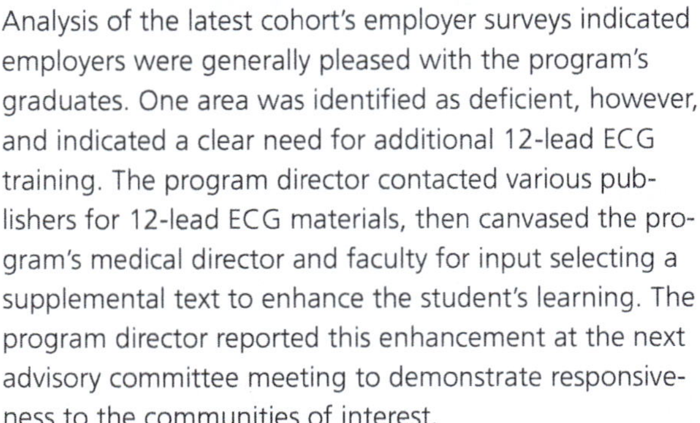

CASE in Point

Analysis of the latest cohort's employer surveys indicated employers were generally pleased with the program's graduates. One area was identified as deficient, however, and indicated a clear need for additional 12-lead ECG training. The program director contacted various publishers for 12-lead ECG materials, then canvased the program's medical director and faculty for input selecting a supplemental text to enhance the student's learning. The program director reported this enhancement at the next advisory committee meeting to demonstrate responsiveness to the communities of interest.

assess the sufficiency of various resources within the program is required and the responses must be entered into the matrix, analyzed, and a specific action plan developed if areas fall below the specified range. The resource categories include program faculty, medical director, support personnel, curriculum, financial resources, facilities, hospital clinical resources, capstone field internship resources, learning resources, and physician interaction. Resource assessment must occur annually. The analysis and action plan must be operationalized and become part of the quality improvement and long-range planning process. This form of resource assessment can also be adapted for other programs offered.

Several other assessment components are recommended at all provider levels, and programs are free to develop tools that are best suited to their program. Instructors in both the classroom and laboratory should be evaluated frequently. It can be tempting to neglect surveying students regarding long-standing faculty who are assumed to be performing adequately; however, all instructional staff should be evaluated at regular intervals, including when new to the role or when signs of potential issues appear. The evaluations should be formal, documented, and reviewed with the educator who was evaluated. Tools for classroom facilitation and skill instruction should be specific and designed to elicit information related to those venues. Comments from the students provide positive feedback, areas for improvements, and often suggestions on ways to further improve the delivery and facilitation of the instructional process. In addition, the Program Director should observe each faculty member in the classroom and skill sessions using a set of criteria directed at professional development as part of an annual review. In some environments where faculty trust level is high, peers evaluate each other and provide constructive feedback. Some institutions have systems in place that preclude or prohibit these types of evaluation processes for a variety of reasons and thus exempt faculty from review, particularly when tenure is involved. In these circumstances the program director and faculty must be creative to find ways to accomplish the goal of obtaining feedback from students and staff in order to continue improving the quality of the educational environment.

Of equal importance at the paramedic level is evaluation of clinical and field internship sites for (1) adequacy of resources to meet the necessary patient contacts and skills and (2) depth and breadth of experiences to allow students to reach entry-level competence. This involves evaluation by the students, but also assessment by the clinical or field internship coordinator. Preceptors and other clinical personnel must provide a learning environment that welcomes the students and encourages participation and skill development. Because organizational culture and staff can change within a facility or agency, it is possible that a site no longer provides the same educational opportunities or environment for the student; therefore, reassessment is necessary to determine whether the site should be maintained as an internship site. The faculty and student evaluations should be tabulated and feedback provided to the clinical and field internship sites. Positive student feedback can contribute to the willingness and interest from the clinical and field sites to continue to place students. Issues with student reception, communication with the students or program staff, and availability of patient care clinical opportunities must also be relayed, and follow-up initiated.

Evaluation of the field internship site is separate from the paramedic student intern's evaluation of the preceptor. Programs can elect to have students evaluate their preceptor each shift or at other specified intervals. It is recommended that students document evaluation frequently to identify issues early, such as student preceptor mismatch, personality conflicts, poor learning environment, unfair bias, unsafe practices, and other concerns. Early identification of potential problems allows the program to make assignment adjustments to benefit the student intern and to deter later concerns that can arise in an unsuccessful internship.

Evaluation is completed at the end of a course of study. The definition of a course varies widely depending on the structure of the education program. Collegiate paramedic programs may consist of numerous 2, 3, or 4 credit-hour courses. EMT and AEMT courses may be one or two semesters. Other programs may be offered in a single block. Evaluation should occur at the end of each delineated course. When the program is considered to be one long course, it is recommended that a course evaluation be completed at least at the midterm point and program end. These evaluations should be summarized, analyzed, and discussed among faculty, the medical director, administrative personnel, and the advisory committee.

Stakeholder feedback is important to all programs and comes from clinical and field internship sites, employers, and advisory committee members. Programs frequently have close relationships with individuals in these arenas and may feel such relationships replace the need for feedback. However, formal discussion at regularly scheduled meetings is vital. These discussions should be documented in detailed minutes. Advisory committee meetings should not be merely an update to the members, but rather a true discussion of the program outcomes, evaluations, surveys, and an opportunity for suggestions and recommendations from the nonprogram members.

Another useful process is **SWOT analysis**, a common practice in business that also works well in the educational environment. It begins with a brainstorming session with personnel and can include faculty, adjuncts, the medical director, and advisory committee members. The group generates lists of program strengths, weaknesses, opportunities, and threats (SWOT). At times the same item may appear in more than one category, such as a threat and an opportunity. Examples of strengths may include faculty, equipment, or clinical opportunities. Weaknesses can be lack of medical director interaction with students, limited clinical opportunities, or no screening process for prospective students. Opportunities could be a new clinical opportunity, such as a cadaver lab or a new pool of preceptors. Threats might include a declining student enrollment or a new competing program. The important element is to be open, honest, and creative. This process can identify potential problems and generate ideas that might not otherwise occur to individuals.

Programs located in a college environment often have access to one or more individuals in the institution responsible for evaluation who can be a resource in the programmatic accreditation process. Typically, colleges also have an individual responsible for coordinating institutional accreditation who can be of valuable assistance. The college may have other assessment and planning tools and processes that are used across all disciplines. These resources can provide further guidance.

Outcomes Measures

Of the various needed outcomes measures, the most challenging for programs is often retention. Programs with open enrollment may feel that they have little control over the admission process, and, of course, all programs must work within their institutional framework. However, it is common for health education programs in colleges to require additional screening and prerequisites. Best practices to increase retention include the following.

1. If the program is required to be open enrollment, the program director should explore with the administration whether it is possible to add prerequisites or screening for the specialized course of study. Various assessment tools exist to evaluate reading, math, and comprehension. Community colleges offer assessment tools and recommendations in each of these key dimensions. Other elements may include prerequisite EMT knowledge and assessment of affective traits.
2. Institute interviews with applicants. Detail the requirements, schedules, rigor, cost, and other specifics to allow the student to make an informed choice regarding admission.
3. Provide a thorough orientation for a new cohort with all of the information identified in the interview.
4. If a new student chooses not to continue with the program after orientation, the program should encourage the drop before the program established add/drop date. From the student perspective, an early drop can provide the maximum tuition refund. For the program, an early drop can affect the attrition rate (the number of students who leave the program).
5. Invite/include student family members to the orientation session to explain the program requirements and how they can support their loved one.
6. Faculty should meet with enrolled students at specified points in the program to review academic status, clinical and field progress toward requirements, areas where the student may be struggling, and potential remediation/resources.
7. Suggest that students form study groups that can provide mutual encouragement and enhance learning.
8. Conduct exit interviews with students who drop/withdraw from the program. Consider using a source outside the program to conduct the exit interview to encourage honest feedback. Faculty may think they know why the student is leaving, but there may be other reasons.
9. Facilitate outside tutoring/resources through faculty, adjunct instructors, or other sources.
10. For programs offered over multiple semesters, it can be easy for a student to just not return. Keep track of the cohort, and make contact with any nonreturning student.

11. If your program administration wants all applicants accepted/enrolled for financial reasons, have a crucial conversation with them about the goals and aims of an EMS career and the paramedic program.
12. Connect with the college's student services office as soon as problems such as learning disabilities are discovered.
13. Provide advising or resources for students regarding personal issues during the program.
14. Recommend that potential applicants complete math, English, and other general education courses to prepare for the rigors of the program, especially if they have been out of the academic environment for some time.
15. Provide frequent evaluation of performance in all domains during the program.

CASE in Point

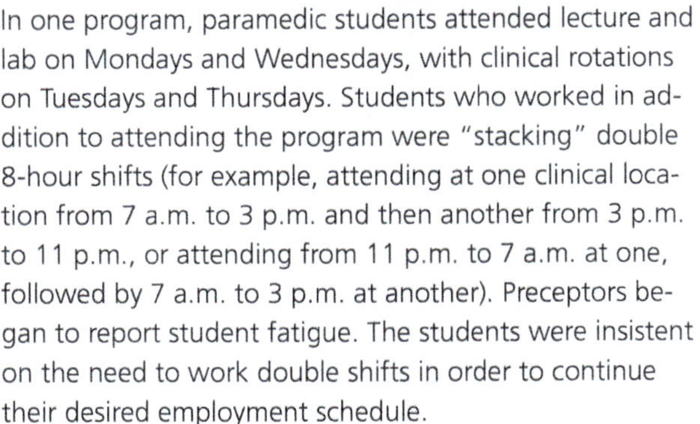

In one program, paramedic students attended lecture and lab on Mondays and Wednesdays, with clinical rotations on Tuesdays and Thursdays. Students who worked in addition to attending the program were "stacking" double 8-hour shifts (for example, attending at one clinical location from 7 a.m. to 3 p.m. and then another from 3 p.m. to 11 p.m., or attending from 11 p.m. to 7 a.m. at one, followed by 7 a.m. to 3 p.m. at another). Preceptors began to report student fatigue. The students were insistent on the need to work double shifts in order to continue their desired employment schedule.

The program director discussed the issue with the advisory committee. The advisory committee members related their policy of not allowing any employee to work more than 12 hours without at least 8 hours of rest. Based on this input, the program director revised the clinical policy to limit students to the same type of scheduling, which provided a lesson in safety as well as a reflection of workplace practice.

Preparation prior to entry into a paramedic program can be an important element in ultimate student success. For example, programs take different approaches to anatomy and physiology regarding when it is offered and the depth and breadth of the content. This topic has been debated and views differ based on whether paramedic education is considered an academic healthcare provider or a technical field, and also whether the education is a degree or certificate track. Programs that require a college-level two-course series of anatomy and physiology anecdotally find that students perform better academically in the paramedic course. This may be due to a solid foundation in anatomy and physiology that leads to better understanding of pathophysiology. A second benefit may be the discipline of study and becoming a student again.

Students who enter an EMS education program may arrive fresh from high school or may have been away from an academic environment for a considerable period of time. Programs can offer information and education on a variety of strategies for success that may include creating a study environment, maintaining a study log, time management, test taking tips, and how to be successful in both the classroom and lab settings. Presentations from former students with their tips for success can be well received and may have more impact than the same information coming from a faculty member.

Another option implemented by some programs is a preparatory (prep) course prior to entry into a paramedic program. The format and content can be tailored to the student population, and topics can include review of basic concepts and skills, basic math review, anatomy and physiology review, medical terminology, skills and scenarios, and an introduction to concepts in the paramedic program, such as pharmacology. The course can be didactic or a combination of didactic and skills, scenarios, and simulations. There is no one key to retention; however, programs have a responsibility to prepare students for success in their chosen field.

Programs that actively participate in ongoing evaluation of quality metrics and implement changes based on those results typically experience minimal challenges with graduate success on credentialing exams. Faculty must monitor student progress in all domains throughout the program, identify potential performance issues early, and work with the student to remediate deficiencies. Performance improvement plans should be implemented to clarify for the student specific deficiencies, improvement expected, metrics used to measure progress, and milestones and required completion date. (See Chapter 23, *Remediation*, for further discussion.) Faculty must monitor the progress and provide additional resources as necessary.

Programs that have fully implemented a portfolio to track skills and patient contacts, and that effectively use scenarios and simulations throughout the course of study, also find improvement in graduate success on credentialing exams. Practice "practical exams" that mimic the National Registry or state exam are also beneficial. Students must also be prepared to complete credentialing exams in a computer-based environment. Programs should help prepare students by administering at least some of the course high-stakes exams using a computer-based format.

Summary

Accreditation is a benefit to students, professional stakeholders, and the public, and the field of paramedic education is no exception. Understanding the rationale for accreditation, the administrative bodies and their roles, and the path to achieving and maintaining accreditation is important to program success. Accreditation provides an opportunity to explore best practices that benefit the student and ultimately the consumer—the patient.

Glossary

accreditation Process in which an educational institution or program is evaluated to determine whether it meets certain standards.

Commission on Accreditation for Prehospital Continuing Education (CAPCE) Accrediting body for continuing education in emergency medical services.

Commission on Accreditation of Allied Health Education Programs (CAAHEP) Approving entity for accreditation of emergency medical services education programs.

Committee on Accreditation of Educational Programs for the Emergency Medical Services Professions (CoAEMSP) Entity that performs accreditation reviews of emergency medical services education programs for CAAHEP.

institutional accreditation Type of accreditation that applies to a college, university, or institution, rather than a specific program of study.

National Emergency Medical Services Educator Certification (NEMSEC) Credentialing body for emergency medical services educators.

programmatic accreditor Accrediting body that serves specialized programs, professions, or schools.

recognition Review of the quality and effectiveness of accrediting organizations.

regional accreditation Type of accreditation that serves public and private institutions, including nonprofit and degree-granting institutions that award 2- and 4-year degrees.

satellite In the context of education, an off-campus location advertised or otherwise made known to individuals outside the sponsor, and which offers all the professional didactic and laboratory content of the program.

self-study report Document created by an institution or program that provides an analysis of that institution or program and that is submitted as part of the accreditation process.

SWOT analysis Analysis method in which a group brainstorms strengths, weaknesses, opportunities, and threats.

References

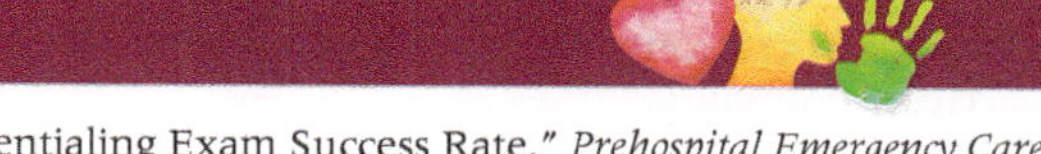

[1] Eaton, Judith S. 2016. "Accreditation Resources." Council for Higher Education Accreditation. Accessed March 5, 2019. http://www.chea.org/userfiles/uploads/AccredRecogUS.pdf.

[2] Eaton, Judith S., and Council for Higher Education Accreditation. 2015, November. "An Overview of U.S. Accreditation." Accessed March 5, 2019. https://www.chea.org/overview-us-accreditation.

[3] Hamm, Michael S. 1997. *The Fundamentals of Accreditation.* Washington, DC: American Society of Association Executives.

[4] Council for Higher Education Accreditation. 2018. "CHEA Homepage." Accessed March 5, 2019. https://www.chea.org/.

[5] U.S. Department of Education. 2019. "Accreditation in the United States." Accessed March 5, 2019. https://www2.ed.gov/admins/finaid/accred/accreditation_pg4.html.

[6] U.S. Department of Education. 2018. "Database of Accredited Postsecondary Institutions and Programs." Accessed March 5, 2019. https://ope.ed.gov/dapip/#/home.

[7] Dickison, Philip, David Hostler, Thomas E. Platt, and Henry E. Wang. 2006. "Program Accreditation Effect on Paramedic Credentialing Exam Success Rate." *Prehospital Emergency Care* 10, no. 2: 224–228. https://doi.org/10.1080/10903120500541126.

[8] Studnek, Jonathan, Antonio R. Fernandez, and Gregg Margolis. 2007. *Factors Affecting the Probability of Passing the National Paramedic Certification Examination.* Columbus, OH: National Registry of Emergency Medical Technicians.

[9] Rodriguez, Severo A., Remle P. Crowe, Rebecca E. Cash, and Ashish R. Panchal. 2017. "Accredited Paramedic Program Graduates Have Higher Student Ability Estimates." *Prehospital Emergency Care* 21, no. 1: 96.

[10] Kutz, Gregory D. 2010, August 4. *For-Profit Colleges: Undercover Testing Finds Colleges Encouraged Fraud and Engaged in Deceptive and Questionable Marketing Practices. Testimony before the Committee on Health, Education, Labor, and Pensions, U.S. Senate. GAO-10-948T.* Washington, DC: U.S. Government Accountability Office. Accessed March 5, 2019. https://eric.ed.gov/?id=ED511120.

[11] Committee on Accreditation of Educational Programs for the Emergency Medical Services Professions. 2018. "CoAEMSP

History / A 40th Anniversary Celebration." Accessed March 5, 2019. https://coaemsp.org/History.htm.

[12] Commission on Accreditation of Allied Health Education Programs and Committee on Accreditation of Educational Programs for the Emergency Medical Services Professions. 2015. *Standards & Guidelines for the Accreditation of Educational Programs in the Emergency Medical Services Professions*. Accessed February 14, 2019. Retrieved https://coaemsp.org/Standards.htm.

[13] EMS.gov. n.d. "Emergency Medical Services Education Agenda for the Future: A Systems Approach." Accessed March 5, 2019. https://www.ems.gov/pdf/education/EMS-Education-for-the-Future-A-Systems-Approach/EMS_Education_Agenda.pdf.

[14] National Registry of Emergency Medical Technicians. 2018, October 7. "National Registry Data, Dashboard, and Maps." Accessed March 5, 2019. https://www.nremt.org/rwd/public/data/maps.

[15] CoAEMSP Database of Accredited Programs. [personal communication].

[16] Committee on Accreditation of Educational Programs for the Emergency Medical Services Professions. 2018, October 7. "Policies & Procedures." Accessed March 5, 2019. https://coaemsp.org/Policy_Procedures.htm.

[17] Committee on Accreditation of Educational Programs for the Emergency Medical Services Professions. 2018, October 7. "Fees." Accessed March 5, 2019. https://coaemsp.org/Fees.htm.

[18] Committee on Accreditation of Educational Programs for the Emergency Medical Services Professions. 2018, January. "Latest News from CoAEMSP." Accessed March 5, 2019. https://myemail.constantcontact.com/Latest-News-From-CoAEMSP.html?soid=1103098668638&aid=QG3rucXtZ4U.

Additional Resources

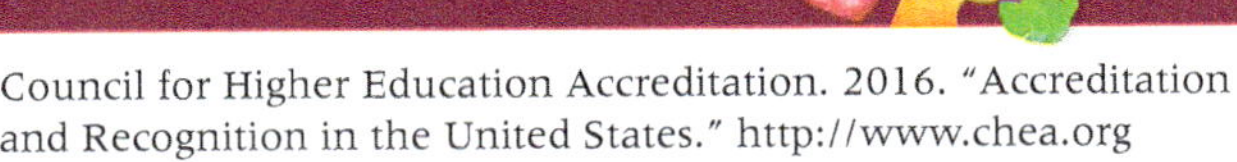

Association of Specialized and Professional Accreditors. n.d. "Quick Reference, Standards, Outcomes, and Quality." https://www.aspa-usa.org/wp-content/uploads/2015/02/ASPA_Standards_Jun12.pdf.

Center for American Progress. 2015, December 14. "Hooked on Accreditation: A Historical Perspective." https://www.americanprogress.org/issues/education-postsecondary/reports/2015/12/14/127200/hooked-on-accreditation-a-historical-perspective/.

Commission on Accreditation of Allied Health Education Programs. n.d. "CAAHEP Accreditation Process." https://www.caahep.org/Accreditation/CAAHEP-Accreditation-Process.aspx.

Commission on Accreditation of Allied Health Education Programs. n.d. "Glossary." https://www.caahep.org/Accreditation/Glossary.aspx.

Commission on Accreditation for Prehospital Continuing Education. 2018. "About CAPCE." https://www.cecbems.org/Home/About.

Committee on Accreditation of Educational Programs for the Emergency Medical Services Professions. n.d. "Letter of Review." https://coaemsp.org/LoR.htm.

Council for Higher Education Accreditation. n.d. "Important Questions about Accreditation, Degree Mills and Accreditation Mills." https://www.chea.org/important-questions-about-diploma-mills-and-accreditation-mills.

Council for Higher Education Accreditation. 2013, June 27. "It's Time to Speak Out: Accreditation, Its Critics and Its Future." https://www.chea.org/its-time-speak-out-accreditation-its-critics-and-its-future.

Council for Higher Education Accreditation. 2016. "Accreditation and Recognition in the United States." http://www.chea.org/userfiles/uploads/AccredRecogUS.pdf.

Council for Higher Education Accreditation. 2017, August. "Ten Ways in Which Accreditation Serves Students, Society and the Public Interest." Accessed March 5, 2019. http://www.chea.org/userfiles/PDFs/ten-ways-accreditation-serves.pdf.

Council for Higher Education Accreditation. 2018, April. "CHEA- and USDE-Recognized Accrediting Organizations." http://www.chea.org/userfiles/Recognition/CHEA_USDE_AllAccred.pdf.

eLearners. n.d. "College Accreditation—Regional vs National Accreditation: A Guide." https://www.elearners.com/colleges/regional-accreditation-vs-national-accreditation/.

National Registry of Emergency Medical Technicians. n.d. "Paramedic Program Accreditation Policy." https://www.nremt.org/rwd/public/document/policy-paramedic.

Renkiewicz, Ginny K., and Michael W. Hubble. 2015. "The Attrition Condition: Use of a Preparatory Course to Reduce EMT Course Attrition and Improve Performance on North Carolina Certification Exams." *Prehospital Emergency Care* 19, no. 2: 260–6. https://doi.org/10.3109/10903127.2014.967429.

U.S. Department of Education. 2018, March 1. "Family Educational Rights and Privacy Act (FERPA)." https://www2.ed.gov/policy/gen/guid/fpco/ferpa/index.html.

U.S. Department of Education. 2019. "Overview of Accreditation in the United States." https://www2.ed.gov/admins/finaid/accred/accreditation.html#overview.

Appendix A: Rubric for Quality Online Education

Organizational Resources to Support Student Learning

	Not Evident	Evident but Needs More Development	Fully Evident	Points Awarded
Information for the online learner				
Introductory				
A statement of introduction and broad description of the purpose of the course	**0**	**1**	**2**	
A list of names and a brief biography of the course developers	**0**	**1**	**2**	
A statement of copyright or disclaimer to identify the owner(s) of the course and the source(s) of the material students are about to use	**0**	**1**	**2**	
Technical				
A list of minimum computer hardware and software requirements for the course	**0**	**1**	**2**	
Special technical requirements are identified such as modem speed, Internet bandwidth, software plug-ins needed, and where to get them.	**0**	**1**	**2**	
Advice about computer settings, Internet security tools such as pop-up blockers and client-based software firewalls	**0**	**1**	**2**	
Guidelines for participating in online discussions (net-iquette) as well as suggestions for handling incoming email, email attachments, viruses, and email filters	**0**	**1**	**2**	
Links to technical assistance resources	**0**	**1**	**2**	

(*continues*)

Developed by the NAEMSE Educational Technology Committee.

Organizational Resources to Support Student Learning (*Continued*)

	Not Evident	Evident but Needs More Development	Fully Evident	Points Awarded
Information for the online learner				
Learning management system instructions				
Instructions for how to use the learning management system tools	0	1	2	
A link to frequently asked questions about the learning management system	0	1	2	
Contact information for technical support or help desk	0	1	2	
A description of the function of each icon or button	0	1	2	
Course support and learning resources				
Instructions for conducting online research	0	1	2	
Guidelines for reference format of papers and citations	0	1	2	
Links to online remedial resources	0	1	2	
Links to library learning resources	0	1	2	
Instructions about how assignments are to be written	0	1	2	

Information for the online learner—comments:

Online Course Organization

	Not Evident	Evident but Needs More Development	Fully Evident	Points Awarded
Course-specific statements				
A statement of requirements for successful course completion	0	1	2	
A statement of instructor expectations of students' participation	0	1	2	
Identification of prerequisites and corequisites of the course	0	1	2	

	Not Evident	Evident but Needs More Development	Fully Evident	Points Awarded
A program map that identifies how the course is related to other courses in the program	**0**	**1**	**2**	
The credit value of the course	**0**	**1**	**2**	
Contact details of the instructor, academic department	**0**	**1**	**2**	
A list of required and recommended reading resources	**0**	**1**	**2**	
Estimated amount of time needed to complete the course	**0**	**1**	**2**	
Information of instructor availability and student contact	**0**	**1**	**2**	
Detailed instructions and tips for completing assignments	**0**	**1**	**2**	
Due dates for all assignments	**0**	**1**	**2**	
Rubrics for all assignments that identify assessment guidelines	**0**	**1**	**2**	
Explanation of the grading scale	**0**	**1**	**2**	
Course-specific resources for learning				
Links to websites that provide information relevant to the course	**0**	**1**	**2**	
Links to websites of organizations or associations related to course content	**0**	**1**	**2**	
A glossary of terms, definitions of new vocabulary	**0**	**1**	**2**	
Content organization and course navigation				
Accurate and up-to-date links to each part of the course and external sources	**0**	**1**	**2**	
Instructional material that is easily located	**0**	**1**	**2**	
Page headers or footers to identify where the student is in the course	**0**	**1**	**2**	
Course content is clear and organized in a logical format.	**0**	**1**	**2**	
Consistent formatting is used throughout the course documents.	**0**	**1**	**2**	
Units of instruction are divided into subunits or subtopics.	**0**	**1**	**2**	
Printer-friendly course materials are available.	**0**	**1**	**2**	
Resources are categorized to identify differences between those that are *required* or *optional*.	**0**	**1**	**2**	

(*continues*)

Online Course Organization (*Continued*)

	Not Evident	Evident but Needs More Development	Fully Evident	Points Awarded
Syllabus includes				
A list of topics to be covered	0	1	2	
A description of the course, the learning objectives, and learning outcomes	0	1	2	
A list of the module objectives	0	1	2	
Summary of the course schedule	0	1	2	
Aesthetic design				
Easy-to-read typeface that is appropriate for the content and common to all programs and computers	0	1	2	
Boldface type is used sparingly, to highlight important terms.	0	1	2	
Underlining is used only for hyperlinks.	0	1	2	
Sufficient contrast between text and background to make information easy to read	0	1	2	
Images are appropriate, support course content, and add visual interest.	0	1	2	
Page layout to keep course pages at a comfortable length	0	1	2	
Layout is appropriate for the content and audience.	0	1	2	
Organized content using headings and subheadings	0	1	2	
The format is uncluttered and includes white space.	0	1	2	
Ragged right margins are used or letters are kerned.	0	1	2	
Effective use of color	0	1	2	
Graphic elements such as diagrams, tables, and photographs illustrate or clarify information presented in the text.	0	1	2	
Illustrations can be viewed easily on a computer screen, and JPEG files are used to accommodate different download speeds.	0	1	2	
Text explaining a graphic is aligned with the nontextual material.	0	1	2	
The material is displayed attractively.	0	1	2	
Learner expectations for download speed are managed particularly for dial-up modem users.	0	1	2	
Consistency in course material includes				
Visual and functional consistency in page layout	0	1	2	
Clear, simple, and user-friendly navigation	0	1	2	
Consistent and accurate spelling and grammar (that models course expectations)	0	1	2	

	Not Evident	Evident but Needs More Development	Fully Evident	Points Awarded
Concisely written material, familiar and common language	**0**	**1**	**2**	
Writing style that is clear, direct, supportive, and friendly	**0**	**1**	**2**	
A conversational tone that employs the second person; the tone is supportive and encouraging.	**0**	**1**	**2**	
Verbs are active, not passive.	**0**	**1**	**2**	
Short sentences and brief paragraphs	**0**	**1**	**2**	
Terms are used consistently.	**0**	**1**	**2**	
Symbols and abbreviations are defined.	**0**	**1**	**2**	
Instructions are stated simply and are easy to understand.	**0**	**1**	**2**	
Writing style does not convey explicit or implicit bias relative to age, culture or ethnicity, race, gender, or sexual preferences.	**0**	**1**	**2**	

Online course design—comments:

Instructional Design and Delivery

	Not Evident	Evident but Needs More Development	Fully Evident	Points Awarded
Promote interaction and communication by including				
An opportunity for students and instructors to introduce themselves and respond to classmate introductions	**0**	**1**	**2**	
Student contact with each other and with instructors is encouraged.	**0**	**1**	**2**	
Student participation is tracked and lower-level participants are drawn in to the discussions.	**0**	**1**	**2**	

(*continues*)

Instructional Design and Delivery (*Continued*)

	Not Evident	Evident but Needs More Development	Fully Evident	Points Awarded
Promote interaction and communication by including				
Instructor incorporates various teaching methods to encourage student interaction.	**0**	**1**	**2**	
Reading and writing assignments are commensurate with course unit load.	**0**	**1**	**2**	
Respect for diverse talents and different ways students learn	**0**	**1**	**2**	
Goals and alignment to learning objectives include				
Managed pace of delivery of course content	**0**	**1**	**2**	
Course content is programmed for appropriate student time on task.	**0**	**1**	**2**	
Instructional activity is made clear (e.g., is it self-paced, or group-paced).	**0**	**1**	**2**	
Expectations of synchronous or asynchronous activities are clearly identified.	**0**	**1**	**2**	
Students are informed about group work activities.	**0**	**1**	**2**	
Learning objectives and activities are integrated and include				
Reading assignments match learning objectives.	**0**	**1**	**2**	
Activities lead to learning the desired concepts.	**0**	**1**	**2**	
Tasks and activities are clarified to determine synchronous or asynchronous, collaborative or cooperative, sequential, or to be completed in any order.	**0**	**1**	**2**	
Instructional material is reviewed frequently.	**0**	**1**	**2**	
Summary of learning is provided periodically to reinforce learning.	**0**	**1**	**2**	
Activities to enhance student learning include				
Video clips of interviews, psychomotor skills	**0**	**1**	**2**	
Screen animations for instructional exercises	**0**	**1**	**2**	
Personal interview reports	**0**	**1**	**2**	
Annotated bibliography	**0**	**1**	**2**	
Student presentations (PowerPoint) as assignments	**0**	**1**	**2**	
PowerPoint presentations with integrated (recorded) narration	**0**	**1**	**2**	
Student-generated podcasts, vodcasts, vignettes	**0**	**1**	**2**	

	Not Evident	Evident but Needs More Development	Fully Evident	Points Awarded
Activities to develop critical-thinking and problem-solving skills include				
Discussions drawn from questions that do not have a single correct answer	0	1	2	
Compare and contrast exercises	0	1	2	
Case studies	0	1	2	
Critique of journal articles	0	1	2	
Collaborative exercises	0	1	2	

Instructional design and delivery—comments:

Assessment and Evaluation of Student Learning

	Not Evident	Evident but Needs More Development	Fully Evident	Points Awarded
Assessment of student learning methods includes				
Acceptable methods for completing assignments are identified (group work, open book).	0	1	2	
A variety of assessment instruments are used (e.g., short/long answer to questions, multiple choice questions, case studies, orals, online quizzes).	0	1	2	
Assessment activities are aligned with learning objectives and include				
Identification of criteria to evaluate participation in online discussion groups	0	1	2	
Clearly written study questions	0	1	2	
Fair and reasonable quantity and scope of graded assignments	0	1	2	
Authentic and validated assessment of learning tools	0	1	2	
Multiple assessment strategies include				
Students' bibliography or reference list that includes a variety of materials such as URLs, books and journals, and videos	0	1	2	

(continues)

Assessment and Evaluation of Student Learning (*Continued*)

	Not Evident	Evident but Needs More Development	Fully Evident	Points Awarded
Multiple assessment strategies include				
Assignment options to allow for different interests, backgrounds, and personal learning styles	**0**	**1**	**2**	
Sample opportunities for students to demonstrate proficiency in different ways	**0**	**1**	**2**	
Assessment feedback includes				
Immediate release of self-graded assignments	**0**	**1**	**2**	
Prompt, frequent, and substantial feedback from the instructor	**0**	**1**	**2**	
Samples of assignments provided to illustrate instructor's expectations	**0**	**1**	**2**	
Instructor modeling of assignment(s)	**0**	**1**	**2**	
Self-assessments and peer feedback include				
Self-tests similar to the final evaluation instruments	**0**	**1**	**2**	
Students generate discussion questions and respond to others' discussion topics.	**0**	**1**	**2**	
Opportunities for peer review	**0**	**1**	**2**	
Opportunities for students to apply a rubric to their own work and describe/defend their score	**0**	**1**	**2**	

Assessment and evaluation of student learning—comments:

Innovative Teaching Technology

	Not Evident	Evident but Needs More Development	Fully Evident	Points Awarded
Tools to facilitate communication include				
Discussion boards	**0**	**1**	**2**	
Synchronous chat	**0**	**1**	**2**	
Email	**0**	**1**	**2**	
Listserv	**0**	**1**	**2**	
Web-conferencing, teleconferencing	**0**	**1**	**2**	

	Not Evident	Evident but Needs More Development	Fully Evident	Points Awarded
Group discussion areas for group activities	**0**	**1**	**2**	
Instant messaging	**0**	**1**	**2**	
Social networking	**0**	**1**	**2**	
Multimedia elements include				
Flash animations	**0**	**1**	**2**	
Tutorials with screen captures and voiceover	**0**	**1**	**2**	
Audio clips, podcasts	**0**	**1**	**2**	
Graphics	**0**	**1**	**2**	
Video clips, vodcasts	**0**	**1**	**2**	
PowerPoint presentations with recorded audio narrations	**0**	**1**	**2**	
CD-ROM or DVD supplemental materials	**0**	**1**	**2**	
Other learning objects, simulations, or interactivities	**0**	**1**	**2**	

Instructor Use of Student Feedback

	Not Evident	Evident but Needs More Development	Fully Evident	Points Awarded
Evaluation of course content				
Evaluation survey is available (actioned) at end of course.	**0**	**1**	**2**	
Student input sought at regular intervals throughout the course	**0**	**1**	**2**	
Open-ended questions to seek student feedback	**0**	**1**	**2**	
Evaluation of online technology used within the course				
Request students to identify flaws of delivery of instruction using technology	**0**	**1**	**2**	
Instructor solicits student feedback to determine improvements for student learning.	**0**	**1**	**2**	
Evaluation of instruction and assessment				
Inadequacies are modified or fixed immediately.	**0**	**1**	**2**	
Instructor modifies elements within the course when identified (e.g., fix bad quiz questions, extend dead-lines, review methods of achieving course objectives)	**0**	**1**	**2**	

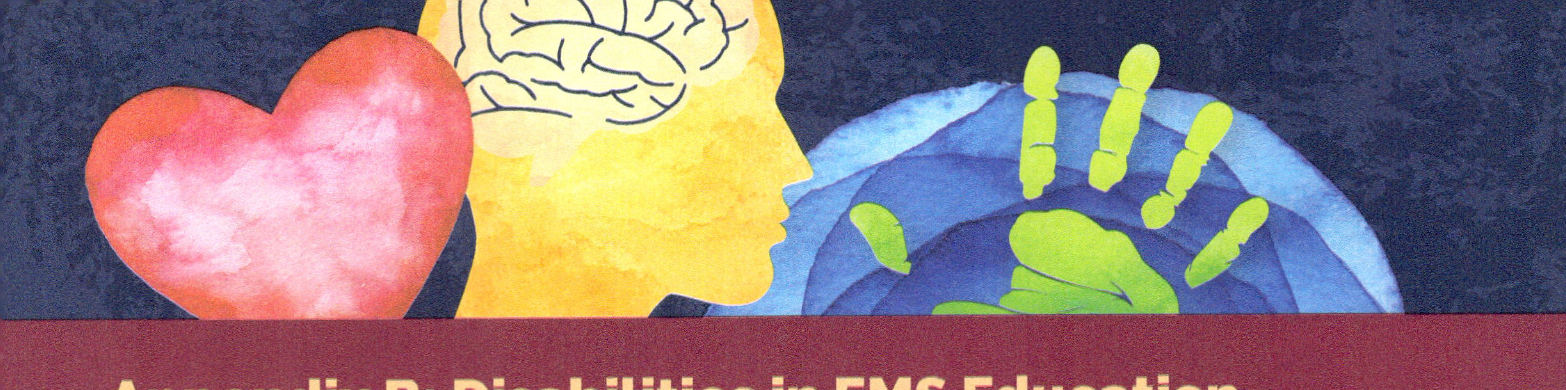

Appendix B: Disabilities in EMS Education

When it comes to addressing disabilities, emergency medical services (EMS) education presents a much more complicated context than the traditional academic classroom. Like many healthcare environments, EMS providers are likely to be in situations where the care they administer makes the difference between life and death. EMS providers use their full sensory, physical, and cognitive capabilities when caring for patients in emergencies, while also utilizing emotional intelligence. Therefore, it may be a natural inclination for the EMS educator to, at first glance, view a student disability as an indicator that the student would be unable to carry out the essential duties of an EMS provider in the classroom, lab, clinical, or field environments.

It is important to keep in mind that not all practicing EMS providers have the same ability to lift heavy patients, the dexterity to start a difficult IV, the emotional control to remain calm in a pediatric code, the ability to auscultate lung sounds in a noisy environment, and the mental ability to quickly calculate a medication drip rate. In every individual, there is a spectrum of underlying physical and mental abilities. It is essential to student success, as well as a legal mandate, that an EMS educator not make assumptions about a disabled student's potential capabilities.

Relevant Laws

The Americans with Disabilities Act of 1990[1] (ADA) and Section 504 of the Rehabilitation Act of 1973[2] are the primary federal laws governing how postsecondary educational institutions must interact with and accommodate students with disabilities. Any educational program or healthcare agency that receives federal funding (including federal student loans) is subject to Section 504, and all public and private institutions are subject to the ADA. Most states also have state-specific laws pertaining to students with disabilities in higher education.

Since the passage of the ADA, EMS educators have gained a greater understanding of the needs of people with disabilities, and equally importantly, have gained a greater appreciation of their capabilities.[3,4] The ADA and Section 504 are intended to combat discrimination against disabled individuals, including ensuring that reasonable accommodations are made for those who have a disability, whether as a consumer, in the workplace, or in an educational setting.

As a result of the increased awareness that came about from the enactment of these laws as well as the removal of architectural barriers and technological advances that permit greater participation in postsecondary education, colleges, universities, and vocational programs have seen an increase in the numbers of enrolled students who identify as having some form of disability. The percentage rose from 2.6% of college freshman in 1978,[5,6] to 11% of the total student body in 2012,[7] and the percentages continue to rise.[8] Accordingly, every EMS educational program must anticipate that it will be confronted with students who self-identify as having a disability. Programs must also have staff who are trained to assess the validity of disability claims and to address student needs by providing appropriate accommodations. Case law, as well as the Department of Education's Office for Civil Rights (OCR), have been very clear that program faculty alone should not make these determinations; instead, individuals trained in administering disability accommodations must undertake this work, with the input of faculty.[9]

Eligibility for Disability Accommodations

The ADA and Section 504 provide the right to disability accommodations to those who have a physical or mental impairment that *substantially* limits one or more *major life activities*.[1,2] These laws also provide protection against discrimination on the basis of disability for those who are perceived as having a disability, even when no impairment exists. However, only individuals who actually have a disability qualify to receive disability accommodations.

The ADA Amendments Act,[10] passed in 2008, broadened the definition of disability, expanding the number of students who are eligible for accommodations, and provided an extensive, but nonexhaustive, list of examples of diagnoses and conditions that trigger ADA protections to provide clarity to those seeking to understand who may be covered by the law. Institutions that are still unsure about a particular student's eligibility should seek outside expertise, including legal counsel or disability experts, as needed, if consultation with school disability specialists does not fully satisfy questions regarding student program participation.

All students enrolled in an EMS program, disabled or not, must meet the *technical standards* of the program. Technical standards are defined in Section 504 as "nonacademic admissions criteria that are essential to participation in the program in question."[11] Technical standards are not the same as learning outcomes, which designate what information students are taught in the program, or essential functions, which relate to employment requirements.[12] Technical standards are drafted by each school; to avoid disability discrimination, it is critical that they delineate the skills required in the program (such as the ability to assess a patient), but not the manner in which students must do so (such as using vision or hearing). Technical standards should be made readily available to students and potential applicants, so they may determine whether they will be able to enter and complete the program.[12] Students may use accommodations to meet the standards, such as using a stethoscope with a visual readout for students without sufficient hearing to use a traditional stethoscope, so the standards should also direct students to the person or office responsible for disability accommodation requests.

EMS educators sometimes express concern that students with disabilities may pose a "direct threat" to their own well-being or to others, particularly patients. A student who poses a direct threat to the health or safety of others may be precluded from participation in a program.[13] An individual's participation may be deemed to pose a direct threat only when combined factors exist: (1) the risk of harm is substantial, current, specific, and nonspeculative; (2) the risk cannot be reasonably eliminated or reduced through disability accommodations; and (3) the risk assessment has been completed based on objective medical or factual information unique to the individual and not based solely on the existence of the disability itself.[14] The direct threat analysis considers not only the classroom component but any required clinical aspect of an EMS program as well. Given the generally risky nature of EMS, the direct threat analysis is always relevant; however, the ADA is clear that concerns must be based on actual student performance and cannot be purely speculative based on the underlying impairment.[15]

Accommodations

If a student is deemed disabled, and otherwise eligible for admission to an EMS program under the Acts as described previously, EMS educational programs are obligated to provide **reasonable accommodation**. That is, if a program *can be* reasonably adapted to accommodate an individual with a disability, it *must do so*. If the program cannot be adapted because to do so would compromise a truly essential aspect of the program, the individual may be disqualified from participation (i.e., admission). Courts have established that education programs are not required to fundamentally alter their curriculum, lower their performance standards, or substantially modify their program requirements in order to accommodate a student's disability, as long as the program can show that it has carefully considered the rejected request and any reasonable alternatives, and that it involved the relevant personnel in the deliberation.[16] The purpose of reasonable accommodation is to ensure equal and full participation of individuals with disabilities to the greatest extent possible.[17] Accommodations must be tailored to the individual student's needs and abilities, and not to the student's general disability.[18] Common accommodations in the academic environment include providing extra time to complete examinations or assignments, separate testing environments that limit distractions, audio recordings of examinations or verbal instructions, large print or braille copies of classroom materials, preferential seating, American Sign Language (ASL) interpreters, and modification of assignments and exams.[19] More specific to the EMS context, practical skills timing and modification to clinical requirements may be requested. There may be some students who are not able to participate in an EMS program; if the technical standards cannot be met, even with disability accommodations, the student may not be qualified to be in the program.

Although there are not many EMS education legal cases to draw from when evaluating what constitutes an unreasonable or a reasonable accommodation, there are many analogous cases from other healthcare professions. In one case involving a profoundly deaf nursing student, the court rejected one-on-one clinical supervision and assistance or removal of the program's clinical component as reasonable accommodations in order to meet the essential requirement of being able to communicate with people wearing a surgical mask, as it was not then possible for the student to read lips.[20] However, in this 1979 decision, the Supreme Court noted that future technological advances may allow the participation of individuals with disabilities in healthcare provision. Indeed, since 2013, most courts considering the issue have required the inclusion of students with disabilities, including ordering a medical school to admit a deaf student,[21] ordering a chiropractic school to allow a student with limited vision to continue in the program,[22] requiring a medical school to provide interpreters and real-time captioning to a student with significant hearing loss,[23] and requiring a hospital to provide sign language interpreters for a nurse employee.[24]

There are limits, however, such as the denial of accommodations for a medical student with debilitating anxiety who requested to complete elements of his residency telephonically.[25] Because technology and educational practices are rapidly evolving, the standard for reasonableness of accommodations is evolving, too. Since these cases were decided, numerous medical and nursing programs have successfully accommodated blind and deaf students. Therefore, based on the methods of accommodation available, a future EMS case may be decided differently.[26]

Programs are not required to provide accommodations that are deemed unduly burdensome or costly.[27] Such accommodations, by definition, are simply not reasonable. An educational institution is given fair deference in determining what accommodations are reasonable; however, it must always be able to establish that any decision to deny an accommodation request is based on a well-reasoned, professional judgment.[28] Furthermore, the determination for what is overly costly rests on the budget for an entire institution or parent entity, not just the program at issue.[29]

Technology will undoubtedly influence future developments in determination of reasonable accommodations in the healthcare environment. The Association of American Medical Colleges published guidelines with specific strategies for enhancing accessibility in 2010, in which it emphasized the role of educational technology, including computerized manikins, as opposed to live-patient practice, in the development of reasonable accommodations.[26,30]

Admissions

The courts have recognized that requirements for healthcare education programs can be related to the requirements of the profession itself.[31] While this connection has been recognized, there is not yet a consistent directive from a majority of courts as to when programs can appropriately condition admission to an academic program on fitness for licensure to practice in the field itself. The ADA expressly forbids inquiring about a student's disability prior to admission to a program.[32] The law generally holds that *if it is possible* for students to participate in the educational program with reasonable accommodations, and they are otherwise eligible for enrollment, *they must be permitted to do so*. Ethically, this situation may obligate the educator to explain to a student candidate with a disability that employment in the profession may not be possible, while not discouraging the student from engaging in the course of study. The key point is that an EMS educator must take great care to ensure any decision to reject admission of any prospective student is not made based on assumptions about a perceived or diagnosed disability.

Certification and Licensure Examinations

Students are able to request and obtain disability accommodations when taking the National Registry of Emergency Medical Technicians (NREMT) exam. Federal disability law states that any public or private entity that administers examinations specifically related to licensure or certification is responsible for ensuring the examinations accurately reflect an individual's aptitude, achievement level, or other factors the examination purports to measure, rather than reflect the individual's impairment.[33] Accordingly, like educational programs, reasonable accommodations on licensing exams must be made available to students who are eligible, so long as they do not create an undue burden or fundamentally alter the examination process.

EMS educators should be familiar with the accommodations policy of the NREMT as well as the specific requirements of their state licensing body. NREMT offers reasonable and appropriate accommodations for the written component of the registration examination for students with documented disabilities.[34] Candidates seeking accommodations must make a written request 4 to 6 weeks before the anticipated testing date. Each accommodation is considered on a case-by-case basis. Accommodations made by EMS programs may differ from those permitted by the NREMT.

Types and Forms of Disability

As discussed previously, the definition of disability under the ADA is intentionally broad, as there are many different forms of impairment, each presenting its own set of unique characteristics.[35] Even within one impairment diagnosis, two students may have different presentations and accommodation needs. Disabilities are commonly divided into two categories: mental and physical. A physical disability can include, but is not limited to, mobility, hearing, speech, and visual impairments.[36] Mental impairments may include any impairment that affects mental, developmental, or cognitive functioning and may include intellectual developmental delays, depression, or specific cognitive, psychomotor, or affective learning disabilities.[36,37] It is important that EMS educators are familiar with the broad range of disabilities.

Learning Disabilities

According to the National Center for Education Statistics, as of the fall of 2017, more than 200,000 students entering college had some form of learning disability.[38] In 2014, the National Center for Learning Disabilities reported that, among high school students with learning disabilities, 54% planned to attend 2- or 4-year college programs, with 43% planning on completing a vocational training course.[39] Although learning disabilities are certainly common, they are not always easy to detect, and it may be assumed, by an untrained educator, that these students are just lazy or low achieving. As it is highly likely that EMS educators will encounter *many* students with learning disabilities during their careers, it is particularly important that EMS educators familiarize themselves with them.

The National Joint Committee on Learning Disabilities (NJCLD) has defined learning disabilities as "a heterogeneous group of disorders manifested by significant difficulties in the acquisition and use of listening, speaking, reading, writing, reasoning, or mathematical abilities."[40] According to Lerner, "These disorders are recognized to be intrinsic to each individual student, often presumed to be due to central nervous system dysfunction, and may occur across a person's life span. While learning disabilities may occur concomitantly with other disabilities (for example, sensory, intellectual, or emotional impairments) or extrinsic influences (cultural or linguistic differences, access to resources, and insufficient instruction), they are not the result of those conditions or influences."[41] The operational portion of the diagnosis, and a common element within many definitions of learning disabilities, is the identification of a gap between a student's potential capability to learn and the learning and achievements of the student.[42] It is important to remember that the presentation of a learning disability is highly individual; therefore, any approach to assisting the learning disabled student must be student-centered, adaptive, and flexible.[41]

While it is far from an exhaustive list, common examples of learning disabilities include dyslexia (a reading and comprehension impairment), dyscalculia (an inability to process numeric calculations), and dysgraphia (an impairment involving an ability to write expressively).[19,43]

Classroom Impact

As discussed previously, there are many forms of disabilities, presenting a wide range of characteristics. It follows that the best methods for addressing these disabilities in the classroom will be equally diverse. A few general recommendations for the EMS educator that are applicable to all disabilities include the following:[19,41,44]

1. If available, develop personal relationships with institutional disability service coordinators as well as those in academic support, medical, wellness, and therapy service programs.
2. At the beginning of the course or program, communicate to the class a willingness to work with students with disabilities, inviting students to go to the designated disability services coordinator to discuss any impairments that may interfere with their performance or a need for accommodations.
3. If a student has approved disability accommodations, you may choose to let the student know that you are available to meet privately with the student regarding their accommodations. Remember to not focus on, or ask questions about, the underlying condition, but rather on how the expressed impairment will impact course participation.
4. Do not make assumptions about a student's ability based on an impairment alone.
5. Encourage the disabled student to keep in touch during the course, so that issues can be addressed as they arise.
6. Be familiar with assistive technology and outside resources that may be available to assist the student during the course.
7. Remain supportive and encouraging. In all interactions, project a willingness to work with students to ensure they are able to be successful in the classroom.
8. Consider communicating information in more than one form—e.g., providing graphics and videos in addition to written slides.
9. Treat students with disabilities as any other student would be treated whenever possible. Do not be overly solicitous, dismiss the student's requirements, or lower expectations.

As stated throughout this section, the best method of addressing a disability is personalized to each student. The educator's approach in the classroom must be individually tailored. Developing a relationship with the students and getting to know them beyond any labels of their disabilities is key to the educator's and the student's success in the EMS program. Likewise, cultivation of a professional relationship with the academic institution's disability services specialists, when available, is invaluable. Relationships with service providers encourage familiarity with the services that are available and give the educator a knowledgeable resource with whom to collaborate. If these services are not available within the EMS education entity, the instructor may attempt to access them through the local community college or consult with an independent education disability specialist. Disability services coordinators have a wealth of experience developing reasonable accommodation plans and an understanding of limitations a particular impairment might impose, and they may be able to recommend assistive technology or other resources and practices to incorporate in the classroom to benefit a particular student. Additionally, it has been demonstrated that students more frequently take advantage of student services at a postsecondary level when they have a personal relationship with the service providers.[45] When the educator develops familiarity with these providers, they can better encourage the student to do so as well. All of these actions reflect an encouraging and supportive attitude toward the student, and an educator's attitude toward a disabled student's participation in a course has a significant impact on performance.[46]

Many actions an educator can take to assist a disabled student reflect standard good classroom practices, such as making lectures and notes readily accessible and easy to understand, making expectations clear, being organized, and providing advance notice of upcoming tasks so that students can make appropriate plans, as well as being adaptable and attentive to individual student progress. An educator should consider their own strengths and weaknesses in the classroom when assessing what they can improve on to assist the disabled student.

Although these are general recommendations, they do not substitute legal advice. Educators who work within a larger institution should contact their institution's disability services coordinator for institution-specific guidance and updates, as the laws and recommendations regarding disabilities and accommodations are ever evolving.

Glossary

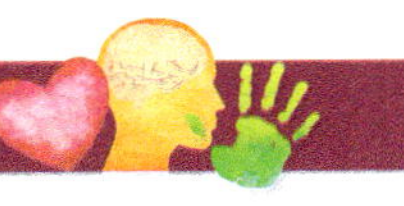

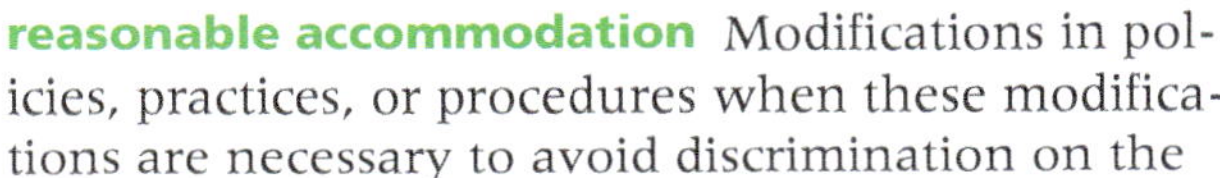

reasonable accommodation Modifications in policies, practices, or procedures when these modifications are necessary to avoid discrimination on the basis of disability, but which do not fundamentally alter an essential aspect of the program.

References

[1] 42 U.S. Code § 12101, *et seq.*

[2] 29 U.S.C. § 701, *et seq.*

[3] Meeks, Lisa M., and Neera R. Jain. 2015. *The Guide to Assisting Students with Disabilities: Equal Access in Health Science and Professional Education*. New York: Springer Publishing Co.

[4] Carey, Brandon M., Grant H. Turnwald, Howard Kallem, Kristi Bleyer, and Barbara Blacklock. 2015. *Meeting the Needs of Students with Disabilities in Health Related Education Programs*. Huntersville, NC: AHEAD.

[5] HEATH Resource Center at the National Youth Transitions Center, Graduate School of Education and Human Development, The George Washington University. n.d. Accessed December 29, 2018. https://www.heath.gwu.edu.

[6] Thomas, Stephen B. 2000. "College Students and Disability Law." *Journal of Special Education*, 33, no. 4: 248–57.

[7] U.S. Department of Education, National Center for Educational Statistics. 2018. "Digest of Educational Statistics: Number and Percentage Distribution of Students Enrolled in Post-Secondary Institutions, Table 311.10." Accessed March 4, 2019. https://nces.ed.gov/programs/digest/d17/tables/dt17_311.10.asp.

[8] Erickson, William, C. Lee, and Sarah von Schrader. 2016. "2015 Disability Status Report: United States." Ithaca, NY: Cornell University Yang Tan Institute on Employment and Disability (YTI). Accessed March 4, 2019. http://www.disabilitystatistics.org/StatusReports/2015-PDF/2015-StatusReport_US.pdf.

[9] Wynne v. Tufts Medical Center, 932 F.2d 19 (1st Cir. 1991); 976 F.2d 791 (1st Cir. 1992); OCR Letter to the University of North Carolina, Greensboro, Case No. 11-17-2001 (2017).

[10] Public Law 110-325.

[11] Section 504 of the Rehabilitation Act of 1973, 45 C.F.R. § 84.3(k)(3) (1978).

[12] Kezar, Laura B., Kristi L. Kirschner, Daniel M. Clinchot, Elisa Laird-Metke, Philip Zazove, and Raymond H. Curry. 2019. "Leading Practices and Future Directions for Technical Standards in Medical Education." *Academic Medicine* 94: 520–7.

[13] Americans with Disabilities Act, 42 U.S.C. § 12182(b)(3).

[14] Bragdon v. Abbott, 524 U.S. 624, 649, 118 S.Ct. 2196, 141 L.Ed.2d 540 (1998).

[15] ADA Regulations, 28 C.F.R. 35.130(h); 28 C.F.R. 36.208.

[16] Wynne v. Tufts University, 976 F.2d 791 (1st Cir. 1992); Guckenberger v. Boston University, 8 F. Supp. 2d 82 (D. Mass. 1998); Zukle v. Regents of Univ.of Cal., 166 F.3d 1041 (9th Cir. 1999); Southeastern Cmty. Coll. v. Davis, 442 U.S. 397 (1979).

[17] Americans with Disabilities Act, 42 U.S.C. § 12101. Findings and purpose.

[18] Pushkin v. Regents of Univ. of Colorado, 165 F.2d 1372 (10th Cir. 1981).

[19] Learning Disabilities Association of America. Accessed May 14, 2019. https://ldaamerica.org.

[20] Southeastern Cmty. Coll. v. Davis, 442 U.S. 397, 99 S. Ct. 2361, 60 L. Ed. 2d 980 (U.S. 1979).
[21] Featherstone v. Pacific Northwest University of Health Sciences, No. 1:CV-14-3084-SMJ (E.D. Wash. 2014).
[22] Palmer College of Chiropractic v. Davenport Civil Rights Commission, 850 NW2d 326 (2014).
[23] Argenyi v. Creighton University, 703 F.3d 441 (8th Cir. 2013).
[24] Searls v. Johns Hopkins Hospital, 158 F. Supp. 3d 427 (D.Md. 2016).
[25] Maczaczyj v. State of New York, 956 F. Supp. 403 (W.D.N.Y. 1997).
[26] Ouellette, Alicia. 2013. "Patients to Peers: Barriers and Opportunities for Doctors with Disabilities." *Nevada Law Journal* 13, no. 3: 645–67.
[27] OCR Regulations, 34 C.F.R. §104.12 (1996).
[28] Bradley v. Univ. of Texas M.D. Anderson Cancer Ctr, 3 F.3d 922 (5th Cir. 1993).
[29] Searls v. Johns Hopkins Hospital, 158 F. Supp. 3d 427 (D.Md. 2016).
[30] Latham, Peter S., and John Hosterman. 2010. *Medical Students with Disabilities: Resources to Enhance Accessibility*. Washington, DC: Association of American Medical Colleges.
[31] Palmer College of Chiropractic v. Davenport Civil Rights Commission, 850 NW2d 326 (2014).
[32] Americans with Disabilities Act: ADA Title III Technical Assistance Manual at III-4.1300.
[33] Disability Law Compliance Manual §10:41.
[34] National Registry of Emergency Medical Technicians. n.d. "Accommodations Policy." Accessed November 25, 2018. https://www.nremt.org/rwd/public/document/policy-accommodations.
[35] Americans with Disabilities Act, 42 U.S.C. § 12102 (2) (A) and (B).
[36] Parry, John W. 1997. *Mental Disabilities and the Americans with Disabilities Act*, 2nd ed. Washington, DC: American Bar Association.
[37] Parry, John W. 1996. *Regulation, Litigation and Dispute Resolution under the Americans with Disabilities Act: A Practitioners Guide to Implementation*, 2nd ed. Washington, DC: American Bar Association; 160.
[38] National Center for Education Statistics. Accessed May 14, 2019. https://nces.ed.gov/.
[39] National Center for Learning Disabilities. Accessed May 14, 2019. https://www.ncld.org.
[40] LD Online. n.d. "National Joint Committee on Learning Disabilities Definition of Learning Disabilities." Accessed May 14, 2019. http://www.ldonline.org/pdfs/njcld/NJCLDDefinitionofLD_2016.pdf
[41] Lerner, Janet W. 1999. *Learning Disabilities: Theories, Diagnosis, and Teaching Strategies*, 8th ed. Boston: Houghton Mifflin College Division.
[42] Mercer, Cecil D., LuAnn Jordan, David H. Allsopp, and Ann R. Mercer. 1996. "Learning Disabilities Definitions and Criteria Used by State Education Departments." *Learning Disability Quarterly* 19, no. 4: 217–32.
[43] Cortiella, Candace, and Sheldon H. Horowitz. 2014. *The State of Learning Disabilities*, 3rd ed. New York: National Center for Learning Disabilities. Accessed March 4, 2019. https://www.ncld.org/wp-content/uploads/2014/11/2014-State-of-LD.pdf.
[44] Keogh, Barbara K. 1994. "A Matrix of Decision Points in the Measurement of Learning Disabilities." In *Frames of Reference for the Assessment of Learning Disabilities*, edited by G. Reid Lyon, 15–26. Baltimore: Paul H. Brookes; Learning Disabilities.
[45] Klem, Adena M., and James P. Connell. 2004. "Relationships Matter: Linking Teacher Support to Student Engagement and Achievement." *Journal of School Health* 74, no. 7: 262–73. https://doi.org/10.1111/j.1746-1561.2004.tb08283.x.
[46] Klehm, Mary. 2013. "Teacher Attitudes: The Effects of Teacher Beliefs on Teaching Practices and Achievement of Students with Disabilities." Dissertation, University of Rhode Island. Accessed March 5, 2019. http://digitalcommons.uri.edu/oa_diss/2.

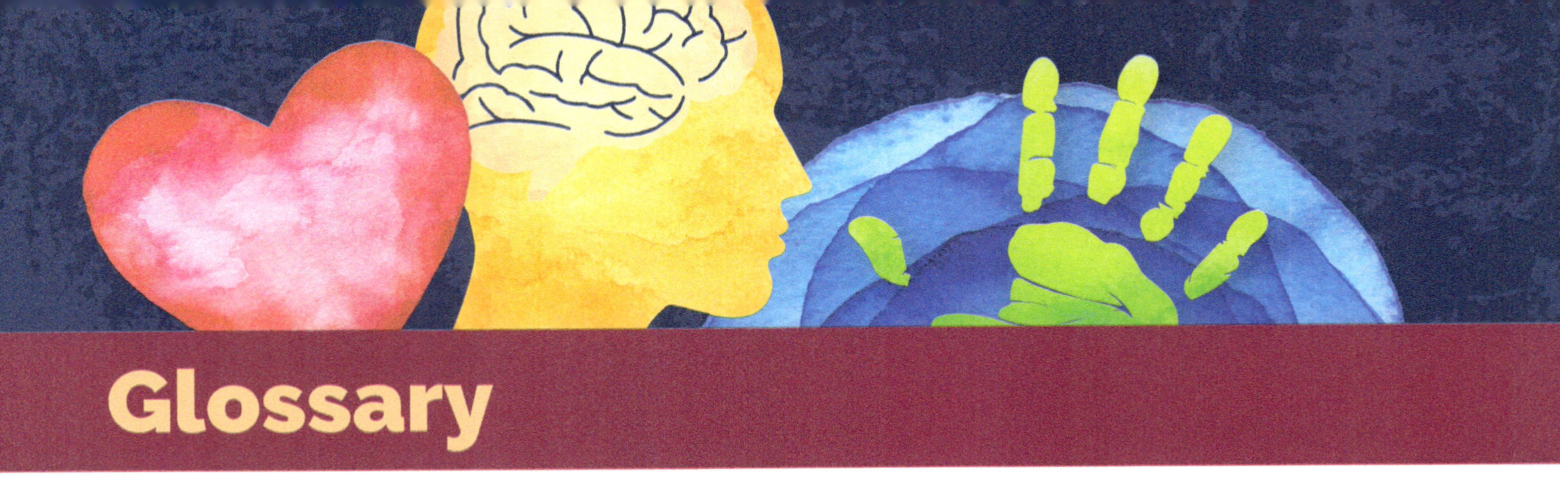

Glossary

3 Es method Model for developing objectives that focuses on emphasis, expectations, and evaluation (assessment).

360-degree evaluation Feedback that utilizes many sources of evaluation, including peers.

ABCD model Model to write objectives in which the audience, behaviors, conditions, and degree required to achieve the objective are clearly defined.

academic dishonesty Breach of the standards of academic integrity, typically including engaging in, assisting in, or condoning lying, cheating, plagiarism, furnishing unauthorized information, unauthorized collaboration on graded work, collusion, falsifying academic records, and any act designed to give unfair advantage to a particular student.

accommodator Experiential learning style in which concrete experience and active experimentation are preferred; favors doing.

accreditation Process in which an educational institution or program is evaluated to determine whether it meets certain standards.

active behavior Student is actively thinking or doing something to learn.

affective domain Learning in terms of feelings, emotions, attitudes, and values.

affiliation agreements Contracts between an EMS facility or program and hospitals or other clinical facilities or individual preceptors.

amygdala Almond-shaped section of the forebrain; this component of the limbic system plays a central role in emotion and learning.

analog technologies Tools such as whiteboards, flip charts, and manipulatives that are used for teaching and learning.

analytic learning Preference for processing information in a logical, sequential manner.

analyze Cognitive domain level that requires separation of whole concepts into individual, smaller parts to determine how the parts interrelate and understand their importance; called Analysis in the 1956 taxonomy.

anchoring Connecting new ideas to concepts already understood through one's prior life experiences.

andragogy The art and science of teaching adults.

Angoff method Expert group consensus process to assign item difficulty, in which the group considers the minimum level of acceptable knowledge, then estimates the percentage of minimally competent candidates who would answer the item correctly.

anticipatory set First activity or item an instructor covers when students arrive, to establish the environment in which learning occurs.

apply Cognitive domain level that relates classroom information to real-life situations; called Application in the 1956 taxonomy.

apps Software programs that are typically downloaded by a user to a mobile device.

articulation Psychomotor domain level that occurs when proficient and competent performance of the skill, with personal style or flair, occurs.

artificial general intelligence (AGI) Machine intelligence that is able to perform the same intellectual work as humans, as opposed to machine ability to perform only certain cognitive tasks.

artificial intelligence (AI) Machine intelligence that is able to perform a specific cognitive task or tasks.

ask, pause, and call Questioning technique wherein the instructor waits for a longer time—up to 30 seconds—before allowing a student to answer a posed question.

assault Occurs when one person places another person in reasonable fear of immediate harm or physical contact.

assessment Process of evaluating whether a student has successfully acquired knowledge, skills, and attitudes.

assimilator Experiential learning style in which a combination of abstract conceptualization and reflective observation are preferred; favors creating theoretical models.

asynchronous learning Student-centered education that utilizes digital/online learning resources to facilitate knowledge sharing independent of time and place.

attribution Root cause of a student's performance deficiency.

audience feedback systems Technological systems that allow a presenter and an audience to interact, for example, by providing feedback or answering questions via an electronic device or clicker.

audience response systems Systems whereby the instructor receives feedback from the audience or class to specific, posed questions through an electronic device that tallies the responses.

auditory learning Preference for learning through sound.

augmentation AMR level at which a technology offers a more effective tool to perform a common task.

augmented reality (AR) Technology in which special eyeglasses usually need to be worn, which superimpose 3-D digital images or holograms on a user's view of the real world.

autonomy Independence.

axon Electrically sensitive fiber of a neuron responsible for the transmission of information away from the nerve cell.

bandwidth In the context of brain-based learning, refers to the available space in the brain for learning.

battery Physical, unlawful touching of another person without consent.

bias Unreasonable judgment.

Bloom's taxonomy Description of the domains of learning developed by Dr. Benjamin Bloom.

blueprinting Planning the exam to facilitate validity with appropriate level of required thinking, content depth, and breadth.

brain-derived neuropathic factor (BDNF) Natural substance released by the brain to improve cognition (thinking) and boost how neurons talk with one another.

branching The number of different directions a simulation may take.

breadth Volume of topics that a student needs to learn to achieve competency in the subject.

briefing Activity immediately preceding the start of a simulation activity where the participants receive essential information about the simulation scenario such as background, information, vital signs, instructions, or guidelines.[1]

budget Financial plan for coordinating revenues (inflows) and expenditures (outflows) over a selected period of time in order to provide a net positive margin.

buzz group Group typically consisting of three to six people who are assigned a specific question or problem to be researched and answered in a short period of time, for example, within a lecture.

central sulcus The longitudinal fissure in the brain that lies on the outside edge of the hemisphere.

cerebellum Region of the brain that is most responsible for producing smooth, coordinated muscle movements.

cerebral cortex Outermost layer of the brain, responsible for creativity, planning, language, and perception.

chaining In the context of education, the process of breaking down the objectives and linking them together in a progression of learning.

characterize Affective domain level that requires development of one's own value system that governs behavior.

charlatans Persons who claim knowledge or skill that they do not possess.

chat rooms Synchronous electronic text communication system that resembles actual real-time conversations.

civil law System of law concerned with ordinary private matters between members of a community.

classroom feedback systems Systems whereby the instructor receives feedback from the audience or class to specific, posed questions through an electronic device that tallies the responses.

clinical coordinator Person who schedules and tracks hospital and other clinical training rotations.

clinical educator Patient care practitioner who guides experiential learning during real patient care.

cloud-based collaborative document Document accessed through the Internet that can be updated by multiple users at the same time.

cloud computing The practice of using remote servers to host and manage computer files.

cognitive domain Learning that takes place through the process of thinking; it deals with facts and knowledge.

cognitive load Effect that results from an overload of information that renders learning ineffective.

cognitive process dimension Dimension that covers the actions in which a learner engages when learning in the cognitive domain.

collaborative learning Group learning model in which the educator poses the learning to small groups and the students divide the labor to find associated details, working toward a common goal.

color of law Implies the mere semblance of legal rights or the appearance of rights; recognition of novel rights that resemble legal rights and adjusts the law to the circumstance.

command response Requirement of the student.

Commission on Accreditation for Prehospital Continuing Education (CAPCE) Accrediting body for continuing education in emergency medical services.

Commission on Accreditation of Allied Health Education Programs (CAAHEP) Approving entity for accreditation of EMS education programs.

Committee on Accreditation of Educational Programs for the Emergency Medical Services Professions (CoAEMSP) Entity that performs accreditation reviews of emergency medical services education programs for CAAHEP.

competency portfolio Documented body of evidence that shows consistently acceptable performance of skills.

computer-adaptive testing Type of testing that is able to adjust the difficulty of items for the candidate based on the candidate's responses.

conceptual knowledge Knowledge type that contains information and an understanding of a subject's principles, generalizations, or theories that are pertinent to a body of knowledge.

confederates Individuals other than the patient (for example, a simulated family member or bystander) who are scripted in a simulation to provide realism, additional challenges, or additional information for the learner.[1]

constitutional protections The U.S. Constitution prohibits the government from violating the constitutional rights of its citizens; U.S. federal civil rights laws allows U.S. citizens to sue governmental actors who violate their constitutional rights; EMS facilities and programs, as well as individual EMS educators themselves, may be considered governmental actors if they receive or benefit (directly or indirectly) from any type of public funding.

content validity Extent to which exam items accurately represent the wider body of knowledge being tested.

context-based learning (situated cognition) Learning strategy that places the lesson within the actual situation in which it will be used.

convergent questions Questions that seek specific information.

converger Experiential learning style in which abstract conceptualization and active experimentation are the dominant preferences; favors practical application of ideas.

cooperative learning Group learning model in which the educator poses the learning to the group and the students work together and are jointly responsible for learning outcomes.

copyright protection Safeguards the original works of authorship fixed in any type of communication material or statements of expression.

corpus callosum Thick band of nerve fibers that connect and allow for communication between the left and right hemispheres of the brain.

create Cognitive domain level in which elements are put together in a new way, to form a logical and functional whole. This is the highest mental function in the new taxonomy; called Synthesis in the 1956 taxonomy.

creativity Activity that is novel and useful and results in contributions to human experience.

crew resource management Team management strategy to ensure safety in environments that have a high acuity for human error.

criminal law System of laws concerned with the punishment and rehabilitation of those who commit crimes that are prohibited by law because their conduct is deemed harmful to society.

criteria-released assessment items Assessment items that are released once certain parameters, such as completion of homework or assignments, have been met.

criterion-referenced grading Grading strategies that assign a grade based on mastery of course objectives.

critical thinking Higher-level cognitive skills or problem-solving skills.

Cronbach's alpha Complex statistical method of assessing internal consistency.

cultural competency Awareness of beliefs and customs of cultures.

cultural humility Understanding of culture in which a person is open to another person's cultural identity and is open to exploring and learning about it.

culture Amalgamation of customs, experiences, languages, attitudes, values, and beliefs common to a defined group.

culture of safety Values and behaviors that prioritize the safety of EMS providers and their patients.

cut score Score required to pass a test; the passing score.

debriefing Session conducted after a simulation event where educators/instructors/facilitators and learners reexamine the simulation experience for the purpose of moving toward assimilation and accommodation of learning to apply in future situations.[1] In the context of small group learning, a session that occurs at the end of a small group activity, in which students reflect on and discuss what was learned.

declarative material Depth and breadth of the content of a lesson; the component of a lesson plan in which objectives and content are arranged and grouped in the order in which they will be taught.

declarative memories Memories of which a person is consciously aware, and which are known to be true, can be seen, and can be measured as fact.

defamation Sharing of true but private information that injures the reputation of another, or the intentional or reckless making of a false statement; two types are libel and slander.

deliberate practice Practice of specific components of psychomotor skills based on specific feedback.

dendrites Branching fibers of axons that act as receptors of information; they receive messages from other neurons and deliver them to the main body of the nerve cell.

depth Amount of detail a student needs to learn or perform within their scope of practice.

dichotomous scoring Type of scoring in which the observable action is either performed or not, to the greatest extent possible.

difficulty level Percentage of students who answer each item correctly.

digital learning Any type of learning that is facilitated by the effective use of technology. It includes the application of a wide range of educational methodologies including blended/hybrid, online, gamification, and virtual/augmented reality.

Digital Millennium Copyright Act (DMCA) Implements treaty obligations of the World Intellectual Property Organization and helps move the U.S. copyright law into the digital age.

discrimination Unjust or prejudicial treatment of different categories of people on the basis of their physical distinctions or any other type of distinction that is based on differences of a group to which persons may perceive themselves to belong.

discussion board Tool used to facilitate threaded discussions within an online course; it is often accessed through a learning management system.

distance education (DE) System of education whereby students and instructors are separated by time and/or location. It includes learning materials delivered in a variety of formats, from paper-based correspondence courses to online digital materials.

distractor Incorrect answer designed to be a plausible alternative to the correct answer.

divergent questions Questions that do not have a single correct answer.

diverger Experiential learning style in which concrete experimentation and reflective observation are preferred; favors observing before experiencing.

domains of learning Categories of learning that include cognitive, affective, and psychomotor.

educational philosophy Set of beliefs that defines the purpose of education.

effectiveness In terms of program evaluation, a measure of the outcome of the program. May be measured by pass/fail rates on credentialing exams, student retention/attrition rates, job placement, satisfaction rates, or quality of patient care by graduates after they transition to the workforce.

Emergency Planning and Community Right-to-Know Act (EPCRA) Helps communities, including facilities or programs, and educators plan for chemical emergencies; requires facilities, programs, and educators to report on the storage, use, and releases of hazardous substances to federal, state, and local governments.

emotional intelligence Type of intelligence in which people is aware of and understands their own emotions.

Equal Employment Opportunity Act (EEOA) Gives the Equal Employment Commission (EEOC) authority to sue in federal courts, when it finds reasonable cause to believe that there has been employment discrimination, including discrimination in or by EMS programs or by EMS educators and students (including any program that leads to or results in employment requiring a certification or licensure).

equating Procedures used to control for examinations of varying difficulty.

equity In the context of education, practices and approaches that set up every student for success and deliberately foster excellence in learning.

evaluate Cognitive domain level in which judgments are made based on existing standards and checking and critiquing content. This is now the fifth level and a precursor to creating; called Evaluation in the 1956 taxonomy.

experiential learning Occurs when a student acquires knowledge and skills from a relevant setting, drawing meaningful lessons from observations, actions, and reflections. Active learning process that engages all senses; learning by doing.

expert Anyone who, through their education and experience, has developed special skills or knowledge of a particular subject, so that they may develop an informed opinion.

extended reality (XR) An umbrella term that refers to the elements of virtual reality, augmented reality, and mixed reality.

F2F Face-to-face classroom learning; also called FTF.

face validity Commonsense validity; when an assessment appears to evaluate what it is intended to evaluate.

facilitation Teaching strategy in which the instructor creates a relaxed atmosphere that makes it easier for the student to learn; assisting a learner in discovering information or their own abilities.

factual knowledge Knowledge type that contains information that is essential to a subject discipline. It includes basic information, terminology, and other elements that are required for a learner to understand the discipline.

Family Educational Rights and Privacy Act (FERPA) Governs the access of confidential information and the data privacy of records to any publicly funded EMS facilities or programs and EMS educator or activity that receives or benefits from government funds; prohibits the release of any type of personally identifiable information about a student or EMS educator except under certain, limited circumstances; this confidentiality and data privacy law is commonly referred to as the Buckley Amendment and named after its principal legislative sponsor, Senator James Buckley of New York.

fiction contract Agreement between the educator and the student to make the simulation as real as possible.

fidelity Degree to which the simulation replicates the real event and/or workplace; this includes physical, psychological, and environmental elements.[1]

field clinical (field experience) Prehospital or outdoor experiences, which may be primarily observation or performing isolated skills as directed by the EMS personnel on the ambulance.

field coordinator Person who schedules and tracks field EMS rotations.

field internship Planned, scheduled educational experience on an advanced life support unit that includes team-leading skills and the management of prehospital patients and scenes. Also, a capstone event in which the student leads the assessment and care, particularly of patients requiring advanced life support care.

fixed cost Cost that is constant (does not fluctuate).

flipped classroom Pedagogical model in which the typical lecture and homework elements are reversed, for example through the use of technology such as a virtual learning environment or learning management system. This student-centered instructional method uses prerecorded lecture and preclass assignments to maximize class time spent on application and problem-solving activities.

formative assessment Ongoing evaluation of student performance throughout a course.

formative course evaluation Course evaluation designed to measure program effectiveness while class is still in progress.

forming stage Group growth stage in which team members encounter one another for the first time, attempt to define the task assigned to them, and start to determine the future course.

fraud Misrepresentation, or the making of a false statement with intent to deceive that causes actual harm to someone who reasonably relies upon the falsification.

Freedom of Information Act (FOIA) Provides that everyone, including EMS educators and students, has the right to request access to government records or information except to the extent the government records or information is protected from disclosure.

gamma-aminobutyric acid (GABA) Most common inhibitory neurotransmitter; it quiets neurons and can exist in up to one-third of synapses.

glial cells Most abundant cell types in the central nervous system; they provide support for and insulation between the surrounding neurons.

global learning Preference for processing information by seeing the whole before the parts.

goal Broad statement of instructional intent.

governmental actor Any person who acts on behalf of the government and is subject to the U.S. Constitution's Bill of Rights, which prohibits the government from violating certain civil rights and freedoms.

grievance Wrong considered as grounds for a claim and potential lawsuit.

Gun-Free Schools Act (GFSA) Directs education programs, including EMS programs in some states, to develop policies requiring referral to the criminal justice or juvenile delinquency system for anyone who brings a firearm or weapon in or around a school campus; mandates expulsion of students for at least 1 year.

harassment Conduct that creates a situation that is hostile or unpleasant, or which makes a person believe they are unsafe; examples include making unwelcome advances, requesting sexual favors, using position or status to intimidate another, insulting another person, interfering with another's ability to do their job, and engaging in bullying behaviors.

Health Insurance Portability and Accountability Act (HIPAA) Establishes national standards for the confidentiality and data privacy and security of healthcare information.

higher-order thinking Relating to Bloom's higher cognitive levels, including analysis, synthesis, evaluation, critical thinking, and problem solving.

high-fidelity In healthcare simulation, refers to simulation experiences that are extremely realistic and provide a high level of interactivity and realism for the learner.[1]

high-stakes assessment Assessment in which the student's continuation in the program depends on successful completion of the exam.

HIPAA Privacy Rule Protects the medical privacy of everyone receiving prehospital intervention services.

hippocampus Area in the limbic system that moves learning from short-term memory into long-term memory.

homeostasis State of equilibrium referring to the body's ability to remain internally stable while external environments vary.

hospital clinical Experiences in a hospital, clinic, or other indoor setting.

hybrid course Course that includes aspects of distance (online) education and traditional education, such as clinical experience or laboratory practice of psychomotor skills.

hypermediality Links to audio, video, graphics, or hyperlinks to other Web pages.

hypothalamus Area in the limbic system that maintains homeostasis by regulating temperature, sleep, and nutrient intake through internal monitoring; also plays a role in the immune system.

imitation Psychomotor domain level that occurs as students repeat and mimic demonstrations.

independent learning Preference for processing information alone rather than in a group setting.

injects Information provided by a simulated dispatcher, a facilitator, or confederates within a simulation that allows the scenario to progress with information that otherwise may not be available to the students.

institutional accreditation Type of accreditation that applies to a college, university, or institution, rather than a specific program of study.

instructional design Process for creating instructional content; key steps include assessing the needs of the learners, writing course objectives, structuring course content, determining assessment strategies, and assessing course effectiveness.

instructor evaluation Formal review of an instructor by their employer for the purposes of forming a basis for contract renewal, pay increase, tenure review, accountability, or union contract requirements.

intentional thinking Process of actively deciding to think about a topic, being aware of one's own thoughts, and shaping thoughts in order to drive toward a specific result.

interrater reliability (IRR) Consistency in scores assigned by different evaluators, for example when grading a particular exam.

item discrimination Degree to which a correct answer for a particular item is associated with high overall scores on the exam; this is essentially a test of reliability.

item-response theory (IRT) Strategy of measuring a test taker's underlying traits or abilities using performance on different test items, which enables computer-adaptive testing to measure ability much more efficiently than classic tests.

Jeanne Clery Disclosure of Campus Security Policy and Campus Crime Statistics Act (Clery Act) Aims to provide transparency around campus crime policy and statistics; EMS programs, educators, and students must understand what this federal safety and security law entails and where their responsibilities lie.

key performance indicators (KPIs) Attributes or functional units that represent core, important aspects and that can be measured to gauge program success.

kinesthetic learning Preference for learning through touch.

knowledge dimension Types of knowledge an educator must consider including within the cognitive domain; includes factual, conceptual, procedural, and metacognitive knowledge.

Kolb's theory Theory that describes two ways that learners can transform experience into knowledge: reflective observation and active experimentation.

Kuder–Richardson Statistical formula to evaluate internal consistency.

large group For the purposes of this text, defined as a greater number of students or audience than can be easily handled for small group activities.

learned helplessness Self-concept that one is not good at something or is unable to achieve something.

learning contract Document mutually agreed to by the student and faculty that defines activities and behaviors that must be met in a specified time frame to achieve specific objectives.

learning management system (LMS) Software application that facilitates the delivery and administration of education courses in an online educational environment.

learning style Preferred method of learning.

lecture Teaching session in which the instructor is the principal teacher.

lecturer Content expert who presents selected didactic material.

longitudinal fissure The anatomical separation between the right and left hemispheres of the cerebrum.

low-fidelity In healthcare simulation, refers to simulation experiences that do not need to be controlled or programmed externally for the learner to participate.[1]

low-stakes assessment Assessment that has relatively little effect on whether a student passes a course.

manipulation Psychomotor domain level that occurs as students practice a skill and begin to create their own styles of performance.

manipulatives Objects or tools that learners can handle and examine during the lesson to increase engagement.

Maslow's hierarchy of needs Theory that identifies an incremental series of human needs. Individuals must satisfy the lower-level needs to achieve the higher levels.

massive open online courses (MOOCs) Courses of study made available over the Internet at minimal to no cost to a very large number of people.

mastery Achieving goals and objectives established for a specific knowledge area; possession of a skill.

measurement error Variation of an exam score due to factors not related to the knowledge the exam intends to measure.

medulla oblongata Spinal cord termination about 1 inch into the lower brain.

mentor Experienced person who actively guides a less experienced person toward a goal.

metacognition Thinking about thinking; literally, "in the midst of knowing"; an awareness and control of one's thinking.

metacognitive knowledge Knowledge type that is an understanding of one's thinking. It uses reflective thinking to strategically improve cognition, solve problems, and think critically.

mirror neurons Neurons that fire when a person performs or thinks of a familiar action, or when seeing another performing that action.

mixed reality (MR) Technology in which special eyeglasses usually need to be worn, which superimpose 3-D digital images or holograms on a user's view of the real world and in which digital elements are able to react to real-life elements.

mnemonics Patterns that are used to assist in recall and that are made from the first letter of each word in a phrase; for example, OPQRST to obtain present and past medical histories in patients with pain.

modification SAMR level at which a technology allows tasks to be done in a completely new way.

moulage Techniques such as use of makeup, props, attachable artifacts, or smells used to simulate injury, illness, disease, aging, and other physical characteristics specific to a scenario.

multiple intelligences Concept that there is more than one type of intelligence.

National Clinicians' Post-Exposure Prophylaxis Hotline Phone line on which consultation is available, or questions are answered about occupational exposures to HIV and other bloodborne pathogens from needlesticks and splashes.

National Emergency Medical Services Educator Certification (NEMSEC) Credentialing body for emergency medical services educators.

naturalization Psychomotor domain level that represents skill performance mastery.

negative discrimination Index that indicates that students who scored well overall did worse on those particular questions than did students who did not score well overall.

negligent referral Latest *new* civil wrong that represents an entire *new* line of litigation that strongly suggests that programs and educators have a duty to be honest in comments made about another educator or student; includes inappropriate recommendations by a program or educator that misrepresents someone's qualifications or character.

neurogenesis Production of new neurons.

neurons Nerve cells; central nervous system cells that generate and transmit information from nerve impulses.

nondeclarative memories Memories of which one is not consciously aware, but which are used to perform motor skills.

normative grading (norm-referenced grading) Grading strategies that compare student performance with the performance of other students; grading on the curve.

norming stage Group growth stage in which the team establishes and maintains ground rules.

objective Specific, measurable learning outcome.

Occupational Safety and Health Act (OSH Act) Federal labor law governing employment-related health and safety.

omnidirectional learning Type of educational environment that is based on an open dialogue in which the instructor serves as facilitator rather than an expert. Discussion responses are directed to everyone in the educational setting, not just to the instructor.

on-the-fly programming Simulation programming that allows the educator to manipulate the program software in response to student decisions and interventions.

operating budget Budget that identifies the expected resources and expenditures of an entity for a given future period, usually spread by month over 1 year.

organize Affective domain level where the learner integrates new, refined, or different beliefs into their existing value system.

passive behavior Student is not engaged or active but only receives information or ideas.

pedagogy The art and science of teaching children.

pedantic bore Instructor who is so concerned with the details, comprehensiveness, and accuracy of a lesson that their content becomes overwhelming and tedious to students.

peer learning networks Groups of social media participants that engage in online learning together, usually without the presence of an instructor.

peer-review activity Type of small group activity in which a student reviews work by another student and provides feedback.

per capita cost per student Total cost of supplies, equipment, and resources needed for each student.

performance alignment Concordance of goals, objectives, content, and assessment tools.

performance gap Difference between actual performance and required performance.

performance stage Group growth stage in which a team develops the ability to work through group problems, and results begin to occur.

podcast Recording of an audio presentation that is made available online and that can be downloaded.

polytomous scoring Type of scoring in which the examiner chooses a number of points indicating how well the step was performed; it is frequently less reliable and more difficult to standardize.

pons Part of the brainstem that serves as a bridge between the medulla and the midbrain and aids the medulla in respiratory regulation.

Power-Load-Margin theory Model that examines the relationship between power (ability) and load (demands on learner).

practical lab instructor Person who teaches in laboratory settings.

prebriefing Information provided by an instructor, for example, verbally at the beginning of a skills session or simulation, which prepares students by explaining what to expect in the session.

preceptor (field training officer) Experienced practitioner (such as a practicing paramedic or health professional) who instructs EMS students in a hospital or the field clinical setting, providing transitional role support and learning experiences.

precision Psychomotor domain level when the skill is performed without mistakes and transfer to other situations or circumstances begins.

predictive validity Ability of an exam to predict performance under other conditions.

prefrontal cortex Region of the brain located in the anterior frontal lobe that is responsible for reasoning, planning, judgment, empathy, abstract ideas, and conscience.

Pregnancy Discrimination Act (PDA) A federal labor law that amended Title VII of the Civil Rights Act that prohibits gender discrimination on the basis of pregnancy; covers discrimination on the basis of pregnancy, childbirth, or related medical conditions.

primary (lead) instructor Person who is qualified to provide leadership or supervision over a series of courses or entire EMS program.

problem-based learning (PBL) Instructional method by which the instructor creates a complex, well-structured problem that a group of students tries to solve.

problem-centered Type of learning in which the student is placed in the context of a real-life situation and must apply knowledge from many subjects in order to resolve an issue at hand.

procedural knowledge Knowledge type that refers to information that assists a student to do something specific within the discipline. This knowledge will typically use algorithms or protocols.

proctoring Act of monitoring the test-taking environment; helps to ensure security of testing materials and to prevent cheating.

productivity Amount of output (service) per unit of input (hours of work), student-contact hours, or semester hours.

program (course) coordinator Educator responsible for program logistics.

program director Person who assumes overall responsibility for program.

program medical director Physician responsible for medical oversight of the program and for ensuring terminal competency through monitoring testing and program evaluation.

programmatic accreditor Accrediting body that serves specialized programs, professions, or schools.

psychomotor domain Learning that takes place through the attainment of skills and bodily, or kinesthetic, movements.

qualitative Nonnumerical observations that show underlying dimensions or patterns of relationships.

quantitative Criteria that identify behaviors through conditions that impose or describe limitations.

receive Affective domain level that occurs as the student acquires awareness of the value or importance of learning information and expresses a willingness to learn.

recognition Review of the quality and effectiveness of accrediting organizations.

redefinition SAMR level at which a technology enables a new task to be performed, which was not possible before.

reflective practice Act of viewing situations and practices through varied lenses, other than from only one's own point of view; in EMS education, involves using a wider mental lens when teaching, considering the views and needs of the institution, future employers, future patients, and other stakeholders.

regional accreditation Type of accreditation that serves public and private institutions, including nonprofit and degree-granting institutions that award 2- and 4-year degrees.

relative lateralization Using both sides of the brain.

reliability Ability of an assessment tool to measure consistently.

remediation Process to analyze and identify performance deficiencies and develop a plan to improve performance.

remember Cognitive domain level that focuses on memorization and recall; called Knowledge in the 1956 taxonomy.

respond Affective domain level where the student actively participates in the learning process and begins to derive satisfaction from it.

reticular activating system (RAS) Area of the brainstem that is responsible for keeping the brain alert by heightening awareness to respond to stimuli related to the sympathetic nervous system's "fight or flight" response.

risk management Process of preventing, or at least minimizing, harm or loss to an EMS facility, program, EMS educator or student, or anyone receiving emergency care.

role-playing Group process that involves students in a dramatization.

rubric Structured grading tool that outlines specific assignment criteria and expected performance, and the value assigned if each is completed. Establishes a framework for assessment.

Safe and Drug-Free Schools and Communities Act (SDFSCA) Encourages the creation of safe, disciplined, and drug-free environments, including support for EMS programs to be free of drugs and violence.

safe classroom Environment in which the student feels little risk of emotional harm while actively participating in learning activities.

SAMR model Taxonomy for categorizing technologies.

satellite In the context of education, an off-campus location advertised or otherwise made known to individuals outside the sponsor, and which offers all the professional didactic and laboratory content of the program.

satisfaction response Voluntary response that brings on a sense of self-esteem.

scaffolding Process of building new learning upon previous learning and knowledge, to aid understanding.

scenarios In healthcare simulation, descriptions of a simulation that includes the goals, objectives, debriefing points, narrative description of the clinical simulation, staff requirements, simulation room set-up, simulators, props, simulator operation, and instructions for standardized patients.[1]

schema of knowledge Patterns of thought and behavior related to categories of information and relationships between and among them.

scholarship High standards and/or quality of academic achievement.

screencast Recording of a computer presentation that is made available online and that can be downloaded.

secondary instructor Person who possesses the appropriate academic or healthcare credentials and an understanding of the principles and theories of education, and is responsible for assisting primary instructors and providing instruction to students.

self-directed learning Learning without instructor presence.

self-efficacy Belief in one's own ability to perform or achieve a goal.

self-regulated learners Learners who are aware of their own motivation and learning skills, and who employ techniques toward self-improvement.

self-study report Document created by an institution or program that provides an analysis of that institution or program and that is submitted as part of the accreditation process.

seminar Recurring small group discussion session comprised of an educator and students.

serotonin Inhibitory neurotransmitter that plays a role in sleep, mood regulation, memory, and learning.

simulation Technique that creates a situation or environment to allow students to experience a representation of a real event for the purpose of practice, learning, assessment, or testing, or to gain an understanding of systems or human actions.[1]

simulation coordinator Person who assists in coordination of simulation opportunities for students. The individual who navigates the technology during the simulation exercise.

SMART method Approach to writing objectives that focuses on objectives being specific, measurable, attainable, relevant, and time-bound.

social intelligence Type of intelligence in which a person has the ability to sense another person's feelings and thoughts, and interpret them correctly.

social learning Preference for processing information effectively while multitasking in a group setting.

Socratic method Method of teaching based on the premise of asking and answering questions with the primary purpose of stimulating critical thinking; from this process, both the educator and students discover other information. Uses the practice of asking, rather than telling, to arouse curiosity in the subject matter so students will arrive at their own conclusions rather than being told the "right" answer.

soma Cell body.

somatosensory cortex Area that receives the bulk of thalamocortical projections from the sensory input fields.

specific feedback Feedback or critique of a skill with enough direction and detail to allow the learner to practice and correct performance without the instructor having to be present.

split-half method Test of internal consistency that divides the exam into halves (commonly odd and even questions), then compares the percentage of correct answers between the two groups of items.

SQ3R Method for enhancing student learning that involves survey, question, read, recall, and review.

staffing plan Documented analysis of the number of educators needed to achieve program goals, and the expertise required for each educator role.

standard of care Prevailing or routine practice patterns; the legal obligation to conform to a minimum level of safe care to protect others from reasonable and foreseeable harm.

standardized patient Individual trained to portray a patient with a specific condition in a realistic, standardized, and repeatable way and where portrayal/presentation varies based only on learner performance.[1]

stem Part of the item that is first offered, which may be written as a question or as an incomplete statement.

storming stage Group growth stage in which team members jockey for position as they struggle to define the team's leadership.

storyboard Document that outlines detailed plans, frame by frame; for example, for the production of an online course.

student-centered learning Instruction that puts the learner at the center of the educational event and incorporates innovative, active teaching strategies such as group work, case studies, role-playing, writing assignments, and so on.

student response system Type of technology in which students answer questions or provide feedback via a technological device, such as a clicker.

substitution SAMR level at which a technology replicates a task that was previously done without a computer or a learning technology; there is no functional change.

summative assessment Evaluation of student performance given to students at the end of a course or unit of learning.

summative course evaluation Retrospective review of the entire program after the class has been completed.

SWOT analysis Analysis method in which a group brainstorms strengths, weaknesses, opportunities, and threats.

syllogism Type of argument in logic that contains a major and minor premise and a conclusion.

sylvian fissure Groove separating the parietal lobe of the brain from the temporal lobe.

synchronous learning Describes forms of teaching and learning that occur at the same time, but not in the same place. In an online environment, this is typically accomplished utilizing a Web-conferencing application.

targeted clinical experience Focused (hospital or field) assignment through which a specific aspect of learning is enhanced or remediated.

task analysis Examination method that provides a comprehensive list of the steps to be performed for a skill or process.

task trainer Model of a part or region of the human body, such as an arm or abdomen, that may use mechanical or electronic interfaces to allow students to practice specific psychomotor tasks such as IV insertion, ultrasound scanning, suturing, etc.[1]

teacher-centered learning Instruction that focuses on the teacher and thus, primarily, the lecture format.

teaching portfolio A collection of documents or other evidence that shows an educator's work over the course of their career, and that can be used for an educator's development and reflection.

team-based learning Learning model in which a longer-term assignment is given to a group of students assigned to a permanent team.

test-enhanced learning Teaching strategy in which frequent formative assessment occurs, in which learners are asked to recall and retain concepts and facts; also called *retrieval practice*.

testing effect Practice in which students read or recall content; are then tested on it so they can retrieve and apply it; and finally, feedback is provided so they can learn from their mistakes.

text to voice Technology that converts written prose to audio.

thalamus Area in the limbic system that organizes cognitive activities, including memory.

T.H.I.N.K. A model or system; a mnemonic used for a model to teach critical-thinking skills that stands for "T," total recall; "H," habits; "I," inquiry; "N," new ideas and creativity; and "K," knowing how you think.

think-pair-share (TPS) Collaborative, student-centered learning strategy in which students pair together to answer a question about lecture content.

time-in-simulation Amount of time spent in a simulation activity.[1]

time-released assessment items Assessment items that are released at a certain point, for example, on a certain calendar day.

Title IX of the Education Amendments Act A comprehensive labor law that prohibits discrimination on the basis of gender in any place or by anyone, including any federally funded EMS facility or program and EMS educator.

tort Private or civil wrong, injury, or legal action that is not necessarily the result of criminal action but for which the law allows a remedy; other than for a breach of contract, the harm in civil torts may be due to negligence, which does not amount to criminal negligence for which the law allows a remedy.

transformational learning Learning theory centered around creating change in perception and thought.

tutorial Discussion-based session led by the educator, which occurs in small group format, in which decisions are made by group consensus, and in which students are expected to provide input.

understand Cognitive domain level that focuses on construction of meaning from types of functions such as written messages; called Comprehension in the 1956 taxonomy.

validity Measuring the knowledge, skills, or abilities that an assessment is intended to evaluate.

value Affective domain level in which the student perceives that a behavior has worth or importance.

variable cost Cost that fluctuates by volume.

variances Differences from the budgeted projections.

video conferencing Meeting that occurs online and that has both visual and audio capability.

virtual reality (VR) Immersive 360-degree, computer-generated environment in which participants interact with objects and the environment through use of a head-mounted display.

visual learning Preference for learning through imagery.

wait time Concept in questioning techniques that gives time to students to think about questions posed to them and to ponder their response.

webinar Live presentation given online, in which an audience can listen and participate through a technological device with Internet access.

whole brain Use of all areas of the brain to process and control all aspects of human interaction.

whole-part-whole method Teaching technique that first provides the big picture, then breaks it into separate parts and steps, then completes the technique with another overview of the big picture.

wiki Website that allows users to collaboratively modify a Web page using their browser. Can be utilized for group projects. The term comes from the Hawaiian/Polynesian word for quick.

willing response Students respond of their own accord.

Reference

[1] Lopreiato, Joseph O. 2016. *Healthcare Simulation Dictionary*. AHRQ Publications No. 16(17)-0043. Rockville, MD: Agency for Healthcare Research and Quality.

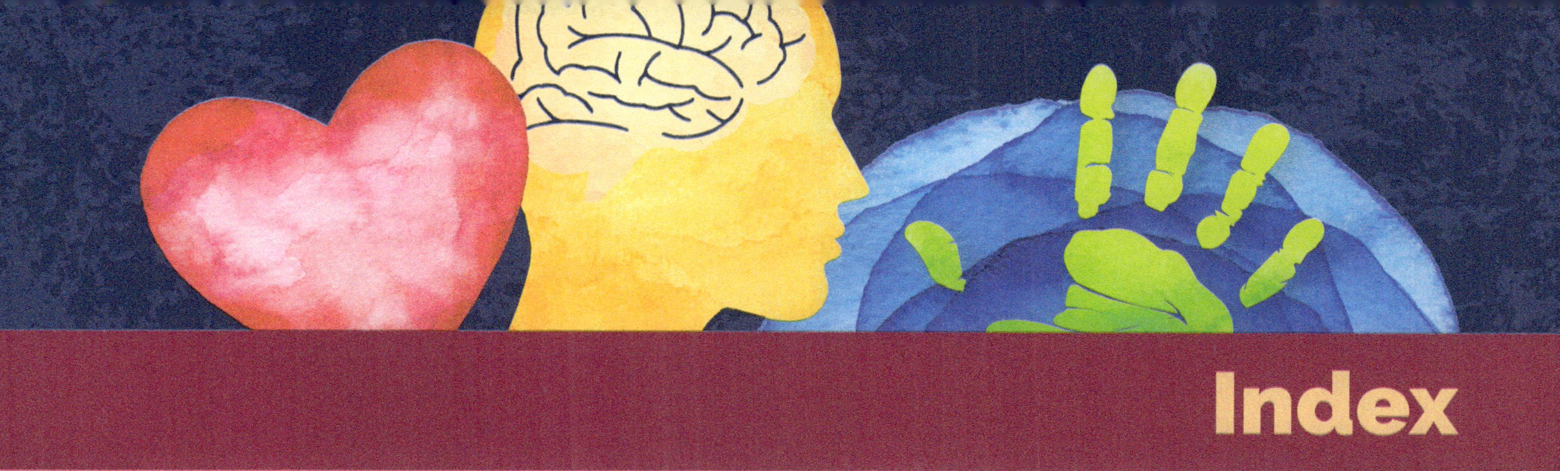

Index

Note: Page numbers followed by *b*, *f*, or *t* indicate material in boxes, figures, or tables, respectively.

A

B

C

D

E

F

G

H

I

J

K

L

M

N

O

P

Q

R

S

Z